Timeline for Application/Admission

This should be considered a general guide for applicants. It is important that an applicant considering medical school consult with his or her prehealth advisor to devise a schedule that works for him or her.

COLLEGE YEAR 1
- **Fall semester**
  - Meet prehealth advisor and investigate prehealth advisory program
  - As applicable, ensure that prehealth advisor receives course directors' evaluations
  - Successfully complete first-semester required premedical coursework and other degree requirements
- **Spring semester**
  - Visit "Considering a Career in Medicine" Web site at *www.aamc.org/students*
  - Identify summer employment/volunteer medically related opportunities
  - Successfully complete second-semester required premedical coursework and other degree requirements
  - Ensure that prehealth advisor receives course directors' evaluations

SUMMER 1
- Complete summer employment/volunteer medically related experience
- Attend summer school, if desired or necessary

COLLEGE YEAR 2
- **Fall semester**
  - Check in with prehealth advisor and participate in prehealth activities
  - Investigate available volunteer/paid medically related clinical or research activities
  - Successfully complete first-semester required premedical coursework and other degree requirements
  - Ensure that prehealth advisor receives course directors' evaluations
- **Spring semester**
  - Check in with prehealth advisor and participate in prehealth activities
  - Participate in volunteer/paid medically related clinical or research activities
  - Identify summer employment/volunteer medically related opportunities
  - Successfully complete second-semester required premedical coursework and other degree requirements
  - Ensure that prehealth advisor receives course directors' evaluations

SUMMER 2
- Complete summer employment/volunteer medically related experience
- Participate in a summer health careers program, if available
- Attend summer school, if desired or necessary

COLLEGE YEAR 3
- **Fall semester**
  - Check in with prehealth advisor and participate in prehealth activities
  - Continue participation in volunteer/paid medically related activities
  - Investigate:
    - Medical education options in MSAR and *www.aamc.org/members/listings/msalphaae.htm*
    - Medical College Admission Test (MCAT®) Web site *www.aamc.org/mcat*
    - Information about the Medical College Admission Test (MCAT®) and American Medical College Application Service (AMCAS) fee assistance on the AAMC Fee Assistance Program Web site *www.aamc.org/fap*, as appropriate
    - AAMC's "Applying to Medical School" Web site *www.aamc.org/students/applying/start.htm*
    - As applicable, information for students from groups underrepresented in medicine on the AAMC Minorities in Medicine Web site *www.aamc.org/students/minorities/start.htm*
  - Begin preparation and register for desired MCAT® administration; visit MCAT® web site *www.aamc.org/mcat* for available test date options
  - Successfully complete first-semester required premedical coursework and other degree requirements
  - Ensure that prehealth advisor receives course directors' evaluations
- **Spring semester**
  - Consult regularly with prehealth advisor regarding:
    - Schedule for completion of school-specific requirements for advisor/committee evaluation
    - Advice about medical education options
  - Continue participation in volunteer/paid medically related activities
  - Prepare for and take desired MCAT® administration; visit MCAT® web site *www.aamc.org/mcat* for available test date options

continued...

continued from page one

COLLEGE YEAR 3	o Continue review of medical education options
	o Take desired MCAT® administration. Registration opens for summer MCAT® administrations
	o Investigate information about medical school application services:
	  • the American Medical College Application Service (AMCAS) on the AMCAS Web site *www.aamc.org/amcas*
	  • the Texas Medical and Dental Schools Application Service (TMDSAS) on the TMDSAS Web site *www.utsystem.edu/tmdsas/*
	  • the Ontario Medical School Application Service (OMSAS) on the OMSAS Web site *www.ouac.on.ca/*
	  • the American Association of Colleges of Osteopathic Medicine Application Service (AACOMAS) on the AACOMAS Web site *https://aacomas.aacom.org/*
	o Investigate as applicable, the AAMC Curriculum Directory Web site *http://services.aamc.org/currdir* for information about medical school curricula and joint, dual, and combined-degree programs
	o Successfully complete second-semester required premedical coursework and other degree requirements
	o Ensure that prehealth advisor receives course directors' evaluations

SUMMER 3	• Participate in a summer health careers program, if available
	• Complete AMCAS application
	• Take desired MCAT® administration
	• Attend summer school, if desired or necessary
	• Become familiar with:
	  o AAMC Recommendations for Medical School Applicants document *www.aamc.org/students/applying/policies*
	  o AAMC Recommendations for Medical School Admission Officers document *www.aamc.org/students/applying/policies*

COLLEGE YEAR 4	• Fall semester
	  o Complete supplementary application materials for schools applied to
	  o Consult regularly with prehealth advisor regarding:
	    • Completion of school-specific requirements for advisor/committee evaluation
	    • Status of application/admission process at medical schools applied to
	  o Continue participation in volunteer/paid medically related activities
	  o Interview at medical schools
	  o Continue review of medical education options
	  o Investigate:
	    ■ Financial aid planning process process
	    ■ Financial aid forms required by school of interest with the AAMC *Financial Aid Forms Required by Medical Schools* searchable database *http://services.aamc.org/msar_reports/*
	  o Successfully complete first-semester elective science and non-science coursework and other degree requirements
	  o Ensure that prehealth advisor receives course directors' evaluations
	• Spring semester
	  o Make interim and final decisions about medical school choice
	  o Immediately notify medical schools which you will not be attending
	  o Ensure that all IRS forms are submitted as early as possible for financial aid consideration
	  o Successfully complete second-semester elective science and non-science coursework and other degree requirements
	  o Graduate

SUMMER 4	o Prepare for medical school enrollment: purchase books and equipment and make appropriate living arrangements o Relax and prepare for medical school o Attend orientation programs and matriculate at medical school

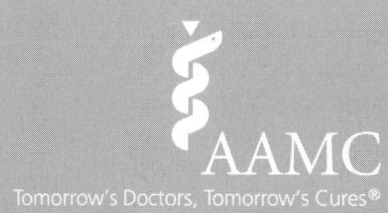
AAMC
Tomorrow's Doctors, Tomorrow's Cures®

Medical School Admission Requirements (MSAR™)

The Most Authoritative Guide to U.S. and Canadian Medical Schools

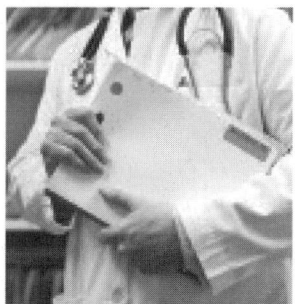
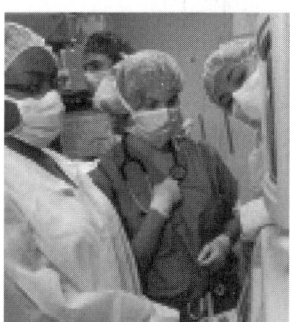
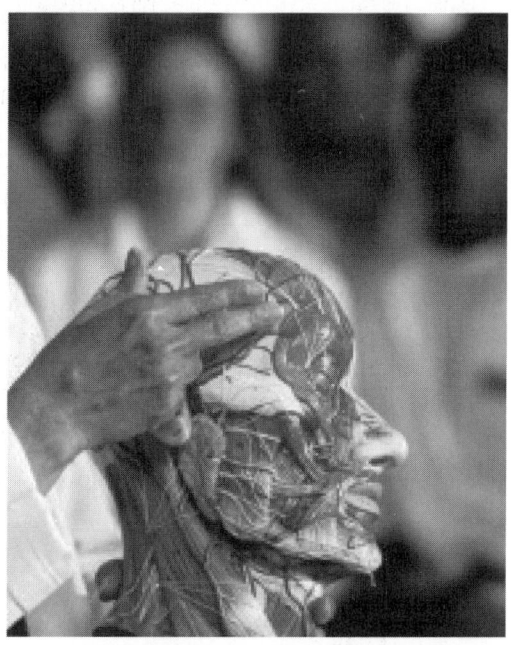

2009–2010

Includes Four Newly-Accredited Medical Schools

- Florida International University College of Medicine
- San Juan Bautista School of Medicine
- Texas Tech El Paso Foster School of Medicine
- University of Central Florida College of Medicine

Association of
American Medical Colleges

AAMC Staff

MSAR Program Administrator
Tami Levin

Content Specialists
Robert F. Sabalis, Ph.D.,
Associate Vice President,
Division of Medical Education

Henry M. Sondheimer, M.D.,
Associate Vice President,
Student Affairs and Programs

Consultants
Gwen Garrison, **Ph.D.**, Director,
Student and Applicant Studies

H. Collins Mikesell, Senior Research
Associate, Division of Medical School
Services and Studies

Karen Mitchell, Associate Vice
President and Director, Medical
College Admission Test

Moira Edwards, Associate Vice
President, Medical School
Application Services

Nancy-Pat Weaver, Associate Director,
Student Financial Services

Lily May Johnson, Manager,
Division of Diversity Policy and Programs

Jack Krakower, Associate Vice
President, Section for Institutional,
Faculty, and Student Services

Susan Gaillard, Technical Support
Analyst, Division of Medical School
Services and Studies

Shelley Yerman, Staff Associate,
Student Affairs and Programs

Revised annually; new edition
available in early spring.

**To order additional copies of
this publication, please contact:**
Association of
American Medical Colleges
Publication Department
2450 N Street, NW
Washington, DC 20037
Phone: 202-828-0416
Fax: 202-828-1123
Email: publications@aamc.org
Web site: *www.aamc.org/publications*

Price: $25.00, plus $8 shipping
(single copy)

ISBN 978-1-57754-072-4

Printed in the United States of America

Group on Student Affairs (GSA)
Steering Committee, 2008–2009

Chair
Georgette Dent, M.D.
University of North Carolina
School of Medicine

Chair Elect
Molly Osborne, M.D., Ph.D.
Oregon Health & Science University
School of Medicine

Vice Chair
Michael G. Kavan, Ph.D.
Associate Dean for Student Affairs
Creighton University
School of Medicine

Immediate Past Chair
Dwight Davis, M.D.
Associate Dean for Admissions
& Student Affairs
Pennsylvania State University
College of Medicine

Chair, GSA-Minority Affairs Section
Cynthia E. Boyd, M.D.
Associate Vice President and Director,
Medical Staff Operations
Rush Medical College of Rush
University Medical Center

Chair, Central Region
Patricia A. Barrier, M.D., M.P.H.
Associate Dean for Student Affairs
Mayo Medical School

Chair, Western Region
Maureen J. Garrity, Ph.D.
Associate Dean Student Affairs
University of Colorado
School of Medicine

Chair, Southern Region
Steven Case, Ph.D.
Associate Dean for Admissions
University of Mississippi
School of Medicine

Chair, Northeast Region
Charles A. Pohl, M.D.
Associate Dean for Student Affairs
& Career Counseling
Jefferson Medical College

Chair, Committee on Admissions
Robert Witzburg, M.D.
Boston University
School of Medicine

Chair, Committee on Student Affairs
Samuel K. Parrish, M.D.
Associate Dean for Student Affairs
Drexel University

**Chair, Committee on
Student Financial Assistance**
Carrie Steere-Salazar
University of California, San Francisco
School of Medicine

Chair, Committee on Student Records
Karen Lewis
Meharry Medical College

Council of Deans Liaison
H. David Wilson, M.D.
Vice President for Health
Affairs and Dean
University of North Dakota
School of Medicine and Health Sciences

**Immediate Past Chair,
Organization of Student
Representatives**
James Littlejohn
Texas A&M University System Health
Science Center College of Medicine

**National Association of Advisors
for the Health Professions**
for the Health Professions
C. Larry Sullivan, Ph.D.
Avila University

Association of American Medical Colleges

The Association of American Medical Colleges (AAMC) has as its purpose the advancement of medical education and the nation's health. In pursuing this purpose, the Association works with many national and international organizations, institutions, and individuals interested in strengthening the quality of medical education at all levels, searching for bio-medical knowledge, and applying these tools to providing effective health care.

As an educational association representing members with similar purposes, the primary role of the AAMC is to assist those members by providing services at the national level that will facilitate the accomplishment of their missions. Such activities include collecting data and conducting studies on issues of major concern, evaluating the quality of educational programs through the accreditation process, providing consultation and technical assistance to institutions as needs are identified, synthesizing the opinions of an informed membership for consideration at the national level, and improving communication among those concerned with medical education and the nation's health. Other activities of the Association reflect the expressed concerns and priorities of the officers and governing bodies.

The AAMC represents all 129 accredited U.S. medical schools; the 17 accredited Canadian medical schools; some 400 major teaching hospitals, including 98 affiliated health systems and 68 Veterans Affairs medical centers; 96 academic and professional societies representing 109,000 faculty members; and the nation's 67,000 medical students and 104,000 residents.

In addition to the activities listed above, the AAMC is responsible for the Medical College Admission Test (MCAT®) and the American Medical College Application Service (AMCAS®) and provides detailed admissions information to the medical schools and to undergraduate premedical advisors.

Important Notice

The information in this book is based on the most recent data provided by member medical schools prior to publication at the request of the Association of American Medical Colleges (AAMC). This material has been edited and in some instances condensed to meet space limitations. In compiling this edition, the AAMC made every reasonable effort to assure the accuracy and timeliness of the information, and, except where noted, the information was updated as of February 2008. All information contained herein, however, especially figures on tuition and expenses, is subject to change and is non–binding for medical schools listed or the AAMC. All medical schools listed in this edition, as with other educational institutions, are also subject to federal and state laws prohibiting discrimination on the basis of race, color, religion, sex, age, handicap, or national origin. Such laws include Title VI of the Civil Rights Act of 1964, Title IX of the Education Amendments of 1972, Section 504 of the Rehabilitation Act of 1973, the Americans with Disabilities Act, and the Age Discrimination Act of 1975, as amended. For the most current and complete information regarding costs, official policies, procedures, and other matters, individual schools should be contacted.

In applying to U.S. or Canadian medical schools, applicants need not go through any commercial agencies. The AAMC neither endorses nor has any relationship with commercial agencies related to medical school admissions.

All URLs in this book can be found at *www.aamc.org/msar*.

AAMC Position on Equal Opportunity

The Association strongly reaffirms the principle of equal opportunity for individuals who are qualified for education and training in, and the practice of, the health professions, without regard to sex, race, creed, color, national origin, age, or handicap. In pursuit of this principle and policy, the AAMC:

1. Requests member institutions to continue to monitor their admission policies and practices to ensure equal opportunity of admission to their educational and training programs.
2. Requests member institutions to continue to undertake and to reinforce programs of affirmative action to increase the diversity of students in the health professions.

Further, recognizing that the underrepresentation of some groups in health professions educational and training programs is but a symptom of broad social and economic problems, the AAMC:

1. Actively supports the organized study of the basic causes of underrepresentation and possible solutions.
2. Actively supports the initiation of new programs, and the broadening of existing programs, which are designed to overcome these problems. These programs include, but are not limited to, those designed to afford women the opportunity to fulfill their educational-professional goals, to eliminate economic barriers to education in the health professions, and to develop increased interest in careers in the health professions at the secondary school and college levels.

Contents

List of Tables and Charts

Alphabetical Listing of Medical Schools

Chapter 12 U.S. Medical Schools

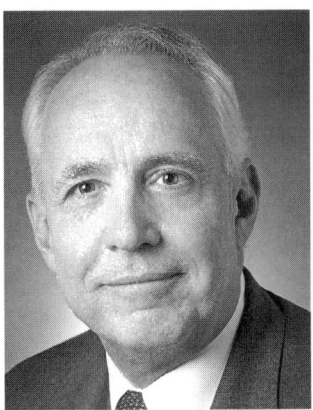

Maybe it was the great feeling you had from volunteering, or the profound concern stirred by a family member's illness that made you think about becoming a doctor. Or, perhaps it was the thrill you experienced in solving a complex research problem that inspired you to dream about finding the next "big cure." Whatever reason led you to consider a career in medicine, you have come to the right place: the Medical School Admissions Requirements (MSAR™) published by the Association of American Medical Colleges (AAMC).

As the national association representing all 129 accredited U.S. and 17 accredited Canadian medical schools, the AAMC publishes the MSAR annually to help aspiring medical students learn about the many options available for their education. The MSAR is the only guide authorized by the schools themselves and, in my view, the best choice for learning more about the myriad programs available.

This book contains data on each school's entrance requirements and selection factors, as well as descriptions of its focus, mission, and curriculum. You also will find details about financial aid and costs, and see the degree of diversity represented by 2007–08 matriculants. And, in what I think is one of the MSAR's best features, you will see the number of accepted applicants at each school who took certain premed courses, performed community service, or worked in research or other medically related positions. In other words, you will see information about students who, only a few years ago, went through the same decision-making process you are undertaking now.

For me, becoming a doctor truly was a life-changing experience. I have no doubt you will find it just as rewarding, and also think you will find it a particularly exciting time to enter medicine. You will be able to use remarkably sophisticated tools to help diagnose and treat patients; collaborate with fellow scientists across the country and around the world to tackle research problems; and contribute your expertise to the critical goal of ensuring all Americans have access to high-quality, affordable health care. And equally important, you will be entering medicine at a time when the country needs your services most, given predicted physician shortages in coming years and plans by medical schools to expand their capacity.

In the end, choosing a medical school is a personal decision that must be based on your own criteria and values. Think about what matters to you, and then take the time to visit each school in which you are interested. Also, visit our Web site, www.aamc.org, for more information about these schools and the resources that can help you do your best on the MCAT® exam. You will also see the many opportunities available to tomorrow's doctors.

I hope you find the MSAR to be an informative and useful guide as you channel your hopes and dreams into a career that truly helps people and makes a difference in their lives. I wish you all the best in your endeavors.

Darrell G. Kirch

Darrell G. Kirch, M.D.
President and CEO
Association of American Medical Colleges

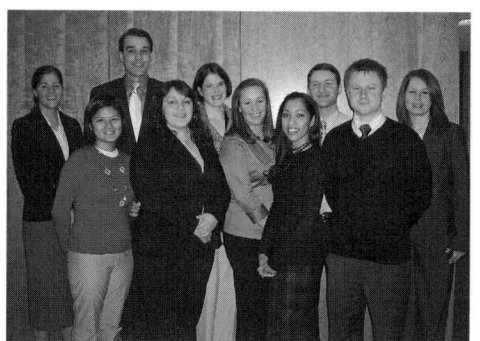

**Organization of Student Representatives
2007–2008**

A philosopher once said, "A journey of a thousand miles begins with a single step." Undoubtedly, you have already taken many steps along the road to medical school. As you take this next step toward a career in medicine, this book will serve as a trustworthy roadmap and guide. Medical School Admission Requirements (MSAR) will provide you with current information of interest for each U.S. and Canadian medical school.

As Chair of the AAMC Organization of Student Representatives (OSR), which is charged with expressing the voice and perspective of 67,000 medical students enrolled in 129 Liaison Committee on Medical Education (LCME)-accredited medical schools in the United States, I would like to congratulate you on the steps that you have already taken and welcome you on the road toward an exciting and rewarding career in medicine.

The mission of the medical education system is to serve the public by educating and training a diverse physician workforce to be engaged in a variety of healthcare functions: clinical medicine, public health, biomedical and health services research, and medical education. In addition, there is a need for physicians who can contribute to the fields of public policy, law, ethics, business, and journalism. We are training in a time of great change, no only in our technical and scientific capabilities but also in the system in which we practice. Opportunities abound within the medical field and are limited only by your imagination and ideals as a medical professional. As the future of medicine unfolds before our eyes, the field is in need of dedicated innovators to lead health care into the next generation. Now is the perfect time to begin considering what your ideals for the future of this profession are and how you would like to play a role in shaping it.

The medical school application process is a challenge in its own right. The demands of time, attention, and finances should not deter you from your ultimate goals, nor should the opinions of others who say it cannot be done. Many resources are available to help with any challenges you might face, such as support for those in need of financial assistance or counseling for those in need of direction. I cannot overemphasize the fact that a career in medicine is available to applicants from all types of backgrounds with all sorts of goals.

Consider your choices broadly and carefully, as each medical school will provide you with unique learning and life experiences. Consult many resources, including your mentors, advisors, and peers, as well as medical school faculty and medical students. Most important, do not underestimate the support and encouragement offered by family and friends. Utilize your medical school interviews to explore the academic and extracurricular opportunities offered at each prospective institution — these are experiences that will enrich your life for years to come.

You have chosen to pursue a fulfilling and important career dedicated to relieving human suffering and improving humanity's health and well-being. I wish you great success on your journey and congratulate you on these first steps toward becoming a doctor.

Diane C. Reis

Diane Crowley Reis
Medical Student
University of Wisconsin School of Medicine and Public Health
2007–2008 Chair, AAMC Organization of Student Representatives

Chapter 1

Medicine as a Career

For those interested in a career in medicine, the choices are almost limitless.

From clinical practice to medical administration, to public health, to military medicine, to medical education, to community health, to biomedical research — medicine is an inclusive profession that offers incredibly varied opportunities to its physician ranks. Ideally, all physicians aspire to be:

- altruistic, compassionate, trustworthy, and truthful in their relationships with patients, patients' family members, and professional colleagues. They understand the history of medicine, medicine's compact with society, their ethical responsibilities as physicians, and their obligations under the law. They act with integrity and honesty; they respect patients' privacy and dignity. They seek to understand the meaning of patients' stories in the context of patients' beliefs and family and cultural values. They avoid being judgmental when patients' beliefs and values conflict with their own. They continue to care for dying patients even when disease-specific therapy is no longer available or desired.

- knowledgeable about the scientific basis of medicine and the normal and abnormal functioning of the body. They have sufficient knowledge of the structure and function of the body, its major organ systems, and the molecular, cellular, and biochemical mechanisms that maintain the body's homeostasis in order to comprehend disease and incorporate modern diagnostic and therapeutic modalities in their practices. They engage in lifelong learning to remain current in their understanding of the scientific bases of medicine.

- skillful in communicating with and providing care to their patients. They obtain from patients an accurate medical history that includes all relevant information, and they perform skillfully a physical examination and those diagnostic procedures warranted by their patients' conditions. They obtain, interpret properly, and manage information from those studies relating to the patients' conditions, and they seek consultation from other physicians and health professionals, when indicated. They understand the etiology, pathogenesis, and various manifestations of the diseases and conditions they are likely to confront in the practice of their specialty. They understand the scientific basis and evidence of effectiveness for each of the therapeutic options available for patients at different times in the course of their conditions, and discuss those options with patients in an honest and objective fashion. They communicate with patients and their families about their concerns regarding the patients' health and well-being. They are sufficiently knowledgeable about both traditional and non-traditional modes of care to provide intelligent guidance to their patients.

- dutiful in working with other physicians and health care professionals to promote the health of individual patients and all community members. They are well-informed about risk factors for disease and injury; they understand disease and injury prevention practices. They promote healthy behaviors through counseling individual patients and their families and public education and action; they actively support traditional public health practices in their communities. They advocate for improving access to care for everyone, especially members of traditionally underserved populations. They understand the economic, psychological, occupational, social, and cultural factors contributing to the development and/or perpetuation of conditions that impair health. They apply principles of evidence-based medicine and cost-effectiveness in making decisions about the utilization of limited medical resources. They collaborate with other physicians, other health care professionals, and individuals representing a wide variety of community agencies. As members of a team addressing individual or population-based health care issues, they lead, when appropriate, and defer to the leadership of others, when indicated. They acknowledge and respect the roles of other health professionals in providing needed services to individual patients, populations, or communities.

Which Path Is Right for You?

Men and women bring to the profession of medicine a broad range of personal interests, educational backgrounds, and occupational histories, as well as unique sets of skills, abilities, experiences, and philosophies. Aspiring physicians seek to achieve lofty, but attainable professional goals in a variety of specialties and clinical settings:

• The satisfaction of enduring patient relationships is one attraction of family medicine or internal medicine, where the "art" of medicine flourishes in each encounter with every patient. Others with a commitment to social justice and the well-being of a community, and an interest in fulfilling the health care needs of the underserved and disadvantaged, can meet these challenges in urban and rural clinics, in community medicine and public health, or as medical missionaries.

• An interest in scientific investigation and the desire to expand the boundaries of medical knowledge are traits of those in the nation's private and public laboratories and research institutions. Physicians interested in communicating their colleagues' laboratory-derived discoveries and interpreting their impact on society enjoy their roles as medical editors, journalists, or experts in medical ethics.

• Careers in general surgery often suit those physicians with a desire for direct feedback about the results of their interventions. Plastic and reconstructive surgery draws others with artistic skills, excellent eye-hand coordination, and aesthetic interests.

• Those interested in mind-body interactions and the emotional lives of their patients might find a home in neurology or psychiatry. Others interested in national defense or the challenges inherent in emergency situations use their skills as flight surgeons or in aerospace or military medicine.

• The economic and public policy aspects of health care guide some physicians to lead think tanks and health-related associations and organizations, as well as to serve in the legislative and executive branches of government. The more visceral aspects of medicine draw some to work with crime and accident victims as emergency medicine physicians or trauma surgeons; others work in orthopedic surgery with patients who have bone, joint, or other musculoskeletal problems.

• For those fascinated by the issues facing groups of patients with age-defined illnesses and problems — from the risks of infancy and early childhood to the challenges of later life — fulfillment can come as pediatricians and geriatricians. Others prefer to pursue detailed knowledge about the intricacies of a single body organ or system, such as that required of ophthalmologists, dermatologists, or neurosurgeons.

• Assisting patients in overcoming complex fertility and gestational problems is the hallmark of the specialties of reproductive endocrinology and obstetrics and gynecology. Those with a long-range interest in reducing the incidence of birth defects and inherited syndromes might find their calling in the field of medical genetics.

• The detection, prevention, and eradication of injury and disease in groups and populations, both in this country and abroad, draw people to preventive medicine and epidemiology at such organizations as the Centers for Disease Control and Prevention or the World Health Organization. Those same interests at the local level can be fulfilled in forensic pathology, coroners' and medical examiners' offices, and state or county health departments.

The possibilities in medicine are almost endless. No matter what your personal interests, skills, or needs may be, medicine encourages and permits you to find your individual niche. Should your interests, abilities, or needs change with time and experience, medicine — because of its emphasis on lifelong learning and its periodic requirements for demonstrating competence — affords ongoing opportunities for refining your skills and reorienting your practice.

Career Guidance and Decision-Making

Medical schools recognize the critical role they play in helping medical students to assess their personal values and interests, identify career options, determine their personal "fit" with those options, and make well-informed decisions about specialty choice. This recognition is reflected in the Careers in Medicine program, created by the AAMC in collaboration with its 129 member medical schools. The four-phase career decision-making format used in this program is similar to that used by premedical students in deciding on medicine as a career, and in deciding which medical schools would be an appropriate match.

In Phase 1 of Careers in Medicine, Understanding Yourself, medical students explore who they are, what activities they enjoy, the values that underlie their lives and work, and the nature of their relationships with other people. During Phase 2, Exploring Options, tools are provided for exploring specialties and other career options. Phase 3, Choosing a Specialty, focuses on comparing the personal information obtained in Phase 1 with the specialty and career options garnered in Phase 2. Finally, in Phase 4, Getting into Residency, plans are laid for application to residency training programs and related activities, such as completing personal statements and interviews.

The process of career-planning and decision-making is dynamic and ongoing. Consider familiarizing yourself with the Careers in Medicine program at *www.aamc.org/careersinmedicine* as you work on plans for application to medical school and a medical education.

Combined, Dual, and Joint Degree Programs

The U.S. medical education system is designed to support the process of identifying and attaining your place in medicine. During both the four years of medical school — known as undergraduate medical education — and in the residency and fellowship training that follows (graduate medical education), opportunities abound for specialized education and training. At medical schools and residency training programs across the country, students and residents are enrolled in combined, dual, and joint degree programs that prepare them well for future careers. Federally funded Medical Scientist Training Programs (MSTPs) assist students in obtaining both the M.D. and Ph.D. degrees in areas related to medical research, and in working with mentors to prepare for careers as academic physicians and physician-scientists (see Chapter 11).

Medical schools on university campuses provide dual M.D./graduate and professional degree programs in a variety of academic disciplines, including the basic sciences, business administration, computer science, education, law, and public health. Graduates of such programs may pursue careers as National Institutes of Health scientists, medical school faculty members, hospital administrators, health care entrepreneurs, medical informatics and diagnostic experts, or forensic scientists and medical examiners; they also become authorities in epidemiology, public health, and community and preventive medicine.

Information about combined college/M.D. programs for high school students can be found in Chapter 10 and on the AAMC Curriculum Directory Web site at *http://services.aamc.org/currdir*. Information about combined, dual, and joint M.D./graduate and professional degree programs (e.g., M.Ed., M.P.H., J.D., M.B.A., and various Ph.D. specializations)

can be found in a database that is searchable by school and program type, also accessible at the AAMC Curriculum Directory Web site. The information in the Curriculum Directory is provided, and periodically updated, by medical school personnel through the AAMC Curriculum Management and Information Tool (CurrMIT).

Characteristics of U.S. and Canadian Medical Schools

The missions of the 129 accredited U.S. and 17 accredited Canadian allopathic medical schools vary as widely as the motivations of individual medical students. (Allopathic medical schools grant the M.D. degree, while osteopathic medical schools grant the D.O. degree.) Each U.S. medical school is periodically required to document that it has met strict accreditation standards set by the Liaison Committee on Medical Education (LCME, *www.lcme.org*), the joint accrediting body of the American Medical Association (AMA, *www.ama-assn.org*), located in Chicago, and the AAMC (*www.aamc.org*), located in Washington, D.C. Canadian medical schools are jointly accredited by the LCME and the Committee on Accreditation of Canadian Medical Schools of the Association of Faculties of Medicine of Canada (*www.afmc.ca*).

Fundamental elements of medical education are shared by all schools: acquisition of basic science knowledge and elementary clinical skills during the first component of the curriculum, and acquisition of more advanced clinical skills under the supervision of attending physician faculty members during the second component of the curriculum. Medical schools also vary on many important characteristics, including institutional mission, curricular emphasis and structure, class size and applicant pool, cost, ownership, and clinical affiliations.

What Kind of School for You?

As an applicant embarks on the path toward a medical career, consideration of the type of medical school is important. Some medical school curricula emphasize the education and training

of primary care physicians, typically meaning general pediatricians, general internists, and family physicians (although obstetrician/gynecologists and others who are the first point of contact for patients are also sometimes included). Some medical schools emphasize the education and training of physicians who will serve the needs of rural patients. Still other schools emphasize the acquisition of research skills and provide opportunities for investigative activities on the part of medical students, with their graduates going on to careers in academic medicine and basic and clinical research. Some schools were founded by state legislatures with a curricular emphasis on the needs of a particular patient population, such as older patients.

Increasingly frequently, medical schools are providing educational opportunities on multiple branch and regional campuses. At some schools, students complete their first two years in classrooms and laboratories on a central campus, then disperse to separate clinical campuses to complete core and elective clinical experiences in their final two years. At other institutions, the opposite occurs.

In 2007, entering class sizes at U.S. medical schools ranged from 42 to 307 students. Applicant pools at U.S. schools also vary greatly. Some public medical schools in smaller states have small pools, with first-year classes selected primarily from among state residents. Other private schools select new entrants from national pools of several thousand applicants, with little regard to applicants' state of legal residence.

In June 2006, the AAMC issued a call for LCME-accredited medical schools to increase their enrollments by 30 percent by 2015, with expansion accomplished by both increasing enrollments in existing schools and establishing new medical schools. This recommendation was based on mounting research and anecdotal data suggesting that current medical school enrollments would result in a shortage of physicians in the United States within the next few decades, unless fundamental changes take place in the demand and need for healthcare and/or in the way healthcare is provided. This recommendation was further supported by data from a growing number of specialty and state-specific studies concluding that shortages exist or will soon exist in particular specialties or states. Additional information about physician workforce projections and the need for more physicians can be found on the AAMC Web site at *www.aamc. org/workforce/*.

Public or Private?

Medical schools generally fall into two categories as a function of their funding sources: public and private. Public medical schools usually receive some of their operating revenue from state or federal governments, while private schools usually generate revenue from other sources, including endowments and tuition. Determining the "real" annual expense associated with attendance at a state-supported or private medical school can be complex. Tuition and fees at public schools are often less than those at private schools, especially for state residents, because educational costs are underwritten with tax revenues. However, this tuition differential usually disappears for students who are not state residents, and tuition at public medical schools for non-residents often equals that of private institutions. On the other hand, some private medical schools with large endowments are able to provide substantial scholarship aid to qualifying students, thus lowering the "effective tuition" rate significantly and permitting those students to graduate with less educational debt than they would have accumulated if they had attended a public medical school in their state of residence.

Some medical schools, both public and private, own and manage their own hospitals, outpatient facilities, and health care systems. Others, sometimes referred to as community-based schools, establish ongoing affiliations with existing inpatient and ambulatory care facilities in their surrounding communities, where students complete the clinical components of their education under the supervision of faculty members.

While all medical schools were established to educate future physicians, they can differ substantially in their educational programs. This and other information about U.S. and Canadian medical schools is presented in greater detail in the school profile pages that begin on page 114. Complete information can also be found on each school's Web site, links to which can be found on the AAMC Web site at *www.aamc.org/medicalschools.htm*, as well as in institutional academic bulletins, brochures, and related publications.

Chapter 2

The Process of Medical Education

The path to medical practice consists of five phases:

- undergraduate premedical education (college)
- undergraduate medical education (medical school)
- graduate medical education (residency and fellowship training)
- licensure and certification
- continuing medical education

While each of these educational elements is separate and distinct from the others, the successful completion of each component is a building block, laying a strong, broad foundation for the eventual independent practice of medicine.

Undergraduate Premedical Education

For future physicians, college affords opportunities for excelling in the natural sciences, the social sciences, and the humanities; for fostering inquiry and problem-solving abilities; for honing communication and interpersonal skills; and for developing intellectual discipline and time-management skills. College begins to prepare students for the academic and personal rigors of a medical education. There they learn to appreciate the continuum of human experience and to learn from the experiences of others — to recognize the impact of culture and family dynamics on human development and thus to value the uniqueness of the doctor-patient relationship.

Medicine is practiced in a social context. Physicians must be able to communicate effectively with people from a variety of backgrounds and life experiences. Medical school admission committees seek to enroll students who bring diverse talents and interests to medicine; their goal is to identify students whose personal and career aspirations are compatible with society's health care needs, whether coping with the international AIDS epidemic, responding to bioterrorism, natural disasters, or other crises, or caring for persons who are medically underserved or economically disadvantaged.

Undergraduate Medical Education

Curricula at U.S. and Canadian medical schools have common elements, although they vary in educational approaches. All medical schools share the goals of preparing students in the art and science of medicine, and providing them with the background necessary to enter a three to seven-year-long period of graduate medical education following receipt of the M.D. degree. A significant amount of periodically updated information about medical school curricula and institutional characteristics can be found in the AAMC databases at *http://services. aamc.org/currdir*.

Each medical school's faculty establishes standards for students' academic performance, personal and professional conduct, clinical proficiency, and promotion and graduation. Many schools have developed comprehensive learning objectives for their educational programs, along with detailed descriptions of the means by which students will be assessed at various stages along the educational continuum. Faculty members determine whether students have met curricular learning objectives by requiring them to demonstrate mastery of both course content and clinical skills — through written tests, oral examinations, and laboratory exercises — and by observing and assessing their clinical acumen. Many schools require students to complete local and national standardized examinations before they can progress to further clinical training. The frequency and methods of evaluation vary from school to school. In recent years medical schools have continued to revise their educational programs, moving from more passive approaches to learning to more active ones and from an emphasis on large-group to small-group learning activities. As possible, lecture formats have been systematically replaced with learning opportunities that promote self-assessment, problem-solving, integration of the basic and clinical sciences, and collaboration with faculty and peers. Increasingly, schools are also requiring students to complete year-end and over-all comprehensive examinations prior to promotion and graduation.

Grading procedures at medical schools vary. Many schools have pass/fail or honors/pass/fail grading systems, while others use letter grades. Whatever the assessment structure, students' knowledge and skills are carefully scrutinized on a periodic basis by members of the faculty. Increasingly, schools are differentiating the assessment of students' academic achievement from that of their personal and professional behavior, with complementary evaluations during each classroom and clinical experience. In the clinical environment, one-on-one relationships between faculty members and students permit close and ongoing observation and feedback.

At three percent, the rate of attrition at U.S. medical schools is remarkably low. Students who are deficient in certain areas often have opportunities for remediation and assistance. Nevertheless, all medical school faculties reserve the right to dismiss any student whose academic or personal characteristics are incompatible with a physician's professional responsibilities.

The first two years. Initially, students learn those basic sciences essential to the practice of medicine. The normal structure and function of human systems are taught through gross and microscopic anatomy, biochemistry, behavioral science, physiology, and neuroscience. Subsequently, the educational focus shifts to abnormalities of structure and function, disease, and general

therapeutic principles through exposure to microbiology, immunology, pathology, and pharmacology.

Throughout the first two years, the clinical significance of basic science material is continuously stressed.

In addition to the core scientific work, students are exposed to a wide variety of topics:

- nutrition
- medical ethics
- genetics
- laboratory medicine
- health care delivery systems
- substance abuse
- human values
- research
- preventive medicine
- community health
- geriatrics
- human sexuality

Lecture-style teaching no longer dominates the classroom; small-group learning, multi-disciplinary clinical conferences, peer-to-peer learning, and case-based and problem-based approaches all have a place in the first two years. These experiences can be with actual patients and with people trained to simulate pathological conditions, known as standardized patients. In addition, interdepartmentally integrated courses are being developed at many schools as an alternative to previous discipline or department-based courses.

By the end of these two years, students have learned the scientific underpinnings of medicine. They also have learned the basics of interviewing and obtaining historical data from patients, as well as of conducting physical examinations, interpreting laboratory findings, and considering diagnostic and treatment alternatives. Students are now prepared to make the transition to the clinical environment on a full-time basis.

The second two years. The second period of undergraduate medical education consists of a series of required clinical rotations, or clerkships, usually lasting from 4 to 12 weeks each, during which medical students work with patients and their families in various inpatient and outpatient settings. Here, they function under the supervision of physician faculty members — known as attending physicians — and residents, and collaborate with other members of the clinical team, including nurses, social workers, psychologists, pharmacists, and technical staff. The pattern, length, and number of rotations differ from school to school, but core clinical training usually includes clerkships in internal medicine, obstetrics/gynecology, pediatrics, psychiatry, and surgery. Depending on the school, required clerkships can also include family medicine, primary care, neurology, a community or rural medicine preceptorship, or an acting internship.

During clinical clerkships, students are assigned to an outpatient clinic or inpatient hospital unit where they assume responsibility for "working-up" a number of patients each week, that is, collecting relevant data and information from them and presenting pertinent findings to a faculty member for diagnosis and treatment planning. Students also participate in the ongoing clinical care of patients assigned to the medical team. Ideally, students follow their patients over time, either during hospitalizations or through the course of outpatient treatment. When appropriate, students also relate to patients' family members — providing information, answering questions, and preparing them for the outcome of patients' care.

During these clinical education experiences, students learn to apply their basic science knowledge and clinical skills in diagnosing and treating patients' illnesses and injuries. They learn clinical decision-making and patient management skills. They interact daily with faculty members, whether at the bedside, during inpatient team discussions ("rounds"), on patient visits, or in case-based lectures and small-group discussions.

Electives. Most medical schools provide curricular opportunities to assist students in pursuing special interests through supplemental educational experiences known as electives, which are offered in the basic, behavioral, and clinical sciences, as well as in basic and clinical research. While electives are typically available during the final year of medical school, they may also be available at other times in the curriculum. Students can complete electives on their own campuses, at other medical schools, through federal and state agencies (such as the Institute of Medicine, *www.iom.edu*; the Indian Health Service, *www.ihs.gov*; and the Centers for Disease Control and Prevention, *www.cdc.gov*), in international settings, and through external non-academic service organizations.

Clinical electives include opportunities in the entire range of medical and surgical specialties and subspecialties. Students seek these experiences for several reasons: to acquaint themselves with additional career options, to broaden and enrich their educational experience, and to expose themselves to areas of specialization that are one-time opportunities.

Residency or specialty. During the fourth year of medical school, students choose a medical specialty and apply to graduate medical education programs (residencies) through such services as the Electronic Residency Application Service (ERAS, *www.aamc.org/eras*) and the National Resident Matching Program (NRMP, *www.nrmp.org*). ERAS is an application service that transmits residency applications, letters of recommendation, transcripts, and other supporting credentials from applicants and medical schools

to internship, residency, and fellowship programs using the Internet. The NRMP is a Web-based program that matches applicants' preferences for specific residency programs with program directors' preferences for specific applicants.

Graduate Medical Education

The third phase of medical training prepares physicians for independent practice in an area of specialization. Residency programs focus on the acquisition of detailed factual knowledge and the development of clinical skills and professional competencies in a particular specialty. These programs are based in hospitals or other health care institutions and, in most specialties, utilize both inpatient and outpatient settings for teaching purposes. Residency programs are accredited by the Accreditation Council for Graduate Medical Education (ACGME, *www.acgme.org*) and its associated Residency Review Committees. Residents, — also known as house officers or house staff, — typically complete educational requirements for certification through a specialty board recognized by the American Board of Medical Specialties (ABMS, *www.abms.org*). Information about medical specialties and subspecialties can also be found on the Careers in Medicine Web site at *www.aamc.org/careersinmedicine*.

For medical students who decide to practice in a medical or surgical specialty, the requirements of that specialty's certifying board will influence the choice of the first-postgraduate-year (PGY1) program. Family medicine, internal medicine, pediatrics, and general surgery encourage students to enter PGY1 programs in that specialty directly, and to continue in these programs until they have completed all specialty board requirements.

Satisfactory completion of three years of training in family practice, internal medicine, or pediatrics or five years of training in general surgery generally qualifies an individual to take the board certification examinations in each of those specialties.

Students seeking careers in other medical or surgical specialties (e.g., dermatology, physical medicine and rehabilitation, radiology) are first exposed to a broad range of clinical experiences during their PGY1 year. Usually these students complete this first residency training clinical year in internal medicine or general surgery or in a diversified "transitional year" program, with the expectation that they will enter a program in the specialty of their choice in the second postgraduate year (PGY2). In some cases, the year of broad clinical exposure may be in the same institution where subsequent subspecialty training occurs. In other instances, specialty training must be completed elsewhere. Education and training in a medical or surgical subspecialty (e.g., cardiology, pulmonology, geriatrics, hematology/oncology, cardiothoracic surgery) take place for varying periods of time after completion of the appropriate preparatory residency training. These trainees in a medical or surgical subspecialty are sometimes referred to as "fellows".

Licensure and Certification

The fourth phase of medical training involves licensure to practice medicine and certification in a specialty. Medical practice is regulated by each individual state or jurisdiction. Each state has a statute, known as a medical practice act, that describes the practice of medicine and identifies the public agency in the state that has responsibility for licensing physicians and regulating medical practice. These agencies protect the public from potentially unprofessional or incompetent physicians.

All states require applicants for a medical license to document that they have both completed appropriate educational and training programs and achieved passing scores on licensure examinations approved by the relevant state agency or board. In 1990, the Federation of State Medical Boards (FSMB, *www.fsmb.org*) and the National Board of Medical Examiners (NBME, *www.nbme.org*) established the United States Medical

Licensing Examination, (USMLE, *www.usmle.org*), a single, three-step licensing examination utilized by all U.S. licensing jurisdictions.

USMLE Step 1 assesses whether the examinee can understand and apply important concepts of the sciences basic to the practice of medicine, with special emphasis on principles and mechanisms underlying health, disease, and modes of therapy. Step 1 ensures mastery of the sciences that provide a foundation for the safe and competent practice of medicine in the present, and the scientific principles required for the maintenance of competence through lifelong learning.

USMLE Step 2 consists of two components: Clinical Knowledge (CK) and Clinical Skills (CS). USMLE Step 2 assesses the examinee's ability to apply medical knowledge, skills, and understanding of clinical science essential for the provision of patient care under supervision, and includes emphasis on health promotion and disease prevention. Step 2 ensures that due attention is devoted to principles of clinical sciences and basic patient-centered skills that provide the foundation for the safe and competent practice of medicine.

USMLE Step 3 assesses whether the examinee can apply medical knowledge and understanding of biomedical and clinical science essential for the unsupervised practice of medicine, with an emphasis on patient management in ambulatory settings. Step 3 provides a final assessment of a physician's ability to assume independent responsibility for delivering general medical care.

In addition to receiving a license from a state medical board, physicians are strongly encouraged to apply voluntarily for certification in a medical or surgical specialty from one of the 24 approved boards of the American Board of Medical Specialties (ABMS, *www.abms. org*). Through comprehensive examinations, these specialty boards determine if candidates have been appropriately prepared in accordance with established educational standards. Those who have satisfied all board requirements are certified and are known as "diplomates" of the specialty board; periodic recertification is offered at intervals of 7 to 10 years. More than 85 percent of licensed physicians in the U.S. have been certified by at least one ABMS member board.

Continuing Medical Education

The fifth and final phase of medical training is continuing medical education, or CME. Physicians continue the educational process in the specific medical specialty in which they completed residency training; CME reflects the commitment to life-long learning that is a hallmark of the medical profession. By attending CME programs regularly, practicing physicians maintain their clinical competence over time and enhance their knowledge and skills. The Accreditation Council for Continuing Medical Education (ACCME, *www.accme.org*) provides a system of voluntary accreditation for providers of continuing medical education programs.

Chapter 3

Undergraduate Premedical Preparation

During college, the successful premedical student completes several important tasks, including:

- the selection of a personally challenging and appealing major
- the timely completion of all required premedical courses
- the pursuit of advanced coursework in areas of special interest
- the establishment of an ongoing relationship with an informed premedical advisor
- participation in a variety of extra-curricular activities and experiences
- the mastery of both course content and academic skills
- the balancing of intellectual development and social and interpersonal growth

Academic Preparation

Choice of major. Medical schools recognize the importance of a strong foundation in the natural sciences — biology, chemistry, physics, and mathematics — and most schools have established minimum course requirements for admission. These courses usually represent about one-third of the credit hours needed for degree completion. This approach deliberately leaves room for applicants from a broad spectrum of college majors, including those in the humanities and social sciences. No medical school requires a specific major of its applicants or matriculants. Admission committee members are aware that medical students can develop the essential skills of acquiring, synthesizing, applying, and communicating information through a wide variety of academic disciplines.

Nevertheless, many premedical students choose to major in a scientific discipline. Ideally, they do so because they are fascinated by science and perceive that such a major can be the foundation for a variety of career options. Choosing science primarily to enhance one's chances for admission to medical school is not in a student's long-term best interest. Medical school admission committees seek students whose intellectual curiosity leads them to a variety of disciplines and whose intellectual maturity assures that their efforts are persistent and disciplined.

Science preparation. The study and practice of medicine are based on modern concepts in biology, chemistry, and physics, and on an appreciation of the scientific method. Hence, mastery of these basic scientific principles is expected of all entering medical students. Medical schools typically require successful completion of one academic year (two semesters or three quarters) of biology and physics and one academic year each of general chemistry and organic chemistry. Each of these courses should be academically rigorous and acceptable for students majoring in those areas.

All science courses should include adequate laboratory experiences.

Although only a few medical schools require applicants to complete a specific course in mathematics, all schools appreciate mathematical competence as a strong foundation for understanding the basic sciences. In addition, a working knowledge of statistics helps both medical students and physicians to become critical evaluators of the medical literature. Familiarity with computers is helpful during the educational experience, as well as in medical practice. Thus, many medical schools recommend coursework in mathematics, statistics, and computer science.

Upper-level science coursework is not typically required by medical schools. Students may choose to take advanced science courses because of their own interests or undergraduate major requirements. Taking additional science courses that duplicate the basic science content of the first two years of medical school is not recommended. In fact, practicing physicians often recommend that premedical students, during their college years, take advantage of what might be their final opportunity for study in non-science areas (e.g., music, art, history, and literature) that might become the basis for avocational interests later in life. Table 3-A gives an overview of the most common courses required by medical schools.

AP and CLEP credit. Premedical students intending to apply college credit earned through Advanced Placement (AP) and College Level Examination Placement (CLEP) to meet premedical requirements should be aware that some medical schools restrict the use of such credit. In most cases, the restrictions involve the official reporting of AP and CLEP credit on the college transcript, establishing an upper limit of such credit toward courses required for admission, or requiring additional upper-level courses in the science areas where AP or CLEP credit was received. Premedical students should carefully review Chapter 7 and pertinent medical school Web sites and publications for additional and current information.

Advanced work. Medical schools encourage honors, independent study, and research work by premedical students. These activities demonstrate in-depth, sustained scholarly exploration and the presence of life-long learning skills that are essential to a career in the medical profession.

Development of Personal Attributes

Academic or scientific accomplishments alone are not sufficient for entry into medical school and the medical profession. Intellectual capacity is obviously important, but it is not sufficient; the most critical aspect of practicing medicine is the physician-patient relationship.

In a publication that outlines learning objectives for all medical students, the AAMC reported that, while physicians are certainly expected to be knowledgeable and skillful, they are also expected to be altruistic and dutiful. The required knowledge and skills are developed in part through the college and medical school educational processes. Dedication to duty, altruism, and the other essential attributes of medical professionals are nurtured through experience — with family, with friends, and with people in need.

In the *Medical School Objectives Program: Learning Objectives for Medical Student Education: Guidelines for Medical Schools* report (*www.aamc.org/meded/msop*), dutifulness is defined as:

- an appreciation of the complex non-biological determinants of poor health
- an awareness of community and public health issues
- the ability to identify risk factors for disease
- a commitment to the early identification and treatment of disease
- an acceptance of the responsibility for making scientifically based medical decisions and for advocating for the care of the underserved
- an understanding of basic issues in health care financing and delivery

Altruism is defined as involving:

- ethical decision-making
- compassion, respect, honesty, and integrity
- collaborative work with other team members
- advocacy on behalf of one's patients
- sensitivity to potential conflicts of interest
- the capacity to recognize one's limits
- the commitment to continuously improve one's knowledge and abilities

These basic elements of the "art" of medicine, along with other important characteristics such as motivation, persistence, and communication and interpersonal skills, evolve over time. Experience in a health-care setting, caring for an ill or elderly family member, participating in basic or clinical science research efforts, working as an emergency medical technician, "shadowing" a physician, or providing emotional support to people in a rape crisis center, emergency room, or social service agency — these types of service activities are recommended to those considering medicine as a career.

TABLE 3-A

Subjects Required by 10 or More U.S. Medical Schools, 2009–2010 Entering Class

Required Subject	No. of Schools (n=129)	Required Subject	No. of Schools (n=129)
Physics	120	Calculus	17
Inorganic (General) Chemistry	119	College Mathematics	35
Organic Chemistry	121	Behavioral Sciences	9
English	84	Humanities	14
Biology	85	Biochemistry	13
Biology/Zoology	40		

NOTE: Figures based on data provided fall 2007.

By participating in such activities, premedical students learn both about the medical profession and about themselves. They learn about their tolerance for stress, their ability to communicate and empathize with people from different backgrounds and cultures, their problem-solving skills, and their willingness to put others' needs before their own. They also come to better understand the nature of medical practice and the daily demands placed upon physicians and their family members. After learning these important lessons, they can decide whether medicine is an appropriate career choice for them.

Finally, premedical students should know how these experiences are assessed by medical school admission committees. At least three criteria are used: length of time invested, depth of the experience, and lessons learned. Short-term experiences such as day-long blood drives or one-time-only shadowing experiences are less enlightening than semester or year-long commitments. Passive activities such as observation are less instructive than those requiring active participation. Most important, admission committees want to know what students derived from these experiences. Applicants should be prepared to answer these kinds of questions about their community, clinical, or research experiences.

For the enrolled medical student, the satisfaction derived from these experiences is often the motivational factor that helps them to "pull through" the challenging demands of medical school, which affect even the best students.

Premedical Advising

Students investigating a career in medicine — no matter where they might be in the process — can get extremely valuable advice from their campus prehealth advisor. Depending on the individual school, prehealth advisors function on either a full or part-time basis. They may be a faculty member (often in a science department), a staff member in the office of an academic dean or the career center, the director of an advising office for pre-professional students, or a physician in part-time practice. Ideally, prehealth advisors are knowledgeable and supportive, as well as well-informed about medical education programs, both locally and nationally. Advisors belong to organizations such as the National Association of Advisors for the Health Professions (NAAHP, *www.naahp.org*) that assist them in their work. They are able to provide information, guidance, and support to interested students and, at times, even challenge students to consider new options or reconsider their decisions.

Prehealth advisors assist premedical students to:

- identify college courses that satisfy premedical requirements
- determine an appropriate sequence for completing those courses
- find tutorial assistance, if needed
- plan academic schedules to accommodate both premedical coursework and other educational objectives, including a study program abroad, a dual major, or a senior honors thesis
- locate volunteer or paid clinical and research experiences
- strengthen the medical school application
- prepare for interviews and standardized tests
- arrange for letters of evaluation and recommendation
- determine the most appropriate career paths based on individual assets, liabilities, values, and life goals

Premedical students usually meet with prehealth advisors when they:

- enter into a premedical curriculum
- join a prehealth student society
- change majors or courses of study
- need information about medical school admission requirements
- prepare to apply to medical school
- get ready for medical school interviews
- seek community, clinical, or research experiences
- require advice about resolving academic problems
- want to discuss future career paths
- plan a postbaccalaureate premedical program or coursework
- prepare for health profession school admission tests
- need letters of evaluation or recommendation

Services provided by a prehealth advisor. Advisors' services typically vary according to the advisor's employment status, the number of premedical students to be served, and the philosophy and organizational structure of the institution. Students should contact their school's advisor to determine what services are available; they generally fall into five categories:

- Academics. Advisors are well informed about premedical coursework on their campuses and about developing suitable academic programs for prehealth students. They collaborate with campus academic staff in designing study, reading skill, and test preparation workshops, and in offering tutoring programs. Advisors publicize regional and national programs of interest to their students.
- Clinical and research experiences. Advisors often work with advisory groups composed of college and medical school teaching and research faculty and community clinicians. These groups help identify part-time jobs, volunteer positions, and opportunities for independent study credit in local laboratories and offices.

- Assistance to student organizations. Advisors often coordinate the activities of the local and national organizations and academic societies that serve prehealth students. These groups plan programs, identify funding sources, and arrange for campus visits from admissions and financial aid personnel, as well as medical school alumni and practicing physicians.
- Advising and support. Advisors help students to pursue realistic individual goals and maximize their potential. They meet with students individually, and they provide group opportunities for students to meet each other and community representatives from various health professions. Advisors establish peer advising and mentoring programs. They are sensitive to the needs of students, including their financial needs, their being a member of a group currently underrepresented in medicine, or their being first in their family to attend college.
- Sharing resources. Prehealth advisors disseminate information and publications from relevant organizations, including the AAMC and the National Association of Advisors for the Health Professions. They provide computer access to Web-based health careers programs and those on educational financing. They distribute information about local, regional, national, and international research and service opportunities. They stock a library of publications related to medical school and medical education, including *Medical School Admission Requirements* (MSAR).

The prehealth committee letter of recommendation. One important service provided by the advisor to prehealth students, and frequently also to alumni, is the prehealth committee letter of recommendation. This is usually a composite letter written on behalf of a medical school applicant by the college or university's prehealth committee. The prehealth advisor may be a committee member or the committee chair, and is usually the liaison between students and the committee, facilitating letter-writing and the distribution of letters to schools.

This letter presents an overview of the student's academic strengths, exposure to health care and medical research environments, contributions to the campus and community, and personal attributes such as maturity and altruism. The letter may also address any extenuating circumstances that may have resulted in deficits in the student's performance during a course or semester, or provide perspective on challenges and problems the student may have encountered. The letter can also explain school-specific courses and programs in which the student has participated.

Some undergraduate institutions do not provide composite letters of recommendation. Instead, they collect individual letters of recommendation and evaluation during the student's enrollment and distribute them at the appropriate time to the medical schools where the student has applied. Students should inquire about the specific services that their institution's prehealth advisor provides.

Finding a prehealth advisor. Students who have difficulty identifying an advisor on their own campus should contact the National Association of Advisors for the Health Professions (NAAHP, *www.naahp.org*). If a student's school does not have a prehealth advisor, volunteer advisors at other institutions may be identified. The NAAHP also offers publications to help students prepare for medical school. You can contact the NAAHP at:

National Association of Advisors for the Health Professions
P.O. Box 1518
Champaign, IL 61824-1518
T (217) 355-0063 F (217) 355-1287
naahpja@aol.com

Special Programs

The majority of medical school applicants are seniors in college. However, numerous schools offer special programs to accommodate "non-traditional" pre-medical and medical students:

Combined college/medical school programs. These programs begin after high school and combine undergraduate and medical school curricula. About five percent of medical students begin their medical education in these programs, which vary by school. Most include the typical eight years of premedical and medical study, although a small number permit students to complete both college and medical school in six to seven years. Several programs limit participation to state residents, and many require prospective medical students to be enrolled at specific affiliated undergraduate institutions. Additional information can be found in Chapter 10.

Deferred entry. Many medical schools consider requests from accepted applicants who wish to defer matriculation, usually for a year, to take advantage of a special opportunity or for other personal reasons. Most schools require a written application and review requests on an individual basis. Some schools require deferred applicants to sign an agreement to attend that school the following year; others will hold a place in the next entering class until a mutually agreed upon date, even if the applicant decides to seek admission to other schools for the next year. Interested applicants are advised to obtain additional information about specific school requirements regarding deferred entry from individual medical schools as they differ from school to school and sometimes change on a year-to-year basis; the school-specific pages in Chapters 12 and 13 also provide relevant information.

Postbaccalaureate premedical programs. Not all medical school applicants are college seniors; some have already completed college. Some embarked on other careers after college, but then decided to apply to medical school. If these graduates were not previously science majors, they must complete required premedical coursework through postbaccalaureate premedical programs, which exist at colleges and universities across the country, both public and private. The programs range from formal, one and two-year programs for full-time students to more informal part-time ones. Some specialize in applicants who are planning to change careers, while others focus on those attempting to enhance their prior academic performance. A searchable database of postbaccalaureate premedical programs can be found on the AAMC Web site at *http://services.aamc.org/postbac*.

Chapter 4

The Application Process

The annual medical school application process begins each spring, as applicants use one of three different processes for applying to U.S. medical schools:

- the American Medical College Application Service (AMCAS) for the 134 U.S. schools and programs (including the M.D./Ph.D. programs of the Texas A&M University System Health Science Center College of Medicine, the University of Texas Southwestern Medical School at Dallas, the University of Texas Medical School at Houston, and the University of Texas Medical Branch at Galveston) that participated in AMCAS for the 2008 entering class (*www.aamc.org/amcas*)
- the Texas Medical and Dental Schools Application Service (TMDSAS) for the seven public allopathic medical schools in Texas (*www.utsystem.edu/tmdsas*)
- school-specific application forms for two medical schools with their own individual application processes. Individual schools often supplement AMCAS and TMDSAS application materials with their own forms and materials, known as "supplemental" or "secondary" application materials.

Application Procedures

AMCAS, TMDSAS, and individual schools manage their application processes and the procedures by which applicant information is made available to medical school admission committee members. The authority and responsibility for selecting individuals who will be admitted to a medical school rest with each school's faculty. Acting through its standing admission committee, the faculty develops and approves criteria for admission. The administrative responsibility for receiving and processing applications rests with admissions officers and members of the admissions office staff. The responsibility for reviewing applicant information, interviewing candidates, and making decisions about admitting candidates rests with admission committee members.

Composition of the admission committee. Medical school admission committees typically include faculty representatives from both basic science and clinical departments. In addition, membership also frequently includes faculty from other colleges and schools in the university, community physicians, other community members, and medical students.

Application processing. Applications are screened and categorized by admissions office staff according to criteria established by the admission committee. Depending on the school, supplemental application materials (including letters of recommendation, an essay, legal residency and other school forms, and a fee) may be requested from all or some applicants, or only from those who meet specific criteria.

As applications are completed, applicants who are of greatest interest to schools are contacted by admissions office staff, and arrangements are made for campus visits and interviews with admission committee members. At some institutions, meetings with off-campus interviewers, including practicing physicians located near an applicant's home or school, may be required. As the process continues, other applicants may also be contacted and interviewed.

Applicants are typically interviewed by more than one committee member, either individually or in a group. After completion of the interview process, interviewers' evaluations are correlated with all other application materials and presented to the admission committee for discussion. Final decisions about admission are usually made by the committee acting as a whole.

All applicants, whether or not they are interviewed, are informed of the admission committee's decision according to the school's individual schedule. Committee decisions can range from an offer of immediate acceptance, to placement of the applicant in a "hold" category or on an alternate list, to non-acceptance. As the admission cycle continues, acceptances are offered until the required number of matriculants have been identified for that year's entering class.

Early Decision Program or regular application? One of an applicant's first decisions is whether to apply to a medical school through the Early Decision Program (EDP) or the regular application process. The fact that candidates applying through the EDP are informed about the outcome of their application at a participating school by October 1 affords them sufficient time to apply to other schools through the regular process if they are not accepted through the EDP.

The decision to apply through the EDP should be made carefully. While criteria for accepting EDP applicants vary among schools, a frequent criterion is that applicants show extraordinary credentials for admission. Applicants considering an EDP application should contact the medical school admissions office for more specific information.

EDP applicants must agree:

• not to apply through the EDP if they have already submitted an initial or secondary (AMCAS or non-AMCAS) application to the M.D. degree program at another U.S. allopathic medical school for the current entering class
• to apply to only one AMCAS medical school through the EDP
• not to submit additional (AMCAS or non-AMCAS) applications until they have received notification of non-acceptance through the EDP, or they have been formally released from the EDP commitment, or the October 1 EDP notification deadline has passed
• to attend the school if offered an EDP acceptance

All EDP applicants accepted by a medical school must adhere to the tenets of the program; any violation will result in an investigation by AMCAS.
With regard to the EDP, medical schools agree to:

• notify each EDP applicant of the admission decision by October 1
• defer each EDP applicant to the regular applicant pool in those instances when an EDP non-acceptance decision is made

Timing of the application process. Each medical school establishes annual deadline dates for receipt of both primary and secondary application materials at the school. These dates are published in medical school bulletins and application materials, on school Web sites, and in Chapters 12 and 13. (Deadline dates range from mid-October to mid-December for receipt of primary application materials at AMCAS-participating schools and November 1 for TMDSAS-participating schools, with varying dates for school-specific applications.) Deadlines for receipt of all secondary application materials at medical schools also vary. Applicants should be aware of all deadline dates for all schools to which they are applying.

The deadline for receipt by AMCAS of the application, fee, and official transcripts for EDP applicants is August 1. (Contact the admissions office or see Chapters 12 and 13 for early decision application deadlines at schools that do not participate in AMCAS.) All secondary application materials must be received at the EDP school by the school's deadline date. EDP candidates may be interviewed by admission committees in late August or September so that final decisions can be made and communicated to EDP candidates by October 1.

Admission committees generally interview candidates for regular admission during the fall, winter, and spring months. Most regular admission offers are made during

the winter months. Medical schools collectively agree to issue, by March 30 of the matriculation year, a number of acceptances at least equal to the size of the first-year entering class. Applicants are therefore encouraged to submit their applications as early in the application process as possible. They are also responsible for ensuring that all required materials are received by the relevant application service and the individual medical school in a timely fashion. Medical schools are not responsible for notifying applicants if parts of their application file are missing.

Notification of acceptance. For the past four decades, AAMC-member medical schools, regardless of the type of application system used, have agreed to observe a set of acceptance procedures for first-year entering students, commonly referred to as the admission "traffic rules." Observing these recommendations (see Page 48 or *www.aamc.org/students/applying/policies*) ensures that applicants and schools know, usually by June, who will be matriculating at each school in the fall. The deadline for notifying EDP applicants of EDP admission decisions is October 1. The earliest and latest dates for notifying regular applicants of acceptance, and the time allowed for applicants to respond to acceptance offers, are indicated in each school's entry in Chapters 12 and 13. The "traffic rules" also recommend that school deposits required of accepted applicants not exceed $100, and that they be refundable until May 15. The deposit amount and refund policy for each school are also indicated in Chapters 12 and 13.

Applicant responsibilities. Just as medical schools agree to a set of "traffic rules" in the application and admission process, applicants are also expected to observe a set of procedures (see Page 50 or *www.aamc.org/students/applying/policies*), thus ensuring an orderly and timely selection process for other applicants and for schools.

Schools' and applicants' observance of these procedures helps to ensure that all applicants are afforded timely notification of the outcome of their medical school applications and timely access to available first-year positions and that schools are protected from having unfilled positions in their first-year entering classes.

Falsifications, omissions, or discrepancies in application materials or irregular behavior during administration of the MCAT® examination will be investigated in accordance with AAMC investigation policies.

The Medical College Admission Test

The Medical College Admission Test (MCAT®) is a standardized examination designed to assist medical school admission committees in assessing applicants' academic preparation, achievement in science, verbal reasoning skills, and written communication skills, and in predicting which applicants will perform adequately in the rigorous medical school curriculum. The MCAT® examination consists of multiple-choice questions and a writing assessment administered as a computerized examination in most parts of the U.S. and Canada and in international locations. Current information about registration, scheduling, testing dates, and testing locations for the computerized MCAT® can be accessed on the MCAT® Web site at *www.aamc.org/mcat*.

The MCAT® provides admission committees with standardized measures of performance for all examinees. The test content outline was developed with input from medical school admissions officers, premedical faculty members, medical educators, practicing physicians, AAMC staff, and a group of testing experts under contract to the AAMC. The MCAT® examination is also designed to encourage those interested in a medical career to pursue broad undergraduate study in the natural and social sciences and in the humanities. It assesses facility with scientific problem-solving, critical thinking skills, and writing ability, as well as the understanding of scientific concepts and principles identified as required for the study of medicine.

The four sections of the MCAT® examination are Physical Sciences, Verbal Reasoning, Biological Sciences, and Writing Sample:

- Physical Sciences and Biological Sciences. These sections are constructed to assess material covered in introductory undergraduate courses in biology; chemistry, including inorganic chemistry and organic chemistry; and general, non-calculus physics. Both sections consist entirely of science problems and may include data presented in graphs, tables, and charts. Both sections are designed to evaluate knowledge of basic concepts, facility with scientific problem-solving, and the ability to interpret data presented in a tabular or graphic format.
- Verbal Reasoning. This section is designed to assess applicants' abilities to comprehend, reason, and think critically. It draws upon material from the humanities, social sciences, and natural sciences. Subject-matter knowledge is not evaluated; the content information necessary to answer test questions is presented in each passage. In preparation for this section, examinees are encouraged to familiarize themselves with the practice of critical thinking and the use of reasoning skills in these disciplines.
- Writing Sample. The essay topics that constitute this section are designed to provide examinees with an opportunity to demonstrate writing and analytic skills. Examinees are allotted 30 minutes to write an essay on a first assigned topic, then another 30 minutes to write an essay on a second assigned topic; each requires an expository response. Essay topics do not pertain to the technical content of biology, chemistry, physics, or mathematics; the medical school application process; reasons for desiring a career in medicine; social or cultural issues not part of the general experience of MCAT® examinees; religious issues; or emotionally-charged subjects.

MCAT® scoring. A total of five MCAT® scores are reported, one for each MCAT® section and a total score. Scores for the Physical Sciences, Verbal Reasoning, and Biological Sciences sections are presented on a numerical scale, ranging from a low of 1 to a high of 15. Scores for the Writing Sample section are presented on an alphabetical scale, ranging from a low of J to a high of T. A total score is also reported, which is the sum of the Physical Sciences, Verbal Reasoning, and Biological Sciences sections, along with the Writing Sample score: for example, 45T.

The MCAT® is administered and scored by the MCAT® Program Office at the direction of the AAMC. Information about the specific content of the examination, its organization, and the scoring system appears on the MCAT® Web site at *www.aamc.org/mcat*.

Test dates. The MCAT® will be administered on 23 days in 2008. On two of these days, the MCAT® will be administered twice, once in the morning and once in the afternoon, for a total of 25 administrations throughout the year. The other 21 days will have either a morning or an afternoon administration.

The first administrations of the year will be in January 2008. In 2008, the MCAT® will also be administered in each month from April to September (for specific dates, see the MCAT® test administration calendar on the MCAT® Web site at *www.aamc.org/mcat*). Most medical schools will utilize MCAT® scores from

2008 MCAT® administrations only for applications to their 2009 entering class. Applicants should check with individual schools to determine their policies regarding utilization of 2009 MCAT® scores for applications to the 2009 entering class. Relevant information can also be found on the school-specific pages in Chapters 12 and 13.

Potential medical school applicants are advised to take the MCAT® about 12-18 months prior to their expected entry into medical school. Many medical schools prefer that applicants take the MCAT® early in the year because of the short time between the availability of late summer and September scores and school application deadlines. Taking the MCAT® early in the calendar year also allows time for students to retake the test later, if necessary. For applicants enrolled in summer courses, a late-summer MCAT® administration may be preferable. Scores will be returned to examinees and available to medical schools approximately 30 days after the test administration. This enables applicants to take the test as late as September and still have their scores available before school application deadlines.

Only those persons who intend to apply to a school of allopathic, osteopathic, podiatric, or veterinary medicine are permitted to take the MCAT®; any other potential examinees must receive special permission prior to taking the examination.

Fees and registration. The examination fee is $210 for each of the 2008 MCAT® administrations. Registration for the 2008 MCAT® is available only online at *www.aamc.org/mcat*. Prior to registering for the MCAT®, potential examinees must familiarize themselves with the information in the publication *2008 MCAT® Essentials*, which is available on the MCAT® Web site.

Testing with accommodations.
Potential examinees with appropriately documented disabilities that meet the definition of a disability under the Americans with Disabilities Act (ADA) may request testing accommodations. Examinees with chronic medical conditions or short-term disabilities that are not covered by the ADA and who have special testing needs should consult with the MCAT® program about accommodations. Information about the documentation that is needed to request testing accommodations and application deadline dates is available at *www.aamc.org/mcat*.

Preparation for the MCAT®. The MCAT® is a "high stakes" achievement test; scores are carefully evaluated by medical school admission committees. Examinees should prepare for the MCAT® by completing premedical introductory biology, general and organic chemistry, and physics coursework (see Chapter 3) prior to taking the MCAT® examination for the first time. If some time has elapsed since the completion of premedical courses, review of course material prior to taking the MCAT® is highly recommended. Potential examinees with ongoing challenges in reading speed or comprehension are advised to address and resolve those issues prior to taking the examination. Campus academic advising or academic skills staff are often well informed about these and related issues.

The MCAT® should not be taken "cold" or for "diagnostic" reasons; the MCAT® Practice Tests can be used for preparation. A variety of MCAT® preparation materials are described at the end of the section.

Retaking the MCAT®. Applicants who are not satisfied with their MCAT® scores should confer with their prehealth advisor about the advisability of retaking the test. Legitimate reasons for retaking the MCAT® can include:

- a significant discrepancy between college grades and MCAT® scores
- having taken the examination prematurely (i.e., without adequate preparation or prior to completion of all relevant premedical coursework)
- serious illness at the time of the examination
- a recommendation from a medical school admissions officer or admission committee member that the MCAT® be retaken

Application procedures for retaking the examination are identical to those for initial testing. The MCAT® may be taken a maximum of three times during each calendar year; there are no exceptions to this policy.

Score reporting. Payment of the MCAT® examination fee includes the reporting of test scores to AMCAS, other application services, and individual medical schools. MCAT® scores are available approximately 30 days after the examination date. Examinees can view MCAT® scores from 1991 to present through the MCAT® Testing History (THx) System (*www.aamc.org/mcat*). Examinees who have tested in 2003 or later and have applied via AMCAS will automatically have their scores released to those institutions designated within the AMCAS application. Scores from tests taken prior to 2003 or any that are to be released to non-AMCAS institutions (regardless of year taken) must be released using the THx System. To request MCAT® scores prior to 1991, examinees must print and complete the request form available on the MCAT® web site (*www.aamc.org/mcat*).

MCAT® examinees are encouraged to request, at the time of registration or through the AMCAS application, that their scores be sent directly to their premedical advisors. This is a free service.

MCAT® publications. The AAMC publishes a variety of practice materials, including a series of official practice tests. MCAT® Practice Online provides previously administered tests. The practice materials feature automated scoring, integrated solutions, diagnostic reports, customized item selection, daily test-taking tips, discussion boards, and enhanced printing options. Free access to a single full-length MCAT® with all the features of MCAT® Practice Online is available at *www.e-mcat.com*.

MCAT® publications are available for purchase online through the MCAT® Web site (*www.aamc.org/mcat*).The MCAT® Web site also contains the *MCAT® Student Manual*, with detailed information about the format and content of the examination and outlines of the science, problem-solving, critical thinking, and communication skills tested by the MCAT®.

American Medical College Application Service (AMCAS)

The American Medical College Application Service (AMCAS) is a non-profit, centralized application processing service for applicants to the first-year entering classes at participating U.S. medical schools. AMCAS policies and procedures are developed in consultation with representatives of participating medical schools. AMCAS benefits both schools and applicants by collecting, verifying, and processing application data and MCAT® scores on behalf of participating medical schools and transmitting those data to them.

AMCAS also assists admission committees by providing rosters and statistical reports regarding the national and individual medical school applicant pools, as well as aggregate data about accepted applicants at medical schools across the nation. AMCAS data are used by the AAMC in various research efforts regarding the medical school applicant and matriculant pools.

AMCAS does not render admission decisions or advise applicants as to the medical schools to which they should apply. Each medical school, through its admission committee and admissions officer, is completely autonomous in its admission decisions.

For the 2009 entering class, 134 U.S. medical schools and programs (including the M.D./Ph.D. program of the Texas A&M University System Health Science Center College of Medicine, the University of Texas Southwestern Medical School at Dallas, the University of Texas Medical School at Houston, and the University of Texas Medical Branch at Galveston) will participate in AMCAS. The nine U.S. medical schools that will not participate in AMCAS for the 2009 entering class include the:

- University of Missouri-Kansas City School of Medicine
- University of North Dakota School of Medicine and Health Sciences
- Texas A&M University System Health Science Center College of Medicine*
- Texas Tech University Health Sciences Center School of Medicine
- Texas Tech University Health Sciences Center, El Paso, Paul L. Foster School of Medicine
- University of Texas Southwestern Medical Center at Dallas Southwestern Medical School*
- University of Texas Medical School at Galveston*
- University of Texas Medical School at Houston*
- University of Texas School of Medicine at San Antonio

The most current listing of participating schools and programs is available at *www.aamc.org/students/amcas/ participatingschools.htm*.

The AMCAS application. The AMCAS application is available via the AMCAS Web site at *www.aamc.org/amcas*. On the AMCAS Web site, applicants will find links to key steps in starting an application, an application worksheet that previews the application content, an application timeline, important FAQs, and other resources to assist them with the application, such as an instruction booklet in PDF format.

The AMCAS application permits applicants to complete, certify, and submit their AMCAS application via the AMCAS Web site. The AMCAS application is accessible 24 hours a day, beginning on or about May 1, 2008, for the 2009 entering class.

AAMC registration. The AAMC has a global registration system. Applicants who have previously registered for the MCAT® THx System, the Fee Assistance Program, AMCAS, or other AAMC services have already selected an AAMC username and password and been assigned an AAMC ID; they should use the same access information to enter the AMCAS application. Those who have not recently registered for AAMC services must complete the AMCAS registration form, select a username and password, and be assigned an AAMC ID. The AAMC secure username, login, and password sequence ensures the confidentiality of their application information.

Transcript requirements and deadlines. Applicants must request that an official transcript be forwarded to AMCAS by the registrar of every post-secondary school at which they have ever been registered.

* The M.D. Programs of the Texas A&M University System Health Science Center College of Medicine, the University of Texas Southwestern Medical School in Dallas, the University of Texas Medical School at Houston, and the University of Texas Medical Branch at Galveston participate in the Texas Medical and Dental School Application Service for the 2009 entering class, but their M.D.-Ph.D. programs participate in the American Medical College Application Service (AMCAS) for the 2009 entering class. Please refer to Chapter 12 for more information.

AMCAS provides a "transcript request form" that expedites the cataloguing and processing of transcripts. To generate a transcript request form, the applicant must complete the "Identifying Information" and "Schools Attended" sections of the AMCAS application and follow the directions for printing the transcript request form. Prior to submitting this form to the registrar's office, the form should be carefully reviewed to ensure that the information is accurate and that the registrar's address is current. Simultaneously, applicants are encouraged to request personal copies of each transcript prior to completing the "Academic Record" section of the AMCAS application.

Transcripts are required from every junior college, community college, trade school, or professional school within the United States, Canada, or U.S. territories, regardless of whether or not credit was earned. This requirement applies also to college courses taken while in high school. Transcripts submitted to AMCAS for prior years' applications cannot be used to verify coursework and grades for an application to the 2009 entering class.

Application materials and official transcripts for the Early Decision Program (EDP) must be received by AMCAS by August 1, 2008. For regular applicants, all official transcripts must be received no later than two weeks following the deadline date for application materials. Refer to the AMCAS online instruction booklet or help text for detailed information about official transcript requirements and deadlines; this information is available at *www.aamc.org/amcas*. AMCAS begins accepting official transcripts on or about May 1, 2008.

Completing the AMCAS application.
The application is divided into different sections, which may be completed during multiple sittings. Extensive on-screen instructions and help text are provided. Payment is also received online.

Applicants are encouraged to print their application after submitting it to AMCAS. To ensure that the submission process was successfully completed, applicants should check the "Date Submitted" field in the upper left-hand corner of the first page of the application. The "Date Submitted" field should have been modified from "N/A" to the current date.

Applicant monitoring responsibilities.
AMCAS provides a dynamic welcome page that details the status of each application. Applicants are responsible for checking this page and addressing identified errors and omissions. Applicants are also expected to thoroughly review changes made by AMCAS during the verification process and alert AMCAS to any issues regarding these changes.

Applicants may change certain information on their application and apply to additional medical schools, using their username, login, and password sequence, after their initial application has been submitted; each add/change requires that the applicant recertify and resubmit the application.

Processing of applications. Regardless of the number of AMCAS-participating schools to which an individual applies, only one application should be submitted to AMCAS. After receipt of the service fee and an official transcript from each postsecondary school at which the applicant has been registered, AMCAS verifies the accuracy of the academic record, as entered by the applicant, by comparing it with the official transcript(s) received in support of the application. Each year, AMCAS surveys postsecondary school registrars for grading system updates, and uses this registrar-provided information to assign AMCAS grades and calculate a normalized GPA for each applicant. Once processing of an application has been completed by AMCAS, AMCAS makes the application available to all designated medical schools. AMCAS also distributes MCAT®

scores, provided that the applicant has released those scores to AMCAS. All 2003 and later MCAT® scores are automatically included in an applicant's AMCAS application. Scores from MCAT® administrations in years prior to 2003 are provided to AMCAS only if the applicant has released those scores to AMCAS.

AAMC Fee Assistance Program (FAP)
The AAMC believes that the cost of applying to medical school should not be a financial barrier to individuals who are interested in becoming physicians. The AAMC Fee Assistance Program (FAP) assists MCAT® examinees and AMCAS applicants who, without financial assistance, would be unable to take the MCAT® or apply to these medical schools that use the AMCAS application.

Applicants who are approved for fee assistance receive the following benefits from the AAMC:

• Reduction of the MCAT® registration fee from $210 to $85 for test administrations in 2008

• Waiver of the application fee of $490 for submitting the completed AMCAS application to up to 13 AMCAS-participating medical schools. Applicants pay $30 for each school beyond the 13 free applications.

In addition, most AMCAS-participating medical schools waive their supplemental application fees for applicants who have been granted fee assistance by the AAMC.

Eligibility
Eligibility decisions are now tied directly to the U.S. Department of Health and Human Services poverty level guidelines. For the 2008 calendar year, applicants whose annual family income is 300% or less of the federal poverty level for their family size will be approved for fee assistance.

How FAP works

Applying for fee assistance is simple. Upon submission of the FAP application online, the FAP program will immediately determine whether or not an applicant meets FAP eligibility requirements. If tentatively approved, the applicant will be asked to submit documentation in support of the application. If the applicant is determined to be ineligible, submission of documentation is not necessary.

Timeline

The FAP application is available online from January through December of each calendar year. However, applicants should note that the FAP application and all required supporting documentation should be received at least three weeks prior to the desired MCAT® registration date and/or AMCAS application deadline.

Additional information about the FAP, including instructions, the application, and information about relevant deadline dates, is available at *www.aamc.org/fap*.

Applicant and Accepted Applicant Data

In 2006-2007, 42,315 persons applied to the 2007 entering class at the 126* allopathic medical schools in the United States. By the fall of 2007, 18,858 applicants had been offered an acceptance to at least one medical school, and 17,759 accepted applicants had matriculated. These accepted applicants possessed a broad range of MCAT® scores and undergraduate grade point averages, as well as a wide variety of personal characteristics and life experiences. Both male and female applicants were distributed across numerous racial and ethnic groups. A small number applied through the Early Decision Program, but the majority used the regular application process.

This chapter contains graphic representations of relevant data for the entire applicant pool, as well as for accepted and non-accepted applicants, for the 2007 entering class. All data presented in this chapter are accurate as of September 25, 2007 [Source: AAMC Data Warehouse; Applicant Matriculant File]. In the following charts:

- "All Applicants" refers to all applicants to the 2007 entering class
- "Accepted Applicants" refers to those applicants accepted to at least one medical school
- "Not Accepted" applicants refers to those applicants not accepted to any medical school

A small number of accepted applicants chose not to matriculate in 2007.

By familiarizing themselves with this information, reviewing the school-specific data in Chapter 12, and comparing themselves with applicants to the 2007 entering class, potential applicants can determine their relative standing on a variety of admission-related factors and can, with their advisors' help, make decisions that are appropriate for them. Extensive information about medical school applicants and matriculants can also be found online at *www.aamc.org/data/facts*.

Performance on the MCAT®

Charts 5-A – 5-E present information about the performance of applicants on the MCAT®:

- Chart 5-A shows that applicants achieved Verbal Reasoning (VR) scores at each score from 1 to 15; the largest number achieved a VR score of 9. Accepted applicants' scores ranged from 1 to 15, although very few had VR scores below 5 (just under 80). At a VR score of 10, the number of accepted applicants exceeded the number not accepted.

Chart 5-A

MCAT® Verbal Reasoning Score Distribution, Year 2007 Applicants

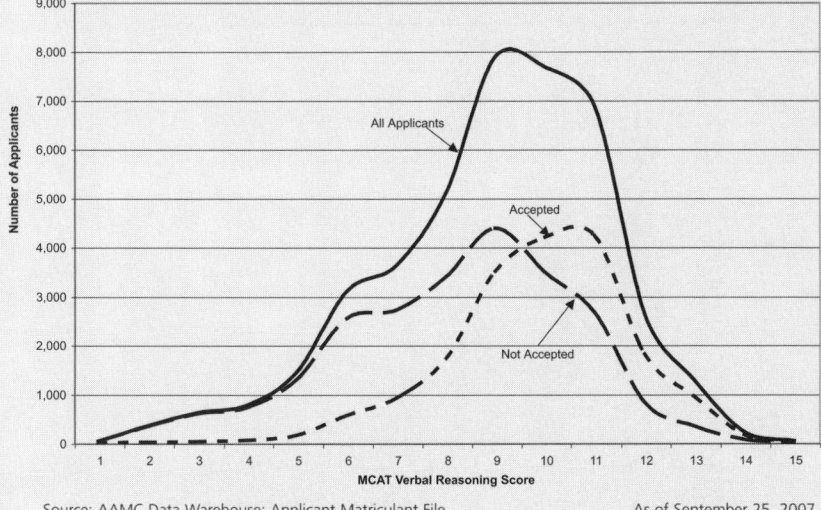

Source: AAMC Data Warehouse: Applicant Matriculant File   As of September 25, 2007

*Acceptance data for medical schools newly accredited in 2007 and 2008 were not included for year 2007 applicants.

Chart 5-B

Physical Sciences Score Distribution, Year 2007 Applicants

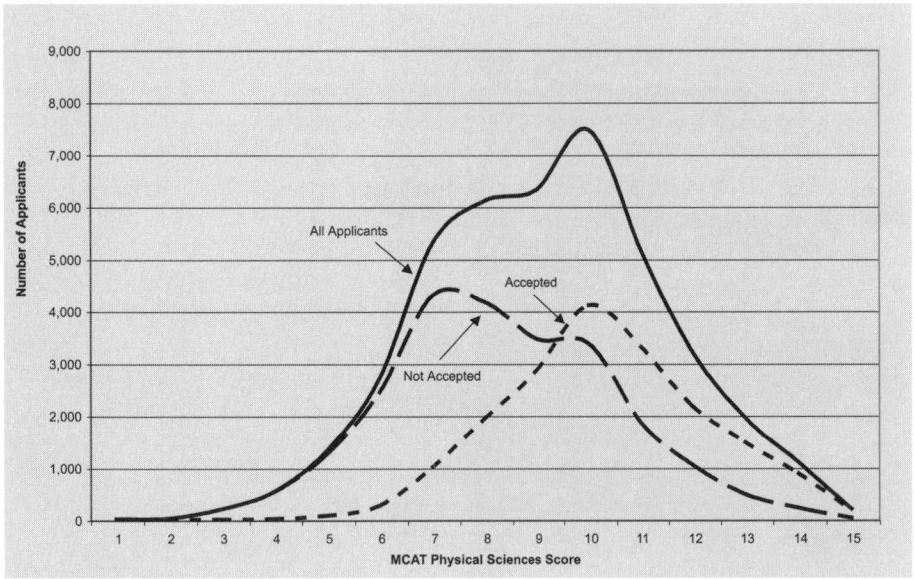

Source: AAMC Data Warehouse: Applicant Matriculant File   As of September 25, 2007

- Chart 5-B shows that applicants achieved Physical Sciences (PS) scores at each score from 1 to 15; the largest number achieved a PS score of 10. Accepted applicants' scores ranged from 3 to 15; fewer than 90 accepted applicants achieved a score of 5 or below. Accepted applicants exceeded not accepted applicants at a PS score of 10.

- Chart 5-C shows that applicants achieved Writing Sample (WS) scores at each score from J to T; the largest number achieved a WS score of Q. Accepted applicants' scores ranged from J to T; the number with scores of K and below was about 130. Accepted applicants exceeded not accepted applicants at a score of Q.

Chart 5-C

MCAT® Writing Sample Score Distribution, Year 2007 Applicants

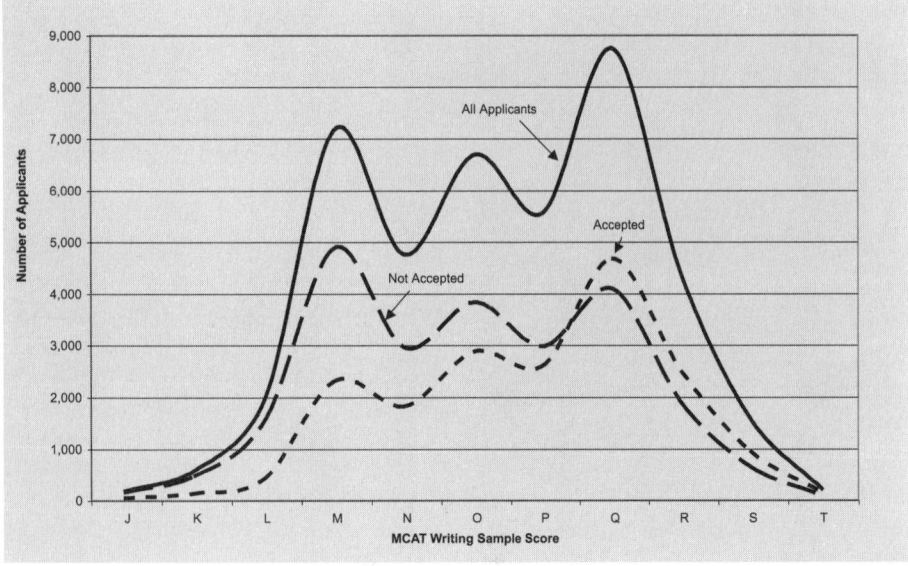

Source: AAMC Data Warehouse: Applicant Matriculant File   As of September 25, 2007

- Chart 5-D shows that applicants achieved Biological Sciences (BS) scores at each score from 1 to 15; the largest number achieved a BS score of 10. Accepted applicants' scores ranged from 2 to 15; about 50 scored 5 or below. Accepted applicants exceeded not accepted applicants at a score of 10.

- Chart 5-E — which shows total scores on the numerically scored sections of Verbal Reasoning, Physical Sciences, and Biological Sciences — reveals that applicants achieved total scores from 4 to 44; the largest number achieved a total score of 29. Accepted applicants achieved total scores from 9 to 44; the number of accepted applicants with total scores of 17 and below (an average of almost 6 on each section) was about 40. Accepted applicants exceeded not accepted applicants at a total score of 29.

No score on a single MCAT® section and no total MCAT® score "guarantees" admission to medical school. Charts 5-A, 5-B, and 5-D reveal that, while applicants with VR, PS, and BS scores of 10 and above had a higher probability of being accepted to medical school, a significant number of applicants with such scores were not accepted. The same holds true for the Writing Sample section; a score of Q and above is a likely, though not definite, barometer for acceptance. Finally, Chart 5-E shows that a substantial number of applicants with total MCAT® scores of 29 and above were not accepted. These findings reveal the importance of factors other than MCAT® performance — including undergraduate academic performance and a variety of personal characteristics and experiential variables — in the medical student selection process.

Chart 5-D
MCAT® Biological Sciences Score Distribution, Year 2007 Applicants

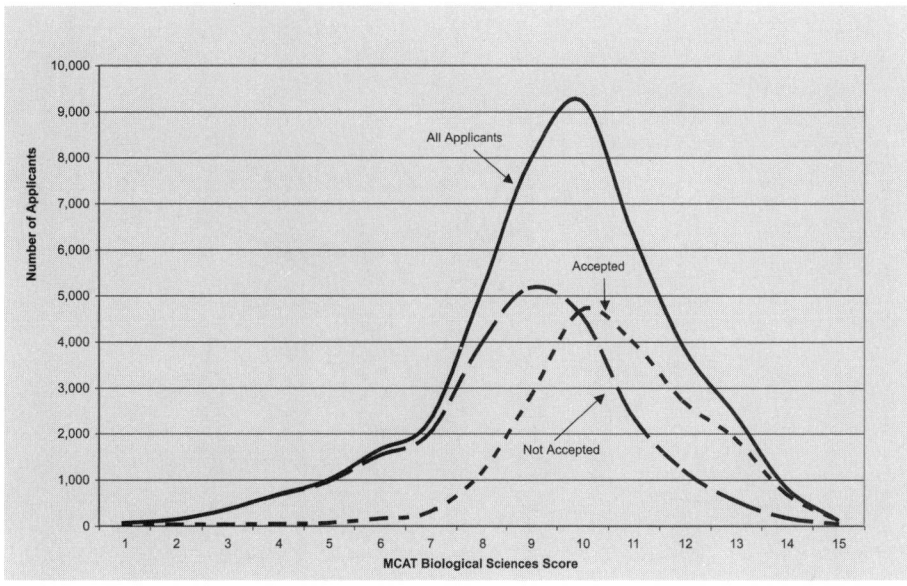

Source: AAMC Data Warehouse: Applicant Matriculant File   As of September 25, 2007

Chart 5-E
MCAT® Total Numeric Score Distribution, Year 2007 Applicants

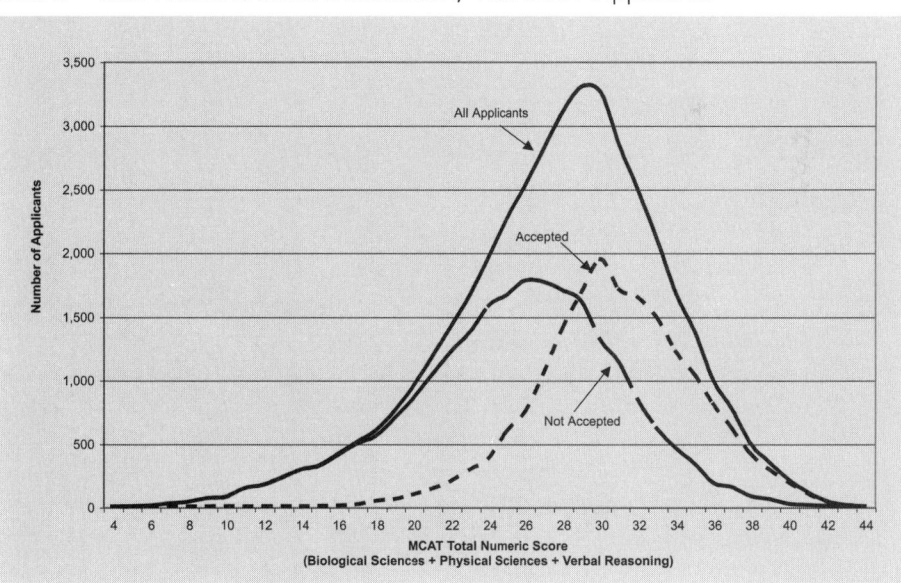

Source: AAMC Data Warehouse: Applicant Matriculant File   As of September 25, 2007

Chart 5-F
Science GPA Distribution, Year 2007 Applicants

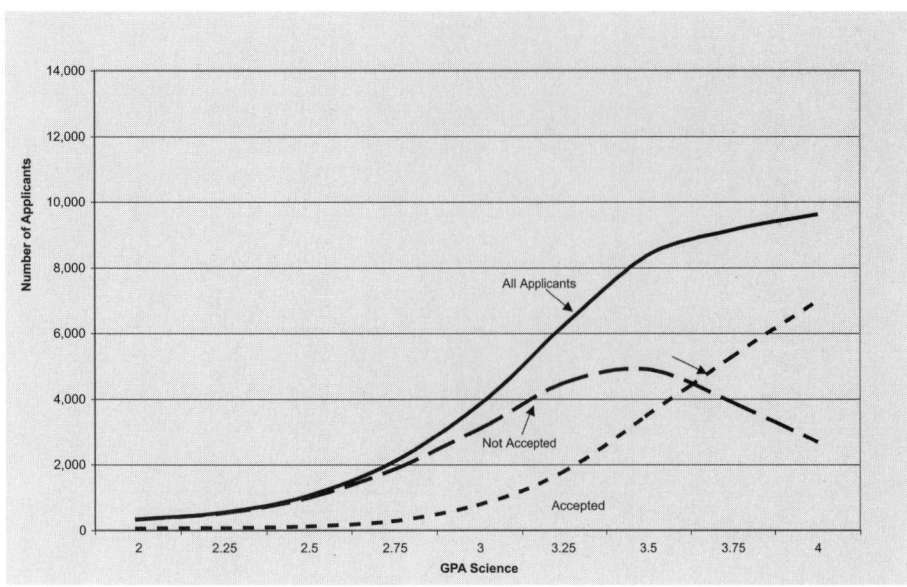

Source: AAMC Data Warehouse: Applicant Matriculant File

As of September 25, 2007

Chart 5-G
Non-Science GPA Distribution, Year 2007 Applicants

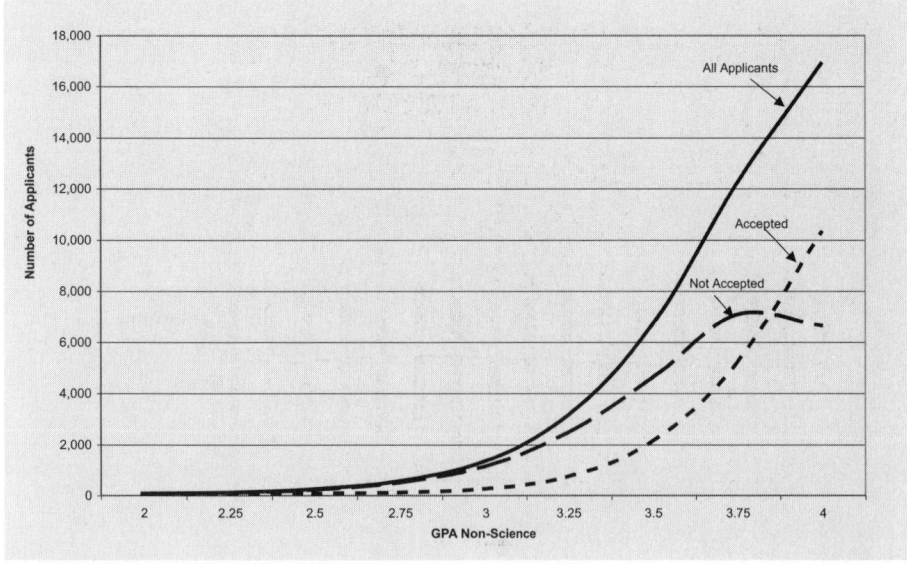

Source: AAMC Data Warehouse: Applicant Matriculant File

As of September 25, 2007

Undergraduate Grade Point Average (GPA)

Charts 5-F — 5-H present information about the undergraduate academic performance of applicants:

• Chart 5-F: undergraduate science GPA (Biology, Chemistry, Physics, and Mathematics)

• Chart 5-G: undergraduate non-science GPA

• Chart 5-H: undergraduate total GPA

Chart 5-F shows that the undergraduate science GPAs of all applicants were on a continuum from 2.0 to 4.0, on a 4.0 scale; most were between 3.75 and 4.0. Accepted applicants also had undergraduate science GPAs across the entire range, but few had GPAs of 2.50 or below (just under 110). The undergraduate science GPA at which accepted applicants exceeded those not accepted was between 3.50 and 3.75.

Chart 5-G shows applicants' undergraduate non-science GPAs along the continuum from 2.0 to 4.0, with most between 3.75 and 4.0. Accepted applicants' undergraduate non-science GPAs also ranged from 2.0 to 4.0, but only about 95 had a GPA of 2.75 or below. At 3.75 to 4.0, accepted applicants exceeded not accepted applicants.

As shown in Chart 5-H, all applicants had total undergraduate GPAs from 2.0 to 4.0, and most were in the range of 3.50 to 3.75. Accepted applicants' total undergraduate GPAs also ranged from 2.0 to 4.0, but only about 120 possessed undergraduate total GPAs of 2.75 or below. Accepted applicants exceeded not accepted applicants at an undergraduate total GPA of between 3.50 and 3.75.

As is the case with MCAT® data, GPA data in Charts 5-F – 5-H show that no undergraduate GPA assures admission to medical school. While applicants with undergraduate science, non-science, and total GPAs in the range of 3.50 to 3.75, 3.75 to 4.0, and 3.50 to 3.75, respectively, were more likely to be accepted to medical school, a significant number of such applicants were not accepted. Again, these findings underscore the importance of a wide variety of personal characteristics and experiential variables in the medical student selection process.

Undergraduate Major

Chart 5-I presents information about the undergraduate majors of all medical school applicants to the 1992-2007 entering classes. Over the past decade, approximately three-fifths of applicants reported undergraduate biological science majors, while the remainder reported a variety of majors, including the humanities, mathematics and statistics, physical sciences, social sciences, other health sciences, and a broad "other" category. The proportion of these majors has remained relatively constant over time, despite annual fluctuations in the applicant pool.

Chart 5-H
Total GPA Distribution, Year 2007 Applicants

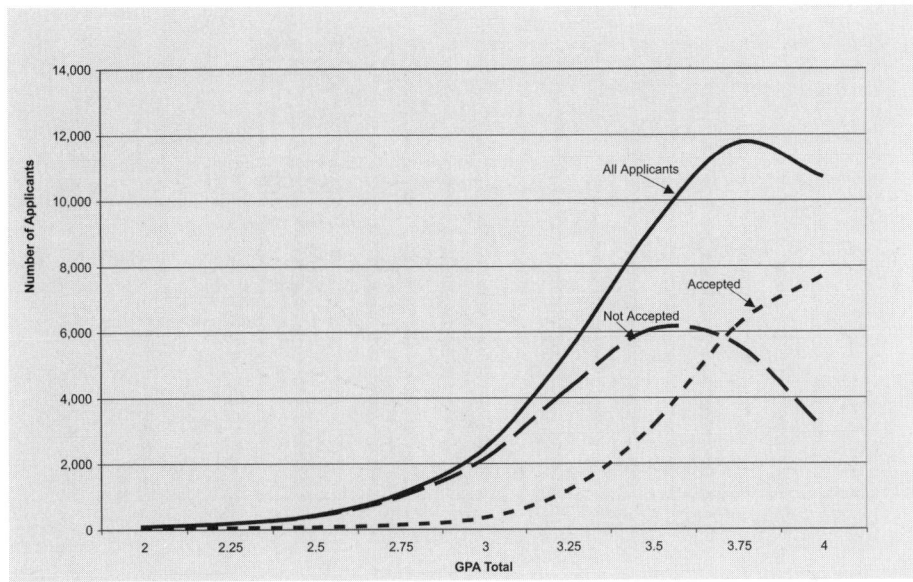

Source: AAMC Data Warehouse: Applicant Matriculant File

As of September 25, 2007

Chart 5-I
Undergraduate Major Distribution, All Applicants, 1992-2007

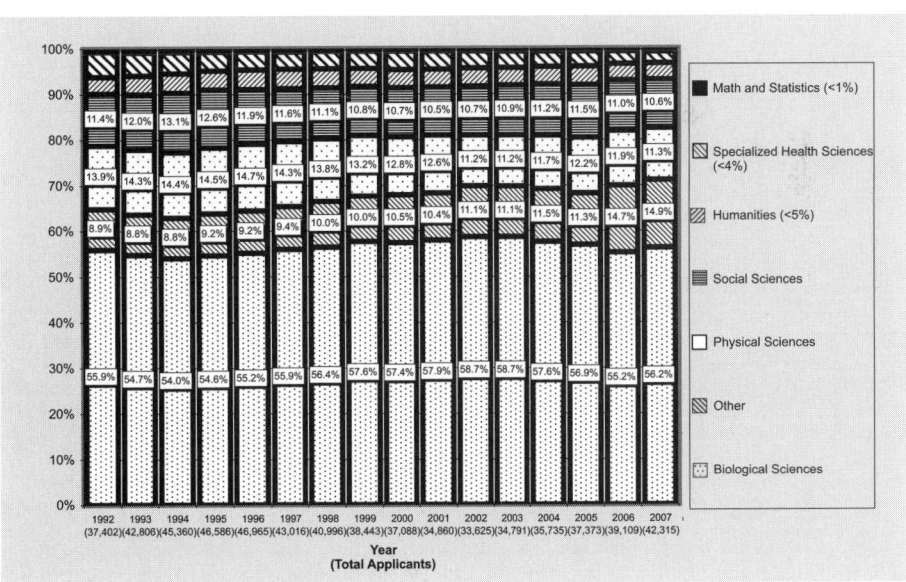

Source: AAMC Data Warehouse: Applicant Matriculant File

As of September 25, 2007

Chart 5-J

Undergraduate Major Distribution, Accepted Applicants, 1992-2007

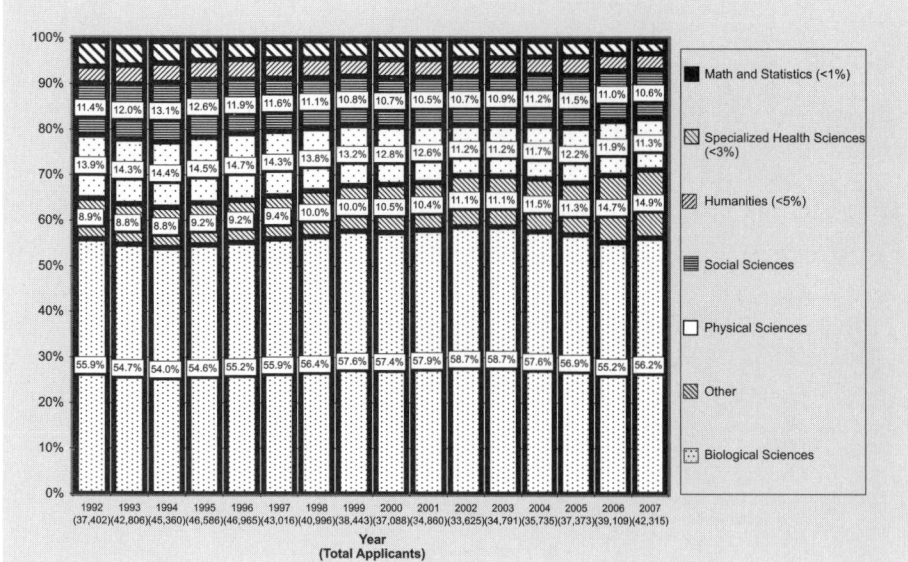

Source: AAMC Data Warehouse: Applicant Matriculant File

As of September 25, 2007

Chart 5-K

Applicants by Gender and Acceptance Status, 1992-2007

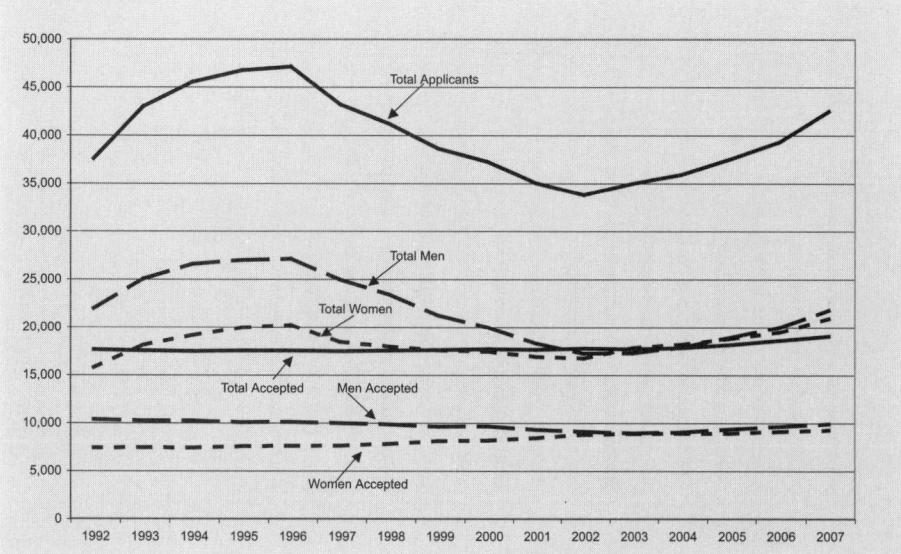

Source: AAMC Data Warehouse: Applicant Matriculant File

As of September 25, 2007

Chart 5-J presents similar information about the undergraduate majors of applicants accepted to the 1992-2007 entering classes. Comparisons of the majors of the total applicant pool with those of accepted applicants reveal acceptance rates, for various science-related majors, ranging from 33.5 percent for applicants with specialized health science majors, to 44.0 percent for biological science majors, to 51.3 percent for physical science majors, the highest rate of acceptance.

Gender

Chart 5-K presents information about the number and gender of the entire applicant pool and of accepted applicants for the 1992-2007 entering classes. The largest annual applicant pool during the past decade was for the 1996 entering class; since that year, the pool gradually declined until 2003, when there was a slight increase (3.5 percent) in applicants. The applicant pool increased again by 2.7 percent in 2004, by 4.6 percent in 2005, by another 4.6 percent in 2006, and by 8.2 percent in 2007. The number of male applicants to the 2007 entering class increased by about 1,700 from the number of male applicants to the previous year's entering class, but that number was still smaller than it had been for any other entering class from 1992 through 1998. The number of female applicants to the 2007 class increased by about 1400 over the number of female applicants to the previous year's entering class, making this cohort the largest number of female applicants on record. While the number of accepted applicants remained fairly constant for 10 years, it has started to increase in recent years, from a low of 17,312 in 1997 to a high of 18,858 in 2007. The number of accepted male applicants has fluctuated from a high of 10,208 in 1992 to a low of 8,810 in 2003. The number of accepted female applicants has increased, with small fluctuations, from a low of 7,255 in the 1994 entering class to a high of 9,107 in 2007. The significant gaps between male and female applicants for the 1992 entering class (6,166) and the 1993 entering class (6,892) have disappeared; 553 and 301 more women than men applied to the 2003 and 2004 entering classes, respectively. In 2005, only 121 more men than women applied. In 2007, 847 more men than women applied to medical school. During the same time span, the gaps between accepted male and female applicants also dropped. Accepted male applicants outnumbered accepted female applicants by 2,951 for the 1992 entering class, but only by 644 for the 2007 entering class. The national ratio of male to female applicants was 49.2 : 50.8 percent for the 2003 entering class, the first time that the number of female applicants was greater than the number of male applicants to medical school. For the 2004 entering class, this trend continued, with a ratio of male to female applicants of 49.6: 50.4. For the 2005 entering class, there were once again more male than female applicants, with a ratio of male to female applicants of 50.2 : 49.8. This trend continued in 2007, with a ratio of male to female applicants of 51.0 : 49.0.

Age

Chart 5-L shows that the age distribution for all applicants to the 2007 entering class was broad, with 17 applicants under the age of 19 at the time of anticipated matriculation, and 68 applicants aged 48 and over. The largest contingent of applicants, 38,247, was between 21 and 28 at the time of anticipated matriculation; the rest of the applicant pool were either under 21 (570) or over 28 (3,498) at the time of anticipated matriculation. Chart 5-L illustrates a similar finding for accepted applicants. Accepted applicants for the 2007 entering class were between 18 and 51 years of age at the time of expected matriculation.

Type of Application

Chart 5-M presents information about application outcomes for Early Decision Program (EDP) and regular applicants to the 2007 entering class: 97.1 percent were

Chart 5-L
Age Distribution, Year 2007 Applicants

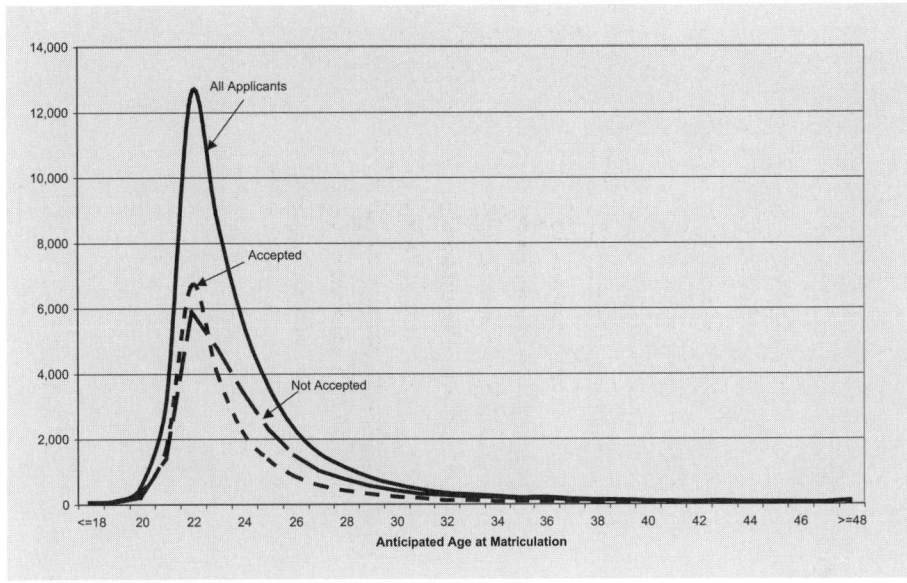

Source: AAMC Data Warehouse: Applicant Matriculant File   As of September 25, 2007

Chart 5-M
Total Applicants by Early Decision Program (EDP) and Acceptance Status, 2007

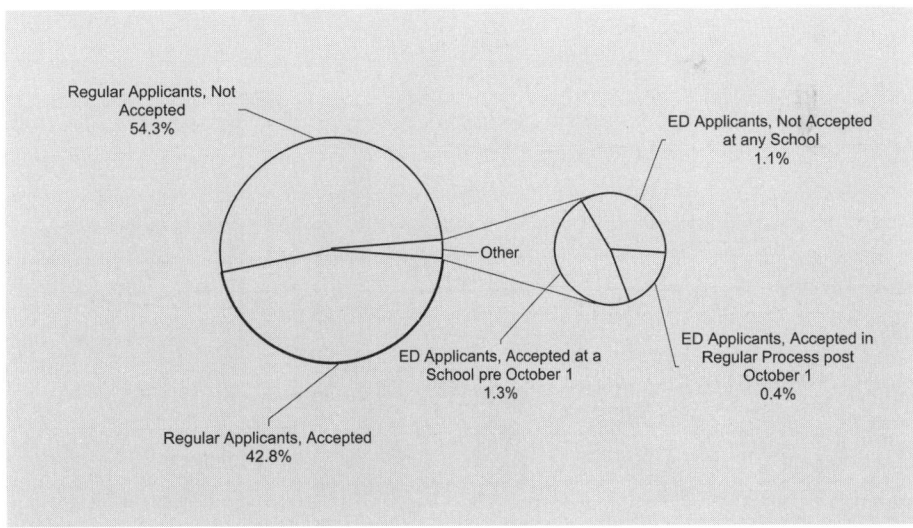

Source: AAMC Data Warehouse: Applicant Matriculant File   As of September 25, 2007

Chart 5-N

Distribution of Self-Reported Ethnicity and Race: All Applicants, 2002-2007

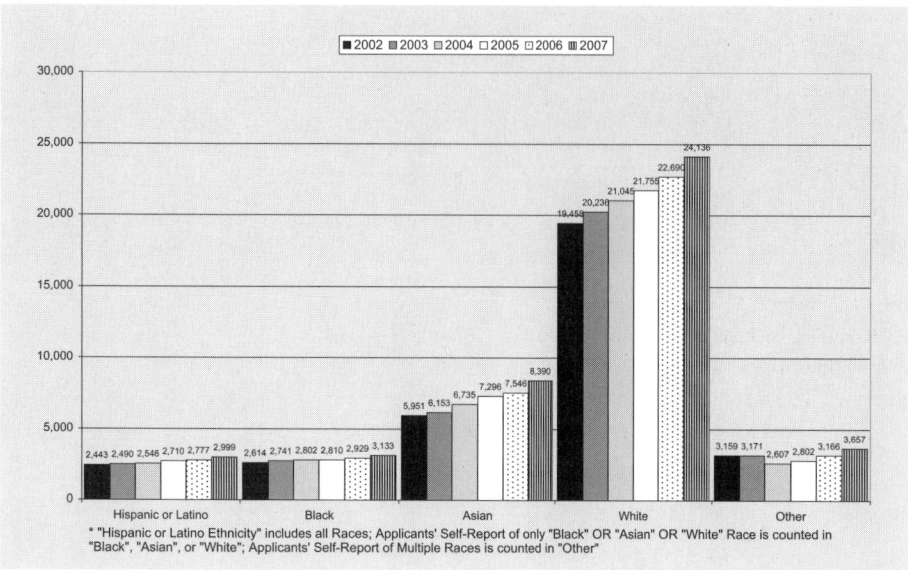

* "Hispanic or Latino Ethnicity" includes all Races; Applicants' Self-Report of only "Black" OR "Asian" OR "White" Race is counted in "Black", "Asian", or "White"; Applicants' Self-Report of Multiple Races is counted in "Other"

Source: AAMC Data Warehouse: Applicant Matriculant File

As of September 25, 2007

Chart 5-O

Distribution of Self-Reported Ethnicity and Race:
All Accepted Applicants, 2002-2007

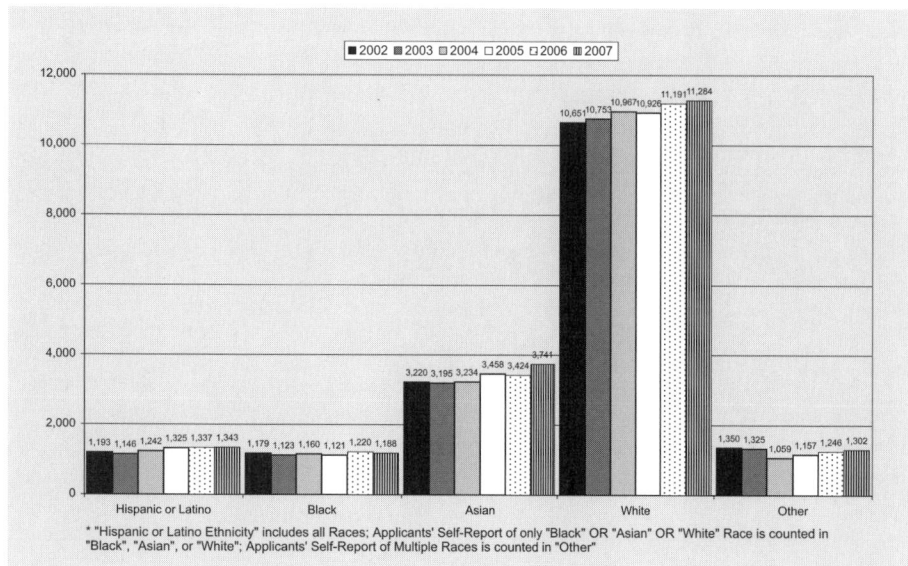

* "Hispanic or Latino Ethnicity" includes all Races; Applicants' Self-Report of only "Black" OR "Asian" OR "White" Race is counted in "Black", "Asian", or "White"; Applicants' Self-Report of Multiple Races is counted in "Other"

Source: AAMC Data Warehouse: Applicant Matriculant File

As of September 25, 2007

regular applicants and 2.9 percent were EDP applicants. Of all applicants, 42.8 percent were accepted to at least one medical school through the regular application process; 1.3 percent were accepted to one medical school through EDP prior to October 1; and 0.4 percent were accepted to at least one medical school after not having been accepted through EDP before October 1. Conversely, 54.3 percent of regular applicants and 38.4 percent of the 2.9 percent of applicants who applied through EDP were not accepted to any medical school for 2007.

Race and Ethnicity

In accordance with the requirements of the U.S. Office of Management and Budget Directive 15, data about race and ethnicity were collected differently by AMCAS for applicants to the 2002 through 2007 entering classes than they were for applicants to prior years' entering classes. For that reason, this section presents applicant race and ethnicity data beginning with 2002 only. Additional applicant data regarding race and ethnicity for prior years are presented on the AAMC Web site at *www.aamc.org/data/facts*.

Chart 5-N shows applicant self-reported race and ethnicity data for all applicants to the 2002 through 2007 entering classes. Chart 5-O shows applicant self-reported race and ethnicity data for all accepted applicants to the 2002 through 2007 entering classes. The following changes occurred in the self-reported racial and ethnic make-up of the applicant pool from 2006 to 2007:

- The number of self-described white applicants in 2006 was 22,690; the number of white applicants in 2007 was 24,136, an increase of 6.4 percent.

- The number of self-described Asian applicants in 2006 was 7,546; the number of Asian applicants in 2007 was 8,390, an increase of 11.2 percent.

- The number of self-described black applicants in 2006 was 2,929; the number of black applicants in 2007 was 3,133, an increase of 7.0 percent.

- The number of self-described Hispanic applicants in 2006 was 2,777; the number of Hispanic applicants in 2007 was 2,999, an increase of 8.0 percent.

- The number of applicants in 2006 whose self-description of their race or ethnicity was in some other category was 3,166; the number of applicants in this cohort in 2007 was 3,657, an increase of 15.5 percent from 2006.

Simultaneously, the following changes occurred among those applicants accepted to the 2006 and 2007 entering classes:

- The number of self-described white accepted applicants in 2006 was 11,191; the number of white accepted applicants in 2007 was 11,284, an increase of 0.8 percent.

- The number of self-described Asian accepted applicants in 2006 was 3,424; the number of accepted Asian applicants in 2007 was 3,741, an increase of 9.3 percent.

- The number of self-described black accepted applicants in 2006 was 1,220; the number of accepted black applicants in 2007 was 1,188, a decrease of 2.6 percent.

- The number of self-described Hispanic accepted applicants in 2006 was 1,337; the number of Hispanic accepted applicants in 2007 was 1,343, an increase of 0.4 percent.

- The number of accepted applicants in 2006 whose self-description of their race or ethnicity was in some other category was 1,246; the number of accepted applicants in this cohort in 2007 was 1,302, an increase of 4.5 percent from 2006.

Additional information of interest to applicants from groups underrepresented in medicine is available in Chapter 6.

Chapter 6

Increasing Diversity in Medical School

The Association of American Medical Colleges (AAMC) believes that both medical education and health care delivery benefit from diversity among medical students, faculty, physicians, researchers, and administrators. The AAMC recognizes that diversity is a broad concept that can encompass a variety of factors, including, among others, race and ethnicity, gender, socioeconomic status, life experiences, and personal characteristics. Individual medical schools determine how best to embrace diversity on their campuses so that their students can obtain the educational benefits that flow from a diverse student body and from diversity among faculty and administrators.

Within this general context, the AAMC has paid particular attention for more than three decades to medical students who are from racial and ethnic populations that are underrepresented in the medical profession. (For more information about the AAMC's definition of "underrepresented in medicine," see *www.aamc.org/meded/urm*.) In particular, the AAMC's Diversity Policy and Programs has been, and continues to be, engaged in a number of programs designed to increase diversity in academic medicine. These programs, while open to all students, are sensitive to the challenges and needs of individuals from racial and ethnic groups underrepresented in medicine, as well as of those persons from disadvantaged backgrounds. Examples of programs that may be useful in exploring medicine as a career are described below.

Enrichment programs. Medical schools nation-wide provide programs and resources specifically designed to assist in preparing and recruiting students for medical education. Some of these programs are held during the school year, while others take place during the summer. Some are designed for high school students, others for college students, and still others for post-baccalaureate students. The AAMC is affiliated with two such opportunities:

- The annual Minority Student Medical Career Awareness Workshops and Recruitment Fair for high school and college students and their family members, which is held each fall during the AAMC's annual meeting. Representatives from all 129 AAMC-member medical schools are invited, and students have the opportunity to talk with them about preparing for medical school, enrichment programs, admission policies and procedures, financial aid, and more. Workshops are also sponsored for family members, guidance counselors, and health professions advisors. The dates and locations of upcoming AAMC annual meetings can be found at *ww.aamc.org/careerfair*.

- Summer Medical and Dental Education Program (SMDEP) is a free, six-week, academic enrichment program for freshman and sophomore students interested in a career in medicine or dentistry. Program activities include science and mathematics-based courses, learning and study skills seminars, career development activities, clinical experiences, and a financial planning workshop. SMDEP is funded by The Robert Wood Johnson Foundation and is offered at 12 U.S. medical and dental schools across the nation. The AAMC's Diversity Policy and Programs, in conjunction with the American Dental Education Association, functions as the national program office. For additional information, visit *www.smdep.org*, or call the toll-free number at 866-56SMDEP.

AspiringDocs.org. The AAMC has also initiated a campaign designed to interest students from groups underrepresented in medicine in careers in medicine by providing information and support. The centerpiece of the campaign, an interactive Web site at *www.AspiringDocs.org*, allows interested individuals to join an online "virtual community" that engages, encourages, and educates through a variety of online features, such as Ask the Experts, Hot Topics, and Inspiring Stories. Students are provided with easy-to-understand

Table 6-A Matriculants by Medical School and Race and Ethnicity 2007*

School State	School Name (Matriculants 2007)	Mexican American	Cuban	Puerto Rican	Other Hispanic or Latino	Total Hispanic or Latino	Chinese	Asian Indian	Pakistani	Filipino	Japanese	Korean	Vietnamese	Other Asian	Total Asian	Native American (incl AK)	Black	Native Hawaiian /OPI	White	Total Matriculants
AL	Alabama	2	2	0	0	2	2	5	16	1	0	0	3	0	26	2	11	0	137	176
	South Alabama	0	0	0	0	0	1	5	0	0	0	0	2	2	9	0	5	1	59	74
AR	Arkansas	1	0	0	1	2	9	6	0	1	1	2	3	2	21	0	5	1	126	155
AZ	Arizona	11	1	1	0	13	5	10	0	2	0	1	1	4	22	2	5	2	98	134
CA	Loma Linda	4	0	4	11	16	18	0	0	5	5	23	1	4	49	1	10	2	94	172
	Southern Cal-Keck	9	1	0	6	16	11	10	0	2	3	7	2	5	38	0	4	2	119	164
	Stanford	6	1	0	2	9	17	12	0	0	0	2	0	4	36	0	2	1	39	86
	UC Berkeley/SF Joint Prog	1	0	0	0	1	1	1	0	0	0	0	1	1	5	1	1	0	10	16
	UC Davis	9	1	0	7	16	15	13	1	3	3	3	3	4	41	1	3	0	54	105
	UC Irvine	5	0	0	6	10	16	5	2	2	2	3	3	5	39	2	3	1	55	104
	UC San Diego	9	0	0	1	10	24	8	0	3	3	6	6	7	53	1	2	0	74	134
	UC San Francisco	18	1	3	6	28	18	6	3	7	7	6	5	3	48	3	21	1	80	147
	UCLA Drew	5	0	0	2	7	2	1	0	0	0	0	2	3	7	1	11	1	3	24
	UCLA-Geffen	10	0	0	7	16	24	9	2	0	3	6	15	7	62	1	4	0	73	145
CO	Colorado	4	0	1	3	8	5	2	0	0	1	1	2	1	11	4	5	0	138	157
CT	Connecticut	2	0	1	4	6	6	6	0	0	0	1	2	1	14	4	8	0	56	81
	Yale	2	2	1	2	7	10	7	0	0	0	2	2	3	24	1	13	0	47	99
DC	George Washington	0	1	1	2	4	8	25	3	2	0	4	0	7	46	2	23	2	100	177
	Georgetown	0	2	1	4	6	11	10	0	0	2	4	3	1	33	0	16	0	135	190
	Howard	1	0	2	7	10	1	4	1	1	0	0	5	1	13	0	96	0	9	130
FL	Florida	0	7	0	6	12	9	20	3	2	0	1	0	3	36	0	7	0	88	132
	Florida State	0	3	0	4	7	2	8	2	2	0	0	1	1	14	0	11	2	95	119
	Miami-Miller	0	10	2	10	23	11	16	2	2	4	3	4	1	38	1	11	0	130	176
	South Florida	4	6	2	4	15	2	16	3	3	0	2	2	5	32	1	8	0	81	120
GA	Emory	1	0	2	5	7	11	13	3	0	1	1	1	4	33	0	5	0	89	130
	MC Georgia	1	0	1	5	7	5	22	2	2	0	5	2	1	36	0	11	0	139	190
	Morehouse	0	0	0	1	1	1	7	0	0	0	0	0	0	8	0	54	0	0	63
HI	Hawaii-Burns	0	0	1	0	1	0	0	0	0	29	2	0	2	9	1	0	11	4	52
IA	Iowa-Carver	6	0	0	0	6	0	1	0	0	0	0	4	1	7	1	0	0	19	62
IL	Chicago Med-Franklin	0	0	1	2	2	17	25	4	3	3	6	3	4	63	3	8	1	101	148
	Chicago-Pritzker	5	0	4	2	11	10	9	1	0	0	5	0	5	30	2	10	2	63	112
	Illinois	22	2	3	14	41	25	42	5	4	2	18	1	5	97	4	26	0	167	307
	Loyola-Stritch	7	0	0	0	10	3	7	0	2	0	4	0	3	19	0	5	0	117	146
	Northwestern-Feinberg	5	1	0	6	10	26	23	1	0	2	4	2	3	54	2	8	0	94	169
	Rush	6	1	1	3	10	8	22	2	1	0	6	1	3	40	1	8	0	88	128
	Southern Illinois	2	1	1	1	4	2	4	2	1	0	1	0	1	10	1	6	0	55	72
IN	Indiana	10	1	0	4	15	9	24	5	2	1	9	1	4	52	3	14	0	224	294
KS	Kansas	9	3	0	2	11	4	3	1	2	2	2	5	4	56	3	14	0	142	176
KY	Kentucky	0	0	1	2	3	4	6	1	1	1	2	5	0	16	2	14	0	85	103
	Louisville	0	0	0	0	0	4	6	0	1	0	1	0	0	13	2	3	0	123	148
LA	LSU New Orleans	3	0	0	1	6	2	13	0	0	0	0	3	2	17	0	10	1	153	179
	LSU Shreveport	1	1	1	3	3	0	8	1	0	1	4	1	2	17	2	11	0	106	117
	Tulane	4	1	0	2	2	13	18	2	2	4	6	0	0	7	0	7	0	106	175
MA	Boston	8	1	0	11	20	14	21	2	2	4	2	8	5	37	0	6	1	132	168
	Harvard	4	3	0	8	14	22	20	2	2	3	2	3	3	45	1	18	1	90	165
	Massachusetts	0	0	1	2	3	7	3	0	2	1	2	3	5	56	2	18	0	77	103
	Tufts	1	0	3	6	11	13	13	1	1	3	1	0	4	13	2	10	0	81	173
MD	Johns Hopkins	1	0	1	3	11	15	13	2	1	2	6	3	4	44	2	5	0	116	118
	Maryland	0	0	0	3	3	3	14	3	1	1	8	1	1	42	1	13	1	62	160
	Uniformed Services-Hebert	4	0	1	4	2	13	8	0	5	0	4	0	8	47	0	19	0	100	173
MI	Michigan	2	1	0	3	7	5	8	0	6	2	6	2	4	33	2	11	0	141	170
	Michigan State	6	0	0	1	7	17	18	0	1	1	4	2	1	43	3	12	0	117	156
	Wayne State	4	1	1	1	4	8	12	4	0	2	5	6	6	30	3	8	1	108	290
MN	Mayo	1	0	2	0	0	4	4	0	1	1	7	3	8	69	3	24	0	206	42
	Minnesota	1	0	0	4	3	1	1	0	0	0	7	0	1	4	1	4	1	32	183
	Minnesota Duluth	0	0	1	4	9	13	4	0	1	1	1	6	6	25	3	5	0	146	58
MO	Missouri Columbia	3	0	0	0	0	0	3	0	0	0	8	0	0	0	8	0	0	52	96
	Missouri Kansas City	1	0	0	1	3	0	0	0	1	1	4	1	1	3	0	19	0	92	94
	St Louis	0	0	0	0	0	5	8	0	6	0	0	0	0	0	0	5	0	0	94
	Washington U St Louis	2	0	0	1	1	9	18	3	1	2	5	6	6	46	1	5	1	128	179
MS	Mississippi	2	0	1	1	4	18	12	0	0	1	6	0	5	39	1	7	0	74	122
NC	Duke	0	0	0	0	0	4	4	0	1	2	4	0	0	11	0	11	0	90	110
	East Carolina-Brody	0	2	0	4	2	11	6	0	1	0	4	1	1	24	1	22	0	51	100
	North Carolina	1	0	1	4	4	8	3	1	0	3	1	2	1	11	2	9	0	53	73
	Wake Forest	3	0	1	1	5	3	6	2	0	0	1	4	0	16	1	20	0	118	161
																				120

Table 6-A Matriculants by Medical School and Race and Ethnicity 2007*

	Matriculants 2007	Mexican American	Cuban	Puerto Rican	Other Hispanic or Latino	Total Hispanic or Latino	Chinese	Asian Indian	Pakistani	Filipino	Japanese	Korean	Vietnamese	Other Asian	Total Asian	Native American (incl AK)	Black	Native Hawaiian /OPI	White	Total Matriculants
ND	North Dakota	0	0	0	0	0	0	0	0	0	0	0	0	0	0	7	0	0	55	62
NE	Creighton	1	1	0	2	4	1	2	0	1	0	5	5	4	19	2	4	1	100	126
	Nebraska	3	0	0	1	4	2	3	0	0	0	0	0	0	5	1	2	1	109	119
NH	Dartmouth	3	0	0	1	5	7	6	0	0	0	0	0	1	17	0	0	0	39	73
NJ	UMDNJ New Jersey	0	8	5	10	22	16	35	6	6	0	11	2	4	78	0	16	1	78	178
	UMDNJ-RW Johnson	0	1	3	9	11	15	29	4	4	2	9	0	7	65	4	14	0	80	166
NM	New Mexico	12	0	0	8	20	3	3	0	0	1	1	0	0	9	4	1	1	55	75
NV	Nevada	2	0	0	2	4	4	3	1	2	1	0	1	0	13	2	5	0	50	62
NY	Albany	0	0	0	4	4	8	22	2	1	1	4	1	3	42	2	5	0	82	144
	Buffalo	0	1	0	1	2	14	9	4	2	0	6	6	3	43	1	4	0	93	139
	Columbia	4	2	2	8	16	14	5	0	0	1	1	0	2	23	0	13	0	107	154
	Cornell-Weill	2	0	0	6	9	9	5	1	2	1	5	0	2	18	0	18	1	118	184
	Einstein	2	1	1	1	5	20	8	0	0	2	6	5	3	42	0	12	1	61	101
	Mount Sinai	3	4	0	6	19	17	9	0	2	0	2	1	1	30	2	8	0	87	141
	New York Medical	0	0	2	2	2	28	15	2	0	3	13	7	9	74	1	2	2	114	195
	New York University	2	2	4	11	17	17	17	4	4	2	17	1	2	45	0	8	0	104	160
	Rochester	2	0	1	1	4	10	4	0	0	2	4	1	1	22	2	11	0	63	101
	SUNY Downstate	2	1	2	9	13	15	17	1	3	1	8	1	9	54	1	17	1	94	169
	SUNY Upstate	0	0	0	0	0	8	16	0	0	0	3	0	5	34	1	17	0	88	160
	Stony Brook	2	1	0	5	7	20	21	3	0	1	10	3	8	46	1	3	0	60	116
OH	Case Western	2	1	2	5	10	20	11	1	1	1	4	0	8	55	0	18	0	103	185
	Cincinnati	0	0	0	0	0	11	11	2	0	1	3	1	5	33	1	11	0	119	161
	Northeastern Ohio	1	1	0	3	5	7	25	4	0	0	1	4	5	40	1	5	1	82	121
	Ohio State	1	0	6	6	8	20	16	1	3	0	6	0	3	43	2	13	0	154	210
	Toledo	2	0	0	0	2	6	17	5	0	0	3	0	7	41	1	8	0	114	165
	Wright State-Boonshoft	1	0	0	1	2	4	7	0	1	0	1	1	1	16	0	3	0	83	100
OK	Oklahoma	1	0	3	0	4	5	10	0	0	1	0	0	5	30	19	3	0	116	164
OR	Oregon	2	0	0	2	4	6	6	0	2	0	2	4	4	18	1	3	1	95	118
PA	Drexel	2	0	1	5	8	22	53	6	1	1	12	0	7	99	10	10	1	167	281
	Jefferson	1	0	0	3	4	17	35	4	5	3	9	8	7	77	2	9	0	168	259
	Penn State	0	2	2	2	6	6	6	1	1	0	0	2	7	22	0	10	2	109	154
	Pennsylvania	0	1	3	3	7	12	10	1	1	0	3	0	2	28	0	15	0	106	153
	Pittsburgh	0	1	2	6	9	13	12	0	0	0	6	3	6	40	2	18	1	92	146
	Temple	3	1	6	6	20	20	13	2	2	2	6	1	2	31	2	13	1	128	178
PR	Caribe	3	6	50	6	61	0	0	0	0	0	0	0	0	0	0	2	0	50	66
	Ponce	0	6	47	5	57	0	0	0	0	0	0	0	0	1	0	2	2	47	63
	Puerto Rico	1	1	100	3	103	0	0	0	0	0	0	0	0	0	1	11	0	46	105
RI	Brown-Alpert	5	1	1	2	9	8	8	0	0	1	4	0	4	25	0	7	0	73	95
SC	MU South Carolina	2	0	0	5	5	5	7	2	1	2	0	3	2	11	3	20	1	127	158
	South Carolina	0	0	0	0	0	0	8	0	0	0	0	0	2	15	0	6	0	65	84
SD	South Dakota-Sanford	0	0	0	0	0	0	0	0	0	0	0	0	0	1	0	3	0	53	54
TN	East Tennessee-Quillen	0	0	1	1	1	1	2	0	0	0	1	0	1	6	0	3	0	52	60
	Meharry	0	0	1	4	7	1	1	0	0	2	1	0	1	6	1	80	0	9	96
	Tennessee	0	2	1	2	2	4	7	0	0	0	1	2	4	18	1	19	0	113	150
	Vanderbilt	0	1	0	4	4	2	10	1	1	0	3	1	6	24	3	7	0	65	105
TX	Baylor	24	2	0	7	31	16	10	2	3	0	2	8	10	50	4	4	0	109	172
	Texas A & M	8	0	0	3	11	8	7	3	0	0	0	7	10	36	1	4	0	60	105
	Texas Tech	13	0	0	7	18	4	7	3	0	1	1	3	18	36	3	7	0	93	140
	UT Galveston	27	2	2	8	37	9	8	0	1	0	1	0	9	33	0	23	0	150	227
	UT Houston	23	2	0	7	34	12	10	0	1	2	2	1	7	39	3	15	1	163	230
	UT San Antonio	28	2	1	7	36	10	8	1	2	0	4	2	16	44	3	12	0	152	220
	UT Southwestern	26	4	2	8	40	20	22	6	0	1	7	1	20	76	0	18	0	105	219
UT	Utah	3	0	1	2	3	5	3	1	0	1	3	4	1	19	0	2	0	82	102
VA	Eastern Virginia	1	0	0	0	1	5	7	3	1	0	4	3	3	24	1	6	0	81	115
	Virginia	2	3	2	5	12	9	8	0	2	0	6	2	1	28	2	8	1	105	143
	Virginia Commonwealth	0	0	0	3	3	6	22	4	3	1	7	4	4	50	0	9	0	123	184
VT	Vermont	1	1	2	2	6	6	0	0	0	4	3	3	0	16	2	3	0	85	112
WA	U Washington	3	0	3	5	9	2	6	1	3	6	4	3	2	24	24	2	2	168	191
WI	MC Wisconsin	5	1	4	2	10	7	21	2	1	1	4	4	3	39	1	7	1	157	204
	Wisconsin	2	0	0	0	5	9	14	0	2	0	6	0	5	37	5	6	0	112	155
WV	Marshall-Edwards	0	0	0	1	1	1	3	1	0	0	0	1	0	9	2	3	0	63	72
	West Virginia	0	1	0	0	3	3	1	0	2	0	2	1	2	15	1	3	0	90	108
	Totals	462	113	323	425	1,277	1,125	1,351	165	160	153	416	284	441	3,890	163	1,281	61	11,881	17,759

Source: AAMC Data Warehouse: Applicant Matriculant File as of 9/25/2007. *Hispanic Ethnicities are alone or in combination with some other Hispanic Ethnicity and include any Race. Ethnicity Counts include U.S. Citizens and Permanent Residents only, and include both Hispanic and Non-Hispanic Ethnicity. The total represents an unduplicated count and also includes matriculants for whom we have no race data or who are foreign. Race Counts include U.S. Citizens and Permanent Residents only. Race Counts include U.S. Citizens and Permanent Residents only, are alone or in combination with some other Race or who are foreign.

information about applying to medical school, financing a medical education, and navigating the medical school application process. AspiringDocs.org includes testimonials from, and question-and-answer opportunities with, practicing physicians, medical students, and real-world experts about what it really takes to get into and succeed in medicine.

Other AAMC resources. The AAMC offers a wide variety of information and hyperlinks in the "Minorities in Medicine" section of the AAMC's Web site at *www.aamc.org/students/minorities/start.htm*, as well as on the AAMC's Diversity Web site at *www.aamc.org/diversity*. Some programs are highlighted below.

• *Minority Student Opportunities in United States Medical Schools* **(MSOUSMS).** Diversity Policy and Programs produces a publication that contains information supplied by individual medical schools about student recruitment and admission, as well as other topics related to enhancing diversity in the academic environment. Information about enrichment programs offered by medical schools is also listed on a school-by-school basis. *MSOUSMS* is designed to be used in conjunction with *Medical School Admission Requirements (MSAR)*. Details about the content of *MSOUSMS* and data tables on Applicants and Graduates are available at *www.aamc.org/msousms*.

• **Enrichment programs online.** Diversity Policy and Programs supports the Web site for "Enrichment Programs on the Web." This site includes a database resource to help undergraduate students locate summer enrichment programs on medical school campuses. Information is available at *http://services.aamc.org/summerprograms/*.

• **Medical School Career Fairs and Events Calendar.** The calendar will allow the AAMC and its constituents, such as the Group on Student Affairs-Minority Affairs Section (GSA-MAS), to coordinate the scheduling of recruitment and other events pertinent to students and constituents to reduce overlap and

allow for maximum attendance. For example, students can easily search for recruitment events at schools in their state or in a specific date range. Information is available at *www.aamc.org/calendar/careerfairs*.

• **Fee Assistance Program (FAP).** The AAMC's FAP helps students with extreme financial limitations whose inability to pay the full Medical College Admissions Test (MCAT®) registration fee or the American Medical College Application Service (AMCAS) fee would prevent them from taking the MCAT® or applying to medical school. Details about the FAP can be found at *www.aamc.org/fap* and in Chapter 4.

• **Medical Minority Applicant Registry (Med-MAR).** Students applying to medical school who self-identify as members of groups that are underrepresented in medicine or who are economically or educationally disadvantaged are given the opportunity to register for Med-MAR at the time they take the MCAT®. The Med-MAR program then circulates basic biographical information about the examinee and the examinee's MCAT® scores to all U.S. medical schools. Details about the registry can be found at *www.aamc.org/students/minorities/resources/medmar.htm*.

• **Data about race and ethnicity in medicine.** The AAMC has a great deal of information about medical education, including detailed data about medical students from an array of racial and ethnic groups.

  • AAMC information about recent matriculant data for each medical school is presented in this publication in Table 6-A, *Matriculants by Medical School and Race and Ethnicity, 2007*.
  • Chapter 5 of this publication includes a section on the self-reported racial and ethnic identification of medical school applicants and accepted applicants for the 2007 entering class.
  • Additional data about medical school applicants, matriculants, and graduates are available on the AAMC Web site at *www.aamc.org/data/facts*.

• Data on medical school faculty—including information on faculty by race and ethnicity—can be found at *www.aamc.org/data/facultyroster/reports.htm*.
• The AAMC publication entitled *Minorities in Medical Education, Facts & Figures 2007* provides race and ethnicity data on medical school applicants, accepted applicants, matriculants, enrollment, graduates, and faculty, along with detailed tables. The full text of *Facts & Figures* can be accessed without charge at *www.aamc.org/students/minorities*.

School-based resources. Students should also take advantage of resources that exist at undergraduate and medical schools. Several examples are listed below.

• **Medical school Web sites.** The AAMC maintains a list of both U.S. and Canadian M.D.-granting medical schools at *www.aamc.org/medicalschools.htm*. This list includes links to each school's Web site.

• **Pre-medical school programs at undergraduate colleges.** Pre-health advisors at undergraduate colleges provide pertinent information on application and admission to medical school or refer students to appropriate contacts. Pre-health advisors also are knowledgeable about programs and resources that students from underrepresented groups and disadvantaged backgrounds are likely to find useful.

• **Medical school minority affairs officers.** Each medical school has a designated minority affairs officer. These individuals are dedicated to increasing diversity among medical students at their schools, and they are an excellent source of information for potential applicants and applicants. To get in touch with a minority affairs officer, students should contact a medical school in their local area or the medical schools in which they have a potential interest.

Directory of Minority Affairs Administrators. The Directory of Minority Affairs Administrators is a searchable database of the Group on Student Affairs-Minority Affairs Section (GSA-MAS) institutional representatives at U.S. medical schools. Students can use this directory to obtain the name of the minority affairs contacts at any of the 129 U.S. medical schools. The directory is searchable by name, location, and institution and is available at *http://services. aamc.org/minorityaffairsdirectory/*.

Financial assistance for medical school. Any individual with an interest in a medical career should not rule out medical school solely because of financial circumstances. Public and private medical schools work hard to offer a variety of financial aid plans to both accepted applicants and already enrolled students. Applicants to medical schools should discuss possibilities for financial assistance with the financial aid officer at the medical schools that interest them, as well as discuss how best to plan effectively for the financing of their medical education. Over four-fifths of medical students nationally receive some type of financial aid to assist them in paying for their medical education. General information about financing a medical education also can be found in Chapter 9 of this publication and at *www.aamc.org/ students/minorities/scholarships.htm*.

Programs at medical schools. Once students enroll in medical school, academic and personal support programs are available to them. These programs assist students from various backgrounds to successfully complete their medical studies, with the ultimate goal of increasing racial and ethnic diversity among physicians entering careers in patient care, teaching, and research, and of eliminating racial and ethnic disparities in health care and health status. The staff members at each medical school who are primarily responsible for these programs are identified in the school-by-school entries in Chapters 12 and 13 of this publication.

Chapter 7

Selection

Decisions about the acceptance and admission of applicants to medical school are based upon multiple criteria that are developed by the faculty of each medical school and are consistent with the school's specific mission and goals. In general, all schools admit applicants who, on the basis of materials presented during the application process, have documented that they possess the personal characteristics desired in future physicians, the ability to successfully complete the academically rigorous curriculum, and the potential to fulfill the institution's mission and goals.

Personal Characteristics

Candidates' personal attributes and experiences are very important factors in selection decisions. All admission committees seek information about the following qualities in an applicant's personal statement, in evaluations and letters of recommendation from premedical advisors and others who know the applicant well, and in personal interviews:

- psychological maturity
- character and integrity
- self-discipline
- altruism
- judgment
- compassion and empathy
- communication skills
- concern for helping others
- intellectual curiosity and enthusiasm
- motivation and persistence
- reliability and dependability
- resilience and adaptability
- accountability
- experience with, and knowledge of, medicine
- leadership skills
- experience in overcoming hardship or disadvantage

Some medical schools supplement these with other characteristics, such as research experience and potential, commitment to caring for the underserved and disadvantaged, volunteer and community service experience, knowledge about health care delivery systems, and potential for enhancing diversity in the educational environment. By "diversity" is meant the contributions that students with different backgrounds, cultures, perspectives, races, ethnicities, characteristics, and personal experiences can make to the educational experience of all students and to the school's cultural, social, and learning milieu.

Letters of Evaluation and Recommendation

Medical schools usually ask applicants to indicate the names of those persons who will be submitting letters of evaluation and recommendation on their behalf. Schools typically require at least one letter from the premedical advisor or committee at the undergraduate school where the applicant completed required premedical coursework. Additional letters are usually sought from college faculty members and other advisors who have both personal knowledge of the applicant's accomplishments and the ability to objectively assess the applicant's abilities, interests, and plans. Admission committee members give less weight to subjective recommendations from personal friends, family members, and political figures. If an applicant had significant employment or military experience during or after college, letters from employers, supervisors, and commanding officers are also appropriate.

Personal and Professional Conduct

An applicant's personal and professional conduct is a crucial factor in admission decisions. Information regarding personal and professional conduct is typically made available to medical schools in three ways:

- **Self-disclosure.** Applicants are expected to disclose any disciplinary action taken against them by an institution of higher learning for violation of institutional regulations or codes of conduct. Applicants are also expected to report any legal action taken against them for violating the law and to submit a straightforward explanation of the circumstances and penalties. Applicants should discuss, as appropriate, the lessons learned and the implications of these incidents for their personal growth.

AMCAS requires an applicant to disclose on the AMCAS application any felony and misdemeanor convictions, any history of dishonorable or general discharge from the Armed Forces of the United States, and any history of institutional action. Those medical schools that do not participate in AMCAS typically require such disclosures, as well.

Failure to disclose or falsification of any official college or legal action is taken very seriously by both the AAMC and medical schools, and can prompt an official AAMC investigation that may result in the withdrawal of an admission offer.

• **Letters of Evaluation and Recommendation.** Information regarding personal and professional history is also often reported in the premedical advisor's or premedical committee's letter. Applicants should be aware that any discrepancies between self-disclosure and disclosure within a letter of evaluation or recommendation will be carefully scrutinized by medical schools.

• **Criminal Background Checks.** In July 2005, the AAMC recommended that a criminal background check be completed on all applicants accepted annually to medical school entering classes. This recommendation resulted from a desire to bolster the public's continuing trust in the medical profession, to ensure the safety and well-being of patients, to ascertain the ability of accepted applicants and enrolled medical students to eventually become licensed physicians, and to minimize the liability of medical schools and their affiliated clinical facilities.

The AAMC is currently working with a group of representative medical schools to test a recently developed AAMC-administered national, centralized process for completing and reporting on criminal background checks to AAMC-member medical schools. It is reasonable to expect that a large proportion of medical schools will choose to participate in this ongoing test for the 2009 entering class. Additional information will be made available to applicants and their premedical advisors as this testing process continues and decisions are made about implementation of policies and procedures for all interested schools.

Academic Ability

Admission committees seek to enroll students who have acquired the academic skills and knowledge necessary to progress successfully through the medical curriculum and who can be active learners throughout their medical careers. Committee members rely on an applicant's academic record and MCAT® scores in evaluating academic ability.

The former measures an applicant's academic competitiveness over time; the latter provides objective information about the applicant's knowledge base compared with others in the national applicant pool.

Academic history. Given the challenges inherent in a medical education, an applicant's academic history allows admission committee members to determine whether the applicant's study skills, persistence, course of study, and grades predict success in medical school. The "Academic Record" on the AMCAS application, containing verified and standardized grades from college transcripts, is carefully reviewed by committee members to determine the:

- grades earned in each course and laboratory
- number of credit hours carried in each academic period
- distribution of coursework among the biological, physical, and social sciences and the humanities
- need for remediation of unsatisfactory academic work
- frequency of Incomplete grades and course withdrawals
- number of years taken to complete the degree program

Although each medical school establishes its own admission criteria, schools usually prefer applicants who have completed their college degrees in a timely manner, carried respectable course loads, balanced science and humanities coursework, and consistently earned 3.0-4.0 grades (on a 4.0 scale). Chapter 5 contains information about the range of science, non-science, and total grade point averages of all applicants for the 2007 entering class.

In assessing an applicant's academic work, admission committees also consider the characteristics of the undergraduate academic institution. Coursework at colleges known for rigorous academic standards frequently get greater weight. Because medical schools vary on accepting high school AP and CLEP credits, the admission policies of individual schools in Chapters 12 and Chapter 13 should be carefully reviewed. Additional information can be achieved on a school's Web site, in its academic bulletin, or from discussions with admissions office personnel.

An applicant who has earned less-than-competitive grades in a given course or academic period should not simply decide to forgo a career in medicine. With the help of a premedical advisor and with additional academic work completed more competitively, an applicant with prior academic problems may still be able to generate a successful application. Just as in medical care and practice, the ability to persist successfully in the face of initial adversity may be perceived as an important attribute in the application and admission process.

MCAT® scores. Scores on the MCAT® can provide supplementary information about a candidate's academic ability and potential. Each medical school decides how MCAT® scores are factored into determining an applicant's ability to accomplish the academic work in the medical curriculum. Some schools average multiple MCAT® scores, some accept the highest score in each section from multiple MCAT® administrations, and others emphasize the most recent set of MCAT® scores. Chapters 12 and 13 present school-specific policies about the oldest and most recent MCAT® scores considered for admission. In addition, the data in Chapters 12 and 13 indicate that the range of MCAT® scores deemed acceptable for admission varies among schools.

MCAT® scores may receive greater attention from admission committees when a candidate's academic record is marginal or when committee members are not familiar with the candidate's undergraduate institution. In addition, a comparison of grades with MCAT® scores can provide committee members with more information than either provides on its own.

Since an applicant's academic ability is a critical selection factor for medical schools, assessing it typically includes a review of both grades and scores on the four sections of the MCAT®. Evaluating the academic preparation and ability of applicants who are not recent college graduates usually includes, in addition to the overall college record, a review of achievement in postbaccalaureate courses. Similarly, the academic abilities of candidates from groups underrepresented in medicine and from educationally and socioeconomically disadvantaged groups require special attention; additional information can be found in Chapter 6 and in the AAMC publication, *Minority Student Opportunities in U.S. Medical Schools* (*www.aamc.org/msousms*).

Interviews

Medical school policies for granting and scheduling admission committee interviews vary. A few public schools in smaller states grant an interview to all candidates who are state residents, while the majority of schools invite candidates only after an extensive screening and prioritizing process. In some instances, the interview is a final step in the assessment process for applicants already deemed to be highly attractive candidates. In other instances, the interview process occurs before any preliminary decision-making by the admission committee. Almost always, an interview is required before a final admission decision is made.

Information about a school's interview policies and procedures is usually provided to applicants in the initial stages of the selection process. Questions and requests for clarification should be directed to staff in the school's admissions office.

Applicant interviews are typically held on the medical school campus. Sometimes an applicant will be asked to interview with a graduate of the school or with a physician in the applicant's area. Some schools have designated interviewers in different geographic regions to minimize time and expense for applicants, but many schools do not offer these off-campus opportunities.

At some schools, interviews are held with individual admission committee members; at others, group interviews are the norm. Some interviewers have prior access to the applicant's information, including grades, MCAT® scores, and letters of evaluation, but other interviewers do not, and they focus instead on the candidate's experiential attributes. The interview can be an excellent opportunity for applicants to visit a campus; view the basic science and clinical facilities; meet faculty, staff, and students; and have their questions answered by members of the faculty and staff who are knowledgeable about the school and its educational and clinical programs.

The interview provides candidates with opportunities to discuss their personal histories and motivation for a medical career, as well as any aspects of their application that merit emphasis or explanation. Candidates should be prepared to discuss all aspects of their application, including their interest in the specific institution. Applicants should be forthright, open, and informative in their meetings with interviewers. Since most admission committee members are experienced interviewers who want to learn about the "real" person, applicants should not try to "game" the interview or paint a picture they believe the interviewer wants to see. For those applicants who are apprehensive about the process, practice interviews with a trusted advisor or friend can help them to present themselves in the best possible light.

AAMC Policies and Procedures For Investigating Reported Violations of Admission and Enrollment Standards

Purpose

Two significant responsibilities of the Association of American Medical Colleges (AAMC) are to promote integrity in the processes associated with entry into medical school or a graduate medical education program, and to encourage high standards during the course of enrollment. These policies and procedures have been developed to advance these purposes by addressing cases that arise in the following areas, while ensuring the rights of all concerned parties.

Policies

The AAMC requires applicants to present accurate and current information at the time application materials are submitted and during all phases of the admission process for entry into medical school or a graduate medical education program.

It is the policy of the AAMC to investigate discrepancies in credentials, attempts to subvert the admission process, and any other irregular matter that occurs in connection with application activities.

Testing Cases

The AAMC requires candidates for the MCAT® examination to present accurate and current information at the time registration materials are submitted and to adhere to all Test Center Regulations and Procedures as outlined in the *MCAT® Essentials*. It is the policy of the AAMC to investigate discrepancies, attempts to subvert eligibility requirements, violations of Test Center Regulations, and irregular behavior exhibited during the administration of the MCAT® or other tests affiliated with the AAMC.

This investigation is distinct from a Score Validity Inquiry conducted by the MCAT® Program, which pertains to the legitimacy of test scores as accurate representations of the individual's performance.

Other Cases

The AAMC may investigate and/or facilitate the reporting of certain cases that occur subsequent to an individual's enrollment in medical school. Such cases include, but are not limited to, academic and ethical violations and criminal activities. In addition, reports documenting cases submitted by other educational agencies may be disseminated by the AAMC to legitimately interested parties after notice and opportunity to comment are afforded the subject of the reports.

Reporting of Cases

The AAMC will prepare and issue a report documenting the nature of a confirmed case and any attachments provided by the individual in accordance with the procedures outlined below. With the issuance of a report, the AAMC makes no judgment as to the culpability of any person with respect to matters reported and does not assess the suitability of an individual to study or practice medicine. Rather, the AAMC strives to communicate complete and accurate information to legitimately interested parties. Evaluation of this information is the responsibility of the recipient of the report.

Procedures

Investigation Proceedings

The subject of any case is informed of the existence of the investigation and is offered an opportunity to respond to the allegations. The individual is also provided with the opportunity to review a draft of any report proposed for distribution prior to issuance. Unless otherwise requested, the final report will include any explanation or justification provided by the individual during the course of the investigation.

A pending investigation may interrupt the processing of application, registration, or testing materials of questionable validity. Such action by the AAMC, however, does not relieve the individual of the responsibility for the payment of normal processing fees.

Arbitration

The AAMC offers the option and reserves the right to request arbitration should the individual conclude that a draft report inaccurately characterizes the matter under investigation or when an agreement between parties on the content and language of the report cannot be reached. Such arbitration must be requested prior to the conclusion of an investigation and the issuance of a final report.

Arbitration is conducted by a neutral arbitrator selected by the Washington, D.C., office of the American Arbitration Association. The arbitrator acts solely on the basis of a written record submitted by both parties and no hearing or oral arguments are held. The arbitrator will have final authority to conclude whether: (1) the report should be distributed as written or (2) the report should be modified in accordance with the arbitrator's directions before distribution or (3) no report should be distributed. In addition, the arbitrator determines which party is responsible for the arbitration fee. All other costs associated with arbitration are borne by the party incurring them.

Report Recipients

The report in final form will be issued to all medical schools or residency programs to which the individual has applied or matriculated during the current cycle and medical schools and residency programs to which the applicant applies or matriculates in the future. If, at the time of the investigation, the individual is enrolled in a medical school or graduate medical education program, the report will be forwarded to the current institution of attendance and will be distributed in response to all future application or matriculation activity.

In addition to its members, the AAMC provides services to other educational institutions. For example, the MCAT® examination is used by a variety of health profession and graduate programs in addition to medicine. The report in final form is therefore subject to issuance in response to application or matriculation at such institutions of which the AAMC has knowledge.

Reports may contain information relevant to academic or disciplinary proceedings, criminal investigations, and decisions relative to entry into graduate medical education programs and professional licensure. It is the position of the AAMC to cooperate with duly constituted agencies by responding to official requests for such reports.

Chapter 8

Acceptance

Medical schools make admission offers to applicants on a continuous basis during the months before the medical school fall semester — as early as September of the year prior to matriculation for Early Decision Program (EDP) applicants, and as late as the first day of class for regular applicants. This process can sometimes become complex, especially when an applicant is admitted to more than one school. Both schools and applicants have rights and responsibilities in this process.

All 129 AAMC-member medical schools agree to observe a set of recommendations on medical school acceptance procedures for first-year entering students (*www.aamc.org/students/applying/policies*), commonly referred to as the admission "traffic rules." Applicants should be familiar with them, as they ensure that application and acceptance processes are timely and fair for all concerned. These recommendations:

- contain important dates all applicants should know

- reserve the right of applicants to hold places at multiple schools without losing an acceptance deposit, usually until May 15

- indicate policies for schools to follow after May 15 regarding applicants who continue to hold multiple places

- set forth prohibitions about a medical school's offering admission to applicants who have already enrolled in, or begun orientation programs at, another medical school. Individual schools' acceptance policies are presented in Chapters 12 and 13, although applicants are encouraged to contact the schools that are of interest to them, as well.

Applicants also have responsibilities (*www.aamc.org/students/applying/policies*). During the application process for the 2007 entering class, 8,095 applicants were accepted to two or more medical schools. Although multiple family, personal, and financial factors can affect applicants' ultimate decisions about which school to attend, they are strongly encouraged to hold only one medical school acceptance at a time. Once applicants make a final decision, they should withdraw their applications promptly from other schools. When possible, applicants holding multiple acceptances should accept their first-choice offer and withdraw from other schools that have made an offer of admission. If a subsequent and more highly preferred admission offer is received, applicants can accept the new offer and withdraw from the school at which they were originally accepted. Immediately upon matriculating at a medical school or participating in an orientation program associated with the beginning of the first-year curriculum, applicants must withdraw their applications to all other medical schools at which they remain under consideration.

Citizenship and Residency

Citizenship. The 2007 entering class at U.S. medical schools included 326 students who were not U.S. citizens or who were not permitted to reside permanently in this country by U.S. Citizenship and Immigration Services, a bureau of the Department of Homeland Security. This relatively small number of international matriculants results from several factors:

- Many public medical schools limit enrollment to state residents.

- State residency statutes require that applicants be either U.S. citizens or permitted to reside permanently or indefinitely in the U.S.

- Many private medical schools require international applicants to document their ability to independently finance a medical education.

- Many countries impose severe restrictions on the exportation of currency.

- Federal financial aid sources generally require students to be either U.S. citizens or permitted to reside permanently or indefinitely in the U.S.

- Many medical schools require completion of premedical coursework at a U.S. college or university.

- Medical schools require documentation of English language proficiency, either from an American undergraduate college or the official agency in the applicant's home country. Information about the Test of English as a Foreign Language (TOEFL) can be found at *www.toefl.org*.

Private medical schools are more likely to accept international students than public schools. However, they frequently require international matriculants to show evidence of a U.S. bank account containing sufficient resources to cover tuition and expenses for one or more years of medical education. International applicants should be aware of these issues and be prepared to meet all special requirements.

State residency. State-supported medical schools generally give preference for admission and transfer to state residents. Some states have additional requirements regarding county or regional residence. Requirements are established by state legislatures and are usually available from school officials or on the school's or state's Web site. For students who are financially independent of their parents, documentation of state residency typically involves:

- payment of state resident income taxes

- voter registration in the state

- physical residence in the state for a prescribed period of time

- possession of a state driver's license

- motor vehicle registration in the state

For students who are financial dependents, the state of residence is usually the same as that of their parents. A school's state residency definition for the purpose of in-state tuition and fee eligibility may differ from definitions for other purposes, such as voting. An applicant can usually have official state residency in only one state at a time. Because of the relationship between state of residence and probability of admission, applicants are strongly encouraged to clarify their official residency status with preferred schools before initiating a formal application.

State residents enrolled in public schools customarily pay lower tuition than non-residents. Some private schools also show preference for state residents for at least some of their places because the school receives state government support. Some states without a public medical school participate in special interstate and regional agreements to provide their residents with access to a medical education. Registrars and residency officers, located either on the medical school or parent institution's campus, can assist applicants with state residency issues.

The individual school entries in Chapter 12 present data about resident and non-resident applicants and matriculants. Nationally, 62.1 percent of 2007 matriculants attended schools in their home states; 80.5 percent of students in public schools and 34.1 percent in private schools were state residents. Public schools are unlikely to admit nonresidents unless they have exceptionally strong credentials or strong ties to the state through prior residency, employment, education, or family members.

Special Regional Opportunities for Applicants

Five interstate agreements provide special opportunities for residents of certain states:

- The Western Interstate Commission for Higher Education (WICHE) supports the Professional Student Exchange Program, enabling students from Montana and Wyoming, after certification by their states and contingent on the availability of funding, to attend a participating medical school and to pay in-state tuition at a public school or reduced tuition at a private school. The student's home state pays a fee to the admitting medical school to help cover costs. Additional information can be obtained from the certifying office in the student's home state; contact information for each state's certifying office can be found on the WICHE Web site at *www.wiche.edu/SEP/PSEP/cert-off.asp*. A student must apply though the home state certifying office by October 15th for priority consideration.

- The WWAMI (Washington, Wyoming, Alaska, Montana, and Idaho) program of decentralized medical education, begun in 1972, provides access to a publicly supported medical education to students from the five participating states. WWAMI students complete their first year at participating institutions in their home states and their second year at the University of Washington School of Medicine in Seattle. Clerkship options are available for third and fourth-year students in community settings throughout the five-state region. Additional information is available at *www.uwmedicine.org/education/wwami*, or from:

Office of Admissions
School of Medicine
University of Washington
A-300 Health Sciences Building
Box 356340
Seattle, WA 98195-6340
(206) 543-7212
askuwsom@u.washington.edu

- Under the auspices of the Southern Regional Education Board (SREB), some students from Alabama, North Carolina, and Tennessee, who have been accepted at Meharry Medical College, can pay reduced tuition at that school. For more information, see the SREB Web site at *www.sreb.org*, or contact the SREB at:

  Southern Regional Education Board
  592 10th St. N.W.
  Atlanta, GA 30318
  (404) 875-9211
  acm-rcp@sreb.org

- The Finance Authority of Maine's (FAME) Maine Access to Medical Education Program — through relationships with participating medical schools, including Dartmouth Medical School and the University of Vermont College of Medicine — ensures preference each year for 20 first-year places for Maine residents certified as eligible by the state. FAME seeks applicants who are most likely to practice primary care in underserved areas of the state. The program pays the school a fee for each student. Although students' tuition and fees are not reduced, they do receive priority for need-based forgivable loans of $5,000 to $25,000 annually.

  Students must commit to completing at least two primary care clinical rotations in Maine following completion of the medical school's core curriculum. Applicants should know that the state of Maine will encourage them to select primary care specialties and to practice in the state following completion of their training. Maine's Advisory Committee on Medical Education reviews all applications, but individual medical schools make final admission decisions. Additional information can be found at *www.famemaine.com*, or from:

Maine Access to
Medical Education Program
Finance Authority of Maine
P.O. Box 949
Augusta, ME 04332-0949
(800) 228-3734

- The Delaware Institute of Medical Education and Research provides payment to Jefferson Medical College of Thomas Jefferson University to reserve at least 20 admissions each year for Delaware residents. To be eligible, applicants must be Delaware residents, meet the premedical academic requirements of Jefferson Medical College, and apply through the American Medical College Application Service (AMCAS). Applicants' undergraduate degrees can be from any accredited U.S. college or university. Additional information is available at *http://dhcc.delaware.gov/information/dimer.shtml*, or from:

Delaware Institute of Medical
Education and Research
The Delaware Higher
Education Commission
Carvel State Office Building
820 North French Street
Wilmington, DE 19801
(302) 577-5240
(800) 292-7935

Deferring Entry into Medical School

An accepted applicant may encounter a special, one-time opportunity that is too attractive to pass up, or be invited to spend an additional year in an ongoing research project, or want to live abroad for a period of time. In recent years, most medical schools have developed delayed matriculation programs that allow applicants to pursue these opportunities without giving up their medical school places.

These deferred-entry programs usually require that the applicant submit a written request, and some schools may also ask for a report at the end of the deferral period. Delays of matriculation are usually granted for one year, although some schools may defer for longer periods of time. Some schools require delayed matriculants to sign an agreement to not apply to other medical schools in the interim, while others permit delayed matriculants to apply to other schools. Deferred matriculants will receive instructions from the school granting the deferral about requirements for another application for the year of actual matriculation. The number of deferrals may be limited, and there may be a deadline date for such applications. Interested applicants should seek specific information from schools that interest them, and schools are encouraged to define their expectations of the deferred applicant in a written document that is signed by both an appropriate school official and the applicant. The school-specific pages in Chapters 12 and 13 also contain information about deferred entrance.

Multiple Acceptances and Final Decisions

Applicants fortunate enough to receive multiple admission offers should not delay their fellow applicants' receipt of an acceptance offer by holding those acceptances for an extended time. Decisions should be made and schools notified as promptly as possible. In the spring, AMCAS shares acceptance information with all medical schools. By mid-May, the AAMC expects that all medical schools will have notified accepted applicants of their financial aid awards and that accepted applicants will have sufficient information to determine which school to attend. May 15 is the deadline for acceptance deposit refunds and for applicants' final decisions about medical schools; after May 15, schools can require applicants to choose the one school that they will attend from among those schools that have offered an acceptance. Under no circumstances should applicants be required to withdraw from other schools' waiting lists as a condition of accepting a medical school place. Ultimately, decisions about where to attend belong to applicants, not schools.

Orientation Programs

Most medical schools hold orientation programs for entering students just prior to the start of the first term. These programs familiarize students with their new environment; provide opportunities to meet fellow students, staff, and faculty; facilitate book and equipment purchases; and start to acculturate students to medicine's professional codes and responsibilities.

Once these orientation periods have begun, students can no longer accept admission offers from other schools, and they should withdraw their names from all waiting lists at other schools.

AAMC Recommendations for Medical School Admission Officers

The following recommendations are promulgated by the Association of American Medical Colleges (AAMC) to ensure that applicants are afforded timely notification of the outcome of their medical school applications and timely access to available first-year positions and that schools are protected from having unfilled positions in their entering classes. These recommendations are being distributed for the information of prospective medical students, their advisors, and personnel at the medical schools to which they have applied.

The AAMC recommends that:
1. Each school:
    a. Publish annually, amend publicly, and adhere to its application, acceptance, and admission procedures.
    b. Utilizing an application service abide by all conditions of its participation agreement with that application service.
2. Each school:
    a. Between August 1 and March 15, notify the AAMC Section for Medical School Application Services of all admission actions within four weeks of those actions being taken.
    b. Between March 16 and the first day of class, notify the AAMC Section for Medical School Application Services of all admission actions within seven days of those actions being taken.
3. Each school notify all applicants — other than combined college/M.D., Early Decision Program (EDP), and deferred matriculation applicants — of acceptance to medical school only after October 15 of each admission cycle. It may be appropriate to communicate notifications of decisions other than acceptance to medical school to applicants prior to October 15.
4. By March 30 of the matriculation year, each school have issued a number of offers of acceptance at least equal to the expected number of students in its first-year entering class and have reported those acceptance actions to the AAMC Section for Medical School Application Services.
5. Prior to May 15 of the matriculation year (April 15 for schools whose first day of class is on or before July 30), each school permit ALL applicants (except for EDP applicants) — including those applying to M.D./Ph.D. programs and those to whom merit or other special scholarships have been awarded:
    a. A minimum two-week time period for their response to the acceptance offer.
    b. To hold acceptance offers from any other schools without penalty.
6. After May 15 of the matriculation year (April 15 for schools whose first day of class is on or before July 30), each school implement school-specific procedures for accepted applicants who, without adequate explanation, continue to hold one or more places at other schools. These procedures:
    a. May require applicants to:
        i. Respond to acceptance offers in less than two weeks.
        ii. Submit a statement of intent, a deposit, or both.
    b. Should recognize the problems of applicants with multiple acceptance offers, applicants who have not yet received an acceptance offer, and applicants who have not yet been informed about financial aid opportunities at those schools to which they have been accepted.
    c. Should permit accepted applicants to remain on other schools' waiting lists and to withdraw if they later receive an acceptance offer from a preferred school.

AAMC Recommendations for Medical School Admission Officers
continued

7. Each school's acceptance deposit not exceed $100 and be refundable until May 15 (except for EDP applicants). If the applicant enrolls at the school, the school is encouraged to credit the deposit toward tuition.

8. After June 1, any school that plans to make an acceptance offer to an applicant already known to have been accepted by another school for that entering class ensure that the other school is advised of this offer at the time that the offer is made. This notification should be made immediately by telephone and promptly thereafter by written correspondence delivered by regular or electronic methods. Schools should communicate fully with each other with respect to anticipated late roster changes in order to minimize inter-school miscommunication and misunderstanding, as well as the possibility of unintended vacant positions in a school's first-year entering class.

9. No school make an acceptance offer, either verbal or written, to any individual who has enrolled in, or begun an orientation program immediately prior to enrollment at, a U.S. or Canadian school. Enrollment is defined as being officially matriculated as a member of the school's first-year entering class.

10. Each school treat all letters of recommendation submitted in support of an application as confidential, except in those states with applicable laws to the contrary. The contents of a letter of recommendation should not be revealed to an applicant at any time.

Approved: AAMC Executive Committee, October 3, 2003

AAMC Recommendations for Medical School Applicants

The following recommendations are promulgated by the Association of American Medical Colleges (AAMC) to ensure that applicants are afforded timely notification of the outcome of their medical school applications and timely access to available first-year positions and that schools are protected from having unfilled positions in their entering classes. These recommendations are being distributed for the information of prospective medical students, their advisors, and personnel at the medical schools to which they have applied.

The AAMC recommends that:

1. Each applicant be familiar with, understand, and comply with the application, acceptance, and admission procedures at each school to which the applicant has applied, as well with as these Recommendations.

2. Each applicant provide accurate and truthful information in all aspects of the application, acceptance, and admission processes for each school to which the applicant has applied.

3. Each applicant submit all application documents (e.g., primary and secondary application forms, transcript[s], letters of evaluation/recommendation, fees) to each school in a timely manner and no later than the school's published deadline date.

4. Each applicant promptly notify all relevant medical school application services and all medical schools with independent application processes of any change, permanent or temporary, in contact information (e.g., mailing address, telephone number, e-mail address).

5. Any applicant who will be unavailable for an extended period of time (e.g., during foreign travel, vacation, holidays) during the application/admission process:
   a. Provide instructions regarding his or her application and the authority to respond to offers of acceptance to a parent or other responsible individual in the applicant's absence.
   b. Inform all schools at which the applicant remains under consideration of this individual's name and contact information.

6. Each applicant respond promptly to a school's invitation for interview. Any applicant who cannot appear for a previously scheduled interview should notify the school immediately of the cancellation of the appointment in the manner requested by the school.

7. Each applicant in need of financial aid initiate, as early as possible, the steps necessary to determine eligibility, including the early filing of appropriate need-analysis forms and the encouragement of parents, when necessary, to file required income tax forms.

8. In fairness to other applicants, when an applicant has made a decision, prior to May 15, not to attend a medical school that has made an offer of acceptance, the applicant promptly withdraw his or her application from that (those) other school(s) by written correspondence delivered by regular or electronic methods.

9. By May 15 of the matriculation year (April 15 for schools whose first day of class is on or before July 30), each applicant who has received an offer of acceptance from more than one school choose the specific school at which the applicant prefers to enroll and withdraw his or her application, by written correspondence delivered by regular or electronic methods, from all other schools from which acceptance offers have been received.

10. Immediately upon enrollment in, or initiation of an orientation program immediately prior to enrollment at, a U.S. or Canadian school, each applicant withdraw his or her application from consideration at all other schools at which he or she remains under consideration.

Approved: AAMC Executive Committee, October 3, 2003

Financing a Medical Education

After being accepted to medical school, a prospective student must finalize an individual plan for covering the significant costs of a medical education, including, among other typical expenses, tuition, fees, books, equipment, living expenses, medical and disability insurance, and transportation. Two major skills are involved: the ability to develop realistic and proactive financing plans and the ability to manage educational debt. There are several factors that a student should consider in making financial decisions:

- Students are typically able to cover the cost of their medical educations with student loans.

- Medical school tuition and fees have increased significantly over the past decade.

- Student educational loans are the most common form of financial assistance.

- Primary financial responsibility for medical school rests with students and their families.

- Most medical students are unable to supplement their income with employment.

- Students with a history of credit problems may not qualify for the private loans that, in some cases, supplement federal borrowing.

- Credit card and other consumer debt obligations cannot be met with student financial aid.

- Available non-loan financial assistance, such as scholarships and grants, is finite, especially for living expenses.

- Criteria for awarding institutional financial aid differ from school to school.

- Funding and eligibility requirements for federal financial aid programs are determined by federal regulations, which can change periodically.

Information about the financial aid forms required by each medical school can be found in the searchable database on the AAMC Web site at *http://services.aamc.org/msar_reports*.

(MD)[2]: Monetary Decisions for Medical Doctors

(MD)[2]: Monetary Decisions for Medical Doctors is a comprehensive, Web-based program (*www.aamc.org/md2*) developed by the AAMC to assist premedical and medical students in their financial planning. Divided into three sections — The Premedical School Years, The Medical School Years, and The

TABLE 9-A

Tuition, Fees and Health Insurance for 2007–2008 First-Year Students in U.S. Medical Schools (in Dollars)

Categories of Students	Range	Private Schools Median	Average
Resident	$15,114 – $50,056	$41,867	$39,696
Nonresident	$0 – $50,056	$42,841	$40,476

Categories of Students	Range	Public Schools Median	Average
Resident	$9,081 – $34,246	$23,065	$22,114
Nonresident	$0 – $68,111	$40,989	$40,869

Figures based on data provided summer 2007. This table excludes the Uniformed Services University of the Health Sciences, a public institution that does not charge tuition or student fees.

TABLE 9-B

Federal Loan Programs for Students

Characteristic	Primary Care Loan	Federal Perkins	Federal Subsidized/ Unsubsidized Stafford	Graduate PLUS Loan
Lender	Medical school financial aid office on behalf of the Department of Health and Human Services	Medical school financial aid office on behalf of the federal government	Bank or other lending institution, the federal government or an eligible institution	Bank or other lending institution, the federal government or an eligible institution
Based on need	Note[1]	Yes	Subsidized – Yes Unsubsidized – No	No
Citizenship requirement	U.S. citizen, U.S. national, U.S. permanent resident, or asylum status	U.S. citizen, U.S. national, U.S. permanent resident, or asylum status	U.S. citizen, U.S. national, U.S. permanent resident, or asylum status	U.S. citizen, U.S. national, U.S. permanent resident, or asylum status
Borrowing limits	Up to cost of attendance (Third- and fourth-year students may receive additional funds to repay previous educational loans received while attending medical school)	$6000/year $40,000 aggregate undergraduate and graduate	$40,500 less subsidized Stafford $8,500 annual maximum; $189,125 less subsidized Stafford $65,500 maximum premed and medical borrowing[2]	Annual Cost of Attendance minus other financial aid
Interest rate	Note[3]	5%	For loans first disbursed since July 1, 2006, 6.8% for the life of the loan	For loans first disbursed since July 1, 2006, 8.5% for the life of the loan
Borrower is responsible for interest during:				
School:	No	No	Subsidized: No Unsubsidized: Yes	Yes
Deferments:	No	No	Subsidized: No Unsubsidized: Yes	Yes
Grace Period:	No	No	Subsidized: No Unsubsidized: Yes	N/A

Residency and Early Practice Years — (MD)[2] provides information that is tailored to the specific needs of students during the different phases of their education. Information covered includes types of financial aid, the financial aid application process, and credit and consumer debt, along with relevant reference materials.

Planning for the Financing of a Medical Education

In 2007, those medical students who graduated with educational debt reported an average educational debt of $139,517. Tuition and other expenses vary from school to school; entries in Chapter 12 provide information about individual schools' tuition and fee schedules, as well as about cost of attendance (minus tuition and fees) and average educational indebtedness for 2007 graduates.

Since most students rely on loans to pay for medical school, they should be aware of two general borrowing concepts:

- Borrowing encumbers future income. When taking an educational loan, the student is obligating future income to pay that loan off, which means that future income may be limited for opening a practice, purchasing a home, buying a car, or starting a family. Some financial analysts estimate that three dollars of future income are needed to pay off every dollar of current borrowing. Medical students should be aware of the implications of borrowing.

TABLE 9-B (continued)

Federal Loan Programs for Students

Characteristic	Primary Care Loan	Federal Perkins	Federal Subsidized/ Unsubsidized Stafford	Graduate PLUS Loan
Grace period	1 year after graduation	9 months after graduation	6 months after graduation	None
Deferments	During school. And primary care residency; check your promissory note or ask your financial aid officer	During school and up to three years of demonstrated economic hardship; check your promissory note or ask your financial aid officer	During school and up to three years of demonstrated economic hardship; check your promissory note or ask your financial aid officer	During school and up to three years of demonstrated economic hardship; check your promissory note or ask your financial aid officer
Repayment requirements	Minimum: $40/month; 10 to 25 years to repay; not eligible for loan consolidation	Minimum: $40/month including interest; maximum 10 years to repay; eligible for loan consolidation	Minimum: $50/month; level, graduated, income sensitive, and extended repayment options available; eligible for loan consolidation	Minimum $50/month; level, graduated, income sensitive and extended repayment options available; eligible for loan consolidation
Prepayment penalties				None
Allowable cancellations				Death or total and permanent disability

- The borrower must decide whether the value of a medical degree is approximately equal to the future income necessary to satisfy educational loans. While borrowing for educational purposes is a good investment in one's future, it has an impact on personal and professional lifestyle choices. Only the individual borrower can assess whether the potential return is worth the initial investment.

Debt Management

Learning to manage money takes constant practice, and formulating and living within a budget are essential elements. Thoughtful spending choices can result in less borrowing now and more disposable income later. Several practices are key to good budgeting:

- Have a spending plan. Prepare a strategy for allocating resources and anticipating periodic expenses, such as car insurance premiums, and unexpected emergencies, such as medical bills.

- Use credit prudently. Possessing one low-interest, no-fee credit card and paying the full balance monthly are highly recommended. Timely payments enhance personal credit ratings and prevent late fees.

- Use financial windfalls wisely. Use the "rule of thirds" for unexpected gifts or tax refunds: one-third to savings, one-third to pay down debt, and one-third to spending.

- Calculate ownership costs. Owning a house or car involves insurance and maintenance costs in addition to mortgage and loan payments.

- Plug spending leaks. Even minor expenditures such as restaurant meals, if they are incurred daily or weekly, add up over time.

- Limit careless shopping. Impulse buying can ruin even the best financial plan. Shop with a list and buy only when specific items are needed.

- Save whenever possible. Saving even a small amount each week can quickly add up.

- Practice delayed gratification. Answering these questions can pare down spending: Is this a "want" or a "need"? Must I have it now? Can I pay less elsewhere? Can I borrow or rent it instead?

- Live on less. Even the essential expenses of housing, transportation, and food can be reduced by living with a roommate, carpooling, using public transportation, or preparing meals at home.

In addition to good budgeting, debt management also requires good record-keeping. The borrower is responsible for maintaining records on monies owed, terms and conditions of each loan, the agencies that service loans, deadline dates, and deferment policies. Copies of application forms and promissory notes should be kept in a safe place. Many loan programs and financial institutions help in this process by providing access to information on their Web sites. Carefully tracking due dates and deadlines is also very beneficial.

Borrowers are also responsible for keeping loan providers and servicers notified of changes in name, contact information, and enrollment status. Borrowers who fail to maintain contact with lenders risk becoming delinquent in their loan payments or defaulting on their loans. Either of these situations can cause serious long-term consequences to the borrower's credit rating and can endanger future borrowing.

Financial Aid Philosophy

Financial aid provides assistance for post-secondary education and opportunities for students to attend schools of their choice. The philosophy of financial aid is that a student's family bears primary responsibility, to the extent possible, for paying educational expenses. From undergraduate to graduate and professional education, there is a decided shift in expectations about who bears the main responsibility for paying educational expenses, as explained below.

Eligibility for financial aid is generally determined by answering three questions:

1. How much does it cost? The answer varies by school and by year in school. Cost is composed of three components: tuition and fees; books, supplies, and equipment; and living expenses. These are frequently referred to as the "cost of attendance" or the "student financial aid budget." Cost of attendance figures by school year should be available from each medical school's financial aid officer.

2. What are the student's resources? The amount that a student's family can contribute to a medical education is called the "expected family contribution." It is determined through a need-analysis formula at the time of the financial aid application, which ensures that all students are treated equitably. Unlike most undergraduate students, graduate and professional students are considered financially independent in determining the expected family contribution for most types of federal financial aid; both income and assets are taken into account. However, eligibility for some types of federal aid requires reporting of family financial information, even though the student is technically considered to be independent. This is also the case at some institutions in determining eligibility for institutional grants, scholarships, and school-based loans. In theory, this approach ensures that certain types of aid are awarded to those students with the greatest need. When school officials request financial information of parents or family members, they are assessing ability, rather than willingness, to pay. In applying for aid, applicants and students should work closely with their medical school financial aid officers.

3. What additional resources are needed? The financial aid officer compares the student's expected family contribution and other resources with the institution's total cost of attendance to determine how much assistance is needed for the academic year. The student then receives an award letter that describes the actual package of financial aid from all available sources.

General Eligibility Criteria

Financial aid programs usually require that the applicant or student is:

- a U.S. citizen, a permanent resident, or permitted to reside indefinitely in the United States by U.S. Citizenship and Immigration Services, a bureau of the Department of Homeland Security.

- making satisfactory academic progress

- in compliance with Selective Service registration requirements

- not in default on other loans

An applicant or student who has defaulted on prior loans will not qualify for most federal programs and may thus be prevented from attending medical school, as the federal government is the most substantial source of financial aid. Some educational financing programs may also require a service commitment, following completion of training, as a condition of assistance.

Types of Financial Aid

In general, there are two types of financial assistance available to medical students:

- **Grants and scholarships.** The type and amount of this support vary by school and may include state and institutional funds. Grants and scholarships do not have to be repaid, but their availability may be very limited. The medical school financial aid officer is the best source of information on which grants and scholarships are available to individual students and how to qualify.

- **Loans.** Most medical student funding is in the form of loans, and details on various loan programs are available from the financial aid officer and from (MD)[2]. There are two types of loans: subsidized and unsubsidized. Subsidized loans carry no interest cost to borrowers during the in-school period, grace period, and any deferment periods, and thus are the most desirable. Unsubsidized loans accrue interest from the date of disbursement. While borrowers are not required to pay interest on unsubsidized loans during school enrollment, grace, and any deferment periods, they will be responsible for the interest costs which will be capitalized (i.e., added back to the loan principal). Private loans, used to supplement other types of aid including federal loans, are examples of unsubsidized loans. Borrowers should seek out private loans very carefully.

While medical students may also be able to work or receive funding through work-study programs offered by sponsoring colleges or universities, participation in these programs is not the norm for medical students.

Credit Issues

Students must not only show a cost of attendance that supports their borrowing from private loan programs, they must also be "credit ready," meaning that they have either a positive credit history or no credit history at all. Students with a history of late payments on consumer obligations are likely to find themselves excluded from private loans until they can resolve their credit problems.

Some medical schools require a credit history as a part of the financial aid application; applicants are advised to request their credit report prior to applying for aid. The applicant may be able to resolve any problems that may be identified before the financial aid application process gets underway. Alternately, the applicant may choose to defer matriculation until these problems can be resolved and expunged from the credit record. Many medical schools will grant a delay of matriculation to an accepted applicant who must address credit problems. Even prospective students with excellent credit histories, but with significant consumer debt, may encounter difficulty in financing medical school.

In all instances, applicants are strongly advised to make early contact with the financial aid officers at medical schools of interest to them to discuss financial aid eligibility and, if necessary, resolve any outstanding credit problems.

Service Commitment Programs

Service commitment programs — awards available through the U.S. Army, Navy, and Air Force, federal agencies, and some state agencies — provide financial assistance to enrolled medical students or residents in return for physician services after completion of medical training. While these programs are not need or cost-based or, strictly speaking, a form of financial aid, they may be of assistance in financing a medical education or in repaying student loans borrowed for medical school expenses.

- **Armed Forces Health Professions Scholarship Program (HPSP) and Financial Assistance Programs (FAP).** The Department of Defense is implementing significant enhancements to the benefits offered in the Armed Forces Health Professions Scholarship Program (HPSP) and Financial Assistance Programs (FAP).

The HPSP provides payment for educational expenses for students enrolled in a course of study leading to a degree in medicine. Educational expenses include tuition, books, equipment, fees and laboratory expenses, as well as a monthly stipend, in exchange for an active duty military service commitment. Effective September 1, 2007, the monthly stipend for all program participants increases from $1,349 to $1,605 per month. Addition-ally, the Navy is presently offering a $20,000 sign on bonus.

The FAP offers monetary benefits to health care professionals in postgraduate specialty training, also in exchange for an active duty service commitment. FAP participants receive the same monthly stipend provided to Health Professions Scholarship Program participants in addition to an annual monetary grant. The current annual grant amount for FAP participants is $28,454.

Persons participating in the HPSP program are commissioned as officers in the Individual Ready Reserve (IRR). While pursuing their course of medical study, they serve for 45 days of active duty at the rank of second lieutenant/ ensign with full pay and allowances during each year they are in the program. FAP members pursuing specialized training serve on active duty in a grade commensurate with their educational level for 14 days during each

TABLE 9-C

Armed Forces Health Professions Scholarship Programs (HPSP)

Characteristic	Navy	Air Force	U.S. Army
Provider	Navy Recruiting Command 5722 Integrity Drive, Bldg 784, Millington, TN 38054 www.navy.com/ healthcareoppor tunities/ 800-USA-NAVY	USAF Recruiting Service Headquarters 550 D Street, Suite 1 Randolph AFB, TX 78150-4527 www.airforce.com/ education/health care/ 800-558-5260	Recruiting Command Attn: RCRO-HS-MC, 1307 Third Avenue, Fort Knox, KY 40121-2726 www.health-care.goarmy.com 800-955-6966
Based on need	No	No	No
Citizenship requirement	U.S. citizen only	U.S. citizen only	U.S. citizen only
Service commitment	Yes	Yes	Yes

Each branch of the Armed Services has a variety of programs. For specific details please see their Web sites or call the above-reference telephone numbers.

year of participation. Active duty service begins after completion of training. For HPSP participants, there is a year-for-year obligation, with a minimum of three years on active duty. For FAP, active duty obligation consists of the length of the FAP benefit plus one year.

Applications are handled by local area military recruiters with contact information listed in telephone books or on the Internet. Prospective applicants also may want to speak with current military physicians who can provide a comprehensive perspective on the practice of military medicine. Applicants for the HPSP/FAP undergo a competitive screening process. Interested medical students are highly encouraged to apply for HPSP since the Armed Forces have not awarded all available scholarships over the past several years. Additional information is provided in Table 9-C.

• **The National Health Service Corps (NHSC).** The NHSC is a part of the federal Health Resources and Services Administration's (HRSA) Bureau of Health Professions. The NHSC's mission is to improve the health of the nation's underserved populations by assisting communities to recruit and retain community-responsive, culturally competent primary care clinicians. The NHSC offers a variety of programs to dedicated students and clinicians interested in pursuing careers in primary care for the underserved, including the NHSC's Scholarship Program and Loan Repayment Program. Both programs offer financial support in exchange for the opportunity to practice in communities of greatest need throughout the nation. The NHSC Scholarship Program is available to qualifying students upon matriculation. Information on NHSC Scholarship and Loan Repayment opportunities, as well as on all NHSC opportunities to serve the underserved, can be found at *http://nhsc.bhpr.hrsa.gov* or obtained by calling 1-800-221-9393; in the AAMC's State and Other Loan Repayment/Forgiveness and Scholarship Programs database, available online at *www.aamc.org/stloan*; from school financial aid officers; and from on-campus faculty NHSC "Ambassadors" in health professions schools across the country.

A list of Ambassadors can be found on the NHSC Web site or obtained by calling 1-800-221-9393.

- **State loan forgiveness or repayment programs.** State programs are frequently available to students and graduates in return for a commitment to serve in the state's areas of need. Most often available to residents and practicing physicians, these programs are sometimes open to enrolled medical students, as well. Information can be found in the searchable database on the AAMC Web site at *www.aamc.org/stloan*, and from school financial aid officers.

Chapter 10

Information on Combined College/M.D. Programs for High School Students

About one quarter of U.S. medical schools offer combined college/M.D. programs for high school students; these programs range in length from six to nine years. The first two to four years of the curriculum consist of undergraduate courses, including required premedical courses; the remaining years are devoted to the medical school curriculum. Graduates receive both a bachelor's degree from the undergraduate institution and an M.D. degree from the medical school.

The purposes of these programs vary by institution:

- to permit highly qualified students to plan and complete a broad liberal arts education before initiating their medical studies

- to attract highly capable students to the sponsoring medical school

- to enhance diversity in the educational environment

- to reduce the total number of years required to complete the M.D. degree

- to educate physicians likely to practice in particular geographic areas or to work with medically underserved populations

- to reduce the costs of a medical education

- to prepare physician-scientists and future leaders in health policy

Potential applicants should familiarize themselves with the mission and goals statement of each combined degree program in which they have an interest in order to ensure a match between their educational and professional goals and those of the program.

These programs typically represent relationships between a medical school and one or more undergraduate colleges located in the same geographic region. They are sometimes part of the same university system, or they can be independent institutions.

Admission is open to highly qualified, mature high school students who are committed to a future career in medicine. State-supported schools generally admit few out-of-state applicants to their combined college/M.D. programs; private schools tend to have greater flexibility regarding state of residency.

While academic requirements vary among the schools sponsoring these programs, they typically include biology, chemistry, physics, English, mathematics, and social science courses. Calculus and foreign-language courses are also frequently required; a computer science course is sometimes recommended. Admission to the medical curriculum may occur immediately or after a student completes a prescribed number of semesters with a minimum grade point average (GPA). In some programs, students are not required to take the MCAT®; in other programs, a minimum MCAT® score must be attained for progression through the program.

Progressing through the program from the undergraduate to the medical curriculum is usually contingent on a student's achieving specific criteria in terms of standardized test scores and GPAs and meeting the school's expectations regarding personal and professional behavior.

High school students interested in a combined college/M.D. program should consult their high school guidance counselor to ensure that they are enrolled in a challenging college preparatory curriculum, one which incorporates the specific courses required for admission to the program. The program descriptions that follow were compiled from responses to a survey sent to all medical schools sponsoring programs of interest to high school students. For additional information, contact each school directly.

The following abbreviations are used in the school entries in this chapter:

ACT
American College Testing Program

AP
Advanced Placement

BCPM
Biology, Chemistry, Physics, and Mathematics

CEEB
College Entrance Examination Board

FAFSA
Free Application for Federal Student Aid

GPA
Grade Point Average

MCAT®
Medical College Admission Test

SAT
Scholastic Aptitude Test

USMLE
United States Medical Licensing Examination

List of Medical Schools Offering Combined College/M.D. Programs for High School Students, 2009–2010

Alabama
University of Alabama School of Medicine

University of South Alabama College of Medicine

California
University of California, San Diego School of Medicine

University of Southern California College of Letters, Arts, and Sciences and Keck School of Medicine

Connecticut
University of Connecticut

District of Columbia
The George Washington University School of Medicine and Health Sciences and The Columbian School of Arts and Sciences

Howard University

Florida
University of Florida College of Medicine

University of Miami

Illinois
Northwestern University Feinberg School of Medicine

University of Illinois at Chicago College of Medicine

Massachusetts
Boston University

Michigan
Michigan State University College of Human Medicine

Wayne State University School of Medicine

Missouri
Saint Louis University School of Medicine

University of Missouri—Kansas City School of Medicine

New Jersey
University of Medicine and Dentistry of New Jersey— New Jersey Medical School

Rutgers University and UMDNJ— Robert Wood Johnson Medical School

New York
Brooklyn College and SUNY Downstate Medical Center

Hobart and William Smith Colleges/SUNY Upstate Medical University

Rensselaer Polytechnic Institute and Albany Medical College

St. Bonaventure University/The George Washington University School of Medicine and Health Sciences

Siena College and Albany Medical College

Sophie Davis School of Biomedical Education/City University of New York

Stony Brook University and Stony Brook University School of Medicine

Union College and Albany Medical College

University of Rochester School of Medicine and Dentistry

Ohio
Case Western Reserve University School of Medicine

Northeastern Ohio Universities College of Medicine

The Ohio State University College of Medicine

University of Cincinnati College of Medicine

Pennsylvania
Drexel University and Drexel University College of Medicine

Lehigh University and Drexel University College of Medicine

Pennsylvania State University and Jefferson Medical College

Temple University School of Medicine

Villanova University and Drexel

University College of Medicine

Wilkes University/SUNY-Upstate
Medical University

Rhode Island
Warren Alpert Medical School
of Brown University

Tennessee
Fisk University and Meharry
Medical College

Texas
Rice University and Baylor
College of Medicine

University of Texas School of
Medicine at San Antonio

Virginia
Eastern Virginia Medical School

Virginia Commonwealth University
School of Medicine

Number of Years Required by Undergraduate and U.S. Medical Schools to Complete the Combined College/M.D. Program, 2009–2010

6 Years
University of Missouri—Kansas City
School of Medicine

6-7 Years
University of Miami

Northeastern Ohio Universities
College of Medicine

Pennsylvania State University and
Jefferson Medical College

7 Years
The George Washington University
School of Medicine and Health
Sciences and The Columbian
School of Arts and Sciences

University of Florida
College of Medicine

Northwestern University
Feinberg School of Medicine

University of Illinois at Chicago
College of Medicine

Boston University*

University of Medicine and Dentistry
of New Jersey—New Jersey
Medical School

Rensselaer Polytechnic Institute
and Albany Medical College

Sophie Davis School of Biomedical
Education/City University of New York

The Ohio State University College
of Medicine

Drexel University and Drexel
University College of Medicine

Lehigh University and Drexel
University College of Medicine

Villanova University and Drexel
University College of Medicine

Fisk University and Meharry
Medical College

University of Texas School of
Medicine at San Antonio

8 Years
University of Alabama
School of Medicine

University of South Alabama
College of Medicine

University of California, San Diego
School of Medicine

University of Southern California
College of Letters, Arts, and Sciences
and Keck School of Medicine

University of Connecticut and
University of Connecticut
School of Medicine

Howard University

Michigan State University
College of Human Medicine

Wayne State University
School of Medicine

Saint Louis University
School of Medicine

Rutgers University and University
of Medicine and Dentistry of
New Jersey—Robert Wood
Johnson Medical School

Brooklyn College and SUNY
Downstate Medical Center

Hobart and William Smith
Colleges/SUNY Upstate
Medical University

St. Bonaventure University/The
George Washington University School
of Medicine and Health Sciences

Siena College and Albany
Medical College

Stony Brook and Stony Brook
University School of Medicine

Union College and
Albany Medical College

University of Rochester
School of Medicine and Dentistry

8 Years cont'd.

Case Western Reserve University
School of Medicine

University of Cincinnati
College of Medicine

Temple University School of Medicine

Wilkes University/SUNY-Upstate
Medical University

Brown Medical School

Rice University and Baylor
College of Medicine

Eastern Virginia Medical School

Virginia Commonwealth University
School of Medicine

9 Years

University of Cincinnati College of
Medicine (College of Engineering—
undergraduate)

*with an 8-year option

University of Alabama School of Medicine

Birmingham, Alabama

Address Inquiries To:
Amelia Johnson
Program Administrator
UAB Honors Academy, HUC 531
University of Alabama at Birmingham
1530 3rd Avenue, South, Birmingham, Alabama 35294-1150
T (205) 996-9842 **F** (205) 996-9838
honorsacademy@uab.edu
www.uab.edu/emsap

Purpose

The UAB Early Medical School Acceptance Program (EMSAP) is designed to give exceptional high school graduates an opportunity to take advantage of the best resources of the undergraduate and medical programs through a mentored relationship with medical school faculty. A medical school professor advises students from high school graduation until the second year of the medical program, establishing a unique relationship.

Requirements for Entrance

Students are selected in their senior year of high school. Both residents and non-residents of Alabama are eligible to apply to the program. Applicants must submit the following documents: (1) a completed EMSAP application; (2) two letters of recommendation from high school administrators, counselors, or teachers describing their suitability for a career in medicine; (3) a brief essay incorporating information about themselves and their career objectives and expectations for contributing to society; and (4) a resume listing their academic achievements, honors received, activities, employment, health-related experience, etc. Applicants must meet the requirements for freshman admission to the university and be admitted to the University by the EMSAP application deadline, January 1, 2009.

Selection Factors

Required high school courses include: four years of English, four years of mathematics, one year of chemistry or physics, and one year of biology. Minimum GPA: 3.5 overall GPA (on a 4.0 scale). Test scores: at least 30 ACT or a minimum 1320 SAT (critical reading + math). Selected applicants are invited for a required interview.

Curriculum

This eight-year program leads to a baccalaureate degree awarded by the University of Alabama at Birmingham (UAB), and to the M.D. degree granted by the University of Alabama School of Medicine. Students must meet the regular undergraduate course requirements for the University of Alabama at Birmingham, complete two required EMSAP (Early Medical School Acceptance Program) seminars and live on campus during their first two years. Applicants may apply to one of three other Honors programs in the Honors Academy. The deadline to apply for both programs is January 1. In order to matriculate to the medical school phase of the program, students must: (1) take the MCAT and receive a minimal total score of 28; (2) maintain an overall GPA of 3.6 and a math and science GPA of 3.5; (3) receive their baccalaureate degree; and (4) meet all requirements and conditions to remain in good standing for their acceptance into the University of Alabama School of Medicine. After the second year of medical school, students must pass the USMLE Step 1 in order to be promoted and graduate. Passing the USMLE Step 2 Clinical Knowledge (CK) examination and sitting for the Step 2 Clinical Skills (CS) examination are required in order to graduate from the medical school. Passing an Observed Structured Clinical Examination (OSCE) is also required for graduation from medical school.

Expenses

	Resident Tuition and Fees	Non-resident Tuition and Fees
Undergraduate	$4,208	$9,296
U.S. Medical School	$16,383	$43,623

Financial Aid

UAB awards comprehensive federal, state, institutional, and private financial aid on the basis of merit, financial need, or both. Each year, the university offers more than 1500 scholarships, including approximately $1.5 million in merit-based awards. Applicants are automatically considered for all academic scholarships when accepted to the university. As academic scholarships are awarded on a first come-first served basis, applicants are encouraged to apply no later than November 1 (prior to EMSAP application deadline) of the senior year of high school.

Application and Acceptance Policies

Filing of application:
    Earliest date: September 1, 2008
    Latest date: January 1, 2009
Application fee: None   Fee Waiver Available: n/a
Acceptance notice:
    Earliest date: Mid-February 2009
    Latest date: Late February 2009
Applicant's response to acceptance offer:
    Latest date: May 1, 2009
Deposit to hold place in class: None
Starting date: Mid-August 2009

Information on 2007–2008 Entering Class

Number of	In-State	Out-of-State	Total
Applicants	59	31	90
Applicants Interviewed	19	7	26
New Entrants	6	4	10
Total number of students enrolled in program: 34			

University of South Alabama College of Medicine

Mobile, Alabama

Address Inquiries To:
Donna Pigg, Assistant Director of Admissons
University of South Alabama Meisler Hall, Room 2500
Mobile, Alabama, 36688-0022
T (251) 460-6141 F (251) 460-7876
dpigg@usouthal.edu
www.southalabama.edu/com/

Purpose

Candidates selected for the program will receive early acceptance from the University of South Alabama and its College of Medicine. Students participating in the program are expected to enter the University of South Alabama College of Medicine in the fall after completion of the baccalaureate degree.

Requirements for Entrance

Students in the senior year of high school or recently graduated individuals who have not yet entered college are eligible to apply for the program. Both residents and non-residents of Alabama may apply.

Selection Factors

Candidates must have a minimum high school GPA of 3.5, as computed by the University of South Alabama, and must present a minimum enhanced composite ACT score of 30 (or comparable SAT score). Candidates must also have demonstrated evidence of leadership qualities, community service, communication skills, and motivation for the study of medicine.

Curriculum

The curriculum will include core requirements for the selected baccalaureate program and prerequisites for matriculation in medical school. Students in the program must maintain a minimum overall GPA of 3.5 and a minimum GPA of 3.4 in the sciences (biology, chemistry, physics) and mathematics. All required courses must be taken at the University of South Alabama unless otherwise approved in advance by the student's undergraduate program director and the Director of Admissions for the College of Medicine. Students will be required to participate in CP-200 (Career Planning; Clinical Observation) for a minimum of four quarters. Students will be given the opportunity to participate in a special summer premedical clerkship. These activities will be planned to give participants a broad exposure to medical education. Students will be required to take the MCAT® for admission to the College of Medicine and will be required to achieve a score above the national average. A formal assessment, including an interview, will be conducted after the student has completed 96 quarter hours of academic work. At this time, students' academic performance and continued interest in a medical career will be assessed.

Expenses

	Resident Tuition and Fees	Non-resident Tuition and Fees
Undergraduate	$6,000	$12,000
U.S. Medical School	$16,082	$29,562

Financial Aid

Information can be obtained from the Office of Financial Aid, Meisler Hall, Room 1200, University of South Alabama, Mobile, Alabama 36688-0002; by phone at (251) 460-6231; or on the school Web site at *www.finaid2.usouthal.edu*.

Application and Acceptance Policies

Filing of application:
    Earliest date: December 15, 2008
    Latest date: January 1, 2009
Application fee: $25   Fee Waiver Available: No
Acceptance notice:
    Earliest date: March 1, 2009
    Latest date: Until program is filled
Applicant's response to acceptance offer:
    Maximum time: Two weeks
Deposit to hold place in class: None
Starting date: August 18, 2009

Information on 2007–2008 Entering Class

Number of	In-State	Out-of-State	Total
Applicants	80	25	105
Applicants Interviewed	30	15	45
New Entrants	10	5	15

Total number of students enrolled in program: 60

University of California, San Diego School of Medicine

La Jolla, California

Address Inquiries To:
Yvonne Coleman, Director of Medical Scholars Program
University of California, San Diego School of Medicine
Office of Admissions, 0621
9500 Gilman Drive, La Jolla, California 92093-0621
T (858) 534-3880 **F** (858) 534-5282
somadmissions@ucsd.edu
http://meded.ucsd.edu/groups/med-scholars/

Purpose

The Medical Scholars Program was established to encourage the recruitment of unusually talented high school students, who would then be attracted to both the University of California, San Diego, (UCSD) undergraduate and medical schools, and to promote the goal of increasing diversity on both campuses.

Requirements for Entrance

Students are selected for this program during their senior year of high school. The program is open to California residents only. Applicants must meet course requirements for UCSD undergraduate admission. They must take either the SAT or ACT and achieve a minimum score of 2250 on the SAT or 34 on the ACT.

Selection Factors

To be eligible for consideration, applicants must have a minimum high school GPA of 4.0 and 2250 on the SAT or 34 on the ACT. The average high school grade-point average for the 2007 entering class was 4.29. Applicants must also demonstrate strong extracurricular involvement, particularly in community service and leadership. Letters of recommendation and an essay are additional considerations. An interview is required. The MCAT® is not required.

Curriculum

This program leads to a baccalaureate degree granted by the University of California, San Diego, and to the M.D. degree granted by the UCSD School of Medicine. It takes eight years to fulfill the requirements for both degrees. The specific course requirements for the baccalaureate degree include a minimum of 6 quarters in either humanities or social sciences and 15 quarters in the natural and physical sciences. Students must take Step 1 of the USMLE after the second year of medical school. Passing Steps 1 and 2 of the USMLE is required in order to be promoted and to graduate.

Expenses

	Resident Tuition and Fees	Non-resident Tuition and Fees
Undergraduate	$8,358	$27,978
U.S. Medical School	$21,465	$33,710

Financial Aid

Sources of financial aid include scholarships, grants, loans, and work-study. Additional information is available from the undergraduate financial aid office: Building 402, University Center, La Jolla, California 92093-0013, or at *www.ucsd.edu/finaid*.

Application and Acceptance Policies

Filing of application:
  Earliest date: February 1, 2009
  Latest date: March 14, 2009
Application fee: None   Fee Waiver Available: n/a
Acceptance notice:
  Earliest date: April 21, 2009
  Latest date: April 28, 2009
Applicant's response to acceptance offer:
  Maximum time: 1 week
Deposit to hold place in class: None
Starting date: September 2009

Information on 2007–2008 Entering Class

Number of	In-State	Out-of-State	Total
Applicants	201	n/a	201
Applicants Interviewed	25	n/a	25
New Entrants	12	n/a	12
Total number of students enrolled in program: 37			

University of Southern California
College of Letters, Arts, and Sciences and Keck School of Medicine

Los Angeles, California

Address Inquiries To:
Karen Rowan-Badger, Director of Admission
College of Letters, Arts, and Sciences
University of Southern California
Los Angeles, California 90089-0152
T (213) 740-5930 **F** (213) 740-1338
admission@college.usc.edu
www.usc.edu/schools/college/admission/baccalaureatemd/

Purpose

The goal of this program is to encourage bright and motivated students to expand the breadth of their education through a diverse liberal arts education. Students accepted into this program have the opportunity to study a wide variety of disciplines beyond the course of the standard premedical curriculum. It is the hope of the university to graduate physicians who are educated in medical science, the arts, and the humanities.

Requirements for Entrance

Students are selected for this program in the senior year of high school. Both residents and non-residents of California and international students are eligible to apply. Although there are no specific high school course requirements, applicants are required to take either the SAT or ACT.

Selection Factors

Academic factors considered include grades and standardized test scores. Participation in extracurricular activities and demonstrated leadership and community service are valued. Students who enrolled in 2007 had a mean high school GPA of 3.88 and a mean SAT score of 2200. An interview is required and is granted by invitation following careful evaluation of an applicant's file.

Curriculum

This program leads to a baccalaureate degree awarded by the University of Southern California, and to the M.D. degree granted by the University of Southern California Keck School of Medicine. This is not an accelerated program; all students must complete four years of undergraduate education and four years of medical school. Students must complete requirements for the bachelor's degree and may pursue any major offered in the university that is compatible with the requirements of the program. There are specific requirements for the bachelor's degree, which include the humanities and social, natural, and physical sciences. Advancement to the medical school phase of the program is based on acceptable academic performance and MCAT® scores as defined by the program. The MCAT® is required and must be taken by the spring of the junior year. Students must take USMLE Steps 1 and 2, and pass Step 1 of the USMLE in order to graduate from the School of Medicine.

Expenses

	Resident Tuition and Fees	Non-resident Tuition and Fees
Undergraduate	$35,810	$35,810
U.S. Medical School	$43,307	$43,307

Financial Aid

Sources of aid include scholarships, grants, work-study programs, and loans. For additional information, contact the Office of Financial Aid, University of Southern California, Los Angeles, California 90089-0912; call (213) 740-1111; or visit *www.usc.edu/dept/fao*.

Application and Acceptance Policies

Filing of application:
  Earliest date: August 1, 2008
  Latest date: December 1, 2008
Application fee: $65   Fee Waiver Available: Yes
Acceptance notice:
  Earliest date: April 1, 2009
  Latest date: April 1, 2009
Applicant's response to acceptance offer:
  Maximum time: 1 month
Deposit to hold place in class: $300; nonrefundable
Starting date: August 2009

Information on 2007–2008 Entering Class

Number of	In-State	Out-of-State	Total
Applicants	457	220	677
Applicants Interviewed	73	38	111
New Entrants	19	11	30
Total number of students enrolled in program: 101			

University of Connecticut
Storrs, Connecticut

Keat Sanford, Ph.D., Assistant Dean for Admissions
Office of Undergraduate Admissions
Special Programs in Medicine & Dental Medicine
University of Connecticut, 2131 Hillside Road, U-88
Storrs, Connecticut 06269-3088
T (860) 486-3137 **F** (860) 486-1476
http://medicine.uchc.edu/prospective/admissions/babs_md.html

Purpose
This program offers gifted and talented high school students, who are focused on a career in medicine, the opportunity to combine a broad-based liberal arts program with a medical education. This program links undergraduate preparation with four years of medical education, resulting in dual degrees: a B.A. or B.S. degree and the M.D. degree.

Requirements for Entrance
Students are selected for this program during the senior year of high school. Both residents and non-residents of Connecticut are eligible to apply. Applicants must take either the SAT I or ACT.

Selection Factors
To be considered for this program, the student should have the following: a high school class ranking in the top five percent; an overall high school grade-point average of 3.5 (4.0 scale); an SAT combined score of 1300 or an ACT composite score of 30; a completed regular undergraduate admission application and a supplemental application for the program in medicine by the January 1 postmark deadline; and, an interview at the School of Medicine. In addition, recommendations from teachers/advisors, as well as evidence maturity, extracurricular activities, and a commitment to the health profession, are considered. To matriculate in the School of Medicine upon completion of undergraduate preparation, the student must meet additional criteria that include: maintaining a college 3.5 cumulative grade-point average (4.0 scale); ordinarily obtaining an MCAT® score of 30+ (with a minimum score of 28), with section scores of 7 or greater; participation in clinical, research, and community service activities; and favorable interviews during the senior undergraduate year. For more information on the medical school program, please contact Dr. Keat Sanford, assistant dean for medical school admissions, at (860) 679-3874 or sanford@nso1.uchc.edu.

Curriculum
Students must complete requirements for a baccalaureate degree from the University of Connecticut. Requirements include courses in the humanities and social sciences. The curriculum typically takes eight years to complete: Years 1 through 4 in the liberal arts and sciences and Years 5 through 8 in the School of Medicine. The MCAT® is required for admission to the medical school phase of the program. Students are required to pass Step 1 of the USMLE for promotion and Step 2 of the USMLE in order to graduate.

Expenses

	Resident Tuition and Fees	Non-resident Tuition and Fees
Undergraduate	$6,456	$19,656
U.S. Medical School	$24,142	$46,778

Financial Aid
All enrolled candidates will be automatically considered for merit scholarships. A full range of financial aid options based on student financial need is available, as well. Candidates for need-based aid must submit the Free Application for Federal Student Aid (FAFSA) by March 1. For more information about student aid programs, contact the University of Connecticut's Office of Student Financial Aid Services at (860) 486-2819; write to U-4116, Storrs, Connecticut 06269; or visit the UConn homepage at *www.uconn.edu*.

Additional Information
Students are provided with enrichment experiences while completing the undergraduate program. Programming includes: courses offered at the main University campus by faculty from the School of Medicine (these have included Mini-Medical School and The Patient and the Healer.); a summer research fellowship opportunity at the School of Medicine; placements to obtain clinical experience; placements to obtain community service experience; and assigned advisory committees for each student including faculty from the School of Medicine.

Application and Acceptance Policies
Filing of application:
    Earliest date: September 1, 2008
    Latest date: n/a
Application fee: $70   Fee Waiver Available: Yes
Acceptance notice:
    Earliest date: March 1, 2009
    Latest date: Until full
Applicant's response to acceptance offer:
    Latest date: May 1, 2009
Deposit to hold place in class: $150; nonrefundable
Starting date: August 2009

Information on 2007–2008 Entering Class

Number of	In-State	Out-of-State	Total
Applicants	83	126	209
Applicants Interviewed	25	15	40
New Entrants	6	3	9
Total number of students enrolled in program: 44			

Chapter 10: Information on Combined College/M.D. Programs for High School Students   69

The George Washington University School of Medicine and The Columbian College of Arts and Sciences

Washington, D.C.

Address Inquiries To:
Office of Undergraduate Admissions
The George Washington University
2121 I Street N.W., Suite 201
Washington, D.C. 20052
T (202) 994-6040; gwadm@gwu.edu
http://gwired.gwu.edu/adm/classroom/honors.html

Purpose

A joint program of The George Washington (GW) University Columbian College of Arts and Sciences and the School of Medicine and Health Sciences, the seven-year B.A.-M.D. program is designed for the high school senior who exhibits academic excellence, leadership in activities, and community service and healthcare experience, and who has confirmed the goal to become a physician. The purpose of the program is to encourage a liberal arts focus in preparation for medical school. Students typically choose majors in a wide variety of fields ranging from economics and psychology to religion and biology. The new, state-of-the-art GW Hospital opened in 2002. Housed on the 6th floor of the new GW Hospital is the GW Clinical Skills Center. Dedicated to education and research, this floor of the hospital features cutting-edge technology in a setting that is among the most innovative in the nation. Through the use of the Surgical Simulation and Demonstration Area and the Standardized Patient Examining Area, medical students gain the comprehensive clinical exposure, feedback, and evaluation they need to become both technically adept and humane caregivers for their patients.

Requirements for Entrance

Students are selected in their senior year of high school. Applicants must be a U.S. citizen, U.S. permanent resident, or Canadian citizen in order to apply. Applicants are expected to complete the SAT or ACT, as well as the SAT Subject Tests in Mathematics, Science, and English. Competitive SAT scores for the program are (equivalent) 2100 and above.

Selection Factors

Academic factors considered in selecting applicants include the strength of the academic program, grades in high school, class rank, and standardized test scores. In addition to academic factors, extracurricular and health-related activities, community service, essays, and letters of recommendation are reviewed. Competitive applicants are those who rank in the top ten percent of their high school class, have shown leadership ability through participation in extracurricular activities, have demonstrated interest in the medical field through experience, and have taken advantage of advanced course offerings. An interview is required and is by invitation only.

Curriculum

A special faculty committee reviews each student's progress throughout the program annually. To continue each year in the program, students must maintain a minimum of a "B" in courses required for admission to the medical school and an overall 3.3 average. Students are not required to take the MCAT®. Students participate in seminars of interest and are involved in community service and health care experiences throughout the undergraduate portion of the curriculum. The review committee will make a final recommendation concerning promotion to the medical school curriculum at the end of the third

year. In the fourth year, students enroll in the School of Medicine and Health Sciences and begin their formal medical training. The baccalaureate degree can be awarded after Year 4 (the first year of medical school) or received before entrance to the M.D. program. The integration of clinical skills begins in the first and second years of medical school, as students spend time with physicians, learning the art and skill of patient interviewing and physical diagnosis. The sixth and seventh years are devoted to developing clinical expertise in a wide variety of hospitals in the D.C. metropolitan area. At the end of the seventh year, students are awarded the M.D. degree.

Expenses

	Resident Tuition and Fees	Non-resident Tuition and Fees
Undergraduate	$ 36,092	$ 36,092
U.S. Medical School	$ 36,092	$ 36,092

Financial Aid

Information may be obtained from The George Washington University, Office of Student Financial Assistance, 2121 "I" Street, N.W., #310, Washington, D.C. 20052. The Office of Student Financial Assistance may be reached by phone at 1-800-222-6242.

Additional Information

A blended tuition is charged for the seven years. This includes an annual $15,000 award.

Application and Acceptance Policies

Filing of application:
    Earliest date: September 1, 2008
    Latest date: December 10, 2008
Application fee: $70   Fee Waiver Available: Yes
Acceptance notice:
    Earliest date: April 2009
    Latest date: April 2009
Applicant's response to acceptance offer:
    Maximum time: May 1, 2009
Deposit to hold place in class: $800; nonrefundable
Starting date: August 2009

Information on 2007–2008 Entering Class

Number of	In-State	Out-of-State	Total
Applicants	n/c	n/c	700
Applicants Interviewed	n/c	n/c	55
New Entrants	n/c	n/c	10
Total number of students enrolled in program: 105			

Howard University College of Medicine

Washington, D.C.

Address Inquiries To:
Dr. Georgiana Aboko-Cole, Director
Center for Preprofessional Education
College of Arts and Sciences, 2225 Georgia Avenue NW, Room 518,
Howard University
Washington, D.C. 20059
T (202) 238-2363
F (202) 588-9820
preprofessional@howard.edu, www.founders.howard.edu/preprof/

Purpose

The goal of this combined-degree program is to encourage talented undergraduate students to choose medicine as a career and to retain these excellent students in the Howard University College of Medicine.

Requirements for Entrance

Students can be selected for this program during the senior year of high school or during the first year of college. There are no state residence requirements. Applicants are expected to have completed the following courses by the time they graduate from high school: at least two years of a foreign language; at least one year each of biology, chemistry, and physics; two years of mathematics; and, four years of English, including literature. They must take either the SAT or the ACT Assessment.

Selection Factors

The academic factors considered in offering admission to an applicant are rank in high school class, GPA, and test scores. Applicants are expected to be in the top five percent of their high school class. In the 2007-2008 entering class, the average GPA was 3.7, and the average SAT combined score was 1950. ACT Assessment cumulative scores ranged from 25 to 29. Personal qualities considered are: superior writing skills, maturity, positive self-confidence, realistic self-appraisal, a realistic assessment of the medical profession, good leadership skills, and sustained demonstration of service to people who are less fortunate. An interview is required.

Curriculum

This program leads to a bachelor's degree awarded by the College of Arts and Sciences at Howard University and to the M.D. degree granted by the Howard University College of Medicine. Students must complete work for a baccalaureate degree. They are expected to complete at least 40 semester hours of humanities and social sciences courses to fulfill general education requirements and at least 46 semester hours of natural and physical sciences courses. Students meet with the director (the advisor) of the Center for Preprofessional Education to design a curriculum tailored to their individual needs. The specific course selection must have the advisor's approval. Students are encouraged to select a major of personal interest. The curricula for both degrees are completed in six years. In the first two years, the curriculum focuses on work toward the bachelor's degree and premedical requirements, and in the last four years the focus is on studies related to medicine. Students in this program must take the MCAT® in April of the second year. The results of the MCAT®,

the GPA, the demonstration of a high level of maturity, and a strong commitment to service in areas where there is a shortage of health professionals are factors in gaining admission to the medical school phase of the combined degree program. Students are also expected to take Steps 1 and 2 of the USMLE while at Howard University College of Medicine; they must pass these examinations prior to promotion and graduation.

Expenses

	Resident Tuition and Fees	Non-resident Tuition and Fees
Undergraduate	$14,020	$14,020
U.S. Medical School	$29,846	$29,846

Financial Aid

Information can be obtained from the Office of Financial Aid, Howard University, Johnson Administration Building, 2400 6th Street, N.W., Washington, D.C. 20059.

Application and Acceptance Policies

Filing of application:
    Earliest date: n/a
    Latest date: March 1, 2009
Application fee: $45   Fee Waiver Available: No
Acceptance notice:
    Earliest date: n/a
    Latest date: May 15, 2009
Applicant's response to acceptance offer:
    Maximum time: July 15, 2009
Deposit to hold place in class: $150; nonrefundable
Starting date: August 2009

Information on 2007–2008 Entering Class

Number of	In-State	Out-of-State	Total
Applicants	5	40	45
Applicants Interviewed	3	17	20
New Entrants	0	10	10
Total number of students enrolled in program: 10			

University of Florida College of Medicine

Gainesville, Florida

Address Inquiries To:
Robyn Sheppard, Director of Admissions
Medical Selection Committee
University of Florida College of Medicine P.O. Box 100216
Gainesville, Florida 32610
T (352) 273-7990 **F** (352) 392-1307
www.med.ufl.edu/oea/admiss/site/Junior.shtml

Purpose

The Junior Honors Medical Program is for undergraduate students who have chosen a career in the medical profession and who have demonstrated superior scholastic ability and personal development during their first two academic years of college enrollment. Experience in health care, community service, and medically related research are extracurricular activities that are considered valuable for these applicants.

Requirements for Entrance

Students are selected for this program during the sophomore year of college enrollment. Admission is open to all possible candidates who are Florida residents. There are no specific high school course requirements. However, admission tests such as the SAT and/or ACT achievement tests are required. The minimum GPA required for application is 3.75 on college coursework; the minimum required SAT score is a 1200. The courses listed must be completed by the spring semester of the applicant's sophomore year: General Chemistry I and II (both with labs), Organic Chemistry I and II (both with labs), and General Physics I and II (both with labs). The following courses may be completed in the junior year: Calculus I and II and Biology I and II (both with labs).

Selection Factors

The academic factors considered in offering admission to an applicant include sophomore standing (two years of college classroom enrollment), competitive SAT or ACT scores, competitive GPA, and completion of prerequisite courses. Involvement in medically related research prior to application is considered positively as well as consistent health care experience and community service. The MCAT® is currently not required. Selected applicants are invited for a required interview held in March and April. Acceptance decisions are not made until grades for the Spring semester are posted and an official transcript is received in the UF COM Admissions Office, usually in May.

Curriculum

The most frequent major for the baccalaureate degree is interdisciplinary biomedical sciences through the College of Liberal Arts and Sciences. Some students choose nutrition as a major through the College of Life Sciences; this option requires approval. The junior year in the program includes undergraduate college required courses and seminars with College of Medicine faculty. During the junior year, JHMP students must complete an Honors Thesis prior to entering medical school. Completion of the thesis earns the designation of honors or high honors in research at graduation for the MD degree. The bachelor's degree is awarded after the fourth year of college enrollment, which is concurrently the first year of medical school.

The University of Florida College of Medicine awards the Doctor of Medicine degree. It takes seven years to complete requirements for both degrees. All courses in the first two years are liberal arts courses. In Year 3, half of the curriculum is in the liberal arts and half in medicine. In Years 4 through 7, all courses are in medicine.

Expenses

	Resident Tuition and Fees	Non-resident Tuition and Fees
Undergraduate	$1,628	$8,921
U.S. Medical School	$23,170	$52,410

Financial Aid

Several sources of financial aid are available to students, including college scholarships and loans, federal Stafford loans, and state National Merit and Robert Byrd Scholarships, if eligible. For more information, contact Eileen Parris, UF COM Office of Financial Aid, P.O. Box 100216 HSC, Gainesville, Florida 32610, (352) 273-7939; or E-mail eparris@ufl.edu.

Additional Information

For the research requirement, the Junior Honors student is assigned a faculty member in a department of interest to the student. The faculty member supervising the research is a mentor to the student. Continued interest in the research area can be continued through the medical school years either through the Research Track Program or the M.D./Ph.D Program.

Application and Acceptance Policies

Filing of application:
    Earliest date: January 15, 2009
    Latest date: January 30, 2009
Application fee: None   Fee Waiver Available: n/a
Acceptance notice:
    Earliest date: May 15, 2009
    Latest date: August 15, 2009
Applicant's response to acceptance offer:
    Maximum time: 2 weeks
Deposit to hold place in class: None
Starting date: August 2009

Information on 2007–2008 Entering Class

Number of	In-State	Out-of-State	Total
Applicants	52	0	52
Applicants Interviewed	21	0	21
New Entrants	12	0	12
Total number of students enrolled in program: 12			

University of Miami

Coral Gables, Florida

Address Inquiries To:
Joe Montgomery, Admissions Officer
Office of Admissions, University of Miami
P.O. Box 248025
Coral Gables, Florida 33124
T (305) 284-4323
webrequest.admission@miami.edu
www6.miami.edu/UMH/CDA/UMH_Main/0,1770,2613-1;14415-3,00.html

Purpose

The Honors Program in Medicine (HPM) offers exceptionally motivated and talented high school students, who have reached a mature and independent decision to study medicine, an opportunity to earn the B.S. and M.D. degrees in seven or eight years.

Requirements for Entrance

Applicants must be U.S. citizens or permanent residents. Both residents and non-residents of Florida are considered for admission. Applicants must be in their last year of high school at the time of application. Applicants must have a minimum combined score of 1400 on the SAT or a composite score of 32 on the ACT, an unweighted GPA of at least 3.75, and take the SAT II Subject Tests in Mathematics, and one science (a minimum score of 600 is required in each). All applicants must have completed eight semesters of mathematics and English and two semesters each of biology and chemistry by the time of graduation from high school.

Selection Factors

Academic factors taken into account include scores on standardized tests, the quality of the high school curriculum (including the number and nature of Advanced Placement courses), and the amount of university-level work already completed. Of equal importance to academic achievements are personal factors such as maturity of thought and action, common sense, empathy, interpersonal skills, appropriate freedom from parental influence, and social cognizance. Most important, the applicant must have made a practical decision to study medicine based on self-initiated patient-contact experiences.

Curriculum

The first three years are spent on the Coral Gables campus taking required science and humanities courses and focusing almost exclusively on work related to the bachelor's degree. The undergraduate portion of the curriculum may be extended to four years if the student is in good academic standing and has established a clear plan of academic and personal growth. HPM students major most frequently in biology, followed by biochemistry. All HPM students must have a 3.7 science GPA and a 3.7 cumulative GPA and an MCAT® composite score of 28 to be promoted to the School of Medicine after three years. Students can be promoted at the end of four years with a cumulative and science GPA of at least 3.5 and a minimum MCAT® score of 26. All students must develop a continuous history of involvement at the undergraduate level in research, campus or community service, patient contact experiences, study abroad, or employment, consistent with a sincere desire to study and practice medicine. HPM students may attend either the parent medical campus in Miami or the regional medical campus located in Boca Raton, Florida, on the campus of Florida

Atlantic University. The missions of the educational programs at both campuses are identical but the regional medical campus emphasizes continuity of care and community medicine. Students at the Miami campus receive their clinical training at Jackson Memorial Hospital and other hospitals affiliated with the Miller School of Medicine, while students at the regional campus receive their clinical training at Boca Raton Community Hospital.

Expenses

	Resident Tuition and Fees	Non-resident Tuition and Fees
Undergraduate	$34,000	$34,000
U.S. Medical School	$30,048	$39,254

Financial Aid

Scholarships, work-study, loans, and state tuition grants are sources of financial assistance. Information on undergraduate financial aid is available from the Office of Admissions on the Coral Gables campus.

Application and Acceptance Policies

Filing of application:
  Earliest date: October 1, 2008
  Latest date: December 31, 2008
Application fee: $65   Fee Waiver Available: No
Acceptance notice:
  Earliest date: April 1, 2009
  Latest date: April 1, 2009
Applicant's response to acceptance offer:
  Maximum time: May 1, 2009
Deposit to hold place in class: $300; nonrefundable
Starting date: August 2009

Information on 2007–2008 Entering Class

Number of	In-State	Out-of-State	Total
Applicants	200	89	289
Applicants Interviewed	70	40	110
New Entrants	8	5	13
Total number of students enrolled in program: 58			

Northwestern University
Feinberg School of Medicine

Evanston, Illinois

Address Inquiries To:
Dr. Marianne Green, Associate Dean for Medical Education
Office of Admission and Financial Aid Northwestern University
1801 Hinman Avenue
Evanston, Illinois 60204-3060
T (312) 503-8915 **F** (312) 503-0840
ug-ad@northwestern.edu
www.medschool.northwestern.edu/hpme

Purpose

The Honors Program in Medical Education (HPME), one of the oldest in the nation, offers a unique opportunity for gifted and highly motivated students who seek careers in medicine or medical science. The HPME provides a broad, flexible and challenging undergraduate education free from many of the pressures related to gaining acceptance to medical school.

Requirements for Entrance

Students are selected for this program during the senior year of high school. Both residents and non-residents of Illinois are eligible to apply. Applicants must meet the following high school course requirements: English, eight semesters; mathematics, including differential and integral calculus, eight semesters; chemistry, two semesters; physics, two semesters; biology, two semesters; and, foreign language, four semesters. They must take either the SAT Reasoning Test or the ACT Assessment with Writing, plus the SAT Subject Tests (in mathematics level 2 and chemistry).

Selection Factors

Academic factors considered in selecting applicants include class rank, grades in high school, and scores on college entrance tests. Average test scores of students in the 2007-2008 entering class were: SAT Critical Reading, 732; SAT Mathematics, 775; SAT Writing 750; CEEB Subject Tests – Chemistry, 764; Mathematics II, 788; ACT plus Writing, 34. Non-academic factors considered are motivation for a career in medicine, concern for others, maturity, team work, and leadership. An interview is required.

Curriculum

The degrees offered in the honors program are a baccalaureate degree (B.A., B.S. in medicine, B.S. in biomedical engineering, or B.S. in communication) and the M.D., all from Northwestern University. Students must complete requirements for a baccalaureate degree in addition to the required science courses (inorganic and organic chemistry, calculus-based physics, biological science sequence). The majority of students in the Feinberg College of Arts & Science major in biological sciences, but have many other options within the college. Students in the McCormick School of Engineering & Applied Sciences major in biomedical engineering and take the basic and advanced engineering courses, in addition to non-science courses. The program in the School of Communication includes special courses in communication sciences and disorders. The curriculum usually takes seven or eight years to complete, and students are encouraged to develop a unique curricular path. During the undergraduate years, the curriculum consists of courses in the liberal arts and sciences, engineering, or speech. After matriculation to Feinberg School of Medicine, the curriculum focuses on medicine. The MCAT® is not required. Students must take Steps 1 and 2 of the USMLE and record passing grades in order to graduate from the medical school.

Expenses

	Resident Tuition and Fees	Non-resident Tuition and Fees
Undergraduate	$35,064	$35,064
U.S. Medical School	$40,313	$40,313

Financial Aid

Sources of aid include Northwestern University and federal, state, and private programs. Undergraduate applicants can receive more information from the Office of Admission and Financial Aid, 1801 Hinman Avenue, Evanston, Illinois 60204-3060; or phone (847) 491-7271. Information about medical school financial aid can be obtained from Financial Aid Professional Schools, Abbott Hall, 710 Superior Street, Chicago, Illinois 60611.

Additional Information

Students are encouraged to explore focused areas of concentration during their undergraduate years that may prepare them personally and professionally for their careers in medicine. Students spend their undergraduate years on the Evanston Northwestern Campus; the medical school curriculum is conducted at the Feinberg School of Medicine Chicago Campus. Tours of the Evanston Campus are given on a regular basis, however, tours are not generally offered for the Chicago Campus. For more detailed information about the program, please see our website: *www.medschool.northwestern.edu/hpme*.

Application and Acceptance Policies

Filing of application:
　Earliest date: n/a
　Latest date: January 1, 2009
Application fee: $65　　　Fee Waiver Available: Yes
Acceptance notice:
　Earliest date: April 1, 2009
　Latest date: n/a
Applicant's response to acceptance offer:
　Latest Date: May 1, 2009
Deposit to hold place in class: $400; nonrefundable
Starting date: September 15, 2009

Information on 2007–2008 Entering Class

Number of	In-State	Out-of-State	Total
Applicants	n/r	n/r	669
Applicants Interviewed	7	15	112
New Entrants	n/r	n/r	22

Total number of students enrolled in program: 110

University of Illinois at Chicago College of Medicine

Chicago, Illinois

Address Inquiries To:
Josephine Volpe, Assistant Director
Academic Affairs/Special Scholarship Programs
University of Illinois at Chicago, 104 Grant Hall, M/C 115
703 S. Morgan Street
Chicago, Illinois 60607
T (312) 355-2477 F (312) 355-1233
gppauic@uic.edu
www.uic.edu/depts/oaa/spec_prog/gppa/

Purpose

The Guaranteed Professional Program Admissions (GPPA) initiative is a combined effort of the University of Illinois at Chicago (UIC) Honors College on the undergraduate campus and the College of Medicine. This program is offered only to high school seniors from Illinois. The GPPA guarantees incoming freshmen a seat in the College of Medicine (provided they qualify upon completion of their undergraduate studies at UIC).

Requirements for Entrance

This program is limited to Illinois residents. Students are selected for this program during the senior year of high school. There are no specific high school course requirements.

Selection Factors

The academic factors considered are rank in high school class, grade-point average, and test scores. Applicants must be in the top 15 percent of their high school class. Applicants must have a minimum ACT composite score of 28, or its SAT equivalent score. In addition to academic factors, extracurricular health-related activities and letters of recommendations are required. Selected applicants are invited for a required interview.

Curriculum

Students in this program are required to complete a baccalaureate degree at the University of Illinois at Chicago (UIC). Students are free to choose any of UIC's majors in eight undergraduate colleges. The Doctor of Medicine degree is awarded by the UIC College of Medicine. It takes at least seven years to fulfill the requirements for both degrees. Students must maintain a 3.5/4.0 cumulative grade-point average. From the freshman year to the junior year, students must take a total of four seminars that will introduce them to various aspects of the medical profession. During the year proceeding expected entry into medical school, students must take the Medical College Admissions Test (MCAT®). Students must earn a MCAT® score of at least the mean of the matriculating students into the College of Medicine in the year prior to expected entry, with no score below 9 in any segment of the exam. If this condition is not met, the student must successfully complete the College of Medicine Pre-matriculation program during the summer before enrolling in medical school. Students will be assessed a fee for participation in the program. Once enrolled in the College of Medicine, students in the program are bound by the policies in force at the time of their entry.

Expenses

	Resident Tuition and Fees	Non-resident Tuition and Fees
Undergraduate	$10,546	$22,936
U.S. Medical School	$27,828	$56,724

Additional Information

All students are assigned a faculty College of Medicine advisor throughout their undergraduate years.

Application and Acceptance Policies

Filing of application:
  Earliest date: September 15, 2008
  Latest date: December 15, 2008
Application fee: $0   Fee Waiver Available: n/a
Acceptance notice:
  Earliest date: March 15, 2009
  Latest date: April 1, 2009
Applicant's response to acceptance offer:
  Maximum time: May 1, 2009
Deposit to hold place in class: None
Starting date: August 2009

Information on 2007–2008 Entering Class

Number of	In-State	Out-of-State	Total
Applicants	294	0	294
Applicants Interviewed	90	0	90
New Entrants	26	0	26
Total number of students enrolled in program: 100			

Boston University School of Medicine

Boston, Massachusetts

Address Inquiries To:
Anthony J. Orlando
Assistant Director of Undergraduate Admissions
Boston University
Office of Undergraduate Admissions, 121 Bay State Road
Boston, Massachusetts 02215
T (617) 353-2300 **F** (617) 353-9695
admissions@bu.edu; www.bu.edu/bulletins/und/item14.html

Purpose

This combined degree program, one of the oldest in the nation, provides an undergraduate premedical preparation that also emphasizes the humanities and social sciences and affords a quality medical education even though the overall period of study is shortened.

Requirements for Entrance

Students are selected for the program at Boston University during the senior year of high school (or after high school if they have not been enrolled in any other degree-granting program). There are no state residence requirements. Students who are completing their high school graduation requirements in three years in order to graduate early are not eligible for this program. Applicants are expected to have completed the following courses by the time they graduate from high school: four years each of English and mathematics (one year of calculus is required); three years each of social sciences and a foreign language; and one year each of biology, chemistry (AP chemistry is strongly recommended), and physics. Applicants must take the SAT or the ACT with Writing. They must take SAT Subject Tests in Mathematics Level 2 and Chemistry. An SAT Subject Test in [a foreign] Language is recommended.

Selection Factors

The academic factors taken into account in offering admission to an applicant include the following: the high school GPA, the SAT or the ACT with Writing score, scores on the SAT Subject Tests, rank in high school class, and the nature of the applicant's high school curriculum. In the 2007-2008 entering class, the average high school GPA was an unweighted 3.9 on a 4.0 scale, and rank in class was in the top two percent. The average combined Critical Reading and Math SAT score was 1521. The average SAT Writing score was 751. SAT Subject Test scores in Chemistry averaged 747. SAT Subject Tests in Mathematics Level 2 averaged 776. Personal characteristics sought in applicants are motivation, maturity, and an understanding of a career in medicine. An interview with College of Arts and Sciences and School of Medicine faculty is required.

Curriculum

This program leads to a baccalaureate degree granted by the College of Arts and Sciences at Boston University and to the M.D. degree awarded by Boston University School of Medicine. Students must complete work for the baccalaureate degree with a major in medical sciences and a minor concentration in a division of the College of Arts and Sciences. Students must also satisfy the course distribution and language requirements of the college. Requirements for this degree include nine one-semester courses in the natural and physical sciences and two one-semester courses in the humanities, mathematics and computer science, and social sciences. The program is seven years in length, with an eight-year option. Students must meet GPA and MCAT® requirements of the program. They are also required to take Step 1 of the USMLE during the medical school portion of the program. Taking Step 2 of the USMLE is not a requirement for graduation, but is strongly recommended.

Expenses

	Resident Tuition and Fees	Non-resident Tuition and Fees
Undergraduate	$35,418	$35,418
U.S. Medical School	$43,234	$43,234

Financial Aid

The usual sources of financial aid are available to students during the undergraduate portion of this program. Once in the medical school, students can qualify for need-based, low-interest, and government-sponsored loans. More information about aid can be obtained from the Office of Financial Assistance, Boston University, 881 Commonwealth Avenue, Boston, Massachusetts 02215, or by phone (617) 353-2965.

Application and Acceptance Policies

Filing of application:
  Earliest date: September 1, 2008
  Latest date: December 1, 2008
Application fee: $75   Fee Waiver Available: Yes
Acceptance notice:
  Earliest date: April 1, 2009
  Latest date: April 15, 2009
Applicant's response to acceptance offer:
  Maximum time: May 1, 2009
Deposit to hold place in class: $650; nonrefundable
Starting date: September 2009

Information on 2007–2008 Entering Class

Number of	In-State	Out-of-State	Total
Applicants	42	509	551
Applicants Interviewed	9	95	104
New Entrants	4	28	32
Total number of students enrolled in program: 75			

Michigan State University
College of Human Medicine

East Lansing, Michigan

Address Inquiries To:
Letitia Fowler, Admissions Senior Counselor
Margo Smith, Program Coordinator
College of Human Medicine
Office of Admissions, A-239 Life Sciences
Michigan State University, East Lansing, Michigan 48824
T (517) 353-9620 **F** (517) 432-0021
mdmsp@msu.edu, http://mdadmissions.msu.edu/main/msapplication.htm

Purpose

The goal of the MD Medical Scholars Program at Michigan State University is to nurture and educate excellent future physicians who will establish caring relationships with patients, who will meet primary healthcare needs in Michigan, especially in underserved rural and inner-city areas, contribute to scientific knowledge, and who will commit to a lifetime of learning and ethical practice.

Requirements for Entrance

Students are selected for this program in the senior year of high school. Both residents and non-residents of Michigan are eligible to apply, with preference given to Michigan residents. Typically 8 of 10 entering students are from Michigan. There are no specific high school course requirements, but applicants are required to have an ACT composite score of 29 or higher, or a combined score on the SAT Mathematics and Critical Reading sections of 1280 or higher. Applicants must have applied to and been accepted by Michigan State University for undergraduate study.

Selection Factors

Academic selection factors include class rank in the top ten percent or a GPA of at least 3.6 achieved in a college preparatory curriculum. Competitive applicants must have strong communication skills, demonstrated leadership, significant work or volunteer experience in the community, and meaningful exposure to the medical setting. Students interested in a career as a primary care physician and in service in physician shortage areas and students from groups underrepresented in medicine are encouraged to apply. Selected applicants are invited for a required interview. In the 2007-2008 entering class, the high school GPA averaged 4.28, and the average mean ACT score was 34; the SAT I score averaged 1458.

Curriculum

The MD Medical Scholars is an enrichment program complimenting the baccalaureate degree awarded by Michigan State University and the M.D. degree granted by Michigan State University College of Human Medicine. It is not an accelerated program; all students must complete requirements for a B.A. or B.S. degree and four years of medical school. Most Medical Scholars participate in the MSU Honors College and many select the Lyman Briggs College, a residential learning community. The most frequent majors are biology and human physiology. Premedical course requirements include eight semesters each of humanities/social sciences, natural sciences, and physical sciences. Medical Scholars complete a liberal arts component that may include a specialization in Health and Humanities. They participate in a research project under the direction of Michigan State University faculty. They complete a year of volunteer community service and at least a year of medical and clinical experience. Students in this program are not required to take the MCAT for promotion or admission to the medical school. While in medical school, they must pass Steps 1 and 2 of the USMLE in order to graduate. The USMLE Step 1 is administered at the completion of Year 2.

Expenses

	Resident Tuition and Fees	Non-resident Tuition and Fees
Undergraduate	$9,897	$23,699
U.S. Medical School	$28,010	$60,890

Financial Aid

A number of options are available for aid. These include college work-study, Pell grants, student aid grants, Supplemental Educational Opportunities Grants, subsidized and unsubsidized Stafford loans, Parent Loans for Undergraduate Students, and private loans. Applicants can receive more information from Michigan State University, Office of Financial Aid, 252 Student Services; East Lansing, Michigan 48824; (517) 353-5940, 432-1155 (Fax); or E-mail: finaid@msu.edu/med.

Application and Acceptance Policies

Filing of application:
  Earliest date: August 15, 2008
  Latest date: November 15, 2008
Application fee: $60   Fee Waiver Available: Yes
Acceptance notice:
  Earliest date: March 15, 2009
  Latest date: June 15, 2009
Applicant's response to acceptance offer:
  Maximum time: 2 weeks
Deposit to hold place in class: $100; nonrefundable
Starting date: August 2009

Information on 2007–2008 Entering Class

Number of	In-State	Out-of-State	Total
Applicants	174	50	224
Applicants Interviewed	39	9	48
New Entrants	8	4	12
Total number of students enrolled in program: 36			

Wayne State University School of Medicine

Detroit, Michigan

Address Inquiries To:
Nancy Galster, Program Coordinator, Honors Program
Wayne State University School of Medicine
2100 Undergraduate Library
Detroit, Michigan 48202
T (313) 577-8523 **F** (313) 577-6425
honors@wayne.edu
www.honors.wayne.edu/medstart.php

Purpose

The MedStart Program is intended to train medical innovators and creative thinkers. As undergraduates, students are treated as part of the medical community, with an emphasis on mentoring and research.

Requirements for Entrance

Students are selected for this program during their senior year of high school. Applicants must be citizens or permanent residents of the United States. Although there are no specific high school course requirements, applicants are required to take the ACT.

Selection Factors

To be considered for this program, applicants must have a minimum ACT score of 25 and a high school GPA of at least 3.5. Community service, team activities, leadership, extracurricular activities, and experience in health care are among the personal attributes and experiential factors sought in applicants. An interview is also required. Once admitted into the program, students are expected to maintain an overall GPA of 3.3 in the freshman year and a 3.50 GPA in the sciences and overall in subsequent years of their undergraduate studies. For subsequent admission to Wayne State University School of Medicine, students in this program must complete all prerequisite courses, take the MCAT® with a minimum percentile (to be determined), and submit an AMCAS application.

Curriculum

The program, eight years in duration, allows students to obtain a baccalaureate degree from Wayne State University and the M.D. degree from Wayne State University School of Medicine. During the four years of their undergraduate studies,100 percent of their coursework will be related to the bachelor's degree. The coursework in the four years of medical school will be spent in achieving the medical degree. Students must meet university requirements for the Honors Program and degree completion. Throughout the eight-year baccalaureate-medical program, monthly seminars are held which are relevant to medical fields and topics in medicine. Students may apply for a ten-week paid clinical research experience in the summer following the junior undergraduate year.

Expenses

	Resident Tuition and Fees	Non-resident Tuition and Fees
Undergraduate	$8,039	$16,790
U.S. Medical School	$28,668	$56,656

Financial Aid

Information about financial aid can be obtained from the Office of Scholarships and Financial Aid, Welcome Center, P.O. Box 4230, Detroit, MI 48202; by telephone (313) 577-3378; or visit *www.financialaid.wayne.edu.*

Application and Acceptance Policies

Filing of application:
  Earliest date: November 1, 2008
  Latest date: January 15, 2009
Application fee: $30   Fee Waiver Available: No
Acceptance notice:
  Earliest date: April 1, 2009
  Latest date: n/a
Applicant's response to acceptance offer:
  Maximum time: May 1, 2009
Deposit to hold place in class: None
Starting date: September 2009

Information on 2007–2008 Entering Class

Number of	In-State	Out-of-State	Total
Applicants	205	13	218
Applicants Interviewed	36	3	39
New Entrants	12	3	15
Total number of students enrolled in program: 66			

Saint Louis University School of Medicine

St Louis, Missouri

Address Inquiries To:
Alexa Barnoski Serfis, Ph.D., Director, Preprofessional Health Studies
PreProfessional Health Studies, Verhaegen Hall Room 314
3634 Lindell Blvd.
St Louis, Missouri 63108-3414
T (314) 977-2840 **F** (314) 977-3660
prehealth@slu.edu
www.slu.edu/colleges/AS/phs/medScholars.html

Purpose

This combined-degree program awards special recognition to exceptional first-year (freshmen) premedical students. It is intended to enhance the educational experience and reduce the stress associated with premedical-medical education.

Requirements for Entrance

Students apply to this program when they apply to Saint Louis University for undergraduate admission. Both residents and non-residents of Missouri are eligible to apply to the program. Applicants are required to complete the following courses prior to graduation from high school: one year of biology, one year of chemistry, and three years of mathematics. In addition to meeting these requirements, applicants must take either the ACT (minimum score of 30) or SAT (minimum score of 1320).

Selection Factors

Outstanding academic achievement in high school is a favorable factor in qualifying for the combined-degree program at Saint Louis University. Selected applicants usually rank in the top ten percent of their high school class. It is required that all candidates achieve a minimum ACT score of 30 or SAT score of 1320. An interview is not required. Students are required to take the MCAT® in April of the junior year (no minimum score required). MCAT® scores are not a factor for promotion or admission to the medical school phase of the program.

Curriculum

This eight-year program leads to a baccalaureate degree awarded by Saint Louis University and to the M.D. degree granted by the Saint Louis University School of Medicine. Students have much flexibility in choosing a major and are encouraged to study in an area of their choice. During the first four years of the curriculum, students will spend 100 percent of their time in coursework related to the bachelor's degree, which includes 42 to 46 semester hours of natural and physical science, 3 to 4 semester hours of mathematics, and 12 semester hours of humanities. There are strict GPA requirements to remain in the program. The remaining four years focus on achieving the M.D. degree.

Expenses

	Resident Tuition and Fees	Non-resident Tuition and Fees
Undergraduate	$28,480	$28,480
U.S. Medical School	$42,783	$42,783

Financial Aid

Information can be obtained from the Office of Financial Aid/Scholarships, DuBourg Hall 121, Saint Louis University, 221 North Grand Boulevard, St. Louis, MO 63103.

Application and Acceptance Policies

Filing of application:
  Earliest date: October 1, 2008
  Latest date: December 1, 2008
Application fee: None   Fee Waiver Available: n/a
Acceptance notice:
  Earliest date: March 1, 2009
  Latest date: n/a
Applicant's response to acceptance offer:
  Maximum time: May 1, 2009
Deposit to hold place in class: None
Starting date: Mid-August 2009

Information on 2007–2008 Entering Class

Number of	In-State	Out-of-State	Total
Applicants	131	411	542
Applicants Interviewed	0	0	0
New Entrants	30	91	121
Total number of students enrolled in program: 234			

University of Missouri-Kansas City School of Medicine

Kansas City, Missouri

Address Inquiries To:
Mary Anne Morgenegg, Admissions Coordinator
Council on Selection
University of Missouri – Kansas City School of Medicine
2411 Holmes, Kansas City, Missouri 64108-2792
T (816) 235-1870 **F** (816) 235-6579
umkcmedweb@umkc.edu
www.med.umkc.edu

Purpose

This combined baccalaureate — M.D. degree program integrates the humanities, social sciences, basic sciences, and clinical medicine throughout the curriculum so that graduates will have the background for lifelong learning in order to meet the needs of their patients, families, and communities.

Requirements for Entrance

The program is primarily designed for high school graduates who are entering college. Residents and non-residents of Missouri are eligible to apply. An applicant's high school curriculum must include, at a minimum, the following: eight semesters of English; eight semesters of mathematics; six semesters of science, including two semesters of biology and two semesters of chemistry; six semesters of social studies; two semesters of fine arts; and, four semesters of a foreign language. One semester of computer science is recommended, but not required. Applicants must meet a minimum academic screen based on the ACT composite score and rank in high school class.

Selection Factors

Applicants' academic potential is judged by the quality of high school courses, rank in high school class, and scores on the ACT. In the 2007-2008 entering class, the average test score was in the 92nd percentile, and the average rank in class was in the 93rd percentile. Personal qualities include maturity, leadership, stamina, reliability, motivation for medicine, range of interests, interpersonal skills, compassion, and job experience. Qualified applicants are invited for a required interview.

Curriculum

The six-year curriculum leads to a baccalaureate degree granted by the University of Missouri, Kansas City (UMKC) College of Arts and Sciences or the UMKC School of Biological Sciences and the doctor of medicine degree granted by the School of Medicine. Students must complete requirements for the bachelor's degree. Students have a choice of majors, but most select liberal arts or psychology. Course requirements for the bachelor's degree in liberal arts include 21 semester hours of humanities, 21 semester hours of social sciences, and 50 semester hours of natural and physical sciences. The curriculum typically takes six years to complete. During the first two years of the curriculum, students spend 75 percent of their time in coursework related to the bachelor's degree. Conversely, in the last four years, students spend 75 percent of their time in courses, clerkships, and electives related to the M.D. degree. Thus, the study of liberal arts, basic sciences, and clinical medicine is integrated throughout the entire curriculum. Students are assigned a faculty advisor (docent), and younger students are paired with older students. During the last four years of the curriculum, students attend a general medicine outpatient clinic for a half-day each week. Students in this program do not take the MCAT®. They must pass Steps 1 and 2 of the USMLE for graduation. An alternate path is available for extended study.

Expenses

	Resident Tuition and Fees	Non-resident Tuition and Fees
Undergraduate	n/a	n/a
U.S. Medical School	$28,228	$56,161

Financial Aid

Contact the UMKC Financial Aid Office at the Administrative Center, 5115 Oak, Kansas City, Missouri 64110, (816) 235-1154.

Application and Acceptance Policies

Filing of application:
  Earliest date: August 1, 2008
  Latest date: November 15, 2008
Application fee: $35   Fee Waiver Available: No
Acceptance notice:
  Earliest date: April 1, 2009
  Latest date: n/a
Applicant's response to acceptance offer:
  Latest date: May 1, 2009
Deposit to hold place in class: $100; refundable by May 14, 2009
Starting date: August 2009

Information on 2007–2008 Entering Class

Number of	In-State	Out-of-State	Total
Applicants	377	321	698
Applicants Interviewed	165	76	241
New Entrants	124	n/a	124

Total number of students enrolled in program: 624

University of Medicine and Dentistry of New Jersey-New Jersey Medical School

Newark, New Jersey

Address Inquiries To:
Lisa Houston, Office of Admissions
UMDNJ – New Jersey Medical School
185 South Orange Avenue, Room C-653, P.O. Box 1709
Newark, New Jersey 07101-1709
T (973) 972-4631 **F** (973) 973-7986
njmsadmiss@umdnj.edu
http://njms.umdnj.edu/education/admissions/seven_year_ba_md.cfm

Purpose

The New Jersey Medical School (NJMS) currently has baccalaureate/M.D. degree programs in collaboration with eight undergraduate institutions. The goal of these programs is to give highly qualified high school students the best opportunity to broaden their premedical preparation, while establishing their career path.

Requirements for Entrance

Applicants must be high school seniors who are in the top ten percent of their class and have a combined SAT Critical Reading and Math test score of 1400 (out of 1600). Please note that we only consider the Critical Reading and Math sections and not the Essay section of the SAT. Applicants must be either U.S. citizens or permanent residents of the U.S. The most qualified and dedicated applicants will receive the highest consideration.

Selection Factors

Applicants are screened on the basis of academic credentials, letters of recommendation, and an essay. Those meeting the criteria are invited for an interview at the undergraduate school. The undergraduate schools then forward credentials of qualified applicants to NJMS for review and selection for a NJMS interview. The application deadline to the undergraduate institution is January 2, 2009.

Curriculum

The program consists of three years at an undergraduate school followed by a four-year medical program. Although not used to determine admission, the MCAT® must be taken prior to medical school matriculation. Promotion to the medical school is contingent upon achieving grades of "B" or better in all premedical courses and maintaining an overall grade point average of at least 3.5 each semester. The baccalaureate degree is awarded by the undergraduate institution upon completion of the first year of medical school. The M.D. degree is awarded by NJMS upon successful completion of all NJMS degree requirements. Students are required to pass Step 1 of the USMLE for promotion to the third year. Passing Step 2 of the USMLE is required for graduation. Nine programs are currently available: Boston University provides an undergraduate emphasis in liberal arts or humanities. This program is open only to residents of New Jersey. For more information, please contact: admissions@bu.edu. Drew University offers premedical preparation in all sciences and liberal arts subjects. For more information, please contact: ksmall@drew.edu. Montclair State University offers premedical preparation in biology, chemistry, biochemistry, molecular biology, computer science, mathematics, psychology, and anthropology. For more information please contact: shillcockj@mail.montclair.edu. New Jersey Institute of Technology offers undergraduate study in the Honors Premedical Curriculum within the Engineering Science Program. For more information,

please contact: honors@njit.edu. Rutgers University-Newark Campus offers premedical preparation in the sciences. For more information, please contact: nyeste@ugadm.rutgers.edu. Stevens Institute of Technology offers premedical preparation in chemical biology. For more information, please contact: efleming@stevens.edu. The College of New Jersey offers preparation in biology, chemistry, history, philosophy, and psychology. For more information, please contact: shevlin@tcnj.edu. The Richard Stockton College of New Jersey offers preparation in chemistry, biology, physics, and liberal arts. For more information, please contact: admissions@stockton.edu. NJMS also offers Articulated Programs, which allow students in their second year of college to apply to matriculate at NJMS after completion of their third year of college through programs with: St. Peter's College (please contact lsciorra@spc.edu). Rutgers University-Newark (please contact jmaiello@andromeda.rutgers.edu) Rutgers University-New Brunswick (please contact hpo@biology.rutgers.edu).

Expenses

	Resident Tuition and Fees	Non-resident Tuition and Fees
Undergraduate	Varies	Varies
U.S. Medical School	$24,121	$37,188

Financial Aid

Financial aid packages for the undergraduate years are determined by the undergraduate schools.

Application and Acceptance Policies

Filing of application:
  Earliest date: Varies by school
  Latest date: Varies by school
Application fee: Varies   Fee Waiver Available: n/a
Acceptance notice:
  Earliest date: Varies by school
  Latest date: April 14, 2009
Applicant's response to acceptance offer:
  Maximum time: Varies by undergraduate school.
Deposit to hold place in class: No
Starting date: Varies

Information on 2007–2008 Entering Class

Number of	In-State	Out-of-State	Total
Applicants	n/a	n/a	292
Applicants Interviewed	n/a	n/a	165
New Entrants	n/a	n/a	27
Total number of students enrolled in program: 134			

Rutgers University and UMDNJ
Robert Wood Johnson Medical School

Piscataway, New Jersey

Address Inquiries To:
Betsi Platt, Administrative Assistant
Rutgers, The State University of New Jersey
Bachelor/Medical Degree Program Nelson Biological
Laboratory, Room A207, 604 Allison Road
Piscataway, New Jersey 08854-8082
T (732) 445-5667 **F** (732) 445-6341
hpo@biology.rutgers.edu
www.lifesci.rutgers.edu/hpo

Purpose

The program permits the early identification and admission of quality medical students. It also integrates medical studies with liberal arts study.

Requirements for Entrance

This program is open to all students enrolled at Rutgers University who are citizens or permanent residents of the United States. Students are selected for this program at the end of their sophomore year. Students must have a 3.50 overall GPA by the end of their third semester and sustain this GPA through the fourth semester at Rutgers University. Residents and non-residents of New Jersey are considered.

Selection Factors

An applicant's high school and college transcripts and faculty recommendations are taken into account in offering admission. In the 2007-2008 entering class, matriculants had achieved an average GPA of 3.9 at the end of the first two years of college. They had an average score of 620 on the SAT Verbal section and 720 on the Mathematics section. Maturity, motivation, and broad interests are personal characteristics sought in applicants. An interview is required. The MCAT is not used.

Curriculum

This program leads to the baccalaureate degree awarded by Rutgers University and to the M.D. degree granted by the University of Medicine and Dentistry of New Jersey-Robert Wood Johnson Medical School. Students must complete requirements for a baccalaureate degree. The most frequent majors for that degree are biological sciences, followed by biochemistry. The program is eight years in duration. The basic sciences and the liberal arts are studied together during a four-year period. While in medical school, students must take and pass Steps 1 and 2 of the USMLE.

Expenses

	Resident Tuition and Fees	Non-resident Tuition and Fees
Undergraduate	$10,841	$20,010
U.S. Medical School	$24,296	$37,363

Financial Aid

Undergraduates should contact the Office of Financial Aid, Rutgers University, 620 George Street, New Brunswick, New Jersey 08901-1175; call (732) 932-7057; or visit the Web site at *http://studentaid.rutgers.edu*.

Application and Acceptance Policies

Filing of application:
    Earliest date: April 1, 2009
    Latest date: May 26, 2009
Application fee: None   Fee Waiver Available: n/a
Acceptance notice:
    Earliest date: July 1, 2009
    Latest date: n/a
Applicant's response to acceptance offer:
    Maximum time: 2 weeks
Deposit to hold place in class: None
Starting date: August 1, 2009

Information on 2007–2008 Entering Class

Number of	In-State	Out-of-State	Total
Applicants	26	2	28
Applicants Interviewed	24	0	24
New Entrants	10	0	10
Total number of students enrolled in program: 19			

Brooklyn College and
SUNY Downstate Medical Center
Brooklyn, New York

Address Inquiries To:
Dr. Raymond Weston, Director, B.A.-M.D. Program
2231 Boylan Hall, Brooklyn College
2900 Bedford Avenue
Brooklyn, New York 11210
T (718) 951-4706 **F** (718) 677-6185
Rweston@brooklyn.cuny.edu http://bamd.brooklyn.cuny.edu/bamd-main.html

Purpose
The aims of this program are to produce physicians who are humanists and who are concerned with the caring, as well as curing, dimensions of medicine and to offer an economically affordable baccalaureate and medical school education.

Requirements for Entrance
Students are selected in their senior year of high school. Admission is limited to New York area residents. Applicants are recommended to have at least a 90 percent CAA (College Admission Average, academic subjects only) and a combined score of at least 1200 on the Mathematics and Critical Reading sections of the SAT Reasoning Test.

Selection Factors
The academic factors taken into account in offering admission to applicants include the high school GPA, SAT scores, New York State Regents Examination scores, and Advanced Placement courses. In the 2007 entering class, most students had a high school average of at least 95, and the sum of SAT Mathematics and Critical Reading scores averaged 1427. Maturity and motivation are personal characteristics sought among applicants. An interview is required.

Curriculum
This program leads to a baccalaureate degree awarded by Brooklyn College and to the M.D. degree granted by the State University of New York (SUNY) Downstate Medical Center College of Medicine. The baccalaureate program includes eight required semester courses in the natural and physical sciences, seven semester courses in the humanities, and three semester courses in the social sciences. Several of these classes are honors sections specifically for students in the B.A.-M.D. program. The most frequent major is psychology. Students may major in any subject, but nonscience majors are encouraged. Students must maintain a 3.5 overall, and 3.5 science, undergraduate GPA to progress to the medical school. Students must take the MCAT® before the end of their senior year at Brooklyn College, achieving a score of at least 9 on each of the sections in one test administration. The program is eight years in length. Students are required to complete three years of community service, as well as a summer clinical internship. The four-year medical school program focuses on the M.D. degree exclusively. It is worth noting, however, that SUNY Downstate Medical College also has an accredited School of Public Health. During medical school, students must take and pass Step 1 of the USMLE.

Expenses

	Resident Tuition and Fees	Non-resident Tuition and Fees
Undergraduate	n/a	n/a
U.S. Medical School	$19,370	$34,070

Financial Aid
Pell grants, Stafford loans, work-study, Hearst Scholarships for minority female students, and Presidential Scholarships are available. Applicants can receive more information from the Financial Aid Office at Brooklyn College, Sherwood Johnson, Director, (718) 951-5045.

Application and Acceptance Policies
Filing of application:
   Earliest date: September 15, 2008
   Latest date: December 31, 2008
Application fee: None   Fee Waiver Available: No
Acceptance notice:
   Earliest date: April 1, 2009
   Latest date: April 1, 2009
Applicant's response to acceptance offer:
   Maximum time: April 20, 2009
Deposit to hold place in class: None
Starting date: August 29, 2009

Information on 2007–2008 Entering Class

Number of	In-State	Out-of-State	Total
Applicants	276	n/a	276
Applicants Interviewed	90	n/a	90
New Entrants	14	n/a	14
Total number of students enrolled in program: 54			

Hobart and William Smith Colleges/ SUNY Upstate Medical University

Geneva, New York

Address Inquiries To:
Dr. Jim Ryan, Professor of Biology
Elizabeth Blackwell Medical Scholars Program
Hobart & William Smith Colleges
Office of Admissions, 629 South Main Street
Geneva, New York 14456
T (800) 852-2256 **F** (315) 781-3914
admissions@hws.edu; www.hws.edu/admissions/adm_apply/firstyear.asp

Purpose

The Elizabeth Blackwell Medical Scholars program is designed for exceptional high school seniors who wish to attend medical school. Applicants to this program must be from a rural community, a group underrepresented in medicine, or be a first generation college student.

Requirements for Entrance

Students apply to the program in their senior year of high school. They must have a minimum SAT I score of 1250 (Mathematics and Critical Reading only) or a 28 ACT score and a high school grade point average of 90 or higher, as well as have demonstrated a commitment to a career in medicine. Students accepted into this program will complete their undergraduate degree at Hobart and William Smith Colleges and are guaranteed admission to Upstate Medical University's College of Medicine, pending all program standards are met.

Selection Factors

This program is for high school students who are from rural areas, from groups underrepresented in medicine, or who are among the first generation in their families to attend college. The following factors are taken into consideration in assessing applicants for admission into this program: grades, rank in class, SAT (ACT) scores, and extracurricular activities. Selected applicants are invited for a required interview.

Curriculum

This eight-year program leads to a baccalaureate degree awarded by Hobart and William Smith Colleges, and to the medical degree awarded by SUNY Upstate Medical University. Students in this program are not required to take the MCAT® for promotion or for admission to the medical school.

Expenses

	Resident Tuition and Fees	Non-resident Tuition and Fees
Undergraduate	$36,718	$36,718
U.S. Medical School	$19,956	$34,656

Financial Aid

Blackwell Scholars are awarded a full-tuition scholarship to attend Hobart and William Smith Colleges. To retain the full-tuition scholarship, awardees must maintain a GPA of at least 3.0 during each semester while at Hobart and William Smith Colleges. More information about financial aid at Hobart and William Smith Colleges can be found at: *www.hws.edu/admissions/adm_finaid.asp* or *www.upstate.edu/prospective/tuition.php.*

Application and Acceptance Policies

Filing of application:
   Earliest date: August 2008
   Latest date: January 15, 2009
Application fee: $45   Fee Waiver Available: Yes
Acceptance notice:
   Earliest date: 2 weeks after March interview
   Latest date: n/a
Applicant's response to acceptance offer:
   Maximum time: 2 weeks after offer is sent
Deposit to hold place in class: $100;
refundable by May 15 of year of entry
Starting date: The fall following graduation from Hobart and William Smith Colleges

Information on 2007–2008 Entering Class

Number of	In-State	Out-of-State	Total
Applicants	32	5	37
Applicants Interviewed	6	0	6
New Entrants	2	0	2
Total number of students enrolled in program: 9			

Rensselaer Polytechnic Institute and Albany Medical College

Troy, New York

Address Inquiries To:
Dean of Undergraduate Admissions
Rensselaer Polytechnic Institute
110 Eighth Street
Troy, New York 12180-3590
T (518) 276-6216 **F** (518) 276-4072
admissions@rpi.edu
www.rpi.edu/dept/admissions/resources/
PhysicianScientistProgramAccelerated.pdf

Purpose

The Accelerated Physician-Scientist Program offers qualified individuals the opportunity to become physicians who are intensively trained in medical research. This innovative approach provides a well-rounded perspective that prepares future practitioners and physician-scientists to perform with confidence and care in a technologically changing environment.

Requirements for Entrance

Students are selected for this program during the senior year of high school. Residents of New York, as well as non-residents of the state, are eligible to apply. Applicants are expected to have completed the following courses by the time they graduate from high school: four years of English; one year each of biology, chemistry, and physics; and four years of mathematics (through pre-calculus). They must take the SAT Reasoning Test and two SAT Subject Area Tests: one mathematics and one science. In lieu of these tests, American College Testing (ACT) Assessment program scores, including the Writing Test, may be submitted. All tests must be completed by the December testing date prior to the proposed September matriculation.

Selection Factors

Academic factors considered in offering admission to an applicant include the quality and nature of coursework in high school, performance in those courses, rank in high school class, and test scores. The 2007-2008 entering class had an average score of 701 on the SAT Critical Reading, 752 on the SAT Mathematics, and 732 on the SAT Writing. Personal qualities sought in applicants are motivation, maturity, and intellectual capacity necessary to pursue the accelerated course of study. An interview is required.

Curriculum

The program leads to a B.S. degree awarded by Rensselaer Polytechnic Institute and the M.D. degree granted by Albany Medical College (AMC). The curriculum for the B.S. and M.D. degrees usually requires seven years to complete. During the first three years of the program spent at Rensselaer, the curriculum involves 70 percent premedical science courses and 30 percent liberal arts courses. Students take 18 courses in the natural and physical sciences and 8 elective courses in the humanities and social sciences. The cornerstone of the program is a mentored research project. During the sixth semester, students split their time between Rensselaer and AMC and begin research that extends over the third and final year at Rensselaer and into the summer preceding the first year of medical school. The research continues throughout the freshman year at AMC and into the following summer. Training in making oral and written scientific presentations is also included. At the medical college, basic and clinical sciences are integrated into themes (primarily organ systems) stressing normal function in Year 1 and pathological processes in Year 2. There are also five longitudinal themes that are integrated throughout the curriculum: clinical skills, ethical and health systems issues, evidence-based medicine, nutrition and informatics. In every theme, student learning is focused on clinical presentations. Basic science seminars reinforce the importance of the basic sciences in Years 3 and 4. Emphasis is placed on primary care throughout the four years, with an increased emphasis on care in ambulatory settings in the clinical rotations of Year 3. Year 4 emphasizes specialty care in various required rotations. Additional electives are available in Year 4. Students admitted to the program are not required to take the MCAT® for admission to Albany Medical College. Students are expected to pass Steps 1 and 2 of the USMLE while at Albany Medical College.

Expenses

	Resident Tuition and Fees	Non-resident Tuition and Fees
Undergraduate	$34,900	$34,900
U.S. Medical School	$43,008	$43,008

Financial Aid

Sources of financial aid are restricted and include endowed scholarships based on need, merit scholarships, work-study, and student loans through federal and institutional programs. Applicants can receive more information by contacting the Financial Aid Office of Rensselaer Polytechnic Institute at (518) 276-6813 or Albany Medical College at (518) 262-5435.

Application and Acceptance Policies

Filing of application:
    Earliest date: September 1, 2008
    Latest date: November 1, 2008
Application fee: $50   Fee Waiver Available: Yes
Acceptance notice:
    Earliest date: March 2009
    Latest date: Until class is filled
Applicant's response to acceptance offer:
    Latest date: May 1, 2009
Deposit to hold place in class: $300; nonrefundable
Starting date: August 2009

Information on 2007–2008 Entering Class

Number of	In-State	Out-of-State	Total
Applicants	91	197	288
Applicants Interviewed	29	45	74
New Entrants	6	4	10
Total number of students enrolled in program: 102			

St. Bonaventure University/George Washington University School of Medicine Dual Degree (BSMD) Program

St. Bonaventure, New York

Address Inquiries To:
Dr. Michael L. Domboski, Director
Franciscan Health Care Professions Programs
Biology Department
De La Roche Hall
St. Bonaventure, New York 14778
T (716)375-2656
prehealth@sbu.edu
www.sbu.edu

Purpose

A joint program of St. Bonaventure University (SBU) and the George Washington University School of Medicine and Health Sciences in Washington, DC (GW), the eight-year B.S.-M.D. program is designed for the high school senior who exhibits academic excellence, leadership in activities, and community service and healthcare experience, all of which have resulted in a passion for a career as a physician. The goal is to prepare the student with a strong background in the natural sciences in preparation for the rigors of medical school. SBU will soon open its new science facilities that will coordinate with the educational processes at GW, utilizing the state-of-the-art GW hospital. The GW Clinical Skills Center is dedicated to education and research with cutting edge technology. Through the Surgical Simulation and Demonstration Area, medical students gain comprehensive and clinical exposure and feedback and skill improvement to enable them to become technically adept and humane caregivers. More information on the GW MD program can be found at *http://www.gwumc.edu/smhs*.

Requirements for Entrance

Students are selected in their senior year of high school. Applicants must be U.S. or Canadian citizens or Permanent Residents of the U.S. Applicants must complete the SAT (Verbal/Mathematics of at least 1300) or ACT (minimal score of 29), as well as the SAT Subject Test in Biology (preferably M).

Selection Factors

Academic factors considered in selecting applicants include high school grades, class rank, and standardized test scores. In addition, extracurricular and health-related activities, community service, volunteerism, research, medical field exposure, personal essays, and letters of recommendation are reviewed. Rank must be in the top 10% of the class, with a GPA of greater than 90 percent. Qualities demonstrating leadership, interest in the medical field through experiences, and AP and Honors courses are considered. An interview is required at SBU and GW and is by invitation only.

Curriculum

The student's progress is reviewed on a regular basis. Students must maintain a minimum of a "B" in courses required for admission to the medical school and an overall 3.3 average. The recommended major is biology, with interests outside of the sciences being encouraged. Students are not required to take the MCAT®. Students are required to remain active in community service, volunteer programs, and internships established through SBU and research components. Students attend presentations and interact with GW MD students on the Medical Center campus. At the end of four years, the student is granted the B.S. degree from SBU. In the first and second years at

GW, the integration of clinical skills begins, as students spend time with physicians, developing patient interviewing skills, conducting physical examinations, and assisting in diagnosis. The third and fourth years at GW are used to develop clinical expertise in a variety of hospitals in the greater D.C. metropolitan area. Upon completion of all requirements, the M.D. degree is awarded by GW.

Expenses

	Resident Tuition and Fees	Non-resident Tuition and Fees
Undergraduate	$23,605	$23,605
U.S. Medical School	$44,915	$44,915

Financial Aid

For information on financial aid, fees, and expenses, please refer to the Web sites for each institution (*www.sbu.edu* and *www.gwumc.edu*) or contact the Financial Aid Offices.

Application and Acceptance Policies

Filing of application:
  Earliest date: September 1, 2008
  Latest date: December 1, 2008
Application fee: $30   Fee Waiver Available: Yes
Acceptance notice:
  Earliest date: March 15, 2009
  Latest date: n/a
Applicant's response to acceptance offer:
  Latest date: May 1, 2009
Deposit to hold place in class: $500; nonrefundable
Starting date: Late August 2009

Information on 2007–2008 Entering Class

Number of	In-State	Out-of-State	Total
Applicants	n/c	175	175
Applicants Interviewed	n/c	35	35
New Entrants	n/c	12	12
Total number of students enrolled in program: 20			

Siena College and Albany Medical College

Loudonville, New York

Address Inquiries To:
Office of Admissions
Siena College
515 Loudon Road
Loudonville, New York 12211-1462
T (518) 783-2423
admit@siena.edu
www.siena.edu/amc

Purpose

The Science, Humanities and Medicine Program offers an eight-year continuum of education that has a special emphasis on the humanities and on community service to the medically underserved, while providing a sound understanding of both the natural and social sciences.

Requirements for Entrance

Students are selected for this program during the senior year of high school. Both residents and non-residents of New York are eligible to apply. Candidates for admission to the Siena/Albany Medical College program must have completed: four years of laboratory science (including biology, chemistry, and physics) and four years of mathematics (including a minimum of pre-calculus [calculus preferred]). Typically, successful candidates will have enrolled in, or completed, advanced-level courses by the end of their senior year in high school. A well-rounded background and demonstrated leadership experience are also important. Of equal significance is the student's proven concern for others and for the community. Applicants must take either the SAT Reasoning Test or ACT Assessment, including the optional Writing test. Tests must be completed by the November testing date prior to the proposed September matriculation.

Selection Factors

Academic factors considered in offering admission to an applicant include: required and elective courses taken, grades earned, class standing, SAT Reasoning Test or ACT scores, including the Writing test, honors received, letters of recommendation, and unique academic experiences. Of great importance to the admission committee are such factors as extracurricular activities, evidence of intellectual curiosity, and interest in the humanities and in the sciences. Students generally rank among the top ten percent of their high school class. The 2007-2008 entering class had an average score of 688 on the SAT Critical Reading section and 695 on the SAT Mathematics section. An interview is required.

Curriculum

This program offers a coordinated eight-year curriculum of premedical and medical education. The undergraduate phase offers an equal distribution of science and non-science courses. Students graduate in four years with a bachelor of arts degree in biology with a minor in the humanities. The undergraduate phase of the program also includes a required summer of human service in a health-related agency, usually in an urban setting or developing nation. Passage from the undergraduate college to the medical school requires achievement of a 3.40 GPA and a continued interest in the human service dimension of the program. At the medical college, basic and clinical sciences are integrated into themes (primarily organ systems) stressing normal function in Year 1 and pathological processes in Year 2. There are also five longitudinal

themes integrated throughout the curriculum: clinical skills, ethical and health systems issues, evidence-based medicine, nutrition, and informatics. In every theme, student learning is focused on clinical presentations. The summer between the sophomore and junior years is dedicated to medically related volunteer service, usually in a rural or inner city clinic. Seminars reinforce the importance of the basic sciences in Years 3 and 4. Emphasis is placed on primary care throughout the four years, with an increased emphasis on care in ambulatory settings in Year 3 clinical rotations. Year 4 emphasizes specialty care in various required rotations. Additional electives are available in Year 4. Students admitted to the program are not required to take the MCAT® for admission to AMC. Students must pass Steps 1 and 2 of the USMLE while at AMC.

Expenses

	Resident Tuition and Fees	Non-resident Tuition and Fees
Undergraduate	$22,510	$22,510
U.S. Medical School	$43,008	$43,008

Financial Aid

Applicants can receive more information by contacting the Siena College Financial Aid Office at (518) 783-2427 or the Albany Medical College Financial Aid Office at (518) 262-5435.

Application and Acceptance Policies

Filing of application:
   Earliest date: September 1, 2008
   Latest date: December 1, 2008
Application fee: $50   Fee Waiver Available: Yes
Acceptance notice:
   Earliest date: March 2009
   Latest date: Until classes are filled
Applicant's response to acceptance offer:
   Latest date: May 1, 2009
Deposit to hold place in class: $200; nonrefundable
Starting date: September 2009

Information on 2007–2008 Entering Class

Number of	In-State	Out-of-State	Total
Applicants	179	125	304
Applicants Interviewed	25	18	43
New Entrants	12	4	16
Total number of students enrolled in program: 91			

Sophie Davis School of Biomedical Education/City University of New York

New York, New York

Address Inquiries To:
Chris Wanyonyi, Director of Admissions
Sophie Davis School of Biomedical Education
Office of Admission, Harris Hall, 160 Convent Avenue
New York, New York 10031
T (212) 650-7718 **F** (212) 650-7708
cwanyonyi@med.cuny.edu
http://med.cuny.edu

Purpose

The purposes of this combined-degree program are to train primary care physicians who will work in medically underserved urban areas, to increase the number of physicians from groups underrepresented in medicine, to intervene in the disparity of access to high quality pre-college science education, and create a medical school pipeline.

Requirements for Entrance

Students are selected for this program in the senior year of high school. Only residents of New York State are eligible to apply. Applicants are expected to have completed the following courses by the time they graduate from high school: two semesters each of chemistry and biology and six to eight semesters of mathematics. They must take the ACT Assessment and SAT tests.

Selection Factors

Academic factors taken into account in offering admission to an applicant are: high school GPA, SAT I scores, ACT Assessment scores, and scores on the New York State Regents Examinations. In the 2007 entering class, high school grades averaged 94 and the sub-score on the Mathematics ACT Assessment averaged 28. The SAT Mathematics average was 645, and the SAT Verbal average was 627. Personal qualities sought in applicants include interest in people, concern for others, initiative, and leadership. An interview is required.

Curriculum

This seven-year program leads to a baccalaureate degree granted by The City College of New York (CCNY) and to the M.D. degree awarded by one of six participating medical schools (Albany Medical College, Dartmouth Medical College, New York Medical College, New York University, SUNY Brooklyn, or SUNY Stony Brook University). During the first five years of the program, students fulfill all requirements for the B.S. degree and study the preclinical portion of the medical school curriculum. After successfully completing the five-year sequence and passing Step 1 of the USMLE, students transfer to one of the participating medical schools for their final two years of clinical training. Students are expected to pass Step 1 of the USMLE to proceed to Years 3 and 4 of medical school. Additionally, students are expected to pass Step 2 of the USMLE to graduate. Students complete the core liberal arts curriculum of CCNY during the first two years. At this time, they also take courses emphasizing the importance of understanding cultural differences for good medical practice and, through community medicine courses, do field work at various community agencies, including many family practice clinics. The final years of the five-year sequence at CCNY include courses necessary in the first two years of medical school, including basic science courses and several community medicine courses. Students also benefit from counseling and academic support services.

Expenses

	Resident Tuition and Fees	Non-resident Tuition and Fees
Undergraduate	$4129	n/a
U.S. Medical School	Varies	Varies

Financial Aid

Pell grants, New York State Tuition Assistance Program Awards, and NYC Merit Awards are all sources of financial aid. The school generally awards several scholarships to incoming students, including The Lois Pope L.I.F.E. scholarships and the William R. Hearst Endowed Scholarship. Scholarships available later in the program include those from the Alan Seelig Memorial Fund, the Aranow Fund, and the Sophie and Leonard Davis Scholarships. Applicants can contact the Financial Aid Office at (212) 650-5819.

Application and Acceptance Policies

Filing of application:
   Earliest date: September 2008
   Latest date: January 8, 2009
Application fee: None   Fee Waiver Available: n/a
Acceptance notice:
   Earliest date: March 25, 2009
   Latest date: April 1, 2009
Applicant's response to acceptance offer:
   Maximum time: May 1, 2009
Deposit to hold place in class: None
Starting date: Late August 2009

Information on 2007–2008 Entering Class

Number of	In-State	Out-of-State	Total
Applicants	732	n/a	732
Applicants Interviewed	238	n/a	238
New Entrants	83	n/a	83
Total number of students enrolled in program: 358			

Stony Brook University and Stony Brook University School of Medicine

Stony Brook, New York

Address Inquiries To:
Undergraduate Admissions, Honors Programs
118 Administration Building
Stony Brook University
Stony Brook, New York 11794-1901
T (631) 632-6868 **F** (631) 632-9898
www.stonybrook.edu/ugadmissions/programs/honors.shtml
Judith.Burke-Berhannan@stonybrook.edu

Purpose

The Scholars for Medicine Program offers conditional acceptance to the Stony Brook University School of Medicine to a select number of outstanding and highly motivated students through one of three programs: The Honors College, WISE (Women in Science and Engineering) and the Engineering Program of Stony Brook University. In addition to acquiring a solid background in the sciences, accepted students have access to a wide array of liberal arts courses through the university. Students also have access to medical school programs in research and a series of health-related seminars.

Requirements for Entrance

Students are selected for this program only during the senior year of high school. There are no state residency requirements. No specific courses are required. Applicants must take the SAT. For non-U.S. citizens, documentation of permanent residency status will be required of accepted students prior to matriculation.

Selection Factors

To be considered for this program, applicants must have a minimum SAT score of 1350 (Critical Reading and Mathematics) and an unweighted high school GPA of 95. The applicant's high school academic record, standardized test reports, essay, history of interests and activities, and required interview at the School of Medicine are factors taken into account in offering admission.

Curriculum

This eight-year program leads to the baccalaureate and M.D. degrees granted by Stony Brook University. Students are expected to complete the requirements for any of the baccalaureate degrees awarded by the university as well as the requirements for either the Honors College, WISE Program or Engineering Program. Undergraduate work taken must include courses required by the School of Medicine, including one year each of biology, physics, inorganic chemistry, organic chemistry (all with lab), and English. No specific major is required for the premedical undergraduate phase. The program provides a seminar series of health-related lectures given by nationally and internationally recognized individuals in health care delivery. In addition, students have an opportunity to engage in cutting-edge research. Admission to the School of Medicine is contingent upon maintaining a minimum GPA of 3.4. The MCAT® is required, and the student should attain a minimum cumulative MCAT® score of 28, with no less than 8 on any section. USMLE Steps 1 and 2 are required for promotion and graduation from the School of Medicine.

Expenses

	Resident Tuition and Fees	Non-resident Tuition and Fees
Undergraduate	$5,760	$12,020
U.S. Medical School	$19,889	$34,589

Financial Aid

Financial aid available to enrolled students includes federal Perkins loans, Equal Opportunity Program, federal work-study, federal Pell Grants, Federal Supplemental Educational Opportunity, NY State Tuition Assistance Program (TAP), and NY State Aid for Part-time Students. Applicants can receive more information by contacting the Office of Financial Aid and Student Employment at Stony Brook University at (631) 632-6840 or visiting the Web site at *http://naples. cc.sunysb.edu/Prov/financial.nsf.* Please contact the programs directly concerning scholarship opportunities.

Application and Acceptance Policies

Filing of application:
    Earliest date: November 1, 2008
    Latest date: December 31, 2008
Application fee: n/a   Fee Waiver Available: n/a
Acceptance notice:
    Earliest date: March 1, 2009
    Latest date: April 4, 2009
Applicant's response to acceptance offer:
    Maximum time: four weeks
Deposit to hold place in class: $100; refundable
Starting date: September 2009

Information on 2007–2008 Entering Class

Number of	In-State	Out-of-State	Total
Applicants	402	94	496
Applicants Interviewed	23	6	29
New Entrants	6	0	6
Total number of students enrolled in program: 23			

Union College and Albany Medical College

Schenectady, New York

Address Inquiries To:
Associate Dean of Admissions
Union College
Schenectady, New York 12308
T (518) 388-6112 **F** (518) 388-8034
admissions@union.edu
www.medicine.union.edu/LIM

Purpose

The Leadership in Medicine Program is specifically designed for students who want to prepare for the challenge of medical leadership by taking advantage of additional educational opportunities as part of their undergraduate education. In addition to offering the standard coursework required for attaining the degrees of B.S., M.S. or M.B.A., and M.D., the integrated program focuses on three areas essential for future leaders in medicine: the economic and financial problems facing medicine, including health policy and health management; the increasing complexity of biomedical ethics; and, the need to maintain a global perspective.

Requirements for Entrance

Students are selected for this program during the senior year of high school. Residents of New York, as well as non-residents of the state, are eligible to apply. Applicants are expected to have completed a challenging curriculum in high school, which must include biology, chemistry, and physics. They must take either the ACT Assessment or the SAT Reasoning Test and two SAT Subject Area Tests (one mathematics and one science). Tests must be completed by the December testing date prior to the proposed September matriculation.

Selection Factors

Academic factors considered in offering admission to an applicant include the quality and nature of coursework in high school, performance in those courses, rank in high school class, and standardized test scores. In the 2007-2008 entering class, the average score was 685 for SAT Critical Reading, 730 for SAT Mathematics, and 717 for SAT Writing. Personal qualities sought in applicants include motivation, maturity, and personal development. Interviews at Union College and Albany Medical College are required.

Curriculum

This program leads to B.S. and M.S. or M.B.A. degrees awarded by Union College and the M.D. degree granted by Albany Medical College. At Union College, students take 30 courses (15 science and 15 non-science) and complete an interdepartmental major in the humanities or social sciences. A special bioethics program supplemented by a health services practicum, a term abroad, and a program in health care management at the Union College Graduate Management Institute are also integral parts of the educational experience. The curriculum for the B.S., M.S., or M.B.A. and M.D. degrees requires eight years to complete. At the medical college, basic and clinical sciences are integrated into themes (primarily organ systems) stressing normal function in Year 1 and pathological processes in Year 2. Five longitudinal themes are integrated throughout the curriculum: clinical skills, ethical and health systems issues, evidence-based medicine, nutrition, and informatics. In every theme, student learning is focused on clinical presentations. Basic science seminars reinforce the importance of the basic sciences in Years 3 and 4. Emphasis is placed on primary care throughout the four years, with an increased emphasis on care in ambulatory settings in Year 3 clinical rotations. Year 4 emphasizes specialty care in various required rotations. Additional electives are available in Year 4. Students admitted to the program are not required to take the MCAT for admission to Albany Medical College. Students are expected to pass Steps 1 and 2 of the USMLE while at Albany Medical College.

Expenses

	Resident Tuition and Fees	Non-resident Tuition and Fees
Undergraduate	$46,245	$46,245
U.S. Medical School	$43,008	$43,008

Financial Aid

Sources of financial aid include various programs based on need, student loans through federal and state assistance, work-study, and merit scholarships. For more information, contact the Financial Aid Office of Union College (518-388-6123) or at Albany Medical College (518-262-5435).

Application and Acceptance Policies

Filing of application:
  Earliest date: September 1, 2008
  Latest date: December 15, 2008
Application fee: $50   Fee Waiver Available: Yes
Acceptance notice:
  Earliest date: March 2009
  Latest date: Until class is filled
Applicant's response to acceptance offer:
  Latest date: May 1, 2009
Deposit to hold place in class: $500; nonrefundable
Starting date: September 2009

Information on 2007–2008 Entering Class

Number of	In-State	Out-of-State	Total
Applicants	155	198	353
Applicants Interviewed	35	39	74
New Entrants	9	6	15
Total number of students enrolled in program: 113			

University of Rochester
School of Medicine and Dentistry

Rochester, New York

Address Inquiries To:
Rochester Early Medical Scholars Coordinator
University of Rochester
Undergraduate Admissions, Box 270251
Rochester, New York 14627-0251
T (585) 275-3221 or (800) 822-2256 **F** (585) 461-4595
http://enrollment.rochester.edu/admissions/
admit@admissions.rochester.edu

Purpose

The Rochester Early Medical Scholars Program (REMS) provides both acceptance to the University of Rochester College of Arts, Sciences, and Engineering and conditional acceptance to the School of Medicine and Dentistry to a group of exceptionally talented and motivated students. REMS allows undergraduates the utmost flexibility in degree programs, mentoring relationships with medical school staff, and early exposure to the medical school curriculum through a series of lectures and seminars.

Requirements for Entrance

Students are selected for this program during their senior year of high school from a large international pool. A recommended high school curriculum includes at least three years of foreign language and social studies, four years each of English, mathematics, and science. A transcript that includes honors, AP and/or IB courses is strongly recommended. Applicants are expected to take the SAT or ACT Assessment. SAT Subject Tests are highly recommended, especially, Mathematics Level 1C or Mathematics Level 2C, and Biology or Chemistry. Interviews are also encouraged.

Selection Factors

Outstanding achievement in a challenging high school curriculum, character, interests, maturity, experience in health care or research settings, and motivation necessary for a career in medicine are required for consideration for entry into the REMS program. Fifty finalists will be invited to interview for REMS, and those interviews are required. In the 2006-2007 entering class, REMS students had an average SAT Verbal (Critical Reading) score of 720 and an average Mathematics score of 721. In order to take their place in the first-year medical school class, REMS students must carry at least a 3.3 overall GPA and a 3.3 biology-chemistry-physics-math GPA by the end of the freshman year, a 3.4 for the sophomore year, and 3.5 thereafter by the time of undergraduate graduation. REMS students do not have to take the MCAT® examination.

Curriculum

The eight-year program leads to a baccalaureate degree and the M.D. degree, both granted by the University of Rochester. Students must complete the baccalaureate degree. The most popular major is biology, followed by chemistry, and health and society. Microbiology, psychology, neuroscience, and cell and developmental biology are also popular majors among REMS students. Undergraduates are encouraged to pursue a variety of academic disciplines in addition to completing their premedical course requirements. The University of Rochester School of Medicine and Dentistry's Double-Helix Curriculum (DHC) is a major innovation in medical education, focusing on a fully integrated basic and clinical science curriculum across all four years of medical school. Students begin their clinical clerkships in January of

their first year and learn in an environment that fosters critical thinking, problem-solving and active learning in small group Problem-Based Learning sessions, lectures, laboratories and clinical skills workshops. See *www.urmc.rochester.edu/SMD/education/medical/curriculum.cfm* for details. As home of the "biopsychosocial model," Rochester values the art and science of medicine as a continuum, and fosters an educational model that is humanistic and patient-centered. REMS students also may apply for any of our combined degree programs, including the MD/PhD, MD/MPH, MD/MBA, and MD/MS programs. A "Take 5" program, offering a tuition-free, fifth undergraduate year, is available to selected REMS students. Summer research programs and extensive international experiences are available at both the undergraduate and medical school levels.

Expenses

	Resident Tuition and Fees	Non-resident Tuition and Fees
Undergraduate	$35,190	$35,190
U.S. Medical School	$38,657	$38,657

Financial Aid

University of Rochester scholarships and loans, plus governmental loans, are available. For more information, write the Financial Aid Office, University of Rochester, Box 270261, Rochester, New York 14627-0261, or phone (585) 275-3226 or (800) 881-8234. Website: *http://enrollment.rochester.edu/financial*.

Application and Acceptance Policies

Filing of application:
    Earliest date: May 15, 2008
    Latest date: December 1, 2008
Application fee: $50   Fee Waiver Available: Yes
Acceptance notice:
    Earliest date: March 1, 2009
    Latest date: April 1, 2009
Applicant's response to acceptance offer:
    Maximum time: May 1, 2009
Deposit to hold place in class: $500; nonrefundable
Starting date: Early September 2009

Information on 2007–2008 Entering Class

Number of	In-State	Out-of-State	Total
Applicants	241	517	758
Applicants Interviewed	13	37	50
New Entrants	3	7	10
Total number of students enrolled in program: 66			

Case Western Reserve University School of Medicine

Cleveland, Ohio

Address Inquiries To:
Christine DeSalvo Miller, Senior Assistant Director
Office of Undergraduate Admission
103 Tomlinson Hall, Case Western Reserve University
10900 Euclid Avenue; Cleveland, Ohio 44106-7055
T (216) 368-4450 **F** (216) 368-5111
admission@case.edu
http://admission.case.edu

Purpose

This program is intended to provide college students with a greater sense of freedom and choice in the pursuit of a premedical baccalaureate degree.

Requirements for Entrance

Students are selected for this program during the senior year of high school. Both residents and nonresidents of Ohio are considered for admission. Applicants are expected to have completed the following courses by the time they graduate from high school: one year each of biology, chemistry, and physics and four years of mathematics. They must take either the ACT Assessment with the Writing Test or the SAT Reasoning Test.

Selection Factors

The applicant's high school academic record, standardized test reports, history of interests and activities, and a required interview are factors taken into account in offering admission. Evidence of strong interpersonal and leadership skills is also sought. While there is no minimum requirement for standardized test scores, in the Fall 2007 entering class, SAT scores ranged from approximately 630-760 on the Critical Reading section and 690-800 on the Math section. The average composite ACT score ranged from 31 to 34.

Curriculum

This eight-year program leads to the baccalaureate and M.D. degrees granted by Case Western Reserve University. Students are expected to complete the requirements for any of the baccalaureate degrees awarded by the colleges of the university. They are expected to satisfy all requirements of, and earn a baccalaureate prior to matriculating in, the School of Medicine. The work taken for the baccalaureate must include the studies specifically required of applicants by the School of Medicine, including one year of biology, two years of chemistry (including organic chemistry), one year of physics, and first-year (freshman) seminar. No specific major concentration is required for the premedical undergraduate phase. To date, the majors most commonly taken have been biology and biochemistry. Psychology, anthropology, chemistry, and biomedical engineering are also popular majors. The first four years of the program are devoted to study for the baccalaureate and the last four years to the curriculum in medicine. Students in the medical phase are required to pass Step 1 of the USMLE for promotion within the program and to pass Step 2 of the USMLE in order to graduate.

Expenses

	Resident Tuition and Fees	Non-resident Tuition and Fees
Undergraduate	$ 33,908	$ 33,908
U.S. Medical School	$ 41,966	$ 41,966

Financial Aid

Sources of aid for the undergraduate phase include merit and need-based aid, college work-study, and university grants and scholarships. For information about aid, contact the Office of University Financial Aid at (216) 368-4530.

Additional Information

The PPSP is intended to include a four-year undergraduate program of study and is not designed as an accelerated program. Matriculation at the School of Medicine will occur no earlier than four years after matriculation into the bachelors degree program at Case Western Reserve University. Students who complete degree requirements in fewer than four years are required to pursue other significant experiences intended to enhance their professional and/or personal development during the terms following the receipt of their bachelors degree and until study at the School of Medicine begins. Examples of this experience may include, but are not limited to: research, study abroad, community service and/or additional undergraduate or graduate coursework. This interim experience must be approved in advance by the Case Western Reserve University School of Medicine Admissions Committee.

Application and Acceptance Policies

Filing of application:
    Earliest date: n/a
    Latest date: December 1, 2008
Application fee: $35   Fee Waiver Available: Yes
Acceptance notice:
    Earliest date: n/a
    Latest date: Mid April 2009
Applicant's response to acceptance offer:
    Maximum date: May 1, 2009
Deposit to hold place in class: $500; nonrefundable
Starting date: August 24, 2009

Information on 2007–2008 Entering Class

Number of	In-State	Out-of-State	Total
Applicants	194	512	706
Applicants Interviewed	6	41	47
New Entrants	1	6	7
Total number of students enrolled in program: 45-50			

Northeastern Ohio Universities College of Medicine

Rootstown, Ohio

Address Inquiries To:
Jill M. Byers, M.Ed., Director of Admissions
Northeastern Ohio Universities College of Medicine
4209 State Route 44, P.O. Box 95
Rootstown, Ohio 44272-0095
T (330) 325-6270 **F** (330) 325-8372
admission@neoucom.edu
www.neoucom.edu/audience/applicants

Purpose

The mission of the Northeastern Ohio Universities College of Medicine (NEOUCOM) is to graduate qualified physicians oriented to the practice of medicine at the community level, with an emphasis on primary care (family medicine, internal medicine, pediatrics, and obstetrics-gynecology). NEOUCOM strives to improve the quality of health care in northeast Ohio. All graduates, regardless of specialty, are provided with a strong background in community and public health.

Requirements for Entrance

Students are selected for the BS/MD program during the senior year of high school. Both residents and non-residents of Ohio are eligible to apply; strong preference is given to in-state applicants. During high school, applicants are expected to pursue a solid college preparatory curriculum, including 4 years of math and 4 years of science. They must take either the ACT or the SAT, and be citizens or permanent residents of the U.S. at the time of application.

Selection Factors

Academic factors considered in admission include standardized test scores, high school GPA and science GPA, extracurricular involvement, medical exposure, coursework, state of legal residence, and interview outcome. In 2007-2008, the mean high school GPA of matriculants was 3.83. The average ACT test score was 29; average SAT was 1299 (verbal and math only). Career maturity and emotional maturity are among the personal qualities weighed by the admissions committee. An interview is required and is offered by invitation only.

Curriculum

Students accepted into the combined BS/MD program pursue the baccalaureate degree by majoring in integrated life sciences at The University of Akron, Kent State University, and Youngstown State University. The accelerated BS/MD program may be completed in six or seven years. The M.D. degree is granted by NEOUCOM. The integrated curriculum is offered in five steps during the four years of medical study. The four-year Doctoring course provides an understanding of professionalism, doctor-patient relationships, and community health. Step 1 courses: Human Development and Structure emphasizes an integrated approach to the study of human anatomy; Molecules to Cells addresses biochemistry, molecular pathology, and genetics. Step 2 courses: Physiological Basis of Medicine emphasizes the physiological concepts in the practice of internal medicine; Brain, Mind, and Behavior includes anatomy, physiology, and chemistry of the nervous system. Step 3: instruction centers on systems and application in clinical settings. Step 4: the core clerkships – family medicine, internal medicine, obstetrics/gynecology, pediatrics, psychiatry, and surgery, an exploratory elective, and an Intersession. Step 5: features electives and a Capstone module focusing on professionalism and humanities and social science disciplines. The Epilogue course provides vital skills needed as interns and residents. Student must pass USMLE Step 1 for promotion, take the USMLE Step 2 Clinical Skills (CS), and pass the Step 2 Clinical Knowledge (CK) to graduate.

Expenses

	Resident Tuition and Fees	Non-resident Tuition and Fees
Undergraduate	Varies	Varies
U.S. Medical School	$28,881	$55,686

Financial Aid

Campus-based financial aid (grants and low interest loans) is awarded on the basis of demonstrated need. Students apply for this aid by completing the FAFSA, the NEOUCOM financial aid application and submitting copies of federal tax returns. To be eligible for campus-based aid, students must submit parent information on the FAFSA and provide federal tax returns. A limited number of grants are available for students who demonstrate need, students who are from a disadvantaged background, and students from groups underrepresented in medicine. Federal educational loans are a major part of the financial aid package. About 80 percent of enrolled students receive some form of financial aid. Financial need is not a factor in admission considerations.

Additional Information

The first class of PharmD students enrolled in the Fall of 2007 and study in an interdisciplinary curriculum with NEOUCOM medical students.

Application and Acceptance Policies

Filing of application:
  Earliest date: August 10, 2008
  Latest date: December 15, 2008
Application fee: $100   Fee Waiver Available: Yes
Acceptance notice:
  Earliest date: December 10, 2008
  Latest date: March 24, 2009
Applicant's response to acceptance offer:
  Latest date: May 1, 2009
Deposit to hold place in class: None
Starting date: June 2009

Information on 2007–2008 Entering Class

Number of	In-State	Out-of-State	Total
Applicants	299	198	497
Applicants Interviewed	208	18	226
New Entrants	105	4	109
Total number of students enrolled in program: 231			

Ohio State University College of Medicine
Early Admission Pathway

Columbus, Ohio

Address Inquiries To:
Lorna Kenyon, Director, Admissions Office
College of Medicine
The Ohio State University
155D Meiling Hall, 370 West 9th Avenue
Columbus, Ohio 43210
T (614) 292-7137 **F** (614) 247-7959
medicine@osu.edu
http://medicine.osu.edu/futurestudents/
medicaleducation/admissions/eap/index.cfm

Purpose

The Early Admission Pathway provides conditional acceptance into the College of Medicine after four years of undergraduate study for a select group of National Merit Finalists, National Achievement Finalists, and National Hispanic Finalists, entering The Ohio State University in Autumn Quarter.

Requirements for Entrance

Students are selected in their senior year of high school. Both residents and nonresidents of Ohio are eligible to apply to the program. In addition to meeting the requirements for freshman admission, applicants are required to submit the results of the ACT Assessment or the SAT I.

Selection Factors

The following factors are taken into consideration in assessing applicants for admission: approval for university honors affiliation; selection as a National Merit, National Achievement, or National Hispanic finalist; grade-point average; high school activities; leadership roles; and extracurricular activities. In the 2007-2008 entering class, the average high school GPA was 4.33 (range of 3.97 to 4.77). The average SAT score was 1527 and the average ACT Assessment score was 33.5.

Curriculum

This eight-year program leads to a baccalaureate degree awarded by The Ohio State University and to the M.D. degree granted by The Ohio State University College of Medicine. The most frequent major for the baccalaureate degree is biology. Regardless of major, students must complete the basic course entry requirements including one year of biological sciences, one year of general chemistry, one year of organic chemistry with lab, and one year of physics with lab. Eligible EAP participants have the option to petition for entry into the College of Medicine after three years of undergraduate course work. Students whose third year option petitions are approved will be able to earn a Bachelor of Science degree in absentia after successful completion of the first year of medical school. Students with a cumulative grade point average of 3.50 or above in all coursework and in all courses in biological sciences, chemistry, physical sciences, and mathematics (BCPM) by the end of Spring Quarter of the second year are not required to take the MCAT®. The MCAT® is required for students with a CPHR and/or BCPM between a 3.00 and 3.49 at the end of Spring Quarter of the second year. They must: complete the baccalaureate degree prior to entry into medical school; register for and take the MCAT® by August 1 of the third year; present a composite MCAT® score of at least 29, with no MCAT® section score less than 8 in order to continue in good standing; work with the EAP academic advisor to determine appropriate course work for the remainder of their undergraduate program; and regain undergraduate college Honors affiliation by the end of Spring Quarter of the third year and maintain

it through the completion of their undergraduate degree program. Students who lose and do not regain college Honors affiliation are no longer eligible for conditional acceptance into the College of Medicine. Students are held to the College of Medicine's standards of honor and professional conduct.

Expenses

	Resident Tuition and Fees	Non-resident Tuition and Fees
Undergraduate	$8,667	$20,562
U.S. Medical School	$27,234	$41,652

Financial Aid

The sources of financial aid available are National Merit/Achievement/Hispanic Distinguished Scholarships valued at the current undergraduate resident tuition rate, plus other merit and need-based aid. For more information, contact the Office of Student Financial Aid, The Ohio State University, 517 Lincoln Tower, 1800 Cannon Drive, Columbus, Ohio 43210; (614) 292-0300.

Additional Information

EAP students have unique opportunities to meet and talk with distinguished College of Medicine faculty and students engaged in clinical and graduate education and research. Faculty and staff meet with EAP students to discuss opportunities for practical experience and the development of desired non-cognitive traits. Mentoring and medical career counseling are also provided. EAP students are encouraged to participate in enrichment activities sponsored by Alpha Epsilon Delta (AED), the pre-medical honor society at The Ohio State University.

Application and Acceptance Policies

Filing of application:
    Earliest date: October 1, 2008
    Latest date: March 1, 2009
Application fee: $40   Fee Waiver Available: No
Acceptance notice:
    Earliest date: April 15, 2009
    Latest date: April 15, 2009
Applicant's response to acceptance offer:
    Latest date: May 1, 2009
Deposit to hold place in class: None
Starting date: September 2009

Information on 2007–2008 Entering Class

Number of	In-State	Out-of-State	Total
Applicants	38	18	56
Applicants Interviewed	27	12	39
New Entrants	13	4	17
Total number of students enrolled in program: 49			

University of Cincinnati College of Medicine

Cincinnati, Ohio

Address Inquiries To:
Nikki Bibler, M.Ed., Assistant Director of Dual Admissions
University of Cincinnati College of Medicine
P.O. Box 670668
Cincinnati, Ohio 45267-0668
T (513) 558-5581 **F** (513) 558-6259
DualAdmissionsProgram@uc.edu
www.med.uc.edu/HS2MD

Purpose

The University of Cincinnati College of Medicine's Dual Admissions Program accepts high school seniors into one of three undergraduate Ohio colleges and into the College of Medicine. The College of Medicine has established a partnership with the following Ohio institutions: the University of Dayton, Miami University, and the University of Cincinnati undergraduate campus. Each undergraduate program will invite selected students already accepted into the university to apply for this program. Once accepted to this special program, students will receive an outstanding education while preparing for medical school and developing the qualities and characteristics to become excellent physicians.

Requirements for Entrance

Students are selected in their senior year of high school. Both residents and non-residents of Ohio are eligible to apply. Priority will be given to Ohio residents. Each university determines its own academic requirements, but the ACT and/or SAT are required.

Selection Factors

In making admissions decisions, the College of Medicine in conjunction with each undergraduate institution considers an applicant's academic record, standardized test performance, examples of leadership, interpersonal skills, and interest in and motivation for medicine. Mature and independent-thinking students who have good decision-making and coping skills are very desirable. Students are strongly encouraged to investigate each of the College of Medicine's undergraduate partners before applying. Only students who have applied to and been accepted by one of the affiliated undergraduate schools will be seriously considered for the Dual Admissions Program. Thus, students are encouraged to apply first to the undergraduate institution and then complete the Dual Admissions Application.

Curriculum

The course of study consists of four years at the undergraduate school, followed by four years in the College of Medicine. University of Cincinnati College of Medicine dual-admissions students are required to satisfactorily fulfill graduation requirements at their undergraduate institution. Students are strongly urged to complete a baccalaureate degree. Students must earn a 3.4 cumulative GPA and a 3.45 BCPM GPA by the beginning of the senior undergraduate year. At this time, they must also earn a composite score of 27 on the MCAT®, with no less than a 9 in Biological Sciences and no less than an 8 in Verbal Reasoning or Physical Sciences. The student must pass Steps 1 and 2 of the USMLE in order to graduate from the College of Medicine. The USMLE Step 1 is administered at the completion of Year 2.

Expenses

	Resident Tuition and Fees	Non-resident Tuition and Fees
Undergraduate	Varies	Varies
U.S. Medical School	$26,910	$46,077

Financial Aid

More information about undergraduate financial aid can be obtained from the undergraduate partners' Office of Admissions.

Application and Acceptance Policies

Filing of application:
   Earliest date: Varies
   Latest date: n/a
Application fee: None   Fee Waiver Available: n/a
Acceptance notice:
   Earliest date: April 1, 2009
   Latest date: Varies for students on the alternate list.
Applicant's response to acceptance offer:
   Latest date: May 1, 2009
Deposit to hold place in class: None
Starting date: Varies by undergraduate program

Information on 2007–2008 Entering Class

Number of	In-State	Out-of-State	Total
Applicants	101	66	167
Applicants Interviewed	33	22	55
New Entrants	19	8	27
Total number of students enrolled in program: 132			

Drexel University and
Drexel University College of Medicine

Philadelphia, Pennsylvania

Address Inquiries To:
Catherine Campbell-Perna, Associate Director
Drexel University
3141 Chestnut Street
Philadelphia, Pennsylvania 19104
T (215) 895-2400 **F** (215) 895-5939
enroll@drexel.edu .
www.drexel.edu/em/undergrad/default.aspx

Purpose

This combined-degree program provides outstanding high school seniors, who are highly motivated toward the medical profession, an opportunity to combine a strong liberal arts undergraduate program in a highly technological environment with a medical education in seven years.

Requirements for Entrance

Students are selected for this program during their senior year of high school. Both residents and non-residents of Pennsylvania are eligible to apply. Prior to graduating from high school, applicants are required to complete one semester of biology, one semester of chemistry, one semester of physics, four years of English, and four years of mathematics. They must take either the SAT or the ACT Assessment.

Selection Factors

The academic factors taken into consideration for admission into the combined-degree program include SAT/ACT scores, high school GPA, and AP and honors courses. The average high school GPA for the 2007-2008 entering class was 4.0, with a mean score of 1470 on the SAT and a 31 Composite on the ACT. Medically related volunteer activities, leadership qualities, and community service are among the personal attributes sought in applicants. An interview at the college of medicine is also required. Once admitted into the program, students are expected to maintain an overall GPA of 3.45 in undergraduate studies; achieve a total minimum MCAT® score of 30, or a score of 9 or better on each section of the MCAT®; apply through AMCAS in the second year; complete all prerequisite courses; and receive no grade less than a C in any course. The MCAT® is a factor in admittance and promotion to the medical school phase of the program.

Curriculum

This seven-year program leads to a baccalaureate degree awarded by Drexel University and to the M.D. degree granted by the Drexel University College of Medicine. The most frequent major is biology, followed by chemistry and biomedical engineering. Students may also choose from a variety of humanities majors. During the first three years of the undergraduate phase, students spend 100 percent of their time in coursework related to the bachelor's degree, which includes 3 semester hours of natural and physical science.

Expenses

	Resident Tuition and Fees	Non-resident Tuition and Fees
Undergraduate	$45,110	$45,110
U.S. Medical School	$42,130	$42,130

Financial Aid

All Students are automatically considered for academic scholarships when applying for admission. Students should complete the FAFSA form by March 1st to be considered for need based financial aid.

Application and Acceptance Policies

Filing of application:
   Earliest date: Rolling
   Latest date: December 1, 2008
Application fee: $75   Fee Waiver Available: Yes
Acceptance notice:
   Earliest date: March 15, 2009
   Latest date: April 15, 2009
Applicant's response to acceptance offer:
   Latest date: May 1, 2009
Deposit to hold place in class: $700; nonrefundable
Starting date: September 22, 2009

Information on 2007–2008 Entering Class

Number of	In-State	Out-of-State	Total
Applicants	88	507	595
Applicants Interviewed	18	162	180
New Entrants	6	25	31

Total number of students enrolled in program: 124

Lehigh University and Drexel University College of Medicine

Bethlehem, Pennsylvania

Address Inquiries To:
Majed Dergham, Assistant Director
Office of Admissions
Lehigh University
27 Memorial Drive West
Bethlehem, Pennsylvania 18105
T (610) 758-3100 **F** (610) 758-4361
www3.lehigh.edu/arts-sciences/cashealth.asp#bacmd

Purpose

This program is designed to give gifted high school students, who are highly motivated for a career in medicine, the opportunity to combine a liberal arts program with a medical education. The baccalaureate degree is awarded after Year 4 (the first year of medical school).

Requirements for Entrance

Applicants are expected to take the SAT Reasoning Test. SAT Subject tests are highly recommended in Mathematics Level 1 or Mathematics Level 2 and Chemistry.

Selection Factors

Generally, a combined SAT score of 1360 (or minimum 31 ACT), a class rank in the top ten percent of the high school class, and a strong motivation for science are necessary for entrance into this program. Most recent matriculants had a high school GPA of 3.7, an SAT Verbal score of 720, and an SAT Mathematics score of 780. Maturity, stability, scholarship, flexibility, independence, and service to others are personal characteristics sought among applicants. An interview is required. Once admitted to the program, students are expected to maintain an overall grade point average of 3.45 or better and a science and math GPA of 3.25 or better with no grade less than a "C" in any courses. Candidates are required to take the MCAT®. All program requirements must be completed at Lehigh University. Scores of either 9 or better on each section of the MCAT® or a combined score of 30 or better (with no score less than a 7 on any section) is required.

Curriculum

This program, seven years in duration, allows students to obtain a bachelor's degree from Lehigh University and the M.D. degree from Drexel University College of Medicine. Students have the flexibility to pursue additional coursework or study abroad during the undergraduate portion of the program. Students are not required to complete work for a bachelor's degree. However, specific course requirements for the degree include two semesters of English, three semesters of mathematics, eight semesters of natural and physical sciences, three semesters each of humanities and social sciences, a freshman seminar, a writing intensive, and four elective courses. All students must pass USMLE Steps 1 and 2 in order to graduate from the medical school.

Expenses

	Resident Tuition and Fees	Non-resident Tuition and Fees
Undergraduate	$44,950	$44,950
U.S. Medical School	$42,130	$42,130

Financial Aid

Institutional scholarships and loans are available, as well as federal loan programs and armed services scholarships. More financial aid information can be obtained from the Financial Aid Office, Lehigh University, 218 W. Packer Avenue, Bethlehem, Pennsylvania 18015.

Application and Acceptance Policies

Filing of application:
   Earliest date: September 1, 2008
   Latest date: November 15, 2008
Application fee: $65   Fee Waiver Available: No
Acceptance notice:
   Earliest date: April 1, 2009
   Latest date: n/a
Applicant's response to acceptance offer:
   Latest date: May 1, 2009
Deposit to hold place in class: $500; nonrefundable
Starting date: August 2009

Information on 2007–2008 Entering Class

Number of	In-State	Out-of-State	Total
Applicants	26	224	250
Applicants Interviewed	12	76	88
New Entrants	1	6	7
Total number of students enrolled in program: 30			

Pennsylvania State University and Jefferson Medical College

University Park, Pennsylvania

Address Inquiries To:
Director of Admissions
Undergraduate Admissions Office
Pennsylvania State University, 201 Shields Building
University Park, Pennsylvania 16802
T (814) 865-5471 **F** (814) 863-7590
www.science.psu.edu/premedmed

Purpose

This accelerated, B.S.-M.D. premedical-medical program, which began in 1963 and has graduated over 900 students, is a cooperative effort between Pennsylvania State University, University Park, and Jefferson Medical College of Thomas Jefferson University in Philadelphia. Accepted students can select either a six- or seven-year schedule, which gives them either two years (with summers) or three years at Penn State before proceeding to four years at Jefferson Medical College. All students selecting the six-year option must begin their studies at the University Park campus in the summer session. Students selecting the seven-year option begin their studies at the University Park campus in the fall semester.

Requirements for Entrance

Students are selected for this program only during the senior year of high school. Both residents and non-residents of Pennsylvania are considered for admission, but preference is given to qualified applicants from Pennsylvania. Applicants are expected to have completed the following courses by the time they graduate from high school: four units of English, 1 ½ units of algebra, one unit of plane geometry, one-half unit of trigonometry, three units of science, and five units of social studies, humanities, and/or the arts.

Selection Factors

To be considered for this program, applicants must be in the top ten percent of their high school class and offer a minimum combined score of 1450 on the critical reading and mathematics section of the SAT Reasoning Test or ACT score of 32. In the 2007-2008 entering class, the average combined score on the SAT was 1530. Motivation, compassion, integrity, dedication, and performance in nonacademic areas are among the personal characteristics sought in applicants. An interview is required. Special attention is given to the student's progress during each semester while at Pennsylvania State University. Students must take a full course load and maintain a minimum GPA of 3.5 in both science and non-science courses. For subsequent admission to Jefferson Medical College, students in this combined-degree program must achieve an average score of 9 or better on each section of the MCAT prior to matriculation in medical school.

Curriculum

This six-year program leads to a baccalaureate degree granted by Pennsylvania State University and to the M.D. degree awarded by Jefferson Medical College. Students begin this program in June immediately after high school graduation. They spend two full years on the Pennsylvania State, University Park, campus; they then proceed to Jefferson Medical College for the regular four-year curriculum. The B.S. degree from Pennsylvania State University is awarded after successful completion of the second year at Jefferson Medical College, and the M.D. degree is awarded after successful completion of the senior year at Jefferson Medical College. Students in the seven-year schedule spend three years at Pennsylvania State, but do not attend summer sessions. Their B.S. degree is awarded after Year 1 at Jefferson Medical College.

Expenses

	Resident Tuition and Fees	Non-resident Tuition and Fees
Undergraduate	$12,284	$23,152
U.S. Medical School	$41,101	$41,101

Financial Aid

At Penn State, scholarships, loans, and grants are the sources of financial assistance available. For more information, write the Office of Student Financial Aid, Pennsylvania State University, University Park, Pennsylvania 16802; or call (814) 865-5471. At Jefferson Medical College, financial aid application materials are mailed in January of the year of medical school matriculation. Students are encouraged to contact the University Office of Student Financial Aid to discuss all financial aid matters.

Application and Acceptance Policies

Filing of application:
    Earliest date: August 1, 2008
    Latest date: November 30, 2008
Application fee: $50   Fee Waiver Available: Yes
Acceptance notice:
    Earliest date: March 15, 2009
    Latest date: March 30, 2009
Applicant's response to acceptance offer:
    Latest date: May 1, 2009
Deposit to hold place in class: $300; nonrefundable
Starting date: Late June 2009

Information on 2007–2008 Entering Class

Number of	In-State	Out-of-State	Total
Applicants	68	321	389
Applicants Interviewed	13	76	89
New Entrants	7	17	24
Total number of students enrolled in program: 46			

Temple University
School of Medicine

Philadelphia, Pennsylvania

Address Inquiries To:
Office of Admissions
Temple University School of Medicine
3400 North Broad Street, SFC Suite 305
Philadelphia, Pennsylvania 19140
T (215) 707-3656 **F** (215) 707-6932
medadmissions@temple.edu
www.temple.edu/medicine

Purpose

The Medical Scholars Program, in conjunction with four undergraduate institutions in Pennsylvania, provides an opportunity for outstanding high school seniors to gain a provisional acceptance to Temple University School of Medicine at the same time that they are accepted into their undergraduate school. The Temple MedScholars Program offers two options: 1) The eight year program offers an enriched undergraduate experience in which the student receives the bachelor's degree after four years and the medical degree after the four years of medical school; 2) The seven year program offers an accelerated experience in which the student begins medical school after three years of undergraduate work, and the medical school degree is received after four years of medical school.

Requirements for Entrance

Students are selected for this program during their senior year of high school. Both residents and non-residents of Pennsylvania are eligible to apply. Although there are no specific high school course requirements, applicants are expected to have a substantial background in science and mathematics. AP coursework is viewed favorably, and students are required to take the SAT or ACT.

Selection Factors

In conjunction with the School of Medicine, each undergraduate institution considers an applicant's GPA, standardized test performance, extracurricular activities (including leadership roles), and interpersonal skills in making admission decisions. Substantial maturity and strong motivation are among the important personal qualities considered by the Admission Committee. The minimum SAT score required is 1350 in the combined Critical Reading and Mathematics sections, with no individual section less than 600 (including the new Writing section). The minimum composite ACT score required is 31. Students are expected to be in the top one to five percent of their high school graduating class. Academic ability should be demonstrated across a wide variety of courses, including AP science coursework. Selected applicants are required to interview with a representative of the undergraduate institution and a medical school admissions officer. Contact the partnering undergraduate institutions directly to obtain additional information about the Medical Scholars Program: Duquesne University, (412) 396-6335; Temple University, (215) 204-2513; Washington and Jefferson College, tklitz@washjeff.edu; and Widener University, (610) 499-4004.

Curriculum

Students in this combined-degree program will complete their baccalaureate degree at one of the four partnering universities listed above. Students offered the accelerated, 7-year experience, will begin medical school after three years of undergraduate work. The medical degree is granted by Temple University School of Medicine. Students

may choose to be a science major, but are free to explore all available options as long as they complete the premedical science requirements. Matriculation to Temple University School of Medicine is conditional upon successful completion of all GPA and MCAT® requirements as outlined by each institution's agreement. Educational innovations are unique at each undergraduate institution. All students are re-quired to complete the M.D. program without deviation from the standard curriculum, including passing USMLE Steps 1, 2CS (Clinical Skills), and 2CK (Clinical Knowledge).

Expenses

	Resident Tuition and Fees	Non-resident Tuition and Fees
Undergraduate	Varies	Varies
U.S. Medical School	$38,502	$47,004

Financial Aid

For information about financial aid, contact the Financial Aid Office of the specific partnering undergraduate institution listed above. Financial aid available to medical students includes grants, scholarships, and student loans. For additional information, visit the School of Medicine Web site at: *www.temple.edu/sfs/med/*.

Application and Acceptance Policies

Filing of application:
  Earliest date: Varies by program
  Latest date: n/a
Application fee: $0   Fee Waiver Available: n/a
Acceptance notice:
  Earliest date: March 15, 2009
  Latest date: April 15, 2009
Applicant's response to acceptance offer:
  Latest date: May 1, 2009
Deposit to hold place in class: None
Starting date: Varies by undergraduate program

Information on 2007–2008 Entering Class

Number of	In-State	Out-of-State	Total
Applicants	n/a	n/a	89
Applicants Interviewed	n/a	n/a	31
New Entrants	n/a	n/a	5
Total number of students enrolled in program: 22			

Villanova University and Drexel University College of Medicine

Villanova, Pennsylvania

Address Inquiries To:
John D. Friede, Ph.D., Health Professions Advisor
Office of University Admission
Villanova University
800 Lancaster Avenue, Villanova, Pennsylvania 19085
T (610) 519-4833 **F** (610) 519-8042
admission@villanova.edu
www.healthprofessions.villanova.edu/

Purpose

This combined-degree program provides outstanding high school seniors, who are highly motivated toward the medical profession, an opportunity to combine a strong liberal arts undergraduate program with a medical education in seven years.

Requirements for Entrance

Students are selected for this program in their senior year of high school. Both residents and non-residents of Pennsylvania are eligible to apply to the program. Applicants are required to complete the following courses prior to graduation from high school: one year of biology, one year of chemistry, one year of physics, four years of English, and four years of mathematics. In addition to meeting these academic requirements, applicants are also required to submit the results of the ACT or SAT. An ACT score of at least 31 or an SAT score of 1360 (Critical Reading and Mathematics, from one test date) is required. SAT II scores are recommended.

Selection Factors

The academic factors taken into consideration for admission into the combined-degree program include: SAT scores, high school GPA and class rank, and letters of recommendation. The average high school GPA for the 2007-2008 entering class was 3.80, unweighted. Extracurricular activities and community service are among the personal attributes sought in applicants. An interview is required. Once admitted into the program, students are expected to maintain an overall GPA of 3.45, and they are required to achieve scores of either a 9 or better on each section of the MCAT® or a combined score of 30 or better (with no score less than 8 on any section of the MCAT®).

Curriculum

Students are required to complete a baccalaureate degree within the first year of medical school. The most frequent major is biology, followed by comprehensive science. This seven-year program leads to a baccalaureate degree awarded by Villanova University and to the M.D. degree granted by the Drexel University College of Medicine. During the undergraduate phase of the program, students will spend 100 percent of their time in coursework related to the bachelor's degree, which includes 41 semester hours of natural and physical science, six semester hours of mathematics, and 51 semester hours of humanities.

Expenses

	Resident Tuition and Fees	Non-resident Tuition and Fees
Undergraduate	$34,320	$34,320
U.S. Medical School	$42,130	$42,130

Financial Aid

For information on financial aid, visit *www.finaid.villanova.edu* and *http://webcampus.drexelmed.edu/admissions/financialaid.asp*.

Application and Acceptance Policies

Filing of application:
    Earliest date: September 1, 2008
    Latest date: November 1, 2008
Application fee: $75   Fee Waiver Available: Yes
Acceptance notice:
    Earliest date: March 15, 2009
    Latest date: March 30, 2009
Applicant's response to acceptance offer:
    Maximum time: May 1, 2009
Deposit to hold place in class: $700; nonrefundable
Starting date: August 24, 2009

Information on 2007–2008 Entering Class

Number of	In-State	Out-of-State	Total
Applicants	26	152	178
Applicants Interviewed	6	53	59
New Entrants	2	6	8
Total number of students enrolled in program: 36			

Wilkes University/SUNY-Upstate Medical University

Wilkes-Barre, Pennsylvania

Address Inquiries To:
Eileen Sharp
Coordinator for Health Science Professional Programs
Wilkes University, 84 West South Street
Wilkes-Barre, Pennsylvania 18766
T (570) 408-7812 **F** (570) 408-7812
eileen.sharp@wilkes.edu
www.wilkes.edu/pages/102.asp

Purpose

This cooperative program is motivated by the need for physicians interested in serving in rural and semi-rural health care delivery systems, as well as the interest of each institution in attracting students of superior ability and accomplishment.

Requirements for Entrance

Students apply to the program in their senior year of high school; applicants must be New York State residents. Candidates for admission must have completed the following high school course requirements: four years each of mathematics, English, science, and social science. Applicants must take the ACT or SAT examination.

Selection Factors

The following factors are taken into consideration in assessing the applicant for admission: grades, rank in class, SAT (ACT) scores, and extracurricular activities. Selected applicants are invited for a required interview.

Curriculum

This eight-year program leads to a baccalaureate degree awarded by Wilkes University and to the M.D. degree granted by SUNY Upstate Medical University. The most frequent major for the baccalaureate degree is biology, followed by chemistry and biochemistry. The M.D. portion of the curriculum does not depart from the "traditional" design. Upstate accepts a special responsibility to provide physicians to New York's underserved rural communities. A student from a rural setting or one subsequently trained there is more likely to practice there. This B.S.-M.D. program attracts students from rural areas who are not likely to otherwise find their way to medical school. Upstate also provides many special opportunities during medical school (Rural Medicine Program, Clinical Campus) to train students in community and rural settings. Students in this program are not required to take the MCAT® for promotion or admission to the medical school. The USMLE Step 1 is required; it must be passed, prior to beginning clinical rotations, to be promoted and in order to graduate. Students must record a score on USMLE Step 2, but passing USMLE Step 2 is not a factor in graduation from the medical school.

Expenses

	Resident Tuition and Fees	Non-resident Tuition and Fees
Undergraduate	$24,080	$34,180
U.S. Medical School	$19,956	$34,656

Financial Aid

The sources of available financial aid are grants, scholarships, and student loans. For more information about financial aid, visit *www.wilkes.edu/pages/132.asp*, or contact the Financial Aid Office at SUNY Upstate Medical University by emailing FinAid@upstate.edu.

Application and Acceptance Policies

Filing of application:
   Earliest date: August 1, 2008
   Latest date: November 10, 2008
Application fee: $35   Fee Waiver Available: Yes
Acceptance notice:
   Earliest date: Within 2 weeks of medical school interview
   Latest date: 2 weeks after medical school interview
Applicant's response to acceptance offer:
   Maximum time: 2 weeks from receiving acceptance offer
Deposit to hold place in class: $100; refundable
Starting date: The Fall following graduation from Wilkes

Information on 2007–2008 Entering Class

Number of	In-State	Out-of-State	Total
Applicants	6	n/a	6
Applicants Interviewed	5	n/a	5
New Entrants	2	n/a	2
Total number of students enrolled in program: 10			

The Warren Alpert Medical School of Brown University

Providence, Rhode Island

Address Inquiries To:
College Admission Office
Brown University, Box 1876
Providence, Rhode Island 02912
T (401) 863-2378
Admissions@Brown.edu
http://bms.brown.edu/plme

Purpose

The Program in Liberal Medical Education (PLME) seeks to graduate physicians who are broadly and liberally educated, and who will view medicine as a socially responsible human service profession. Designed as an eight-year program, the PLME combines liberal arts and professional education. Great flexibility is built into the program. Working with PLME advising deans who are physicians, each student develops an individualized educational plan consistent with his or her particular interests. The PLME is a primary route of admission to The Warren Alpert Medical School.

Requirements for Entrance

Students are selected for the PLME in the senior year of high school. The Brown Admission Office recommends that applicants should have completed the following courses: four years of English, with significant emphasis on writing; three years of college preparatory mathematics; three years of a foreign language; two years of laboratory science above the freshman level; two years of history, including American history; at least one year of coursework in the arts; and at least one year of elective academic subjects. Prospective science or engineering majors should have taken physics, chemistry, and advanced mathematics. Familiarity with computers is recommended for all applicants. Applicants must take the SAT Reasoning Test and any two SAT Subject Tests (except for the SAT II Writing Test), or the ACT. (PLME applicants are encouraged to include a science SAT Subject Test).

Selection Factors

Students are selected on the basis of scholastic accomplishment and promise, intellectual curiosity, emotional maturity, character, motivation, sensitivity, caring, and particularly the degree to which they seem adapted to the special features of the program. In the 2007-2008 entering class, students, on average, were in the top one percent of their high school class and had achieved, on average, a score of 718 Verbal, 737 Mathematics, and 720 Writing on the SAT Reasoning Test. An interview is not required.

Curriculum

The PLME leads to a baccalaureate degree and to the M.D. degree granted by The Warren Alpert Medical School. Students must complete a baccalaureate degree in the field of their choice. Each student's educational plan is highly individualized. The PLME combines the flexibility and opportunities of an undergraduate education at Brown University with effective preparation for participation in an equally innovative medical education program.

Expenses

	Resident Tuition and Fees	Non-resident Tuition and Fees
Undergraduate	$41,542	$36,174
U.S. Medical School	$38,672	$38,672

Financial Aid

For undergraduates in the first four years of the PLME, financial aid is awarded by the Financial Aid Office at Brown University as a package. Students are awarded monies via scholarships, work-study, and loans. During the last four years of the PLME, financial aid is administered by the The Warren Alpert Medical School Office of Admissions and Financial Aid. Both loans and scholarships are available, although loans are the most common form of assistance.

Application and Acceptance Policies

Filing of application:
    Earliest date: November 1, 2008
    Latest date: January 1, 2009
Application fee: $70   Fee Waiver Available: No
Acceptance notice:
    Earliest date: December 15, 2008
    Latest date: Early April 2009
Applicant's response to acceptance offer:
    Latest date: May 1, 2009
Deposit to hold place in class: None
Starting date: September 2009

Information on 2007–2008 Entering Class

Number of	In-State	Out-of-State	Total
Applicants	48	1926	1974
Applicants Interviewed	n/a	n/a	n/a
New Entrants	1	49	50
Total number of students enrolled in program: 223			

102   *Medical School Admission Requirements, 2009–2010*

Fisk University and Meharry Medical College

Nashville, Tennessee

Address Inquiries To:
Keith Chandler, Dean of Admissions
Fisk University, Office of Admissions
1000 17th Avenue North
Nashville, Tennessee 37208
T (615) 329-8666 **F** (615) 329-8774 fax
lcampbell@fisk.edu
www.mmc.edu

Purpose

The Joint Program in Biomedical Sciences is designed to address America's need to train bright young students from groups under-represented in medicine who are dedicated to finding solutions to biomedical problems through research and who will be future health care providers.

Requirements for Entrance

Students are selected at the end of their first semester of undergraduate coursework on the Fisk University campus. There are no specific high school course requirements. Applicants must have competitive scores on the ACT and/or the SAT. They must have completed at least one semester at Fisk University. Participates must submit an application with a personal statement which details their career goals and letters of recommendation from two college science or mathematics professors to the Office of Admissions.

Selection Factors

The courses taken and grades earned at Fisk University, plus ACT and/or SAT scores, are considerations for eligibility for this program. Applicants must rank in the top 20 percent of their high school class. Students must take the MCAT® prior to admission into the clinical phase of the program, and a satisfactory score is required for medical school admission.

Curriculum

The Joint Program in Biomedical Sciences, seven years in duration, allows students to obtain a baccalaureate degree from Fisk University and the M.D. degree from Meharry Medical College. Course requirements for the baccalaureate degree include 8 semesters of natural and physical sciences and 12 semesters each in the humanities and social sciences. Students are required to spend two summers in a structured academic enrichment program. Students must take Steps 1 and 2 of the USMLE during the medical school portion of the program. Passing these examinations is a factor in promotion and graduation from medical school. The most frequent major chosen by students is biology, followed by chemistry.

Expenses

	Resident Tuition and Fees	Non-resident Tuition and Fees
Undergraduate	n/a	n/a
U.S. Medical School	$32,336	$32,336

Financial Aid

Applicants and students can apply for institutional scholarships and grants, U.S. Department of Education Title IV Federal Student Aid (work-study and loans), U.S. Department of Health and Human Services Student Aid Programs (loans and scholarships), Southern Regional Education Board Grants, and Tennessee Black Conditional Grants. Meharry's Office of Student Financial Aid makes available most federal, regional, and state financial aid applications and brochures on numerous funding opportunities. See Meharry's Web site at *www.mmc.edu* (index to financial assistance) for sources of financial aid. The Meharry Medical College Library and local public libraries have publications on most sources of student financial aid. Applicants can receive more information from the Office of Student Financial Aid, Meharry Medical College, 1005 D.B. Todd Boulevard, Nashville, Tennessee 37208.

Additional Information

All students who are selected for the program are on scholarship while enrolled at Fisk University.

Application and Acceptance Policies

Filing of application:
    Earliest date: September 15, 2008
    Latest date: February 1, 2009
Application fee: None   Fee Waiver Available: n/a
Acceptance notice:
    Earliest date: February 15, 2009
    Latest date: March 15, 2009
Applicant's response to acceptance offer:
    Maximum time: 1 week
Deposit to hold place in class: None
Starting date: Retroactive second semester, undergraduate year one

Information on 2007–2008 Entering Class

Number of	In-State	Out-of-State	Total
Applicants	4	6	10
Applicants Interviewed	2	7	9
New Entrants	2	2	4
Total number of students enrolled in program: 8			

Rice University and Baylor College of Medicine

Houston, Texas

Address Inquiries To:
Rice University, Office of Admissions—MS-17
P.O. Box 1892
Houston, Texas 77251-1892
T (713) 348-RICE **F** (713) 348-5323
admi@rice.edu
www.bcm.edu/medschool/baccmd.htm

Purpose

To promote the education of future physicians who are scientifically competent, compassionate, and socially conscious in order to apply insight from the extensive study of liberal arts and other disciplines to the study of modern medical science.

Requirements for Entrance

Students are selected for this program during their senior year of high school. Both residents and non-residents of Texas are considered for admission. Applicants are expected to have had a varied and rigorous high school program with high academic achievement. They must take the SAT Reasoning Test or ACT, plus three SAT Subject tests.

Selection Factors

The high school academic record, standardized test scores, course selection, extracurricular activities, and letters of recommendation are some of the factors taken into account in offering admission to an applicant. In the 2007-2008 entering class, students averaged above the top five percent in their high school class.

Curriculum

This is not an accelerated program; all students are expected to complete four years of undergraduate education and four years of medical school. Students earn a baccalaureate degree from Rice University, and are awarded the M.D. degree by Baylor College of Medicine. Minimum course requirements for this program include at least two semesters each in the humanities and social sciences and eight semesters in the natural and physical sciences. The medical part of the curriculum devotes approximately 1 1/2 years to the basic sciences with clinical experience, and 2 1/2 years to clinical science with some basic science coursework. The MCAT® is not required for promotion or admission to the medical school. Students are required to take Step 1 of the USMLE in their second or third years. They are also required to take Step 2 of the USMLE, but passing these examinations is not a graduation requirement.

Expenses

	Resident Tuition and Fees	Non-resident Tuition and Fees
Undergraduate	$28,900	$28,900
U.S. Medical School	$12,782	$25,882

Financial Aid

Sources of financial aid include academic, athletic, and need-based scholarships. Applicants can receive more information from the Rice University Admission Office, M.S. 17, 6100 Main Street, Houston, Texas 77035.

Application and Acceptance Policies

Filing of application:
    Earliest date: November 1, 2008
    Latest date: December 1, 2008
Application fee: $60   Fee Waiver Available: Yes
Acceptance notice:
    Earliest date: n/a
    Latest date: Mid-April 2009
Applicant's response to acceptance offer:
    Latest date: May 1, 2009
Deposit to hold place in class: $300; refundable by August 2009
Starting date: August 2009

Information on 2007–2008 Entering Class

Number of	In-State	Out-of-State	Total
Applicants	264	204	468
Applicants Interviewed	21	22	43
New Entrants	8	4	12
Total number of students enrolled in program: 56			

University of Texas
School of Medicine at San Antonio

San Antonio, Texas

Address Inquiries To:
David Jones, Ph.D.
University of Texas School of Medicine at San Antonio
7703 Floyd Curl Drive, Mail Code 7790
San Antonio, Texas 78229
T (210) 567-6080 **F** (210) 567-6962
medadmissions@uthscsa.edu
http://som.uthscsa.edu/admissions/index.asp

Purpose

In partnership with the University of Texas-Pan American this program offers the opportunity to achieve conditional acceptance to medical school as early as the junior year at UT Pan American. Participants are provided mentorship by medical school faculty and educational enrichment and clinical experiences in the Summer Premedical Academy. Frequent meetings with medical school faculty during the year provide encouragement and support toward matriculation into medical school. Acceptance to medical school after three years of undergraduate school is possible.

Requirements for Entrance

Students are selected during their senior year of high school. The program is only open to residents of Texas who are citizens or permanent residents of the United States. While there are no specific high school course requirements, applicants are required to take the SAT and/or ACT. Concurrent or AP coursework is encouraged.

Selection Factors

Academic factors considered in selecting applicants include SAT/ACT scores and strength in science and mathematics coursework. In addition to an impressive academic portfolio, applicants must also demonstrate a sincere interest in medicine and present letters of recommendation from their high school counselors or teachers. An interview by members of the School of Medicine Admissions Committee is also required. Students are admitted to medical school based on a sliding scale of the ratio of MCAT® scores and science GPA, an interview with the Admissions Committee as well as a demonstrated continued commitment to study medicine.

Curriculum

Students must maintain a science and overall GPA of 3.25 or better and are required to complete all medical school prerequisite coursework with a grade of "C" or better. Students also participate in six-week Summer Premedical Academies for which scholarships are provided. During each summer starting after their freshman year, students come to the medical school campus in San Antonio to participate in academic enrichment programs, as well as twice weekly clinical preceptorships. The program is designed to increase the students' academic preparedness for the next year's coursework and for an MCAT® review course during the summer between their junior and senior years. The clinical preceptorships are designed to increase students' awareness of issues in clinical medicine and to develop a clear understanding of performance expectations while in medical school.

Expenses

	Resident Tuition and Fees	Non-resident Tuition and Fees
Undergraduate	$5,016	$12,716
U.S. Medical School	$12,443	$27,627

Financial Aid

Financial aid is not available from the medical school during the undergraduate years.

Additional Information

The Summer Premedical Academy provides academic enrichment coursework along with clinical preceptorships. Students are also mentored by faculty and students of the medical school. There is also an opportunity to meet with education specialists to assist with learning disabilities.

Application and Acceptance Policies

Filing of application:
Earliest date: December 1, 2008
Latest date: February 1, 2009
Application fee: None   Fee Waiver Available: n/a
Acceptance notice:
Earliest date: April 1, 2009
Latest date: April 30, 2009
Applicant's response to acceptance offer:
Maximum time: 2 weeks
Deposit to hold place in class: None
Starting date: April 30, 2009

Information on 2007–2008 Entering Class

Number of	In-State	Out-of-State	Total
Applicants	15	n/a	15
Applicants Interviewed	11	n/a	11
New Entrants	5	n/a	5
Total number of students enrolled in program: 13			

Eastern Virginia Medical School
Norfolk, Virginia

Address Inquiries To:
Office of Admissions, Mail Code 3
Eastern Virginia Medical School
700 W. Olney Road
Norfolk, Virginia 23507-1607
T (757) 446-5812 **F** (757) 446-5896
www.evms.edu/admissions

Purpose

Eastern Virginia Medical School currently has combined programs with nine colleges and universities: Christopher Newport University, The College of William and Mary, Old Dominion University, Hampton University, Norfolk State University, Hampden-Sydney College, Saint Paul's College, Virginia State University and Virginia Wesleyan College. The purpose of these programs is to enlist outstanding undergraduate students into a track that provides great freedom and choice in the pursuit of a baccalaureate degree.

Requirements for Entrance

Students are selected during their sophomore year of college. Both residents and non-residents of Virginia are eligible to apply. There are no specific high school course requirements, but students must take the SAT.

Selection Factors

Applicants will be evaluated on their academic performance during their freshman year of college and the first semester of their sophomore year of college. An emphasis is placed on leadership skills and extra-curricular activities, including medical volunteering. Selected applicants are invited for an interview.

Curriculum

The eight-year curriculum leads to a baccalaureate degree awarded by Christopher Newport University, The College of William and Mary, Old Dominion University, Hampton University, Norfolk State University, Hampden-Sydney College, Saint Paul's College, Virginia State University or Virginia Wesleyan College. The M.D. degree is granted by Eastern Virginia Medical School. Course requirements for the baccalaureate degree vary at each undergraduate institution. The most frequent major is biology. This early assurance program does, however, permit the student the opportunity for academic diversity. Students selected who have combined SAT scores greater than 1250 will not be required to take the MCAT. Step 1 of the USMLE must be taken at the completion of the second year of medical school. Students must pass Steps 1 and 2 of the USMLE to complete the program and receive the M.D. degree.

Expenses

	Resident Tuition and Fees	Non-resident Tuition and Fees
Undergraduate	Varies	Varies
U.S. Medical School	$24,204	$43,400

Financial Aid

For information about financial aid during the undergraduate phase, contact the Office of Financial Aid at the undergraduate institutions identified. Eight programs are available: Christopher Newport University, Harold Grau, Ph.D., (757) 594-7946; The College of William and Mary, Beverley T. Sher, Ph.D., (757) 221-2852; Old Dominion University, Terri Mathews, (757) 683-5201; Hampton University, Karen Davis, Ph.D., (757) 727-5150; Norfolk State University, Alicia McClain, Ph.D., (757) 823-8991; Hampden-Sydney College, H.O. Thurman, Ph.D., (434) 223-6177; Saint Paul's College, Sunday Adesuyi, Ph.D., (434) 848-6484; Virginia State University, Pamela Leigh-Mack, Ph.D., (804) 524-5285 and Virginia Wesleyan College, Victor Townsend, Ph.D., (757) 455-3392. For information about financial aid during the medical school phase, contact the Office of Financial Aid at Eastern Virginia Medical School at (757) 446-5804.

Application and Acceptance Policies

Filing of application:
    Earliest date: Varies
    Latest date: Varies
Application fee: $35   Fee Waiver Available: No
Acceptance notice:
    Earliest date: Varies
    Latest date: Varies
Applicant's response to acceptance offer:
    Maximum time: Varies
Deposit to hold place in class: $100; refundable by May 15, 2009
Starting date: August 2009

Information on 2007–2008 Entering Class

Number of	In-State	Out-of-State	Total
Applicants	18	20	38
Applicants Interviewed	15	13	28
New Entrants	5	0	5

Total number of students enrolled in program: n/a

Virginia Commonwealth University School of Medicine

Richmond, Virginia

Address Inquiries To:
Dr. Anne L. Chandler
Senior Associate Dean
The Honors College
Virginia Commonwealth University
P.O. Box 843010 Richmond, Virginia 23284-3010
T (804) 828-1803 **F** (804) 827-1669
achandle@vcu.edu
www.pubinfo.vcu.edu/honorscollege/prostudents/guaranteedadm-reqmed.asp

Purpose

The Guaranteed Admission Program of the Honors College offers academically capable, highly focused students an opportunity to pursue diverse, intellectually challenging programs of study. Students who successfully complete the Guaranteed Admission Program will be able to enter the medical school without the pressure of further competition. Close contact with the School of Medicine throughout the undergraduate program aids students in testing their career choice and in preparing for a lifelong commitment to learning in the profession.

Requirements for Entrance

Students are selected during their senior year of high school, and there are no state residency restrictions. All candidates are considered. The specific minimum high school course requirements are as follows: four units in English; three units in mathematics (to include algebra I and either geometry or algebra II); two units in science (at least one a laboratory science); and three units of history or social sciences or government. Students are strongly encouraged to present at least two units in a modern or ancient foreign language. Also required are standardized test scores on the ACT or SAT. The ACT composite score must be at or above 29. The combined SAT1 score must be at or above 1910 and obtained in a single sitting, with no score below 530. An unweighted GPA of 3.5 (on a 4.0 scale) is also required.

Selection Factors

Academic factors considered in offering admission to an applicant include: GPA, letters of reference, test scores, well-rounded and rigorous academic preparation, health care-related experience, and written and oral communication skills. The average GPA for students accepted for the 2007-2008 class was 3.85 (unweighted scale of 4.0), and the average SAT score was 2140. Selected applicants are invited for a required interview.

Curriculum

Students are required to complete a baccalaureate degree. The most frequent major is biology; the next most frequent major is chemistry. The undergraduate degree is awarded by Virginia Commonwealth University. Specific course requirements vary, depending upon the major. During the medical school program, there is a longitudinal clinical experience (Foundations of Clinical Medicine) in a community primary care practice that meets weekly for both of the first two years. Students are required to take Step 1 of the USMLE at the end of their second year. They must also take USMLE Step 2, but passing these examinations is not a promotion or graduation requirement. The doctor of medicine degree is also awarded by Virginia Commonwealth University. It takes eight years to fulfill the requirements for both degrees.

Expenses

	Resident Tuition and Fees	Non-resident Tuition and Fees
Undergraduate	$6,196	$18,740
U.S. Medical School	$27,188	$40,858

Financial Aid

There are several sources of financial aid available to students, including scholarships, loans, grants, and work-study. For more information, contact the Virginia Commonwealth University Financial Aid Office, P.O. Box 842506, Richmond, Virginia 23284-2506; (804) VCU-MONY.

Application and Acceptance Policies

Filing of application:
    Earliest date: September 1, 2008
    Latest date: November 15, 2008
Application fee: $30   Fee Waiver Available: Yes
Acceptance notice:
    Earliest date: April 1, 2009
    Latest date: n/a
Applicant's response to acceptance offer:
    Maximum time: May 1, 2009
Deposit to hold place in class: $100; nonrefundable
Starting date: August 2009

Information on 2007–2008 Entering Class

Number of	In-State	Out-of-State	Total
Applicants	48	113	161
Applicants Interviewed	23	37	60
New Entrants	9	9	18
Total number of students enrolled in program: 74			

Chapter 11

Training of Physician-Scientists: MD-PhD Programs

While most medical students will ultimately decide to devote their medical careers primarily to the care and treatment of patients, a smaller group of students at each medical school will choose a different career goal — to become physician-scientists (also referred to as research physicians and physician-investigators). Physician-scientists use their research and clinical skills both in the laboratory and at the bedside. They engage in basic and clinical research to advance medical knowledge, promote health, solve medical problems, combat disease, and improve medical care. They also attempt to bridge the gap between laboratory research and clinical medicine. They frequently are faculty members at academic medical centers and other research institutions; they also play important roles in biotechnology and at pharmaceutical companies.

Educational and Training

One path to a career as a physician-scientist is enrollment in a combined M.D.-Ph.D. program, which can be completed in a total of seven to eight years. An M.D.-Ph.D. student can complete the Ph.D. degree in any of a variety of scientific specializations. These include, among others, biochemistry, cell biology, biomedical engineering, developmental biology, genetics, immunology, pathology, pharmacology, physiology, biophysics, bioinformatics, epidemiology, molecular biology, and neuroscience. However, not every medical school offers each area of specialization. Another route to a career in medical research is through completion of a Ph.D. degree or a research fellowship following receipt of the M.D. degree, either in lieu of, or after completing, a residency in a medical specialty. However, the opportunity to complete both the M.D. and Ph.D. degrees in a shorter time period than it would take to complete both degree programs separately, as well as to integrate research and clinical training, makes the combined M.D.-Ph.D. program

option very attractive to many students who have decided to pursue careers in medical research.

Such programs are frequently referred to as "joint," "combined," or "dual" degree programs. It is important to note that some schools also use these terms to describe other educational programs linked to the M.D. degree, including Master's degree programs (e.g., in education, public health, and business administration) and other doctoral-level programs (e.g., in law, computer science, and history).

A complete and up-to-date listing of M.D.-Ph.D. programs at AAMC-member medical schools, including information about available areas of specialization, can be found on the AAMC Curriculum Directory Web site at *http://services.aamc.org/currdir*. Currently, almost all U.S. and Canadian medical schools have organized M.D.-Ph.D. programs in one or more areas of specialization. Some are relatively small in size (1-2 new students per year, with a dozen total students), while others are much larger (up to 20 new students annually, with a total enrollment of 150 students).

The typical M.D.-Ph.D. program is completed in a total of seven to nine years and includes:

- completion of the first two years of combined medical and graduate school coursework, followed by

- three to five years of doctoral research, including the completion of a thesis project, and

- a return to medical school for core clinical training and electives during the final years of the medical curriculum.

At some schools, integrated approaches to graduate and medical education and training have been introduced. These integrated approaches involve, among other educational innovations, interdisciplinary and interdepartmental seminars, summer research opportunities, and planned interactions with teams composed of both basic science and clinical investigators. While the national trend involves a move toward more integrated curricula, there is currently an array of curricular choices available.

Following receipt of both the M.D. and Ph.D. degrees, the physician-scientist then completes residency training in a medical specialty, often followed by additional clinical and/or research training in a fellowship program, prior to initiating a career as a physician-scientist.

Application and Admission

The application and admission processes for M.D.-Ph.D. programs are handled in different ways at different schools. While, at some schools, persons interested in enrolling in M.D.-Ph.D. programs apply to these programs through the usual M.D.-only application process, there are school-specific variations in application processes (see Chapter 4). Potential applicants should investigate the M.D.-Ph.D. program Web site at each medical school of interest and review written materials prior to initiating an application. At some schools, the application may first be referred to the admission committee for the regular M.D. program for assessment and an acceptance decision, with the applications of accepted students only then referred for further consideration by Ph.D. program faculty members. Other schools have a separate admission committee for M.D.-Ph.D. applicants. Still other schools will consider applicants for the Ph.D. component of the program only after their successful completion of the first year (or more) of medical school.

Because M.D.-Ph.D. applicants plan to become both physicians and scientists, admission committee members will review primary and secondary application materials for evidence of the usual attributes and experiences that are important for admission of students to the M.D.-only program (see Chapter 7). In addition, however, they will seek, in the applicants' statement of career goals as a physician-scientist and in letters of recommendation from faculty members or investigators with whom the applicant has previously worked, additional evidence of:

- relevant and substantive research interest and experience during or after college

- an appreciation for, and understanding of, the work of physician-scientists, and

- intellectual drive, research ability and acumen, and perseverance

Some medical schools will accept applications from M.D.-Ph.D. candidates only for both degree programs, and will not consider applicants whose credentials are not deemed sufficient for enrollment in either program. Other schools permit the applicant who is not accepted to the M.D.-Ph.D. combined degree program to continue to pursue admission to the M.D.-only curriculum. Since school policies differ on this matter, applicants are well advised to clarify relevant application and admission policies at each school of interest prior to making application. Generally, an applicant who is not accepted to a combined M.D.-Ph.D. program, but who wishes to attend the M.D.-only educational program should express his or her continuing interest in the M.D.-only program to admission office staff.

Financing M.D.-Ph.D. Program Enrollment

The sources of funding for M.D.-Ph.D. students vary from school to school. During the award period from July 1, 2007 through June 30, 2008, the National Institute of General Medical Sciences at the National Institutes of Health (NIH) reports support of 40 M.D.-Ph.D. programs at 45 degree-granting institutions. These programs are identified as Medical Scientist Training Programs (MSTP). A full listing is available at *www.nigms.nih.gov/ Training/InstPredoc/PredocInst-MSTP.htm*. (There are approximately 75 other medical schools that do not have NIGMS MSTP training grants, but that also offer opportunities for M.D.-Ph.D. studies.)

At schools with MSTP programs, M.D.-Ph.D. students might receive full support for both the M.D. and Ph.D. components of their education, including a stipend, tuition waivers, and health insurance. At schools without MSTP funding, varying degrees of partial support may also be available from other federal and non-federal sources, although frequently in lesser amounts and sometimes only for the Ph.D. components of the combined degree program. Applicants should ascertain from program officials the nature of financial support for students enrolled in the M.D.-Ph.D. program prior to making application and accepting a position in the program.

Careers in Academic Medicine and Medical Research

Approximately four-fifths of M.D.-Ph.D. graduates are employed as faculty members in academic medical centers, where they engage in substantial research activity and compete for available research funding from governmental, foundation, and other sources. One quarter of these graduates are faculty members in basic science departments, while three quarters are faculty members in clinical departments. They are also employed in clinical medicine, government, and industry, as well as in basic, clinical, translational, and epidemiological research.

Some physician-scientists at academic medical centers devote the majority of their time to their research, with the remainder of their time devoted to the other responsibilities of academic faculty members: clinical service, teaching, committee membership, and administration.

Advantages and Disadvantages of M.D.-Ph.D. Programs

One advantage of enrollment in a combined M.D.-Ph.D. program is the time saved from completing both programs separately. M.D.-Ph.D. students also enjoy opportunities for excellent research experiences and superb faculty mentoring frequently unavailable to the M.D.-only student. By virtue of these experiences, M.D.-Ph.D. students can significantly enhance their understanding and mastery of the basic science background underlying patients' clinical problems, and use that information to generate improvements in clinical diagnosis and treatment. Funding for the M.D.-Ph.D. student from MSTP and other federal and non-federal sources can result in a reduction in educational debt at program completion, although the long duration of training means that this type of support should not be a determinant of the decision to pursue admission to a combined M.D.-Ph.D program.

One disadvantage of M.D.-Ph.D. training is the length of enrollment in the program, followed by required residency and fellowship training, resulting in delayed onset of a professional career relative to M.D.-only peers. On average, however, M.D.-Ph.D. graduates begin their independent careers at about the same age as M.D.-only faculty. Another disadvantage is the several-year interval between the basic science and clinical years of medical school, during which classmates go on to complete their medical educations and which may require some M.D.-Ph.D. students to refresh their basic clinical skills before starting clinical clerkships.

Additional Information

For additional information and advice about application to, and enrollment in, a combined M.D.-Ph.D. program and the work of physician-scientists, contact your pre-health advisor and the M.D.-Ph.D. program director at medical schools of interest.

Chapter 12

Information About U.S. Medical Schools
Accredited by the LCME

Information about individual U.S. medical schools is given in the following two-page entries for the 129 schools (125 in the fifty states, four in Puerto Rico) that will be considering applications for the summer 2009 entering class. The schools presented here are accredited as of February 2008 by the Liaison Committee on Medial Education (LCME), which is sponsored by the Association of American Medical Colleges (AAMC) and the American Medical Association (AMA).

Individual school entries are each two pages, one devoted to narrative information and the other devoted to data and tabular information:

Page one: Narrative Information

- **Contact Information** — Admissions office staff, mail and email addresses, phone and fax numbers, and Web site addresses for the medical school, admissions office, and financial aid office.

- **General Information** — Background and basic information about the medical school and its program.

- **Curricular Highlights** — Information about the medical education curriculum and educational philosophy and methodologies.

- **USMLE Step 1 and Step 2 Clinical Knowledge (CK) and Clinical Skills (CS) Policies** — United States Medical Licensing Examination (USMLE) policies and requirements for promotion and/or graduation. For the most current policies, see the AAMC Curriculum Directory Web site at *http://services.aamc.org/currdir/ section1.*

- **Selection Factors** — Basic information regarding coursework, personal characteristics and experiences, and general requirements for applicants to be considered for acceptance and matriculation.

- **Financial Aid** — General information about the financial aid programs provided by the school, as well as additional contact information.

- **Information about Diversity Programs** — Information about the school's diversity initiatives and programs for students from groups underrepresented in medicine, as well as additional contact information.

- **Campus Information** — Information about total enrollment figures, campus setting, housing, special features, and satellite and/or regional campuses.

Page two: Data and Tabular Information

- **Application Process and Requirements for 2009–2010**

  - Primary Application Service — Notation of which type of application the school utilizes for primary applications (the American Medical College Application Service [AMCAS], the Texas Medical and Dental School Application Service [TMD-SAS], or a school-specific application) and about the earliest and latest filing dates for the primary application.

  - Secondary Application — This section notes if a secondary application is required, to whom the secondary application is submitted, required fees, the potential availability of a fee waiver, and the earliest and latest filing dates for secondary application materials.

  - Latest MCAT® Considered — The most recent MCAT® administration from which an MCAT® score can be submitted in support of an application.

  - Oldest MCAT® Considered — The earliest MCAT® administration from which an MCAT® score can be submitted in support of an application.

  - Early Decision Program — This section notes if the school participates in an Early Decision Program (EDP), when EDP applicants are notified about acceptance decisions, and if the Early Decision Program is available only to state residents or to both state residents and non-residents.

- Regular Acceptance Notice — The earliest and latest dates on which acceptance notices are sent to applicants. These dates do not refer to those applicants who have applied to special programs.

- Applicant's Response to Acceptance Notice – Maximum Time — The maximum period of time applicants are provided to respond to the acceptance offer.

- Requests for Deferred Entrance Considered — Information about deferred entrance opportunities at the school.

- Deposit — Information on the amount of the deposit required to hold a place in the next entering class, when the deposit is due, if the deposit is applied to tuition, if the deposit is refundable, and final date for requesting a deposit refund.

- Estimated Number of New Entrants — The number of regular, EDP and special program applicants expected to matriculate in the next year's entering class.

- Start Month/Year — The anticipated starting date in 2009 for the program.

- Interview Format — General information on how interviews are conducted and about the availability of regional interviews.

- **Other Programs** — Information regarding the availability of postbaccalaureate premedical, summer, and combined degree programs. Web sites and contact information are provided, as available.

- **Premedical Coursework** — Coursework and laboratories that applicants are either required or recommended to complete prior to matriculation.

- **MCAT® Information for Accepted Applicants** — This chart displays, for each section of the MCAT®, the National Median MCAT® score for all 2007 accepted applicants to all U.S. medical schools (the number in the shaded

circle), the individual school's median MCAT® scores for all 2007 applicants accepted to the school (the number in the white circle), and the range of scores on each MCAT® section for all 2007 applicants accepted to the school (the gradient line behind the circled numbers). Where applicable, schools have noted if it is their policy to average an applicant's MCAT® scores from various MCAT® administrations. Note: Chart 5-E (Chapter 5) presents information about the likelihood of acceptance for applicants whose scores on all MCAT® sections are at the lower end of the score range. Additionally, schools have noted whether the MCAT® is required for admission and the percentage of accepted applicants who took the MCAT®. Note: Several schools have special programs that do not require applicants to provide MCAT® scores. Therefore, although the MCAT® may be required for admission to the regular M.D. program, the percentage of accepted applicants who took the MCAT® may be less than 100%.

The national median scores for each MCAT® section published in this chapter represent median scores for the entire pool of accepted applicants to all medical schools. Thus, based on the fact that each acceptance of an applicant reflects an independent decision by each medical school, when an applicant has been accepted by more than one medical school, that applicant's MCAT® scores are included in the calculation of the national median more than once.

- **Overall GPA Median and Science GPA Median** — These data are for all applicants accepted to the medical school's 2007-2008 entering class.

- **Selection Factors** — Proportion of Accepted Applicants with Relevant Experience – These percentages were derived from applicant self-reports on the 2007 AMCAS application. They represent the percentage of accepted applicants who reported experiences

in the categories of Community Service/Volunteer Work, Medically-Related Work, and Research Experience. Data provided from schools that participate in the TMDSAS application or that use a school-specific primary application were calculated in the same manner as those derived from the AMCAS application.

- **Acceptance & Matriculation Data for 2007–2008** — Data in this chart reflect verified applications, not initiated applications. The top half of the chart notes the number of applicants (resident, non-resident, international, and total) who applied, were interviewed, and/or deferred entrance.

The lower portion of the chart displays information about the number of resident, non-resident, international, and total matriculants who were accepted through any Early Assurance Program (EAP), the Early Decision Program (EDP), and any college/M.D. or M.D./Ph.D. program, as well as the total number of matriculants from any application process in the school's 2007–2008 entering class. Information is also noted regarding the school's ability to accept applications from international applicants.

- **Matriculant Demographics** — Information about the number of men and women who matriculated in the 2007 first-year class for the first time.

- **Matriculants' Self-Reported Race/Ethnicity** — This information reflects data that were self-reported by applicants on their applications. Note: The sum of the columns may not reflect the actual number of matriculants. Applicants are permitted to select, in their racial and ethnic self-descriptions, more than one race and/or ethnicity. Each selection is counted. Therefore, if a given matriculant selects three races and/or ethnicities, that matriculant will be counted in three different columns. The total number of matriculants is presented in the row labeled "unduplicated."

- **Matriculants who were Science and Math Majors** — In this calculation, "Science and Math Majors" include: Aerospace Engineering, Agriculture, Anatomy, Astronomy, Biochemistry, Biology, Biomathematics, Biomedical Engineering, Biomedical Science, Biophysics, Botany, Chemical Engineering, Chemistry, Chemistry and Biology, Civil Engineering, Computer Science, Double Major Science, Electrical Engineering, Engineering, Environmental Studies, Forestry, Genetics, Geology, Geophysics, Human Biology, Mathematics, Mechanical Engineering, Meteorology, Microbiology, Molecular Biology, Natural Science, Neuroscience, Oceanography, Pathology, Pharmacology, Physics, Physiology, Premedicine, Psychobiology, Science General, Science-Other, Biology, Science-Other Physics, Statistics, and Zoology. These definitions reflect applicants' self-report on their AMCAS application; assistance was also provided by members of the National Association of Advisors for the Health Professions (NAAHP).

- **Matriculants with Baccalaureate and/or Graduate Degrees** — Information about the percentage of matriculants with baccalaureate and/or graduate degrees at the time of matriculation.

- **Specialty Choice** — The information in this chart was derived from program directors' reports to the National Graduate Medical Education (GME) Census in GME Track™ for 2003, 2004, and 2005 graduates of each medical school.

- **Financial Information** — Cost of Attendance, Tuition and Fees, Other Expenses and Health Insurance information is derived from the 2007–2008 AAMC Tuition and Student Fees Questionnaire. Regarding health insurance, "can be waived" means that this fee may be waived for any student with existing and comparable health insurance coverage (e.g., through a parent or a spouse).

Data about % of Enrolled Students Receiving Financial Aid and Average 2007 Graduate Indebtedness are derived from the 2006–2007 Liaison Committee on Medical Education (LCME) 1B Survey. Note: Scholarship and Grant amounts include funding from programs with a service commitment.

Abbreviations

Listed below are the abbreviations used in the school entries in this chapter.

AMCAS — American Medical College Application Service

CACMS — Committee on Accreditation of Canadian Medical Schools

CLEP — College Level Examination Program

EAP — Early Assurance Program

EDP — Early Decision Program

FAF — Financial Aid Form

FAFSA — Free Application for Federal Student Aid

FAP — AAMC Fee Assistance Program

GPA — Grade Point Average

LCME — Liaison Committee on Medical Education

LCME 1B — Liaison Committee on Medical Education 1B Survey

MCAT® — Medical College Admission Test

NA — Non-Applicable

NC — Not Collected

NR — Not Reported

REC — Recommended

REQ — Required

TMDSAS — Texas Medical and Dental School Application Service

TSF — Tuition and Student Fees Questionnaire

USMLE — United States Medical Licensing Examination

WICHE — Western Interstate Commission for Higher Education

WWAMI — WWAMI is an enduring partnership between the University of Washington School of Medicine and the states of Wyoming, Alaska, Montana, and Idaho. Its purpose is to provide access to publicly supported medical education across the five-state region. "WWAMI" is derived from the first letter of each of the five cooperating states.

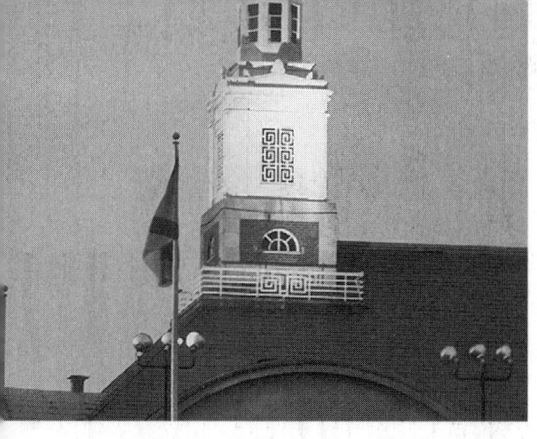

University of Alabama School of Medicine
Birmingham, Alabama

Medical Student Services/Admissions
University of Alabama School of Medicine
VH 100, 1530 3rd Ave. S.
Birmingham, Alabama 35294-0019
T 205 934 2433   **F** 205 934 8740

Admissions www.uab.edu/uasom/admissions
Main www.uab.edu/uasom/
Financial www.uab.edu/uasom/financialaid
Email medschool@uab.edu

Public Institution

Dr. Robert R. Rich, Dean

Dr. Nathan B. Smith, Assistant Dean for Admissions

Marsha Kelley Sutton, Program Administrator for Diversity Programs

Mark H. Martin, Associate Director of Financial Aid

General Information
The School of Medicine was founded in Mobile in 1859 and has been located in Birmingham since 1945. The main campus is in Birmingham, with branch campuses, created in 1969, in Huntsville and Tuscaloosa.

Mission Statement
The School of Medicine is dedicated to the education of physicians and scientists in all of the disciplines of medicine and biomedical investigation for careers in practice, teaching, and research. Necessary to this educational mission are the provision of outstanding medical care and services and the enhancement of new knowledge through clinical and basic biomedical research.

Curricular Highlights
Community Service Requirement: Optional.
Research/Thesis Requirement: Optional.

The four-year program emphasizes the fundamentals underlying clinical medical practice, with attention to the emotional, cultural, and social characteristics of patients and to the importance of adapting care to meet their needs. In addition to the pre-clinical science courses, the first two years include an Introduction to Clinical Medicine course providing training in medical professionalism, interviewing, and physical examination. The third and fourth years consist of required rotations and electives, with clinical experiences in both hospital and ambulatory settings. There are structured opportunities for research. Students must pass an Observed Structured Clinical Examination (OSCE) prior to graduation. There are three special degree programs: MD/PhD, MD/MPH, and a BA-BS/MD program (EMSAP), as well as a program for rural

Alabama residents. Each program has special curricular requirements.

USMLE
Step 1: Required. Students must record a passing score for promotion.
Step 2: Clinical Skills (CS): Required. Students must record a passing total score to graduate.
Step 2: Clinical Knowledge (CK): Required. Students must record a passing total score to graduate.

Selection Factors
The Admissions Committee is committed to admitting those applicants who possess the intelligence, skills, attitudes, and other personal attributes to become excellent physicians and to meet the health care needs of the state of Alabama. Desirable attributes include: solid academic performance, effective communication and interpersonal skills, evidence of service to others, empathy, emotional maturity, personal resilience, honesty, leadership ability, sense of purpose, and experiences to promote an understanding of what it means to be a physician (shadowing). Commitment and ability to meet the healthcare needs of Alabama's underserved populations (urban and rural), to biomedical research/academic careers, and to primary care careers are desirable. There is a special acceptance program for state residents committed to rural practice in Alabama. Transfers from other LCME-accredited medical schools are considered for students in good academic standing, who have a compelling reason to transfer and who have ties to Alabama. AP or CLEP coursework appearing on the AMCAS application will be accepted to meet a premedical requirement, although further coursework in biology and chemistry are desirable and may be necessary to be a competitive applicant. Other requirements: minimal total MCAT of 24 on the most recent exam, minimum grade of "C" on all required coursework, and completion of 90 hours of undergraduate credit from an accredited US college or university. With rare exceptions, completion of an undergraduate degree is required; all work toward current degrees must be completed prior to matriculation to the medical school.

Financial Aid
There are financial resources to fund an entire medical education. Resources include scholarships and low and higher interest loans. State merit scholarships are available in limited numbers to Alabama residents with exceptional academic records. State residents committed to rural practice in specific areas of Alabama may qualify for a loan forgiveness program.

Information about Diversity Programs
Through the Office for Diversity Programs, the Admissions Committee attempts to identify and provide career counseling to students from groups under-represented in medicine.

Campus Information

Setting
The Birmingham campus is part of the UAB Medical Center, a world-renowned academic medical center with more than 70 research centers across 82 city blocks. All students complete the Pre-Clerkship Phase in Birmingham. For required clinical rotations, students are assigned to Birmingham or one of two branch campuses.

Enrollment
For 2007, total enrollment was: 720

Special Features
Students are encouraged to participate in mentored research opportunities, ranging from one-month projects to degree programs (MPH and MS). Students are required to complete a Scholarly Activity extending across all four years.

Housing
About 1,400 spaces are available in campus residence halls. Most medical students live off-campus and find affordable housing within a 15-minute commute to the campus.

Satellite Campuses/Facilities
Both the Huntsville and Tuscaloosa campuses offer students opportunities for community-based education, as well as rotations in regional medical centers offering a full range of medical specialties. Both campuses have new clinical education facilities.

Application Process and Requirements 2009–2010

Primary Application Service: AMCAS

Earliest filing date: June 1, 2008
Latest filing date: November 1, 2008

Secondary Application Required?: Yes
Sent to: Screened applicants
URL: www.uasom.uab.edu/secondaryapplication
Fee: Yes, $75
Fee waiver available: Yes
Earliest filing date: August 1, 2008
Latest filing date: November 15, 2008

Latest MCAT® considered: September 2008
Oldest MCAT® considered: 2006

Early Decision Program
School does have EDP
Applicants notified: October 1, 2008
EDP available for: Residents only

Regular Acceptance Notice
Earliest date: October 15, 2008
Latest date: Until class is full

Applicant's Response to Acceptance Offer – Maximum Time: Two weeks

Requests for Deferred Entrance Considered: Yes

Deposit to Hold Place in Class: Yes
Deposit (Resident): $50
Deposit (Non-Resident): $100
Deposit due: With acceptance offer
Applied to tuition: Yes
Deposit refundable: Yes
Refundable by: May 15, 2009

Estimated number of new entrants: 176
EDP: 15, special program: 44

Start Month/Year: July 2009

Interview Format: Individual interviews are held only on Thursdays, September through March. Regional interviews are not available.

Other Programs

PREPARATORY PROGRAMS
Postbaccalaureate Program: No
Summer Program: Yes,
www.uasom.uab.edu/shep
Rural Medicine Programs: Yes,
https://www.uasom.uab.edu/secondaryapplication/RMSPHome.html
Summer Health Enrichment Program: Yes,
www.uasom.uab.edu/shep

COMBINED DEGREE PROGRAMS
Baccalaureate/MD: Yes, www.uab.edu/emsap
MD/MPH: Yes, http://138.26.144.80/websites/uab_soph_V2_0/content.asp?ID=727
MD/MBA: No
MD/JD: No
MD/PhD: Yes, www.uab.edu/uasom/mstp/

Premedical Coursework

Course	Req.	Rec.	Lab.	Hrs.
Inorganic Chemistry	•		•	8
Behavioral Sciences				
Biochemistry		•		
Biology				
Biology/Zoology	•		•	8
Calculus				
College English	•			6
College Mathematics	•			6

Course	Req.	Rec.	Lab.	Hrs.
Computer Science				
Genetics				
Humanities				
Organic Chemistry	•		•	8
Physics	•		•	8
Psychology				
Social Sciences				
Other				

Selection Factors: 2007 Accepted Applicants

Proportion of Accepted Applicants with Relevant Experience (Data Self-Reported to AMCAS®)		
Community Service/Volunteer		77%
Medically-Related Work		77%
Research		70%

Shaded bar represents accepted scores ranging from the 10th percentile to the 90th percentile. School Median ● National Median ●

Overall GPA	2.0	2.1	2.2	2.3	2.4	2.5	2.6	2.7	2.8	2.9	3.0	3.1	3.2	3.3	3.4	3.5	3.6	3.7	(3.8)	3.9	4.0
Science GPA	2.0	2.1	2.2	2.3	2.4	2.5	2.6	2.7	2.8	2.9	3.0	3.1	3.2	3.3	3.4	3.5	3.6	3.7	(3.8)	3.9	4.0

MCAT® required: Yes, 100% of 2007 accepted applicants took MCAT®

Verbal Reasoning	3	4	5	6	7	8	9	(10)	11	12	13	14	15
Physical Sciences	3	4	5	6	7	8	9	(10)	(11)	12	13	14	15
Biological Sciences	3	4	5	6	7	8	9	(10)	(11)	12	13	14	15
Writing Sample			J	K	L	M	N	O	(P)	(Q)	R	S	T

Acceptance & Matriculation Data for 2007–2008 First Year Class

	Resident	Non-Resident	International	Total
Applied	443	1517	30	1990
Interviewed	254	119	0	373
Deferred	4	1	0	5
Matriculants				
Early Assurance Program	0	0	0	0
Early Decision Program	12	0	0	12
Baccalaureate/MD	8	0	0	8
MD/PhD	1	7	0	8
Matriculated	157	19	0	**176**

Applications accepted from International Applicants: No

Matriculant Demographics: 2007–2008 First Year Class

Men: 104 **Women:** 72

Matriculants' Self-Reported Race/Ethnicity

Mexican American	2	Korean	2
Cuban	0	Vietnamese	3
Puerto Rican	0	Other Asian	0
Other Hispanic	0	Total Asian	26
Total Hispanic	2	Native American	2
Chinese	5	Black	11
Asian Indian	16	Native Hawaiian	0
Pakistani	1	White	137
Filipino	0	Unduplicated Number	
Japanese	0	of Matriculants	176

Science and Math Majors: 72%
Matriculants with:
Baccalaureate degree: 99%
Graduate degree(s): 10%

Specialty Choice

2003, 2004, 2005 Graduates, Specialty Choice (As reported by program directors to GME Track™)	
Anesthesiology	7%
Emergency Medicine	5%
Family Practice	8%
Internal Medicine	17%
Obstetrics/Gynecology	8%
Orthopaedic Surgery	3%
Pediatrics	12%
Psychiatry	3%
Radiology	4%
Surgery	8%

Financial Information

Source: 2006–2007 LCME I-B survey and 2007–2008 AAMC TSF questionnaire

	Residents	Non-Residents
Total Cost of Attendance	$41,573	$68,813
Tuition and Fees	$16,608	$43,848
Other (includes living expenses)	$23,598	$23,598
Health Insurance (can be waived)	$1,367	$1,367

Average 2007 Graduate Indebtedness: $110,040
% of Enrolled Students Receiving Aid: 79%

Criminal Background Check

This medical school requires a criminal background check prior to matriculation.

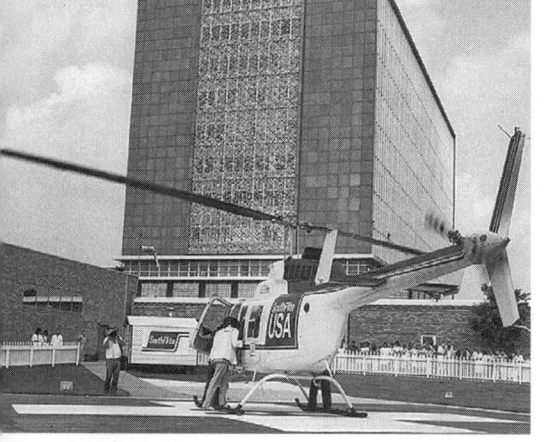

University of South Alabama College of Medicine
Mobile, Alabama

Office of Admissions, 2015 MSB
University of South Alabama
College of Medicine
Mobile, Alabama 36688-0002
T 251 460 7176   F 251 460 6278

Admissions www.southalabama.edu/com/admissions.shtml
Main www.southalabama.edu/com/
Financial www.finaid2.usouthal.edu/
Email mscott@usouthal.edu

Public Institution

Dr. Samuel J. Strada, Dean

Mark Scott, Director for Admissions

Dr. Margaret O'Brien, Associate Dean, Student Affairs

Dr. Hattie M. Myles, Assistant Dean, Special Programs and Student Affairs

General Information

The College of Medicine of the University of South Alabama was approved by the Board of Trustees of the university in 1967; the Alabama state legislature passed a resolution authorizing the college on August 19, 1967. The college admitted a charter class in January 1973. The basic medical sciences are housed on the university campus. The University of South Alabama Medical Center, operating continuously since 1831, has provided clinical medical education for more than a century. It is the major physician-staffed emergency facility in South Alabama and has been named a Level I trauma center by the Alabama Committee on Trauma. Other clinical training facilities include the U.S.A. Children's and Women's Hospital.

Mission Statement

To prepare talented, highly qualified students to become physicians, providing them the opportunity to develop basic science and clinical skills that will carry them successfully through residency and their career in medicine.

Curricular Highlights

Community Service Requirement: Optional.
Research/Thesis Requirement: Optional.

The first year is devoted to the basic sciences of anatomy, physiology, biochemistry, neuroanatomy, and embryology. Early introduction to clinical problems is also offered in courses such as Correlation Conferences and Medical Practice and Society. The second year includes pathology, physical diagnosis, microbiology-immunology, pharmacology, and behavioral science. Public health/epidemiology and medical genetics round out the second-year curriculum.

The third year has six clinical clerkships: medicine, surgery, pediatrics, psychiatry/neurology, obstetrics-gynecology, and family practice. The fourth year is composed of nine rotations of four weeks each. Students are required to select one rotation each in clinical neuroscience, surgical subspecialties, ambulatory care, primary care, subspecialty in medicine, pediatrics or obstetrics-gynecology, an acting internship, and an in-house elective. Three of the rotations may be used for approved extramural experiences. Letter grades are given until the fourth year, where a pass/fail/honors system is used.

USMLE

Step 1: Required. Students must record a passing score for promotion.
Step 2: Clinical Skills (CS): Required. Students must record a passing total score to graduate.
Step 2: Clinical Knowledge (CK): Required. Students must record a passing total score to graduate.

Selection Factors

The Committee on Admissions will consider all candidates whose undergraduate grades and scores on the MCAT® indicate that they can handle the rigorous curriculum of the College of Medicine. However, admission is based on more than scholastic achievement. Applicants will be considered on their potential to become conscientious and capable physicians. The University of South Alabama provides equal educational opportunities and is open to all qualified students without regard to race, creed, national origin, sex, or handicap with respect to all of its programs and activities. Because the college is state-supported, preference is given to Alabama residents. However, highly qualified out-of-state applicants are seriously considered. Disadvantaged, rural, and minority residents are strongly encouraged to apply. Fee waivers, based solely on economic need, are granted, when documented.

Financial Aid

The Office of Financial Aid coordinates the programs of assistance available to medical students demonstrating financial need. Scholarships are also available for entering freshmen and medical students who have demonstrated academic excellence and/or financial need.

Information about Diversity Programs

The school is committed to the enrollment and education of individuals from all disadvantaged groups. For information, contact Dr. Hattie M. Myles, assistant dean of special programs and student affairs.

Campus Information

Setting

The medical school is located in a suburban setting with easy access to restaurants, shopping, and the city's largest park system, which has both affordable golf and tennis facilities. Gulf Shores and Dauphin Island are less than an hour away, where students can enjoy some of the finest beaches in the United States. The hospitals and clinics are located throughout Mobile County and serve the health care needs of the community. These facilities include the only Level I trauma center in the region, as well as the latest in cancer treatments offered through the University of South Alabama Cancer Institute.

Enrollment

For 2007, total enrollment was: 280

Special Features

With only 74 students in each class and a large research-based clinical system consisting of four hospitals, students are exposed to significant procedural opportunities.

Housing

Very few, if any, students choose to live on campus due to the many safe and affordable housing options within a 5-mile radius of the campus. With the relative low cost of home ownership in the Mobile area, many students have found buying a small house or condo more cost-effective than leasing.

Satellite Campuses/Facilities

Students do their hospital training in any one of four hospitals, depending on the rotation. The College of Medicine also has clinic-based training with preceptors in facilities located throughout Alabama.

Application Process and Requirements 2009–2010

Primary Application Service: AMCAS
Earliest filing date: June 1, 2008
Latest filing date: November 15, 2008

Secondary Application Required?: Yes
Sent to: Screened applicants
URL: www.usouthal.edu
Contact: D. Mark Scott, (251) 460-7176
mscott@usouthal.edu
Fee: Yes, $75
Fee waiver available: Yes
Earliest filing date: June 15, 2008
Latest filing date: December 31, 2008

Latest MCAT® considered: September 2008
Oldest MCAT® considered: 2005

Early Decision Program
School does have EDP
Applicants notified: October 1, 2008
EDP available for: Residents only

Regular Acceptance Notice
Earliest date: November 15, 2008
Latest date: Until class is full

Applicant's Response to Acceptance
Offer – Maximum Time: Two weeks

Requests for Deferred
Entrance Considered: Yes

Deposit to Hold Place in Class: Yes
Deposit (Resident): $50
Deposit (Non-Resident): $50
Deposit due: With response to acceptance offer
Applied to tuition: Yes
Deposit refundable: Yes
Refundable by: May 15, 2009

Estimated number of new entrants: 74
EDP: 10, special program: 5

Start Month/Year: August 2009

Interview Format: Students meet one-on-one with three interviewers. Regional interviews are not available.

Other Programs

PREPARATORY PROGRAMS
Postbaccalaureate Program: No
Summer Program: Yes,
Dr. Hattie Myles, (251) 460-7313,
hmyles@usouthal.edu

COMBINED DEGREE PROGRAMS
Baccalaureate/MD: Yes, www.usouthal.edu
(251) 460-6141
MD/MPH: No
MD/MBA: No
MD/JD: No
MD/PhD: Yes,
www.southalabama.edu/com/programs.shtml,
D. Mark Scott, (251) 460-7176,
mscott@usouthal.edu

Premedical Coursework

Course	Req.	Rec.	Lab.	Hrs.	Course	Req.	Rec.	Lab.	Hrs.
Inorganic Chemistry	•		•	8	Computer Science				
Behavioral Sciences					Genetics				
Biochemistry		•			Humanities		•		6
Biology	•		•	8	Organic Chemistry	•		•	8
Biology/Zoology					Physics	•		•	8
Calculus		•			Psychology				
College English	•			6	Social Sciences				
College Mathematics	•			6	Other				

Selection Factors: 2007 Accepted Applicants

Proportion of Accepted Applicants with Relevant Experience (Data Self-Reported to AMCAS®)		Community Service/Volunteer	77%
		Medically-Related Work	74%
		Research	60%

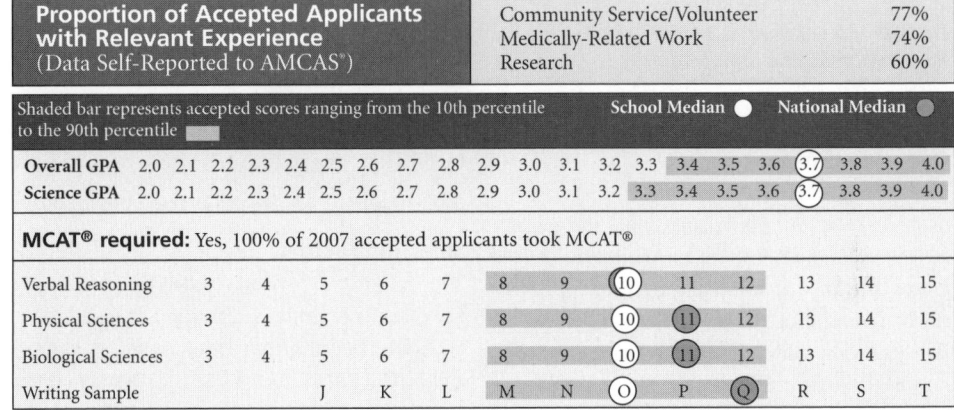

Shaded bar represents accepted scores ranging from the 10th percentile to the 90th percentile. School Median ● National Median ●

Overall GPA	2.0	2.1	2.2	2.3	2.4	2.5	2.6	2.7	2.8	2.9	3.0	3.1	3.2	3.3	3.4	3.5	3.6	(3.7)	3.8	3.9	4.0
Science GPA	2.0	2.1	2.2	2.3	2.4	2.5	2.6	2.7	2.8	2.9	3.0	3.1	3.2	3.3	3.4	3.5	3.6	(3.7)	3.8	3.9	4.0

MCAT® required: Yes, 100% of 2007 accepted applicants took MCAT®

Verbal Reasoning	3	4	5	6	7	8	9	(10)	11	12	13	14	15
Physical Sciences	3	4	5	6	7	8	9	(10)	(11)	12	13	14	15
Biological Sciences	3	4	5	6	7	8	9	(10)	(11)	12	13	14	15
Writing Sample			J	K	L	M	N	(O)	P	(Q)	R	S	T

Acceptance & Matriculation Data for 2007–2008 First Year Class

	Resident	Non-Resident	International	Total
Applied	374	623	57	1054
Interviewed	188	22	0	210
Deferred	1	0	0	1
Matriculants				
Early Assurance Program	n/a	n/a	n/a	n/a
Early Decision Program	2	0	0	2
Baccalaureate/MD	0	0	0	0
MD/PhD	0	0	0	0
Matriculated	65	8	1	**74**

Applications accepted from International Applicants: Yes

Matriculant Demographics: 2007–2008 First Year Class

Men: 42   **Women:** 32

Matriculants' Self-Reported Race/Ethnicity

Mexican American	0	Korean	0
Cuban	0	Vietnamese	1
Puerto Rican	0	Other Asian	2
Other Hispanic	0	Total Asian	9
Total Hispanic	0	Native American	0
Chinese	1	Black	5
Asian Indian	5	Native Hawaiian	0
Pakistani	0	White	59
Filipino	0	Unduplicated Number	
Japanese	0	of Matriculants	74

Science and Math Majors: 78%
Matriculants with:
    Baccalaureate degree: 100%
    Graduate degree(s): 8%

Specialty Choice

2003, 2004, 2005 Graduates, Specialty Choice
(As reported by program directors to GME Track™)

Anesthesiology	3%
Emergency Medicine	4%
Family Practice	7%
Internal Medicine	25%
Obstetrics/Gynecology	8%
Orthopaedic Surgery	6%
Pediatrics	12%
Psychiatry	1%
Radiology	5%
Surgery	5%

Financial Information

Source: 2006–2007 LCME I-B survey and 2007–2008 AAMC TSF questionnaire

	Residents	Non-Residents
Total Cost of Attendance	$39,432	$52,912
Tuition and Fees	$16,082	$29,562
Other (includes living expenses)	$20,850	$20,850
Health Insurance (can be waived)	$2,500	$2,500

Average 2007 Graduate Indebtedness: $119,696
% of Enrolled Students Receiving Aid: 90%

Criminal Background Check

This medical school does not require a criminal background check prior to matriculation.

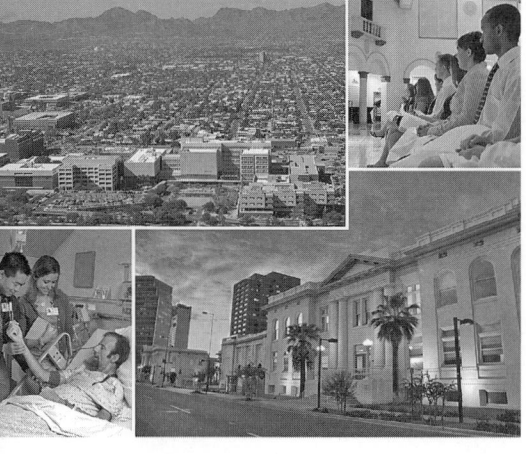

University of Arizona College of Medicine

Tucson, Arizona

Admissions Office, University of Arizona
College of Medicine
P.O. Box 245075
Tucson, Arizona 85724-5075
T 520 626 6214(T), 602 827 2005(PX)
F 520 626 3777(T), 602 827 2212(PX)

Admissions www.admissions.medicine.arizona.edu
Main www.medicine.arizona.edu/
Financial www.medicine.arizona.edu/financial-aid
Email medapp@email.arizona.edu (T)
phxmed@email.arizona.ed (PX)

Public Institution

Dr. Keith A. Joiner, Dean

Dr. Edward H. Shortliffe, Dean, Phoenix Campus

Dr. Ana Maria Lopez, Associate Dean, Office of Outreach & Multicultural Affairs

Maggie Gumble, Associate Director, Financial Aid

General Information

The College of Medicine enrolled its first class of students in 1967. As a professional and graduate college of the University of Arizona, its programs provide education and training for both the M.D. and Ph.D. degrees. UACOM has two four-year campuses: The Tucson Campus, adjacent to the main campus of the University of Arizona, and the newly opened Phoenix Campus, located in downtown Phoenix.

Mission Statement

The Tucson (TUS) and Phoenix (PHX) campuses offer distinct, but related four-year educational programs leading to the Doctor of Medicine degree. Both are designed for student achievement in the following six core competencies: (1) Medical Knowledge; (2) Patient Care; (3) Interpersonal and Communication skills; (4) Professionalism; (5) Practice-based Learning and Improvement; and (6) Systems-based Practice & Population Health.

Curricular Highlights

Community Service Requirement: Optional.
Research/Thesis Requirement: Optional.

The Tucson and Phoenix educational tracks utilize a similar core structure, while each track contains distinct elements. The first two years of each curriculum is structured in integrated blocks that focus on organs systems or disease states. The second two years consist of required clinical clerkships in key disciplines and significant time for elective work. Basic and clinical science are interwoven with threads, such as behavioral science and humanism, health and society, and interprofessional education. Both curricula emphasize active learning, guided independent learning, working in teams, and early clinical experience. Nearly all students take part in our robust co-curricular activities, including medical student research programs, rural health programs and service learning programs.

USMLE

Step 1: Required. Students must record a passing score for graduation, but not promotion.
Step 2: Clinical Skills (CS): Required. Students must only record a score.
Step 2: Clinical Knowledge (CK): Required. Students must record a passing total score to graduate.

Selection Factors

The University of Arizona College of Medicine accepts only Arizona residents, highly qualified WICHE applicants from Montana and Wyoming, and Native Americans who reside on reservations contiguous with the state of Arizona. The Admissions Committee considers many factors in evaluating applicants, including the entire academic record, performance on the MCAT®, the applicant's personal statement, interviews, and letters of recommendation. Applicants are chosen on the basis of their career goals, motivation, academic ability, integrity, maturity, altruism, communication skills, and leadership abilities. Clinical, research, or community service experience is viewed favorably. The Admissions Committee strives to accept a student body with diverse backgrounds in order to best meet the medical needs of the people of Arizona. Priority consideration is given to applicants who demonstrate a willingness to practice in medically underserved areas of Arizona. No preference is given to any particular type of undergraduate major. Since many of the patients who receive care at the Arizona Health Sciences Center and its affiliated clinics and hospitals speak Spanish as their primary language, it would be useful for the University of Arizona medical students to be conversant in Spanish.

Financial Aid

Federal and local scholarships and loans are available to students with financial need. All determinations of need are made after an applicant is accepted for enrollment.

Information about Diversity Programs

The University of Arizona College of Medicine believes in the educational benefits of diversity. We actively recruit and admit students with diverse backgrounds and experiences and our educational programs include activities where the diversity of the student body contributes to the educational experience. We foster a supportive environment for students of all backgrounds.

Campus Information

Setting

The Tucson campus is located on the campus of the University of Arizona, with all the facilities and services expected of a major university. The College of Medicine is contiguous with University Medical Center and faculty clinics. It is adjacent to the Colleges of Nursing, Pharmacy, and Public Health and to the interdisciplinary Bio5 Research Institute. The Phoenix campus, named the University of Arizona College of Medicine, Phoenix-in Partnership with Arizona State University is located on the Phoenix Biomedical Campus in downtown Phoenix. The University of Arizona shares the Phoenix Biomedical Campus with the Arizona State University's Department of Biomedical Informatics and with the Translational Genomics Research Institute. The Phoenix Biomedical Campus is near ASU's Downtown Campus, which includes ASU's College of Nursing and Healthcare Innovation and School of Social Work. The University of Arizona College of Medicine has numerous affiliated hospitals and clinical sites and many research affiliations throughout Arizona.

Enrollment

For 2007, total enrollment was: 477

Satellite Campuses/Facilities

The UA College of Medicine-Phoenix, in partnership with Arizona State University expanded from a two-year clinical experience to a full, four-year curriculum. Over the next decade, the College of Medicine-Phoenix will add educational, research and clinical facilities to the Phoenix Biomedical Campus, also home to the Translational Genomics Institute (TGen).

Application Process and Requirements 2009–2010

Primary Application Service: AMCAS
Earliest filing date: June 1, 2008
Latest filing date: November 1, 2008

Secondary Application Required?: Yes
Sent to: Selected Applicants
URL: n/a
Fee: Yes, $75
Fee waiver available: Yes
Earliest filing date: July 1, 2008
Latest filing date: January 15, 2009

Latest MCAT® considered: September 2008
Oldest MCAT® considered: 2005

Early Decision Program
School does not have EDP
Applicants notified: n/a
EDP available for: n/a

Regular Acceptance Notice
Earliest date: March 2, 2009
Latest date: Until class if full

Applicant's Response to Acceptance
Offer – Maximum Time: Two weeks

Requests for Deferred
Entrance Considered: Yes

Deposit to Hold Place in Class: No
Deposit (Resident): n/a
Deposit (Non-Resident): n/a
Deposit due: n/a
Applied to tuition: n/a
Deposit refundable: n/a
Refundable by: n/a

Estimated number of new entrants: 158
EDP: n/a, special program: n/a

Start Month/Year: August 2009

Interview Format: Two 30 to 50-minute interviews. Regional interviews are not available.

Other Programs

PREPARATORY PROGRAMS
Postbaccalaureate Program: Yes
Summer Program: No

COMBINED DEGREE PROGRAMS
Baccalaureate/MD: No
MD/MPH: Yes,
Lane Johnson, M.D. , M.P.H., (520) 626-6029
lpj@u.arizona.edu
MD/MBA: Yes,
Tanisha N. Price-Johnson, (520) 626-6214
tanishap@email.arizona.edu
MD/JD: No
MD/PhD: Yes,
Maureen Driscoll, (520) 626-6097
maureend@email.arizona.edu

Premedical Coursework

Course	Req.	Rec.	Lab.	Sems.
Inorganic Chemistry	•			2
Behavioral Sciences				
Biochemistry				
Biology				
Biology/Zoology	•			2
Calculus				
College English	•			2
College Mathematics				

Course	Req.	Rec.	Lab.	Sems.
Computer Science				
Genetics				
Humanities				
Organic Chemistry	•			2
Physics	•			2
Psychology				
Social Sciences				
Other				

Selection Factors: 2007 Accepted Applicants

Proportion of Accepted Applicants with Relevant Experience (Data Self-Reported to AMCAS®)		
Community Service/Volunteer		67%
Medically-Related Work		92%
Research		74%

Shaded bar represents accepted scores ranging from the 10th percentile to the 90th percentile   School Median ● National Median ●

Overall GPA	2.0	2.1	2.2	2.3	2.4	2.5	2.6	2.7	2.8	2.9	3.0	3.1	3.2	3.3	3.4	3.5	3.6	3.7	(3.8)	3.9	4.0
Science GPA	2.0	2.1	2.2	2.3	2.4	2.5	2.6	2.7	2.8	2.9	3.0	3.1	3.2	3.3	3.4	3.5	3.6	(3.7)	3.8	3.9	4.0

MCAT® required: Yes, 100% of 2007 accepted applicants took MCAT®

Verbal Reasoning	3	4	5	6	7	8	9	(10)	11	12	13	14	15
Physical Sciences	3	4	5	6	7	8	9	(10)	(11)	12	13	14	15
Biological Sciences	3	4	5	6	7	8	9	(10)	(11)	12	13	14	15
Writing Sample			J	K	L	M	N	O	(P)	(Q)	R	S	T

Acceptance & Matriculation Data for 2007–2008 First Year Class

	Resident	Non-Resident	International	Total
Applied	658	152	4	814
Interviewed	602	14	0	616
Deferred	7	0	0	7
Matriculants				
Early Assurance Program	n/a	n/a	n/a	n/a
Early Decision Program	0	0	0	0
Baccalaureate/MD	n/a	n/a	n/a	n/a
MD/PhD	1	0	0	1
Matriculated	132	2	0	**134**

Applications accepted from International Applicants: No

Specialty Choice

2003, 2004, 2005 Graduates, Specialty Choice (As reported by program directors to GME Track™)	
Anesthesiology	7%
Emergency Medicine	10%
Family Practice	10%
Internal Medicine	14%
Obstetrics/Gynecology	5%
Orthopaedic Surgery	2%
Pediatrics	15%
Psychiatry	4%
Radiology	5%
Surgery	9%

Matriculant Demographics: 2007–2008 First Year Class

Men: 51   **Women:** 83

Matriculants' Self-Reported Race/Ethnicity

Mexican American	11	Korean	1
Cuban	1	Vietnamese	1
Puerto Rican	1	Other Asian	4
Other Hispanic	2	Total Asian	22
Total Hispanic	13	Native American	2
Chinese	5	Black	5
Asian Indian	10	Native Hawaiian	2
Pakistani	2	White	98
Filipino	2	Unduplicated Number	
Japanese	0	of Matriculants	134

Science and Math Majors: 74%
Matriculants with:
    Baccalaureate degree: 100%
    Graduate degree(s): 10%

Financial Information

Source: 2006–2007 LCME I-B survey and 2007–2008 AAMC TSF questionnaire

	Residents	Non-Residents
Total Cost of Attendance	$35,275	$0
Tuition and Fees	$17,736	$0
Other (includes living expenses)	$16,147	$0
Health Insurance (not applicable)	$1,392	$0

Average 2007 Graduate Indebtedness: $104,616
% of Enrolled Students Receiving Aid: 91%

Criminal Background Check

This medical school does not require a criminal background check prior to matriculation.

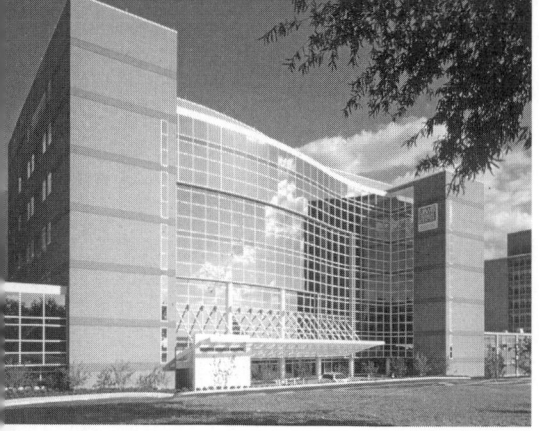

University of Arkansas College of Medicine

Little Rock, Arkansas

Office of the Dean, University of Arkansas for
Medical Sciences College of Medicine
4301 West Markham Street, Slot 551
Little Rock, Arkansas 72205-7199
T 501 686 5354   **F** 501 686 5873

Admissions www.uams.edu/com/applicants/
Main www.uams.edu/com/
Financial www.uams.edu/com/fin-aid/default.asp
Email southtomg@uams.edu

Public Institution

Dr. Debra Fiser, Vice Chancellor and Dean

*Tom G. South, Director, Admissions
and Financial Aid*

*Dr. Billy R. Thomas, Associate Dean,
Office of Diversity*

*Dr. Richard P. Wheeler, Executive Associate
Dean, Academic Affairs*

General Information

In 1879, eight visionary physicians had the fore-
sight to each invest $625 to secure a charter from
the Arkansas Industrial University. On October
7, 1879, the medical school opened its doors to
22 eager students. From these humble begin-
nings grew the excellence and prestige now
embodied in the College of Medicine. Today, the
College of Medicine has over 1000 full-time and
part-time faculty, over 600 residents, and almost
600 medical students. UAMS is Arkansas' only
institution of professional and graduate education devoted solely to the health and biological
sciences. In fulfilling its educational mission, the
College of Medicine, in conjunction with the
UAMS Medical Center, provides the environment and opportunities for students and
practitioners alike to learn and maintain the
knowledge and skills required in the 21st century. Comprehensive services are delivered in an
interdisciplinary environment to all Arkansans,
regardless of their ability to pay. The school is in
the planning phase for a major expansion initiative: a replacement hospital, new student housing, new psychiatry center, an addition to both
the Jones Eye Institute and the Outpatient
Center, and a new affiliated state psychiatric hospital. The university's commitment is to facilitate
discovery through applied research and to teach
the best science and compassionate care to
tomorrow's caregivers. As much as the school is
proud of its past achievements, it believes that its
best still lies ahead.

Mission Statement

"In relentless pursuit of excellence, every day"
summarizes the essence of the school's fourfold
mission to teach, to heal, to search, and to serve.

Curricular Highlights

Community Service Requirement: Optional.
Research/Thesis Requirement: Optional.

Along with the standard courses in anatomy, biochemistry, and physiology, the first year includes
a program to introduce the student to clinical
contacts and concepts. This is accomplished with
formal lectures in medico-socioeconomic topics,
small-group discussions, faculty-supervised
interviews with patients, and the extensive use of
standardized patients. The third year is a full 48
weeks with rotation through the major clinical
services. This expanded clinical year provides
substantial preparation for the predominantly
elective fourth year, which consists of a minimum of 36 weeks to a maximum of 48 weeks of
courses selected with the assistance of a faculty
advisor. On- and off-campus electives are available to round out preparation for each student's
career goals. Opportunities are provided for students to engage in research activities and to pursue graduate courses leading to the M.D./Ph.D.
and M.D./M.P.H. degrees. The number of
M.D./Ph.D. scholarships has increased significantly in recent years. Students are also provided
with expanded opportunities through the
M.D./M.B.A. and M.D./J.D. degree programs.

USMLE

Step 1: Required. Students must record a passing
score for promotion.
Step 2: Clinical Skills (CS): Required. Students
must record a passing total score to graduate.
Step 2: Clinical Knowledge (CK): Required. Students must record a passing total score to graduate.

Selection Factors

Selection is based on scholastic attainment, performance on the MCAT, personal interviews with
members of the faculty, and recommendations,
particularly evaluations by college pre-professional advisory committees. Applicants should

also demonstrate time and effort devoted to volunteerism and community service. Selection is
made without regard to race, sex, creed, national
origin, age, or handicap. Unsuccessful applicants
may reapply without prejudice. Non-Arkansas
residents who have strong ties to Arkansas are
encouraged to apply.

Financial Aid

An applicant's financial status is not a factor in
selection for admission. The Rural Practice
Programs allow students who commit to practice
primary care medicine in rural communities in
Arkansas to receive loans during medical school.
The student is obligated to return to a rural community following residency training and to practice full time for the same number of years the
student was assisted during medical school. For
each year of service, one year of loans is forgiven
until the debt is retired. A unique feature of the
Rural Practice Programs allows Arkansas resi-
dents on the Alternate List, who are willing to
practice full-time in a rural community in
Arkansas, to interview with the Arkansas Rural
Medical Practice Student Loan and Scholarship
Board. If the Board approves the alternate's
Rural Practice Program application, the applicant
is advanced to the top of the alternate list.
For additional details, contact the Financial
Aid Office.

Information about Diversity Programs

Students from groups underrepresented in medicine are encouraged to apply. The Office of
Diversity has developed an active recruitment
and retention program. The five-week Summer
Science Program offers an introduction to the
medical school curriculum, along with reading
and study skill enrichment sessions designed to
strengthen students' mastery of these areas. A
pre-matriculation program is available to all
students accepted for admission.

Campus Information

Enrollment

For 2007, total enrollment was: 571

Application Process and Requirements 2009–2010

Primary Application Service: AMCAS
Earliest filing date: July 1, 2008
Latest filing date: November 1, 2008

Secondary Application Required?: Yes
Sent to: All applicants
URL: www.uams.edu
Contact: Tom South, (501) 686-5354
SouthTomG@uams.edu
Fee: Yes, $100
Fee waiver available: Yes
Earliest filing date: July 1, 2008
Latest filing date: November 1, 2008

Latest MCAT® considered: September 2008
Oldest MCAT® considered: 2006

Early Decision Program
School does not have EDP
Applicants notified: n/a
EDP available for: n/a

Regular Acceptance Notice
Earliest date: December 15, 2008
Latest date: Until class is full

Applicant's Response to Acceptance Offer – Maximum Time: Two weeks

Requests for Deferred Entrance Considered: Yes

Deposit to Hold Place in Class: No
Deposit (Resident): n/a
Deposit (Non-Resident): n/a
Deposit due: n/a
Applied to tuition: n/a
Deposit refundable: n/a
Refundable by: n/a

Estimated number of new entrants: 160
EDP: 160, special program: n/a

Start Month/Year: August 2009

Interview Format: Team interviews on scheduled interview dates. All interviews are conducted on campus.

Other Programs

PREPARATORY PROGRAMS
Postbaccalaureate Program: No
Summer Program: Yes, www.uams.edu/
physiology/eduadv/main.htm
Dr. James Pasley, (501) 686-5128

COMBINED DEGREE PROGRAMS
Baccalaureate/MD: No
MD/MPH: Yes, www.uams.edu
MD/MBA: Yes, www.uams.edu
MD/JD: Yes, www.uams.edu
MD/PhD: Yes, www.uams.edu

Premedical Coursework

Course	Req.	Rec.	Lab.	Sems.	Course	Req.	Rec.	Lab.	Sems.
Inorganic Chemistry	•			2	Computer Science		•		
Behavioral Sciences		•			Genetics		•		
Biochemistry		•			Humanities		•		
Biology	•			2	Organic Chemistry	•			2
Biology/Zoology		•			Physics	•			2
Calculus		•			Psychology				
College English	•			2	Social Sciences				
College Mathematics	•			2	Spanish & Speech Comm.				

Selection Factors: 2007 Accepted Applicants

Proportion of Accepted Applicants with Relevant Experience (Data Self-Reported to AMCAS®)		Community Service/Volunteer	74%
		Medically-Related Work	72%
		Research	72%

Shaded bar represents accepted scores ranging from the 10th percentile to the 90th percentile   School Median ● National Median ●

Overall GPA	2.0	2.1	2.2	2.3	2.4	2.5	2.6	2.7	2.8	2.9	3.0	3.1	3.2	3.3	3.4	3.5	3.6	(3.7)	3.8	3.9	4.0
Science GPA	2.0	2.1	2.2	2.3	2.4	2.5	2.6	2.7	2.8	2.9	3.0	3.1	3.2	3.3	3.4	3.5	(3.6)	3.7	3.8	3.9	4.0

MCAT® required: Yes, 100% of 2007 accepted applicants took MCAT®

Verbal Reasoning	3	4	5	6	7	8	9	(10)	11	12	13	14	15
Physical Sciences	3	4	5	6	7	8	9	(10)	(11)	12	13	14	15
Biological Sciences	3	4	5	6	7	8	9	(10)	(11)	12	13	14	15
Writing Sample			J	K	L	M	N	(O)	P	(Q)	R	S	T

Acceptance & Matriculation Data for 2007–2008 First Year Class

	Resident	Non-Resident	International	Total
Applied	323	888	19	1230
Interviewed	298	94	0	392
Deferred	13	4	0	17
Matriculants				
Early Assurance Program	0	0	0	0
Early Decision Program	0	0	0	0
Baccalaureate/MD	n/a	n/a	n/a	n/a
MD/PhD	3	0	0	3
Matriculated	129	26	0	**155**

Applications accepted from International Applicants: No

Specialty Choice

2003, 2004, 2005 Graduates, Specialty Choice (As reported by program directors to GME Track™)	
Anesthesiology	7%
Emergency Medicine	4%
Family Practice	19%
Internal Medicine	12%
Obstetrics/Gynecology	7%
Orthopaedic Surgery	5%
Pediatrics	7%
Psychiatry	7%
Radiology	4%
Surgery	4%

Matriculant Demographics: 2007–2008 First Year Class

Men: 100   **Women:** 55

Matriculants' Self-Reported Race/Ethnicity

Mexican American	1	Korean	2
Cuban	0	Vietnamese	3
Puerto Rican	0	Other Asian	2
Other Hispanic	1	Total Asian	21
Total Hispanic	2	Native American	0
Chinese	9	Black	5
Asian Indian	6	Native Hawaiian	1
Pakistani	0	White	126
Filipino	1	Unduplicated Number	
Japanese	1	of Matriculants	155

Science and Math Majors: 77%
Matriculants with:
   Baccalaureate degree: 98%
   Graduate degree(s): 10%

Financial Information

Source: 2006–2007 LCME I-B survey and 2007–2008 AAMC TSF questionnaire

	Residents	Non-Residents
Total Cost of Attendance	$33,940	$49,472
Tuition and Fees	$16,430	$31,962
Other (includes living expenses)	$15,650	$15,650
Health Insurance (can be waived)	$1,860	$1,860

Average 2007 Graduate Indebtedness: $117,036
% of Enrolled Students Receiving Aid: 93%

Criminal Background Check

This medical school requires a criminal background check prior to matriculation.

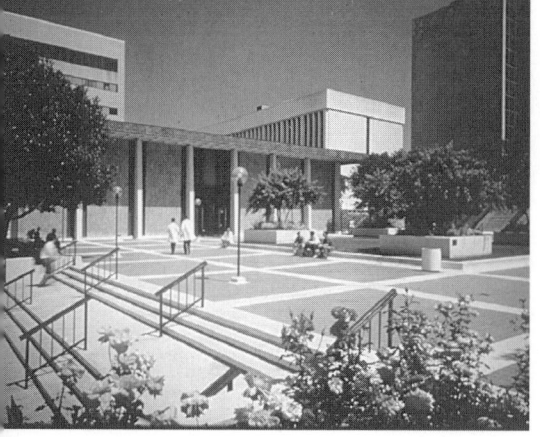

Keck School of Medicine of the University of Southern California
Los Angeles, California

University of Southern California
Keck School of Medicine, Office of Admissions
1975 Zonal Avenue, KAM 100-C
Los Angeles, California 90089-9021
T 323 442 2552 **F** 323 442 2433

Admissions www.usc.edu/schools/medicine/education/admissions
Main www.usc.edu/schools/medicine
Financial www.usc.edu/schools/medicine/education/financial_aid
Email medadmit@usc.edu

Private Institution

Dr. Carmen A. Puliafito, Dean

Dr. Erin A. Quinn, Associate Dean for Admissions

Althea Alexander, Assistant Dean for Minority Student Affairs

Gina Camello, Director of Admissions

Alicia M. Rugley, Scholarships and Grants Coordinator

General Information

The Keck School of Medicine of the University of Southern California was established in 1885 as the region's first medical school. All Keck students train at the Los Angeles County+USC Medical Center, one of the largest medical teaching centers in the United States. Through affiliations with over a dozen other private and public hospitals, Keck students have a highly diverse clinical training experience.

Mission Statement

The mission of the Keck School of Medicine is to improve the quality of life for individuals and society by promoting health, preventing and curing disease, advancing biomedical research, and educating tomorrow's physicians and scientists.

Curricular Highlights

Community Service Requirement: Optional.
Research/Thesis Requirement: Optional.

Students are progressively involved with regular patient contact beginning the first week of medical school. An important feature in the curriculum is the Introduction to Clinical Medicine course. The doctor-patient relationship and interviewing are presented during the first year, and physical diagnosis and history-taking are taught in the second. Groups of six to seven students are led by a faculty member who serves as a clinical tutor for their first two years. The curriculum is designed to enhance students' understanding of the basic sciences and their relevance to clinical medicine. Curricular themes are guided by select Pathways and delivered in a case-centered format with the integration of small-group learning sessions,

directed-independent study, and innovative instructional technologies. The first year of the Year I-II continuum begins with 18 weeks of Core Principles of Health and Disease, followed by 49 weeks of organ system review, ending with a 10-week Integrated Case Study section. Each week of the academic year is composed of approximately 20 hours of lecture and small-group sessions, with an additional 20 hours of directed-independent study or Introduction to Clinical Medicine. Examinations in all systems throughout the first two years are graded pass/fail. Dean's Recognition is awarded on the basis of year-end comprehensive examinations and special projects. The final two years are designed as a continuum of two academic calendar years. Each student's program is individually designed to include 50 weeks of required clerkships, 16 weeks of selective clerkships, 16 weeks of elective clerkships, and required senior seminars. Grading for the final two years is on an honors, high pass, pass, and fail basis.

USMLE
Step 1: Required. Students must record a passing score for promotion.
Step 2: Clinical Skills (CS): Required. Students must only record a score.
Step 2: Clinical Knowledge (CK): Required. Students must only record a score.

Selection Factors
The Admissions Committee seriously considers candidates whose academic achievement and MCAT® performance indicate the ability to satisfactorily complete the rigorous demands of the medical school curriculum. Also, the committee evaluates various non-academic factors, including personal motivations, evidence of qualities deemed desirable for the study and practice of medicine, significant achievements in extracurricular pursuits, and demonstrated commitment to service and community.

Financial Aid
A variety of university scholarships and loans are available to supplement federal and state programs. Awards are based on need as demonstrated through a financial statement.

Information about Diversity Programs
The Office of Diversity at the Keck School of Medicine strives to recruit, enroll, and retain students of all socioeconomic, cultural, and ethnic backgrounds. For additional information and opportunities, please visit *www.usc.edu/schools/medicine/school/offices/diversity.html.*

Campus Information

Setting
Located on USC's Health Sciences Campus, the 31-acre medical campus is part of an ethnically diverse community in northeast Los Angeles. The campus is a short drive away from many of the recreational, cultural, and entertainment activities that Los Angeles has to offer.

Enrollment
For 2007, total enrollment was: 679

Special Features
The Keck School of Medicine ranks in the top 25 U.S. medical schools in terms of federal research support. Its affiliations with Los Angeles County Hospital, one of the nation's largest teaching hospitals, and a number of state-of-the-art private hospitals and centers, provide students with an unparalleled hands-on clinical education in a broad range of diseases and settings.

Housing
On-campus housing is available at Seaver Residence Hall. A majority of students live off-campus in nearby communities, many of which are within five miles of campus. During the summer months, the Student Services Office compiles and posts listings of available housing and roommate announcements to assist students in finding housing.

Satellite Campuses/Facilities
Supervised by Keck School faculty, medical students play a key role in patient care in more than a dozen affiliated hospitals, including the adjacent LAC+USC Medical Center.

Application Process and Requirements 2009–2010

Primary Application Service: AMCAS
Earliest filing date: July 1, 2008
Latest filing date: November 1, 2008

Secondary Application Required?: Yes
Sent to: All AMCAS-certified applicants
URL: www.usc.edu/schools/medicine/ksomnfl.html
Fee: Yes, $90
Fee waiver available: Yes
Earliest filing date: July 1, 2008
Latest filing date: December 1, 2008

Latest MCAT® considered: September 2008
Oldest MCAT® considered: 2006

Early Decision Program
School does have EDP
Applicants notified: September 15, 2008
EDP available for: Both Residents and Non-Residents

Regular Acceptance Notice
Earliest date: November 1, 2008
Latest date: Until class is full

Applicant's Response to Acceptance Offer – Maximum Time: Ten Days

Requests for Deferred Entrance Considered: Yes

Deposit to Hold Place in Class: Yes
Deposit (Resident): $100
Deposit (Non-Resident): $100
Deposit due: Within ten days after notification of acceptance
Applied to tuition: Yes
Deposit refundable: Yes
Refundable by: May 15, 2009

Estimated number of new entrants: 168
EDP: 10, special program: n/a

Start Month/Year: August 2009

Interview Format: On-campus interviews only, closed-file. Regional interviews are not available.

Other Programs

PREPARATORY PROGRAMS
Postbaccalaureate Program: Yes,
http://chem.usc.edu/undergraduate/premed.html
Summer Program: No

COMBINED DEGREE PROGRAMS
Baccalaureate/MD: Yes,
www.usc.edu/schools/medicine/ksomnfl.html
MD/MPH: Yes,
www.usc.edu/schools/medicine/ksomnfl.html
MD/MBA: Yes,
www.usc.edu/schools/medicine/ksomnfl.html
MD/JD: No
MD/PhD: Yes,
www.usc.edu/schools/medicine/ksomnfl.html
Master of Science in Clinical & Biomedical Investigations: Yes,
www.usc.edu/schools/medicine/ksomnfl.html

Premedical Coursework

Course	Req.	Rec.	Lab.	Sems.
Inorganic Chemistry	•		•	2
Behavioral Sciences				
Biochemistry	•			1
Biology	•		•	2
Biology/Zoology				
Calculus		•		
College English	•			
College Mathematics				

Course	Req.	Rec.	Lab.	Sems.
Computer Science		•		
Genetics				
Humanities	•			
Organic Chemistry	•		•	1
Physics	•		•	2
Psychology				
Social Sciences	•			
Molecular Biology	•			1

Selection Factors: 2007 Accepted Applicants

Proportion of Accepted Applicants with Relevant Experience (Data Self-Reported to AMCAS®)	
Community Service/Volunteer	69%
Medically-Related Work	89%
Research	86%

Shaded bar represents accepted scores ranging from the 10th percentile to the 90th percentile   School Median ●   National Median ●

Overall GPA	2.0	2.1	2.2	2.3	2.4	2.5	2.6	2.7	2.8	2.9	3.0	3.1	3.2	3.3	3.4	3.5	3.6	(3.7)	3.8	3.9	4.0
Science GPA	2.0	2.1	2.2	2.3	2.4	2.5	2.6	2.7	2.8	2.9	3.0	3.1	3.2	3.3	3.4	3.5	3.6	(3.7)	3.8	3.9	4.0

MCAT® required: Yes, 100% of 2007 accepted applicants took MCAT®

Verbal Reasoning	3	4	5	6	7	8	9	(10)	(11)	12	13	14	15
Physical Sciences	3	4	5	6	7	8	9	10	(11)	(12)	13	14	15
Biological Sciences	3	4	5	6	7	8	9	10	(11)	(12)	13	14	15
Writing Sample			J	K	L	M	N	O	P	(Q)	R	S	T

Acceptance & Matriculation Data for 2007–2008 First Year Class

	Resident	Non-Resident	International	Total
Applied	3541	2585	304	6430
Interviewed	488	214	14	716
Deferred	1	3	0	4
Matriculants				
Early Assurance Program	n/a	n/a	n/a	n/a
Early Decision Program	1	1	0	2
Baccalaureate/MD	7	2	0	9
MD/PhD	2	1	0	3
Matriculated	116	44	4	**164**

Applications accepted from International Applicants: Yes

Matriculant Demographics: 2007–2008 First Year Class

Men: 91   **Women:** 73

Matriculants' Self-Reported Race/Ethnicity

Mexican American	9	Korean	7
Cuban	1	Vietnamese	2
Puerto Rican	0	Other Asian	5
Other Hispanic	6	Total Asian	38
Total Hispanic	16	Native American	1
Chinese	11	Black	4
Asian Indian	10	Native Hawaiian	2
Pakistani	0	White	119
Filipino	2	Unduplicated Number	
Japanese	3	of Matriculants	164

Science and Math Majors: 63%
Matriculants with:
Baccalaureate degree: 100%
Graduate degree(s): 9%

Specialty Choice

2003, 2004, 2005 Graduates, Specialty Choice (As reported by program directors to GME Track™)	
Anesthesiology	4%
Emergency Medicine	5%
Family Practice	6%
Internal Medicine	17%
Obstetrics/Gynecology	6%
Orthopaedic Surgery	4%
Pediatrics	9%
Psychiatry	7%
Radiology Diagnostic	4%
Surgery General	6%

Financial Information

Source: 2006–2007 LCME I-B survey and 2007–2008 AAMC TSF questionnaire

	Residents	Non-Residents
Total Cost of Attendance	$67,100	$67,100
Tuition and Fees	$43,307	$43,307
Other (includes living expenses)	$22,860	$22,860
Health Insurance (can be waived)	$933	$933

Average 2007 Graduate Indebtedness: $168,903
% of Enrolled Students Receiving Aid: 89%

Criminal Background Check

This medical school does not require a criminal background check prior to matriculation.

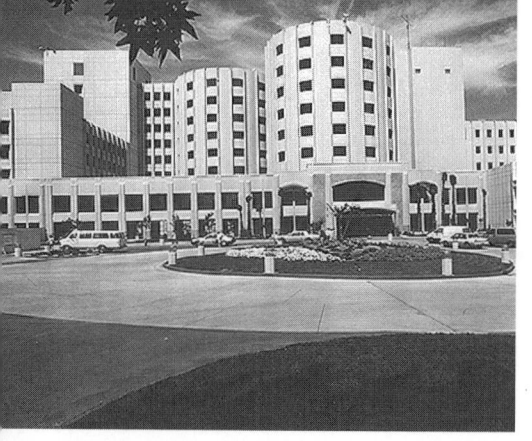

Loma Linda University School of Medicine

Loma Linda, California

Associate Dean for Admissions
Loma Linda University
School of Medicine
Loma Linda, California 92350
T 909 558 4467   F 909 558 0359

Admissions www.llu.edu/llu/academics/admissions.htm
Main www.llu.edu/llu/medicine
Financial www.llu.edu/ssweb/finaid
Email admissions.sm@llu.edu

Private Institution

Dr. H. Roger Hadley, Dean

Dr. Stephen A. Nyirady, Associate Dean for Admissions

Dr. Daisy Deleon, Assistant to the Dean for Diversity

Verdell Schaefer, MBA, Financial Aid Director

Lenoa Edwards, Assistant Dean for Admissions

General Information

The School of Medicine was established in 1909. It consists of basic science facilities and the Loma Linda University Medical Center. Also used for clinical instruction are local, regional, county, community, and Veterans Affairs hospitals. The School of Medicine's objectives include providing the student with a solid foundation of medical knowledge, assisting the student to attain professional skills, motivating investigative curiosity, and instilling a desire to participate in the advancement of knowledge. The school reinforces interest in the practical application of Christian principles through service to humanity.

Mission Statement

The school's overriding purpose is the formation of Christian physicians, educated to serve as generalists or specialists and providing whole-person care to individuals, families, and communities.

Curricular Highlights

Community Service Requirement: Optional.
Research/Thesis Requirement: Optional.
Numerous opportunities available

The School of Medicine seeks to prepare students who will be well grounded in the science and art of medicine. The first two years involve an organ systems-based approach to the study of the biomedical sciences, including their application to clinical medicine. The last two years provide clinical rotations in the major areas of medical practice: surgery, internal medicine, pediatrics, obstetrics-gynecology, family medicine, emergency medicine, ambulatory care, psychiatry, and preventive medicine. Elective time is available for additional experience in clinical or research areas. Qualified students interested in a career in academic medicine may earn an M.S. or Ph.D. degree along with the M.D. degree in a total of six to eight years. Student performance is evaluated by standard or scaled scores. The grading system is on a pass/fail basis.

USMLE

Step 1: Required. Students must record a passing score for promotion.
Step 2: Clinical Skills (CS): Required. Students must record a passing total score to graduate.
Step 2: Clinical Knowledge (CK): Required. Students must record a passing total score to graduate.

Selection Factors

The MCAT and a minimum of three years (90 semester hours or 135 quarter hours) of collegiate preparation in an accredited college or university in the U.S. or Canada are required. Preference is given to applicants who will have completed the baccalaureate degree prior to matriculation. No specific major is preferred. Demonstrated ability in the sciences is important. CLEP and pass/fail credits are not acceptable for required courses. Applicants are urged to take the MCAT by the spring of the application year. The Admissions Committee seeks candidates who have demonstrated the greatest potential for becoming capable physicians. A strong academic background is needed in preparation for medical studies. While special attention is given to performance in science courses, candidates should also have a solid foundation in the humanities, social sciences, and human behavior. The Admissions Committee seeks applicants who demonstrate problem-solving skills, critical judgment, and the ability to pursue independent study and thinking. For nonacademic qualifications, the committee looks for a commitment to medicine, sound judgment, a positive attitude, the ability to make decisions, participation in meaningful extracurricular activities, emotional stability, and integrity. The School of Medicine is owned and operated by the Seventh-day Adventist Church. While, therefore, preference for admission is given to members of this church, it is a firm policy of the Admissions Committee to admit a number of applicants from other faith traditions who have demonstrated a strong commitment to Christian principles. No candidate is accepted on the basis of religious affiliation alone. The school does not discriminate on the basis of race, sex, age, or handicap. After receipt of the AMCAS application, each applicant is requested to submit a supplementary form and supply preprofessional faculty evaluations and/or personal letters of recommendation. Invitations for an interview are extended to selected applicants. Applicants with an outstanding academic record and with a particular interest in Loma Linda University School of Medicine are encouraged to apply through the Early Decision Program (EDP). Final selections are made by the Admissions Committee on the basis of overall scholastic record, personal character and qualifications, and promise of success as a physician.

Financial Aid

The School of Medicine has loan funds available through the Student Finance Office. All aid is awarded on the basis of a uniform needs analysis. Financial aid information is provided to all accepted students. In view of the costs of a medical education, students are urged to plan their financial programs carefully.

Information about Diversity Programs

The School of Medicine encourages applications from persons from groups underrepresented in medicine. The Assistant to the Dean for Diversity works closely with the Office of Admissions to facilitate the admissions process for these applicants.

Campus Information

Enrollment

For 2007, total enrollment was: 686

Application Process and Requirements 2009–2010

Primary Application Service: AMCAS
Earliest filing date: June 1, 2008
Latest filing date: November 1, 2008

Secondary Application Required?: Yes
Sent to: All applicants
URL: Made available upon receipt
of verified AMCAS application
Contact: Office of Admissions, (909) 558-4467
admissions.sm@llu.edu
Fee: Yes, $75
Fee waiver available: Yes
Earliest filing date: July 1, 2008
Latest filing date: November 15, 2008

Latest MCAT® considered: September 2008
Oldest MCAT® considered: 2006

Early Decision Program
School does have EDP
Applicants notified: October 1, 2008
EDP available for: Both Residents
and Non-Residents

Regular Acceptance Notice
Earliest date: December 15, 2008
Latest date: Until class is full

Applicant's Response to Acceptance
Offer – Maximum Time: 30 days

Requests for Deferred
Entrance Considered: Yes

Deposit to Hold Place in Class: Yes
Deposit (Resident): $100
Deposit (Non-Resident): $100
Deposit due: With acceptance offer
Applied to tuition: Yes
Deposit refundable: Yes
Refundable by: May 15, 2009

Estimated number of new entrants: 175
EDP: 10, special program: n/a

Start Month/Year: August 2009

Interview Format:
Regional interviews are not available.

Other Programs

PREPARATORY PROGRAMS
Postbaccalaureate Program: No
Summer Program: No

COMBINED DEGREE PROGRAMS
Baccalaureate/MD: No
MD/MPH: No
MD/MBA: No
MD/JD: No
MD/PhD: Yes,
www.llu.edu/llu/medicine/basicsciences/msp.html
Lawrence Sowers, PhD, (909) 558-4480
lsowers@llu.edu

Premedical Coursework

Course	Req.	Rec.	Lab.	Hrs.
Inorganic Chemistry	•	•		8
Behavioral Sciences				
Biochemistry		•		
Biology				
Biology/Zoology	•		•	8
Calculus				
College English	•			
College Mathematics				

Course	Req.	Rec.	Lab.	Hrs.
Computer Science		•		
Genetics				
Humanities				
Organic Chemistry	•		•	8
Physics	•		•	8
Psychology				
Social Sciences				
Intro to Basic Statistics		•		

Selection Factors: 2007 Accepted Applicants

Proportion of Accepted Applicants with Relevant Experience (Data Self-Reported to AMCAS®)		
Community Service/Volunteer		72%
Medically-Related Work		74%
Research		66%

Shaded bar represents accepted scores ranging from the 10th percentile to the 90th percentile ▪   School Median ● National Median ●

Overall GPA	2.0	2.1	2.2	2.3	2.4	2.5	2.6	2.7	2.8	2.9	3.0	3.1	3.2	3.3	3.4	3.5	3.6	(3.7)	3.8	3.9	4.0
Science GPA	2.0	2.1	2.2	2.3	2.4	2.5	2.6	2.7	2.8	2.9	3.0	3.1	3.2	3.3	3.4	3.5	3.6	(3.7)	3.8	3.9	4.0

MCAT® required: Yes, 100% of 2007 accepted applicants took MCAT®

Verbal Reasoning	3	4	5	6	7	8	9	(10)	11	12	13	14	15
Physical Sciences	3	4	5	6	7	8	9	(10)	(11)	12	13	14	15
Biological Sciences	3	4	5	6	7	8	9	(10)	(11)	12	13	14	15
Writing Sample				J	K	L	M	N	O	(P)	(Q)	R	S	T

Acceptance & Matriculation Data for 2007–2008 First Year Class

	Resident	Non-Resident	International	Total
Applied	1993	2064	270	4327
Interviewed	196	168	27	391
Deferred	5	2	4	11
Matriculants				
Early Assurance Program	0	0	0	0
Early Decision Program	4	4	1	9
Baccalaureate/MD	n/a	n/a	n/a	n/a
MD/PhD	0	1	1	2
Matriculated	83	74	15	**172**

Applications accepted from International Applicants: Yes

Matriculant Demographics: 2007–2008 First Year Class

Men: 97   **Women:** 75

Matriculants' Self-Reported Race/Ethnicity

Mexican American	4	Korean	23
Cuban	0	Vietnamese	1
Puerto Rican	4	Other Asian	4
Other Hispanic	11	Total Asian	49
Total Hispanic	18	Native American	1
Chinese	18	Black	10
Asian Indian	0	Native Hawaiian	0
Pakistani	0	White	94
Filipino	5	Unduplicated Number	
Japanese	1	of Matriculants	172

Science and Math Majors: 68%
Matriculants with:
Baccalaureate degree: 98%
Graduate degree(s): 6%

Specialty Choice

2003, 2004, 2005 Graduates, Specialty Choice (As reported by program directors to GME Track™)	
Anesthesiology	10%
Emergency Medicine	8%
Family Practice	17%
Internal Medicine	13%
Obstetrics/Gynecology	3%
Orthopaedic Surgery	3%
Pediatrics	5%
Psychiatry	6%
Radiology	2%
Surgery	8%

Financial Information

Source: 2006–2007 LCME I-B survey
and 2007–2008 AAMC TSF questionnaire

	Residents	Non-Residents
Total Cost of Attendance	$58,046	$58,046
Tuition and Fees	$35,506	$35,506
Other (includes living expenses)	$21,100	$21,100
Health Insurance (can be waived)	$1,440	$1,440

Average 2007 Graduate Indebtedness: $150,190
% of Enrolled Students Receiving Aid: 89%

Criminal Background Check

This medical school requires a criminal background check prior to matriculation.

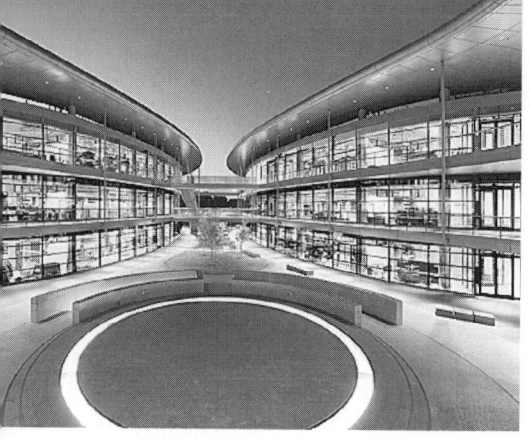

Stanford University School of Medicine

Stanford, California

Office of MD Admissions
Stanford University School of Medicine
251 Campus Drive, MSOB X3C01
Stanford, California 94305-5404
T 650 723 6861   F 650 725 7855

Admissions http://med.stanford.edu/md/admissions
Main http://med.stanford.edu
Financial http://med.stanford.edu/md/financial_aid
Email mdadmissions@stanford.edu

Private Institution

Dr. Philip A. Pizzo, Dean

Dr. Gabriel Garcia, Associate Dean of Medical School Admissions

Dr. Ronald D. Garcia, Assistant Dean of Minority Affairs

Charlene Hamada, Assistant Dean of Student Affairs

Jonnie Perez, Assistant Director of Medical School Admissions

General Information

The School of Medicine is an integral part of Stanford University. The history of Stanford Medical School begins in 1858 with the founding in San Francisco by Dr. Elias Samuel Cooper of the first medical school on the Pacific Coast. Stanford's School of Medicine is the lineal descendent of this pioneer medical school. In 1908, Stanford University adopted the Cooper Medical College in San Francisco as its medical school and moved it to the university campus in 1959. The Stanford School of Medicine is consistently ranked in the top ten of all research university medical centers in the country.

Mission Statement

Stanford is committed to being a premier research-intensive medical school that improves health through leadership, collaborative discoveries, and innovation in patient care, education, and research. In particular, Stanford seeks individuals whose leadership will result in significant advances in the ability to care for patients. We strive to admit a diverse body of students who are interested in the intellectual substance of medicine and are committed to advancing the field of medicine, broadly defined (i.e. clinical medicine, biomedical sciences, health policy, medical education, and community health).

Curricular Highlights

Community Service Requirement: Optional. Opportunities available and encouraged.
Research/Thesis Requirement: Optional. Opportunities available and encouraged.

Stanford is committed to ensuring that each graduate has fully explored his/her potential as a student and as a scholar. Key goals of the curriculum are the melding of 21st century laboratory and medical sciences, and helping each student build in-depth expertise in an area of personal interest through our Scholarly Concentrations program. While traditional courses and clerkships are required for graduation, the duration of study leading to the M.D. degree may vary from four to six years. All M.D. candidates must satisfactorily complete at least 13 quarters of academic work. Fees for additional quarters are nominal. Courses are graded pass/fail.

USMLE

Step 1: Required. Students must record a passing score for promotion.
Step 2: Clinical Skills (CS): Required. Students must record a passing total score to graduate.
Step 2: Clinical Knowledge (CK): Required. Students must record a passing total score to graduate.

Selection Factors

Stanford does not discriminate on the basis of race, religion, national origin, sex, marital status, age, or disability. The applicant's state of residence is not relevant in the selection process. Applicants whose MCAT® scores are below the national mean are highly unlikely to be admitted to the medical school. Transfer Students: For information on the transfer policy, see the Stanford Web site.

Financial Aid

Available grant and loan funds are awarded to students on the basis of demonstrated need. Our generous financial aid program allows our students to graduate with one of the lowest educational debts for any medical school, private or public. For federal aid, students are considered to be independent. For university-based aid, students are considered to be dependent up until the age of 30, and the school will consider the student's parents' ability to contribute to the cost of financing the student's education in determining eligibility for loans and grants. Foreign students must complete a certification of finances reflecting an account of funds to cover the cost of education for the M.D. degree.

Information about Diversity Programs

Stanford takes pride in its highly diverse and exceptionally qualified student body and is committed to increasing the representation of members of groups underrepresented in medicine. It particularly encourages applications from such candidates and others that will contribute to the diversity of the learning environment.

Campus Information

Setting

The school is located on the 8,800 acre campus of Stanford University (second largest university complex in the world) and is situated in Northern California, approximately 35 miles south of San Francisco and 25 miles north of San Jose.

Enrollment

For 2007, total enrollment was: 463

Special Features

The combination of scientists who pursue basic science research questions and clinicians closely involved in patient care leads to innovative, fruitful collaboration. An example is Bio-X, a unique program designed to promote interdepartmental bioscience research. The program fosters the convergence of leading-edge research in basic, applied and clinical sciences across the spectrum from molecules to organisms. The program involves the schools of Humanities and Sciences, Engineering, and Medicine and is housed in the James H. Clark Center for Biomedical and Engineering Sciences.

Housing

On-campus housing is guaranteed for the first year.

Satellite Campuses/Facilities

Student rotations take place in the major clinical teaching facilities: Stanford Hospital (663 beds), Lucile Packard Children's Hospital (152 beds), Santa Clara County Valley Medical Center (791 beds), the Palo Alto Veterans Affairs Hospital (1,000 beds), and Kaiser Santa Clara Medical Center (327 beds).

Application Process and Requirements 2009–2010

Primary Application Service: AMCAS
Earliest filing date: June 1, 2008
Latest filing date: October 15, 2008

Secondary Application Required?: Yes
Sent to: All applicants
URL: https://med.stanford.edu/aes/
Fee: Yes, $85
Fee waiver available: Yes
Earliest filing date: July 1, 2008
Latest filing date: November 15, 2008

Latest MCAT® considered: September 2008
Oldest MCAT® considered: August 2006

**Early Decision Program
School does have EDP
Applicants notified:** October 1, 2008
EDP available for: Both Residents
and Non-Residents

**Regular Acceptance Notice
Earliest date:** December 2008
Latest date: Varies

**Applicant's Response to Acceptance
Offer – Maximum Time:** Two weeks

**Requests for Deferred
Entrance Considered:** Yes

Deposit to Hold Place in Class: Yes
Deposit (Resident): $100
Deposit (Non-Resident): $100
Deposit due: n/a
Applied to tuition: Yes
Deposit refundable: Yes
Refundable by: May 16, 2009

Estimated number of new entrants: 86
EDP: 1, special program: n/a

Start Month/Year: August 2009

Interview Format: One faculty and one
student interview. Regional interviews are
not available.

Other Programs

**PREPARATORY PROGRAMS
Postbaccalaureate Program:** No
Summer Program: Yes,
http://coe.stanford.edu/

**COMBINED DEGREE PROGRAMS
Baccalaureate/MD:** No
MD/MPH: Yes, http://med.stanford.edu/md-mph/
MD/MBA: No
MD/JD: No
MD/PhD: Yes, http://mstp.stanford.edu

Premedical Coursework

Course	Req.	Rec.	Lab.	Sems.
Inorganic Chemistry	•		•	2
Behavioral Sciences		•		
Biochemistry				
Biology	•		•	2
Biology/Zoology				
Calculus		•		
College English				
College Mathematics				

Course	Req.	Rec.	Lab.	Sems.
Computer Science				
Genetics				
Humanities			•	
Organic Chemistry	•		•	2
Physics	•		•	2
Psychology				
Social Sciences			•	
Other 1 & 2			•	

Selection Factors: 2007 Accepted Applicants

Proportion of Accepted Applicants with Relevant Experience (Data Self-Reported to AMCAS®)		
Community Service/Volunteer	69%	
Medically-Related Work	87%	
Research	95%	

Shaded bar represents accepted scores ranging from the 10th percentile to the 90th percentile. School Median ● National Median ●

Overall GPA	2.0	2.1	2.2	2.3	2.4	2.5	2.6	2.7	2.8	2.9	3.0	3.1	3.2	3.3	3.4	3.5	3.6	3.7	(3.8)	3.9	4.0
Science GPA	2.0	2.1	2.2	2.3	2.4	2.5	2.6	2.7	2.8	2.9	3.0	3.1	3.2	3.3	3.4	3.5	3.6	3.7	(3.8)	3.9	4.0

MCAT® required: Yes, 100% of 2007 accepted applicants took MCAT®

Verbal Reasoning	3	4	5	6	7	8	9	(10)	(11)	12	13	14	15
Physical Sciences	3	4	5	6	7	8	9	10	(11)	12	(13)	14	15
Biological Sciences	3	4	5	6	7	8	9	10	(11)	12	(13)	14	15
Writing Sample				J	K	L	M	N	O	P	(Q)	R	S	T

Acceptance & Matriculation Data for 2007–2008 First Year Class

	Resident	Non-Resident	International	Total
Applied	2460	3661	336	6457
Interviewed	207	356	22	585
Deferred	8	13	1	22
Matriculants				
Early Assurance Program	n/a	n/a	n/a	n/a
Early Decision Program	0	0	0	0
Baccalaureate/MD	n/a	n/a	n/a	n/a
MD/PhD	4	8	0	12
Matriculated	35	48	3	**86**

Applications accepted from International Applicants: Yes

Specialty Choice

2003, 2004, 2005 Graduates, Specialty Choice (As reported by program directors to GME Track™)	
Anesthesiology	7%
Emergency Medicine	6%
Family Practice	7%
Internal Medicine	13%
Obstetrics/Gynecology	3%
Orthopaedic Surgery	4%
Pediatrics	8%
Psychiatry	7%
Radiology	6%
Surgery	5%

Matriculant Demographics: 2007–2008 First Year Class

Men: 55   **Women:** 31

Matriculants' Self-Reported Race/Ethnicity

Mexican American	6	Korean	2
Cuban	1	Vietnamese	3
Puerto Rican	0	Other Asian	4
Other Hispanic	2	Total Asian	36
Total Hispanic	9	Native American	0
Chinese	17	Black	2
Asian Indian	12	Native Hawaiian	1
Pakistani	0	White	39
Filipino	0	**Unduplicated Number**	
Japanese	0	**of Matriculants**	86

Science and Math Majors: 86%
Matriculants with:
          Baccalaureate degree: 100%
          Graduate degree(s): 23%

Financial Information

Source: 2006–2007 LCME I-B survey
and 2007–2008 AAMC TSF questionnaire

	Residents	Non-Residents
Total Cost of Attendance	$67,400	$67,400
Tuition and Fees	$41,850	$41,850
Other (includes living expenses)	$23,498	$23,498
Health Insurance (can be waived)	$2,052	$2,052

Average 2007 Graduate Indebtedness: $76,650
% of Enrolled Students Receiving Aid: 77%

Criminal Background Check

This medical school does not require a criminal
background check prior to matriculation.

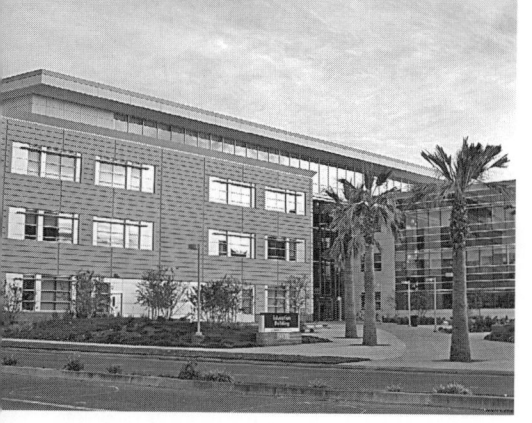

University of California, Davis, School of Medicine
Sacramento, California

Office of Admissions and Outreach
School of Medicine University of California
4610 X Street, Suite 1202
Sacramento California 95817
T 916 734 4800

Admissions www.ucdmc.ucdavis.edu/ome/admissions/
Main www.ucdmc.ucdavis.edu/medschool
Financial www.ucdmc.ucdavis.edu/ome/finaid/
Email medadmsinfo@ucdavis.edu

Public Institution

Dr. Claire Pomeroy, Dean

*Edward D. Dagang,
Director of Admissions and Outreach*

*Dr. Mark Henderson, Associate Dean,
Admissions & Outreach*

Lauren Snow, Financial Aid Director

General Information
With a new, state-of-the-art home on the Sacramento campus, the UC Davis School of medicine prides itself in offering a rich and diverse academic environment. The school grooms students for leadership roles in medicine, research, health policy, medical education and management/administration. Distinctions include: ranking in the top 50 schools for research and primary care, strong, dual-degree programs (M.P.H., M.B.A., Ph.D.), and a new five-year program for students interested in telecommunications-enhanced rural medicine. The school admitted its first class in 1968.

Mission Statement
With a mantra of, "Learn. Discover. Share.", the school's educational mission is to create a supportive and collaborative environment which empowers students to develop skills, knowledge and attitudes to become tomorrow's leaders in patient care, public service, research and education. The mission of the larger UC Davis Health System is "discovering and sharing knowledge to advance health."

Curricular Highlights
Community Service Requirement: Optional.
Research/Thesis Requirement: Optional.

UC Davis believes that acquiring and perfecting the skills needed to become a compassionate, culturally-competent and knowledgeable physician requires a combination of hands-on experiences, didactic instruction and problem-based challenges. With an emphasis on self-directed and small group learning, our curriculum is designed to encourage students to evaluate, think and formulate decisions to provide the highest level of patient care. Basic and clinical science courses are designed to illuminate situations that arise in the clinical setting as well as to spark interest in biomedical research, public health and other areas. A cutting-edge Clinical Skills Center in our new medical education building maximizes technology's role in learning from standardized patients. Finally, our students gain valuable experience through their leadership roles in the community, including our five student-run free health clinics which benefit various underserved populations in the diverse Sacramento area.

USMLE
Step 1: Required. Students must record a passing score for promotion.
Step 2: Clinical Skills (CS): Required. Students must record a passing total score to graduate.
Step 2: Clinical Knowledge (CK): Required. Students must record a passing total score to graduate.

Selection Factors
Academic strengths in both physical/biological sciences and humanities are valued, as are experiences in both research and clinical care. We look for a broad array of life experiences which align with our institutional values of diversity, equality, community engagement and accessible healthcare.

Financial Aid
Most financial aid is based on demonstrated need, and a wide range of scholarships, fellowships, grants and loans are available. All students are considered for university-awarded, merit and need-based scholarships.

Information about Diversity Programs
Our curriculum's emphasis on cultural competency aligns well with our diverse medical student body, which reflects the diversity of California. The health system often hosts and/or sponsors local, state and regional meetings of medical student organizations including the Latino Medical Student Association and the Student National Medical Association. The UC Davis Health System's Office of Diversity is committed to fostering a supportive environment that maximizes the learning and working experiences for all medical students, residents, faculty and staff.

Campus Information

Setting
The new Medical Education building is located on UC Davis' growing Sacramento campus. The 140-acre area is adjacent to downtown Sacramento and is home to our level-one trauma teaching hospital (UC Davis Medical Center), our Children's Hospital, our NCI-designate Cancer Center, a leading national autism facility called the MIND Institute, our outpatient clinics, and a variety of research labs, including our stem cell research center. In the coming year, the Sacramento campus will also be home to the New California Telemedicine Resource Center and the new UC Davis Betty Irene Moore School of Nursing.

Enrollment
For 2007, total enrollment was: 400

Special Features
The school continues to rise quickly in NIH rankings and was awarded one of the first twelve prestigious NIH Clinical and Translational Science Awards in 2006. In 2005, the school won the AAMC's Outstanding Community Service Award.

Housing
Most students reside in communities surrounding the Sacramento campus, including the thriving urban Midtown area. Sacramento residents benefit from a variety of recreational, cultural, political and nightlife activities while living in one of California's more manageable and navigable cities.

Satellite Campuses/Facilities
Most clinical rotations take place at the UC Davis Medical Center in Sacramento and other facilities in the UC Davis Health System. Others take place at Sacramento's Kaiser, Sutter and Methodist hospitals as well as David Grant Medical Center at Travis Air Force Base and San Joaquin General Hospital in Stockton. Students enrolled in our new Rural-PRIME program have opportunities to rotate through our rural hospital network sites and some students gain credit at hospitals and clinics abroad.

Application Process and Requirements 2009–2010

Primary Application Service: AMCAS
Earliest filing date: June 1, 2008
Latest filing date: October 1, 2008

Secondary Application Required?: Yes
Sent to: Screened applicants
Contact: Terri Hall
(916)734-4800, terri.hall@ucdmc.ucdavis.edu
Fee: Yes, $60
Fee waiver available: Yes
Earliest filing date: July 1, 2008
Latest filing date: February 1, 2009

Latest MCAT® considered: September 2008
Oldest MCAT® considered: August 2005

Early Decision Program
School does not have EDP
Applicants notified: n/a
EDP available for: n/a

Regular Acceptance Notice
Earliest date: October 15, 2008
Latest date: Until class is full

Applicant's Response to Acceptance
Offer – Maximum Time: Two weeks

Requests for Deferred
Entrance Considered: Yes

Deposit to Hold Place in Class: No
Deposit (Resident): n/a
Deposit (Non-Resident): n/a
Deposit due: n/a
Applied to tuition: n/a
Deposit refundable: n/a
Refundable by: n/a

Estimated number of new entrants: 105
EDP: n/a, special program: n/a

Start Month/Year: End of July 2009

Interview Format: Open file, two interviews. Regional interviews are not available.

Other Programs

PREPARATORY PROGRAMS
Postbaccalaureate Program: Yes,
www.ucdmc.ucdavis.edu/ome/postbacc/index.html
Summer Program: No

COMBINED DEGREE PROGRAMS
Baccalaureate/MD: No
MD/MPH: Yes, http://mph.ucdavis.edu
Stephen McCurdy, M.D.
(530) 752-8051, samccurdy@ucdavis.edu
MD/MBA: Yes, www.gsm.ucdavis.edu/students
David L. Woodruff, (530) 752-0515
dlwoodruff@ucdavis.edu
MD/JD: No
MD/PhD: Yes, http://mdphd.ucdavis.edu
Michael F. Seldin, M.D., Ph.D.
(530) 754-6016, mfseldin@ucdavis.edu

Premedical Coursework

Course	Req.	Rec.	Lab.	Qtrs.
Inorganic Chemistry	•		•	15
Behavioral Sciences		•		
Biochemistry		•		4
Biology	•		•	15
Biology/Zoology				
Calculus	•			6
College English	•			12
College Mathematics				

Course	Req.	Rec.	Lab.	Qtrs.
Computer Science				
Genetics		•		4
Humanities				
Organic Chemistry		•	•	12
Physics	•		•	12
Psychology				
Social Sciences		•		
College Statistics		•		4

Selection Factors: 2007 Accepted Applicants

Proportion of Accepted Applicants with Relevant Experience (Data Self-Reported to AMCAS®)		
Community Service/Volunteer		71%
Medically-Related Work		89%
Research		83%

Shaded bar represents accepted scores ranging from the 10th percentile to the 90th percentile — School Median ○ National Median ○

Overall GPA	2.0	2.1	2.2	2.3	2.4	2.5	2.6	2.7	2.8	2.9	3.0	3.1	3.2	3.3	3.4	3.5	3.6	(3.7)	3.8	3.9	4.0
Science GPA	2.0	2.1	2.2	2.3	2.4	2.5	2.6	2.7	2.8	2.9	3.0	3.1	3.2	3.3	3.4	3.5	(3.6)	3.7	3.8	3.9	4.0

MCAT® required: Yes, 100% of 2007 accepted applicants took MCAT®

Verbal Reasoning	3	4	5	6	7	8	9	(10)	11	12	13	14	15
Physical Sciences	3	4	5	6	7	8	9	10	(11)	12	13	14	15
Biological Sciences	3	4	5	6	7	8	9	10	(11)	12	13	14	15
Writing Sample			J	K	L	M	N	O	P	(Q)	R	S	T

Acceptance & Matriculation Data for 2007–2008 First Year Class

	Resident	Non-Resident	International	Total
Applied	3774	929	158	4861
Interviewed	439	30	1	470
Deferred	4	1	0	5
Matriculants				
Early Assurance Program	n/a	n/a	n/a	n/a
Early Decision Program	0	0	0	0
Baccalaureate/MD	n/a	n/a	n/a	n/a
MD/PhD	3	0	0	3
Matriculated	103	2	0	**105**

Applications accepted from International Applicants: Yes

Specialty Choice

2003, 2004, 2005 Graduates, Specialty Choice (As reported by program directors to GME Track™)	
Anesthesiology	3%
Emergency Medicine	10%
Family Practice	12%
Internal Medicine	17%
Obstetrics/Gynecology	3%
Orthopaedic Surgery	4%
Pediatrics	13%
Psychiatry	9%
Radiology	6%
Surgery	7%

Matriculant Demographics: 2007–2008 First Year Class

Men: 43   **Women:** 62

Matriculants' Self-Reported Race/Ethnicity

Mexican American	9	Korean	3
Cuban	1	Vietnamese	3
Puerto Rican	0	Other Asian	4
Other Hispanic	7	Total Asian	41
Total Hispanic	16	Native American	0
Chinese	15	Black	3
Asian Indian	13	Native Hawaiian	0
Pakistani	1	White	54
Filipino	3	Unduplicated Number	
Japanese	3	of Matriculants	105

Science and Math Majors: 62%
Matriculants with:
   Baccalaureate degree: 100%
   Graduate degree(s): 13%

Financial Information

Source: 2006–2007 LCME I-B survey and 2007–2008 AAMC TSF questionnaire

	Residents	Non-Residents
Total Cost of Attendance	$44,475	$56,720
Tuition and Fees	$24,299	$36,544
Other (includes living expenses)	$18,721	$18,721
Health Insurance (can be waived)	$1,455	$1,455

Average 2007 Graduate Indebtedness: $106,322
% of Enrolled Students Receiving Aid: 93%

Criminal Background Check

This medical school does not require a criminal background check prior to matriculation.

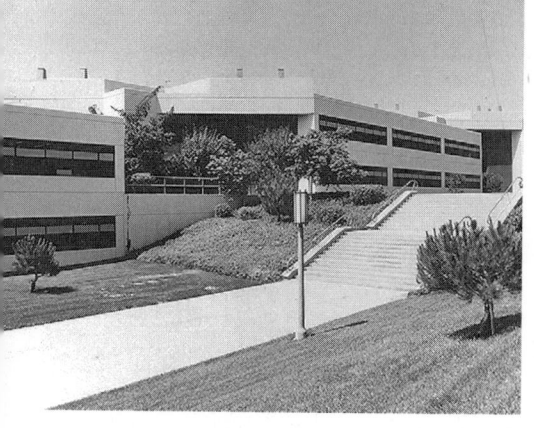

University of California, Irvine, School of Medicine

Irvine, California

University of California Irvine School of Medicine
Office of Admissions and Outreach
Berk Hall, Room 100
Irvine, California 92697-4089
T 800 824 5388   **F** 949 824 2485

Admissions www.ucihs.uci.edu/admissions
Main www.ha.uci.edu/som/meded/
Financial www.ofas.uci.edu/content/Medical
Entering.aspx
Email medadmit@uci.edu

Public Institution

Dr. David Bailey, Vice Chancellor for Health Affairs and Dean

Dr. Ellena M. Peterson, Associate Dean for Admissions and Outreach

Luis Medina, Director of Financial Aid

Gayle J. Pierce, Director of Admissions and Outreach

General Information

The UC Irvine School of Medicine is located in Orange County between Los Angeles and San Diego. Approximately 425 medical students are enrolled; the faculty includes 650 full-time and 1,500 voluntary members in 25 academic departments. Areas of research emphasis include: neurosciences, oncology, cardiovascular and pulmonary diseases, infectious diseases and molecular biology. Educational facilities are located on the main UC Irvine campus and approximately 10 miles north on the Orange campus is the UC Irvine Medical Center. In addition to the Medical Center, clinical facilities include off-site outpatient facilities and numerous affiliated hospitals and clinics. Special programs within the medical school include MD/MBA and MD/PhD (MSTP) programs and the Program in Medical Education for the Latino Community (PRIME-LC) that incorporates a MD and Master's degree emphasizing Latino heath care issues.

Mission Statement

The UC Irvine School of Medicine is dedicated to advancing the knowledge and practice of medicine for the benefit of society. This mission will be achieved through programs of excellence in education, research, clinical care, and service to the public.

Curricular Highlights

Community Service Requirement: Optional.
Research/Thesis Requirement: Optional.

The UC Irvine School of Medicine is dedicated to the nurturing of humanistic, caring physicians with state-of-the-art clinical expertise and

skills. In addition to the basic sciences in the first two years, substantial clinical material has been integrated into the curriculum through the development of the Clinical Foundations/Introduction to Medicine course. In the first year, students work with standardized patients to develop interview and physical examination skills. These clinical skills are further strengthened in the second year by working in the community with patients. In addition, clinically oriented courses are designed to complement the material covered in basic science courses. During the clinical years, students rotate through the core clinical services of internal medicine, family medicine, surgery, obstetrics and gynecology, psychiatry, pediatrics, emergency medicine, radiology, and neurology. Clinical advisors guide students in the selection of 20 weeks of electives tailored to the students' career goals and educational needs.

USMLE

Step 1: Required. Students must record a passing score for promotion.
Step 2: Clinical Skills (CS): Required. Students must record a passing total score to graduate.
Step 2: Clinical Knowledge (CK): Required. Students must record a passing total score to graduate.

Selection Factors

The Admissions Committee screens for applicants whose academic records indicate that they will be able to handle the medical school curriculum. In addition to scholastic achievement, attributes deemed desirable in prospective students include leadership and participation in extracurricular activities, including exposure to clinical medicine, research, and community service. Consideration is given to applicants from disadvantaged backgrounds. Preference is given to California residents and applicants who are either U.S. citizens or Permanent Residents. The School of Medicine does not accept transfer students.

Financial Aid

The Financial Aid Office coordinates financial aid application materials; reviews and evaluates information provided by applicants; secures, manages, and provides funds in the form of scholarships,

grants, and loans to assist in meeting students' educational expenses; and provides debt management counseling.

Information about Diversity Programs

UC Irvine is a multicultural community, composed of individuals from diverse backgrounds. Activities, programs, classes, workshops, lectures, and everyday interactions are enriched by acceptance of one another. The university community strives to create an atmosphere of positive engagement and mutual respect.

Campus Information

Enrollment

For 2007, total enrollment was: 429

Special Features

The UC Irvine Medical Center offers a full scope of acute and general medical care. A new state-of-the-art acute care inpatient facility is scheduled for completion by Spring 2009. The Medical Center houses the most sophisticated neonatal unit in the county, the University Children's Hospital, an Emergency Department which is designated as Orange County's only Level I Trauma Center, a Neuropsychiatric Center, and the Chao Family Comprehensive Cancer Center. In addition, as part of its focus on family and preventive health, the UC Irvine Medical Center has five neighborhood health centers located throughout Orange County. The new Medical Education Building is scheduled to open on the UC Irvine campus by Fall 2009. Included in this facility will be a simulation and clinical skills suite, lecture halls and small group teaching rooms, all with telemedicine and video conferencing capability.

Housing

On-campus apartment communities are available to single and married students with families. Services are also available to assist students looking for off-campus housing.

Application Process and Requirements 2009–2010

Primary Application Service: AMCAS
Earliest filing date: June 1, 2008
Latest filing date: November 1, 2008

Secondary Application Required?: Yes
Sent to: Screened applicants
URL: n/a
Fee: Yes, $60
Fee waiver available: Yes
Earliest filing date: July 15, 2008
Latest filing date: January 15, 2009

Latest MCAT® considered: September 2008
Oldest MCAT® considered: 2006

Early Decision Program
School does not have EDP
Applicants notified: n/a
EDP available for: n/a

Regular Acceptance Notice
Earliest date: November 15, 2008
Latest date: Until class is full

Applicant's Response to Acceptance Offer – Maximum Time: Two weeks

Requests for Deferred Entrance Considered: Yes

Deposit to Hold Place in Class: No
Deposit (Resident): n/a
Deposit (Non-Resident): n/a
Deposit due: n/a
Applied to tuition: n/a
Deposit refundable: n/a
Refundable by: n/a

Estimated number of new entrants: 104
EDP: n/a, special program: n/a

Start Month/Year: August 2009

Interview Format: Selected applicants are interviewed by both a faculty member and a student. Regional interviews are not available.

Other Programs

PREPARATORY PROGRAMS
Postbaccalaureate Program: Yes
outreach@uci.edu
www.ucihs.uci.edu/admissions
Summer Program: No

COMBINED DEGREE PROGRAMS
Baccalaureate/MD: No
MD/MPH: No
MD/MBA: Yes,
www.ucihs.uci.edu/com/mdmba
MD/JD: No
MD/PhD: Yes,
http://mstp.uci.edu
Additional Program: Yes,
www.ucihs.uci.edu/PRIMELC

Premedical Coursework

Course	Req.	Rec.	Lab.	Sems.
Inorganic Chemistry	•	•		2
Behavioral Sciences		•		
Biochemistry	•			1
Biology	•	•		2
Biology/Zoology				
Calculus				1
College English	•			1
College Mathematics				

Course	Req.	Rec.	Lab.	Sems.
Genetics		•		
Humanities		•		
Organic Chemistry	•		•	2
Physics	•			2
Psychology				
Social Sciences				
Upper Division Biology	•			1
Statistics		•		1

Selection Factors: 2007 Accepted Applicants

Proportion of Accepted Applicants with Relevant Experience (Data Self-Reported to AMCAS®)		
Community Service/Volunteer	71%
Medically-Related Work	94%
Research	91%

Shaded bar represents accepted scores ranging from the 10th percentile to the 90th percentile — School Median ● National Median ●

Overall GPA	2.0	2.1	2.2	2.3	2.4	2.5	2.6	2.7	2.8	2.9	3.0	3.1	3.2	3.3	3.4	3.5	3.6	(3.7)	3.8	3.9	4.0
Science GPA	2.0	2.1	2.2	2.3	2.4	2.5	2.6	2.7	2.8	2.9	3.0	3.1	3.2	3.3	3.4	3.5	3.6	(3.7)	3.8	3.9	4.0

MCAT® required: Yes, 100% of 2007 accepted applicants took MCAT®

Verbal Reasoning	3	4	5	6	7	8	9	(10)	11	12	13	14	15
Physical Sciences	3	4	5	6	7	8	9	10	(11)	12	13	14	15
Biological Sciences	3	4	5	6	7	8	9	10	(11)	12	13	14	15
Writing Sample			J	K	L	M	N	O	P	(Q)	R	S	T

Acceptance & Matriculation Data for 2007–2008 First Year Class

	Resident	Non-Resident	International	Total
Applied	3749	726	61	4536
Interviewed	455	18	0	473
Deferred	3	0	0	3
Matriculants				
Early Assurance Program	0	0	0	0
Early Decision Program	0	0	0	0
Baccalaureate/MD	n/a	n/a	n/a	n/a
MD/PhD	3	3	0	6
Matriculated	101	3	0	**104**

Applications accepted from International Applicants: No

Specialty Choice

2003, 2004, 2005 Graduates, Specialty Choice (As reported by program directors to GME Track™)	
Anesthesiology	7%
Emergency Medicine	9%
Family Practice	10%
Internal Medicine	17%
Obstetrics/Gynecology	8%
Orthopaedic Surgery	3%
Pediatrics	6%
Psychiatry	8%
Radiology	4%
Surgery	5%

Matriculant Demographics: 2007–2008 First Year Class

Men: 53　　　　**Women:** 51

Matriculants' Self-Reported Race/Ethnicity

Mexican American	5	Korean	2
Cuban	0	Vietnamese	9
Puerto Rican	0	Other Asian	5
Other Hispanic	6	Total Asian	39
Total Hispanic	11	Native American	2
Chinese	16	Black	3
Asian Indian	5	Native Hawaiian	1
Pakistani	2	White	55
Filipino	2	Unduplicated Number	
Japanese	3	of Matriculants	104

Science and Math Majors: 74%
Matriculants with:
　　Baccalaureate degree: 100%
　　Graduate degree(s): 8%

Financial Information

Source: 2006–2007 LCME I-B survey and 2007–2008 AAMC TSF questionnaire

	Residents	Non-Residents
Total Cost of Attendance	$44,986	$57,231
Tuition and Fees	$21,823	$34,068
Other (includes living expenses)	$20,657	$20,657
Health Insurance (can be waived)	$2,506	$2,506

Average 2007 Graduate Indebtedness: $115,362
% of Enrolled Students Receiving Aid: 90%

Criminal Background Check

This medical school requires a criminal background check prior to matriculation.

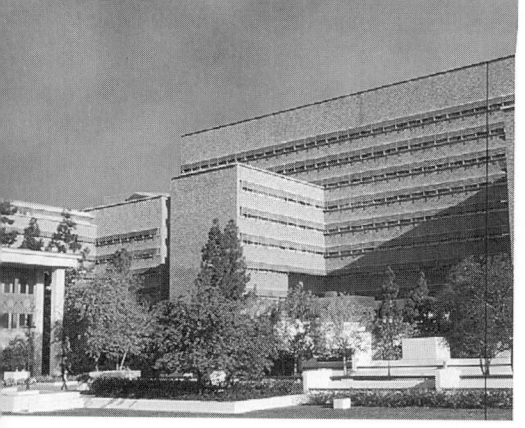

University of California, Los Angeles
David Geffen School of Medicine at UCLA
Los Angeles, California

David Geffen School of Medicine at UCLA
Office of Admissions
10833 Le Conte Avenue
Los Angeles, California 90095-7035
T 310 825 6081

Admissions www.medstudent.ucla.edu/ prospective/
Main http://dgsom.healthsciences.ucla.edu/ms-resources
Financial www.medstudent.ucla.edu/current/fao/
?pgID=210
Email somadmiss@mednet.ucla.edu

Public Institution

Dr. Gerald Levey, Dean

Lili Fobert, Director of Admissions

Patricia Pratt, Director of Outreach

Teddie Milner, Director of Financial Aid

Dr. Neil Parker, Dean for Admissions and Students

General Information

The David Geffen School of Medicine at UCLA is on the UCLA campus. The University Medical Center, Ambulatory Plaza, Mattel Children's and Neuropsychiatric Hospital and Eye Institute are adjacent. These institutions, together with the Schools of Dentistry, Nursing, and Public Health, are integral parts of the environment. Major affiliations include LA County Harbor and Oliveview Medical Centers, Veterans Affairs Medical Centers West LA and Sepulveda, Cedars-Sinai Medical Center and Kaiser Permanente. The decision of which medical school to attend is extremely important. We provide applicants with critical information through our websites. Applicants may check their status on the Admission Web site. Students invited for interviews participate in student tours, meet faculty, students, staff, and members of the Admissions Committee.

Mission Statement

The school seeks students who will be future leaders, have distinguished careers in clinical practice, teaching, research, and public service. The school strives to create an environment in which students prepare for a future where scientific knowledge, societal values and human needs are ever-changing.

Curricular Highlights

Community Service Requirement: Optional. Student-run Clinics are numerous; 80% do service.

Research/Thesis Requirement: Optional. Over 75% participate in research.

The first two years present a thorough grounding in the science basic to medicine. An integrated approach to basic & clinical sciences is enhanced through problem-based learning in small groups. Students are introduced to a holistic approach to patient care from the beginning through the nationally recognized Doctoring course. The first two years center on processes of disease, with emphasis on organ system-oriented instruction. The third year core clerkships encompass internal medicine, surgery, obstetrics and gynecology, pediatrics, psychiatry, family practice, radiology, and neurology. The senior year, through a set of Colleges, provide a unique mentoring and educational experience bringing together student and faculty with similar interests. Senior electives are designed to provide students with a foundation to develop and fulfill personal interests, broaden clinical knowledge, and provide an advantage in securing desired residencies. UCLA has a pass/fail grading system, allowing students to actively participate in school and student-organized activities. There are student run clinics at the Salvation Army Homeless Center, Mobile Clinic, Health Fairs, and activities teaching high school students preventive health, and work with the underserved. Student use summers for research, community work, and international work. The MSTP programs leads to MD-PhD degrees for those interested in research. This program requires 3-5 additional years to the MD study. Stipends are provided for this program. The school also offers joint MD-MBA and MD-MPH programs chosen in the junior year. The program is designed for students interested in organization leadership roles. Our Drew program is for those interested in the underserved. Our UCR/UCLA Program is a cooperative venture with the University of California, Riverside. Students spend their first two years at UCR with the same curriculum as UCLA, followed by their final two clinical years at the UCLA School of Medicine.

USMLE

Step 1: Required. Students must record a passing score for promotion.

Step 2: Clinical Skills (CS): Required. Students must record a passing total score to graduate.

Step 2: Clinical Knowledge (CK): Required. Students must record a passing total score to graduate.

Selection Factors

Preference is given to those showing evidence of broad training and high achievement in college education and those who possess those traits of personality and character essential to the success in medicine and the provision of quality, professional and humane medical care. We look for through coursework, school activities, community service and research for evidence of maturity, intellect, scholarship, and service to their communities and to those who are underprivileged and disadvantaged, are culturally aware and are able to speak a second language, especially Spanish. Final selections are made on the basis of individual qualifications and not on the basis of race, ethnicity, sex, age, sexual orientation, national origin or disability.

Financial Aid

Scholarships and loan are available to US citizens and are awarded on the basis of financial need and academics. Every effort is made to provide as much aid as needed.

Information about Diversity Programs

We pride ourselves on the diversity of our student body. Multiple programs to celebrate our diversity are part of student life and are integral to the learning environment.

Campus Information

Setting

We are located on the main UCLA campus offering numerous opportunities for theatre, recreation, athletics and cultural events.

Enrollment

For 2007, total enrollment was: 668

Special Features

UCLA hospital has been ranked by US News & World Report "Best in the West" for 17 years and third in the nation. A new state of the art medical center opens this year.

Housing

Graduate housing in walking distance is available for the first two years.

Application Process and Requirements 2009–2010

Primary Application Service: AMCAS
Earliest filing date: June 1, 2008
Latest filing date: November 1, 2008

Secondary Application Required?: Yes
Sent to: Screened applicants
URL: Supplied after screening
Fee: Yes, $60
Fee waiver available: Yes
Earliest filing date: n/a
Latest filing date: within 45 days of request

Latest MCAT® considered: September 2008
Oldest MCAT® considered: 2006

Early Decision Program
School does not have EDP
Applicants notified: n/a
EDP available for: n/a

Regular Acceptance Notice
Earliest date: December 15, 2008
Latest date: Until class is full

Applicant's Response to Acceptance
Offer – Maximum Time: Two weeks

Requests for Deferred
Entrance Considered: Yes

Deposit to Hold Place in Class: No
Deposit (Resident): n/a
Deposit (Non-Resident): n/a
Deposit due: n/a
Applied to tuition: n/a
Deposit refundable: n/a
Refundable by: n/a

Estimated number of new entrants: 183
EDP: n/a, special program: n/a

Start Month/Year: August 2009

Interview Format: One-on-one with faculty. Regional interviews are not available.

Other Programs

PREPARATORY PROGRAMS
Postbaccalaureate Program: Yes, www.medstudent.ucla.edu/prospective
Summer Program: Yes, Patrica Pratt (310) 825-5375, ppratt@mednet.ucla.edu

COMBINED DEGREE PROGRAMS
Baccalaureate/MD: No
MD/MPH: Yes, www.medstudent.ucla.edu/prospective
MD/MBA: Yes, www.medstudent.ucla.edu/prospective
MD/JD: No
MD/PhD: Yes, www.medstudent.ucla.edu/prospective

Premedical Coursework

Course	Req.	Rec.	Lab.	Sems.	Course	Req.	Rec.	Lab.	Sems.
Inorganic Chemistry	•		•	2	Computer Science		•		
Behavioral Sciences					Genetics				
Biochemistry					Humanities		•		
Biology	•		•	2	Organic Chemistry	•		•	2
Biology/Zoology					Physics	•		•	2
Calculus		•			Psychology				
College English	•			2	Social Sciences				
College Mathematics	•			2	Other 1 & 2		•		

Selection Factors: 2007 Accepted Applicants

Proportion of Accepted Applicants with Relevant Experience (Data Self-Reported to AMCAS*)		
Community Service/Volunteer		66%
Medically-Related Work		92%
Research		92%

Shaded bar represents accepted scores ranging from the 10th percentile to the 90th percentile. School Median ● National Median ●

Overall GPA	2.0	2.1	2.2	2.3	2.4	2.5	2.6	2.7	2.8	2.9	3.0	3.1	3.2	3.3	3.4	3.5	3.6	3.7	(3.8)	3.9	4.0
Science GPA	2.0	2.1	2.2	2.3	2.4	2.5	2.6	2.7	2.8	2.9	3.0	3.1	3.2	3.3	3.4	3.5	3.6	3.7	(3.8)	3.9	4.0

MCAT® required: Yes, 100% of 2007 accepted applicants took MCAT®

Verbal Reasoning	3	4	5	6	7	8	9	(10)	11	12	13	14	15
Physical Sciences	3	4	5	6	7	8	9	10	(11)	12	13	14	15
Biological Sciences	3	4	5	6	7	8	9	10	(11)	(12)	13	14	15
Writing Sample				J	K	L	M	N	O	P	(Q)	R	S	T

Acceptance & Matriculation Data for 2007–2008 First Year Class

	Resident	Non-Resident	International	Total
Applied	5013	2548	263	7824
Interviewed	500	215	2	717
Deferred	2	1	0	3
Matriculants				
Early Assurance Program	0	0	0	0
Early Decision Program	0	0	0	0
Baccalaureate/MD	n/a	n/a	n/a	n/a
MD/PhD	8	3	0	11
Matriculated	148	21	0	169

Applications accepted from International Applicants: Yes

Specialty Choice

2003, 2004, 2005 Graduates, Specialty Choice (As reported by program directors to GME Track™)	
Anesthesiology	6%
Emergency Medicine	9%
Family Practice	8%
Internal Medicine	12%
Obstetrics/Gynecology	5%
Orthopaedic Surgery	4%
Pediatrics	11%
Psychiatry	4%
Radiology	7%
Surgery	6%

Matriculant Demographics: 2007–2008 First Year Class

Men: 94   **Women:** 75

Matriculants' Self-Reported Race/Ethnicity

Mexican American	15	Korean	6
Cuban	0	Vietnamese	15
Puerto Rican	0	Other Asian	8
Other Hispanic	9	Total Asian	69
Total Hispanic	23	Native American	2
Chinese	26	Black	15
Asian Indian	10	Native Hawaiian	1
Pakistani	2	White	76
Filipino	3	Unduplicated Number	
Japanese	3	of Matriculants	169

Science and Math Majors: 74%
Matriculants with:
 Baccalaureate degree: 100%
 Graduate degree(s): 8%

Financial Information

Source: 2006–2007 LCME I-B survey and 2007–2008 AAMC TSF questionnaire

	Residents	Non-Residents
Total Cost of Attendance	$49,715	$61,960
Tuition and Fees	$22,551	$34,796
Other (includes living expenses)	$25,970	$25,970
Health Insurance (can be waived)	$1,194	$1,194

Average 2007 Graduate Indebtedness: $85,397
% of Enrolled Students Receiving Aid: 86%

Criminal Background Check

This medical school requires a criminal background check prior to matriculation.

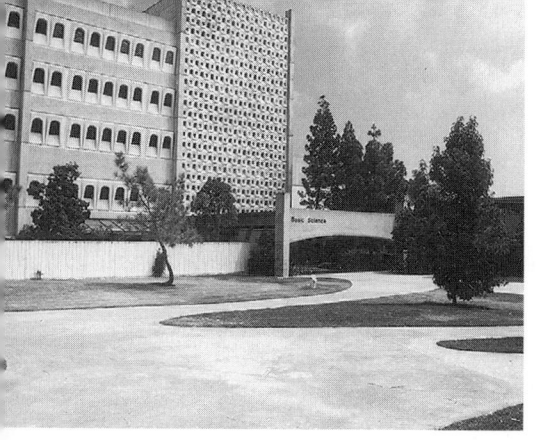

University of California, San Diego, School of Medicine

La Jolla, California

Office of Admissions, 0621, Medical Teaching Facility
UC San Diego School of Medicine
9500 Gilman Drive
La Jolla, California 92093-0621
T 858 534 3880   F 858 534 5282

Admissions http://meded.ucsd.edu/admissions
Main http://meded-portal.ucsd.edu
Financial http://meded.ucsd.edu/hsfao
Email somadmissions@ucsd.edu

Public Institution

Dr. David A. Brenner, Vice Chancellor and Dean

Dr. Carolyn Kelly, Associate Dean for Admissions and Student Affairs

Carol Hartupee, Director of Financial Aid

Brian Zeglen, Director of Admissions

General Information

Students at the University of California, San Diego (UCSD) benefit from a diverse faculty and access to a wide variety of research and clinical opportunities.

Mission Statement

The overall objective of the medical school curriculum is to instill graduates with the knowledge, skills, and attributes that will lead to their becoming capable and compassionate physicians. Our educational philosophy is to give students an opportunity to go beyond the core curriculum and pursue electives and independent study that take full advantage of the resources available at UCSD and in the surrounding region, helping them to become expert clinicians and scientists who are aware of, and responsive to, community needs.

Curricular Highlights

Community Service Requirement: Optional. Many community service activities are available.
Research/Thesis Requirement: Optional. Independent Study Project is required.

The goal of the medical curriculum and faculty-student interactions is to develop critical, objective, conscientious physicians prepared for changing conditions of medical practice and continuing self-education. The integrated core curriculum of the first two years provides entering students with an essential understanding of the fundamental disciplines underlying modern medicine. The core curriculum of the last two years is composed of the major clinical specialties taught in hospital and out-patient settings, and relevant extended-care facilities. Elective opportunities are pursued during both the pre-clinical and clinical years. Several combined M.D.-Master's degree programs are

available. A new Program in Medical Education in Health Equity has been developed. The Medical Scientist Training Program provides the opportunity to earn both the M.D. and Ph.D. degrees over a seven to eight-year period of study. A Medical Scholars Program at UCSD (B.S.-M.D.) is available for outstanding California high school seniors planning careers in medicine. A second B.S.-M.D. program is available between UCSD School of Medicine and California Institute of Technology.

USMLE

Step 1: Required. Students must record a passing score for promotion.
Step 2: Clinical Skills (CS): Required. Students must record a passing total score to graduate.
Step 2: Clinical Knowledge (CK): Required. Students must record a passing total score to graduate.

Selection Factors

The Admissions Committee selects applicants who have demonstrated intelligence, maturity, integrity, and dedication to the ideal of service to society. The school is seeking a student body with a broad diversity of backgrounds and interests. The Admissions Committee seeks students with broad training and in-depth achievement in a particular area of knowledge, whether in the humanities, social sciences, or natural sciences. Other evaluation factors include evidence of meaningful involvement in extracurricular activities, performance on the MCAT®, letters of recommendation, and personal interviews. The Admissions Committee interview evaluates the applicant's abilities and skills necessary to satisfy the non-academic or technical standards established by the faculty and the personal characteristics necessary to become an effective physician. Preference is afforded to California residents, and consideration is given only to applicants who are either U.S. citizens or permanent residents. The UCSD School of Medicine participates in the WICHE Professional Student Exchange Program. The School of Medicine does not accept transfer students.

Financial Aid

Financial aid in the form of scholarships,

grants, loans, and work opportunities is offered to help students in need of financial assistance. Medical Scientist Training Program participants may receive full tuition and stipend support during their combined degree training.

Information about Diversity Programs

The UCSD School of Medicine is committed to expanding the educational opportunities for applicants coming from disadvantaged educational or economic backgrounds. This institutional commitment is expressed through a pre-matriculation summer program, a conditional acceptance program, tutorial support programs, and financial aid assistance.

Campus Information

Setting

UCSD School of Medicine is located in La Jolla, California.

Enrollment

For 2007, total enrollment was: 521

Special Features

UCSD is a hub both for outstanding clinical programs and cutting-edge research. Recognized regional clinical programs include a Level 1 trauma center, an innovative Stroke Center, a leading AIDS/HIV treatment program, and a Regional Burn Center. Other specialized resources include the UCSD Cancer Center, the functional MRI facility, the Institute for Molecular Medicine, and the Stein Institute for Research on Aging. Both the prestigious Ludwig Institute for Cancer Research and the Howard Hughes Medical Institute have significant presences on campus.

Housing

Medical students at UCSD live both in on- and off-campus housing.

Satellite Campuses/Facilities

Clinical rotations are conducted at the UCSD Medical Centers, VA San Diego Healthcare System, San Diego Children's Hospital, Scripps-Mercy Hospital, Balboa Naval Medical Center, and a variety of ambulatory care sites throughout San Diego.

Application Process and Requirements 2009–2010

Primary Application Service: AMCAS
Earliest filing date: June 1, 2008
Latest filing date: November 1, 2008

Secondary Application Required?: Yes
Sent to: Screened applicants
(858) 534-3880, somadmissions@ucsd.edu
Fee: Yes, $60
Fee waiver available: Yes
Earliest filing date: July 1, 2008
Latest filing date: One month after receiving Secondary Application invitation

Latest MCAT® considered: September 2008
Oldest MCAT® considered: 2006

Early Decision Program
School does not have EDP
Applicants notified: n/a
EDP available for: n/a

Regular Acceptance Notice
Earliest date: October 15, 2008
Latest date: Until class is full

Applicant's Response to Acceptance Offer – Maximum Time: Two weeks

Requests for Deferred Entrance Considered: Yes

Deposit to Hold Place in Class: No
Deposit (Resident): n/a
Deposit (Non-Resident): n/a
Deposit due: n/a
Applied to tuition: n/a
Deposit refundable: n/a
Refundable by: n/a

Estimated number of new entrants: 134
EDP: n/a, special program: n/a

Start Month/Year: August 2009

Interview Format: Two open-file interviews. Regional interviews are not available.

Other Programs

PREPARATORY PROGRAMS
Postbaccalaureate Program: Yes,
http://meded.ucsd.edu/postbac
Summer Program: Yes,
http://meded.ucsd.edu/somi220/

COMBINED DEGREE PROGRAMS
Baccalaureate/MD: Yes,
http://meded.ucsd.edu/asa/admissions/
Yvonne Coleman, (858) 534-3880
somadmissions@ucsd.edu
MD/MPH: Yes,
http://meded.ucsd.edu/ugme/goddp/
MD/MBA: No
MD/JD: No
MD/PhD: Yes,
http://meded.ucsd.edu/ugme/goddp/
Additional Program: Yes,
http://meded.ucsd.edu/ugme/goddp/

Premedical Coursework

Course	Req.	Rec.	Lab.	Hrs.
Inorganic Chemistry	•			8
Behavioral Sciences		•		
Biochemistry		•		
Biology	•			8
Biology/Zoology		•		
Calculus		•		
College English		•		
College Mathematics	•			8

Course	Req.	Rec.	Lab.	Hrs.
Computer Science		•		
Genetics		•		
Humanities		•		
Organic Chemistry	•			8
Physics	•			8
Psychology		•		
Social Sciences		•		
Other				

Selection Factors: 2007 Accepted Applicants

Proportion of Accepted Applicants with Relevant Experience (Data Self-Reported to AMCAS®)		
Community Service/Volunteer		65%
Medically-Related Work		85%
Research		88%

Shaded bar represents accepted scores ranging from the 10th percentile to the 90th percentile   School Median ● National Median ●

Overall GPA	2.0	2.1	2.2	2.3	2.4	2.5	2.6	2.7	2.8	2.9	3.0	3.1	3.2	3.3	3.4	3.5	3.6	3.7	(3.8)	3.9	4.0
Science GPA	2.0	2.1	2.2	2.3	2.4	2.5	2.6	2.7	2.8	2.9	3.0	3.1	3.2	3.3	3.4	3.5	3.6	3.7	(3.8)	3.9	4.0

MCAT® required: Yes, 98% of 2007 accepted applicants took MCAT®

Verbal Reasoning	3	4	5	6	7	8	9	(10)	(11)	12	13	14	15
Physical Sciences	3	4	5	6	7	8	9	10	(11)	(12)	13	14	15
Biological Sciences	3	4	5	6	7	8	9	10	(11)	(12)	13	14	15
Writing Sample				J	K	L	M	N	O	P	(Q)	R	S	T

Acceptance & Matriculation Data for 2007–2008 First Year Class

	Resident	Non-Resident	International	Total
Applied	3611	1821	68	5500
Interviewed	484	85	0	569
Deferred	6	4	0	10
Matriculants				
Early Assurance Program	0	0	0	0
Early Decision Program	0	0	0	0
Baccalaureate/MD	7	0	0	7
MD/PhD	4	4	0	8
Matriculated	123	11	0	**134**

Applications accepted from International Applicants: No

Specialty Choice

2003, 2004, 2005 Graduates, Specialty Choice (As reported by program directors to GME Track™)	
Anesthesiology	7%
Emergency Medicine	8%
Family Practice	8%
Internal Medicine	16%
Obstetrics/Gynecology	4%
Orthopaedic Surgery	3%
Pediatrics	11%
Psychiatry	6%
Radiology	5%
Surgery	5%

Matriculant Demographics: 2007–2008 First Year Class

Men: 66   **Women:** 68

Matriculants' Self-Reported Race/Ethnicity

Mexican American	9	Korean	6
Cuban	0	Vietnamese	6
Puerto Rican	0	Other Asian	7
Other Hispanic	1	Total Asian	53
Total Hispanic	10	Native American	1
Chinese	24	Black	2
Asian Indian	8	Native Hawaiian	0
Pakistani	0	White	74
Filipino	3	Unduplicated Number	
Japanese	3	of Matriculants	134

Science and Math Majors: 84%
Matriculants with:
　　Baccalaureate degree: 98%
　　Graduate degree(s): 13%

Financial Information

Source: 2006–2007 LCME I-B survey and 2007–2008 AAMC TSF questionnaire

	Residents	Non-Residents
Total Cost of Attendance	$45,568	$57,813
Tuition and Fees	$21,465	$33,710
Other (includes living expenses)	$22,609	$22,609
Health Insurance (can be waived)	$1,494	$1,494

Average 2007 Graduate Indebtedness: $89,102
% of Enrolled Students Receiving Aid: 91%

Criminal Background Check

This medical school requires a criminal background check prior to matriculation.

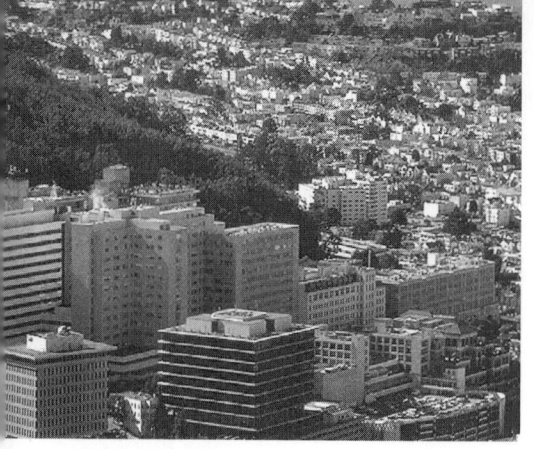

University of California, San Francisco, School of Medicine

San Francisco, California

School of Medicine, Admissions
C-200, Box 0408
University of California, San Francisco
San Francisco, California 94143
T 415 476 4044

Admissions http://medschool.ucsf.edu/admissions
Main http://medschool.ucsf.edu
Financial http://saawww.ucsf.edu/
financial/welcome.htm
Email admissions@medsch.ucsf.edu

Public Institution

Dr. Sam Hawgood, Interim Dean

Carrie Steere-Salazar, Director, Student Financial Services

Hallen Chung, Director

Dr. David Wofsy, Associate Dean for Admissions

General Information

One of the top medical schools in the nation, the UCSF School of Medicine is dedicated to excellence in education, research, and patient care. Woven throughout all of these pursuits is a strong commitment to public service, a collaborative work ethic, and providing care for diverse communities. Ranked among the top ten medical schools in the nation, the UCSF School of Medicine earns its greatest distinction from the outstanding faculty — including three Nobel laureates, 34 National Academy of Sciences members, 38 American Academy of Arts and Sciences members, 72 Institute of Medicine members, and 17 Howard Hughes Medical Institute investigators. The school is comprised of 26 academic departments, 10 organized research units, and seven interdisciplinary centers at sites throughout San Francisco.

Mission Statement

The UCSF School of Medicine strives to advance human health through a four-fold mission of education, research, patient care, and public service.

Curricular Highlights

Community Service Requirement: Optional.
Research/Thesis Requirement: Optional.

The first two years consist of integrated core instruction in the basic, behavioral, social, and clinical sciences; clinical experience is introduced within the first week of classes. Emphasis is placed on small-group teaching. Students begin longitudinal patient experiences during the Foundations of Patient Care course. In the last two years, the various clinical departments provide 54 weeks of Clinical Core, which teach students the basic skills of clinical medicine. The fourth year includes Advanced Studies, which

encompasses elective rotations, research, and specific fields of inquiry that prepare students for post-graduate training. For more detailed information, visit the School of Medicine Web site at *www.medschool.ucsf.edu/curriculum/overview/index.aspx.*

USMLE

Step 1: Required. Students must record a passing score for promotion.
Step 2: Clinical Skills (CS): Required. Students must only record a score.
Step 2: Clinical Knowledge (CK): Required. Students must only record a score.

Selection Factors

UCSF students must have demonstrated the ability to perform at a very high level in their prior academic pursuits. Among the many applicants who meet this essential criterion, the school seeks to create a student community that is characterized by diversity in background, extra-curricular talents, academic interests, and career aspirations. There is no single mold that defines a UCSF student. UCSF wants some students who aspire to become terrific doctors, some who will become great scientists, some who will be leaders in health policy, and so on. The goal is to create the most stimulating and enjoyable possible environment in which to live and learn. For further details regarding the admissions process, please visit the School of Medicine's Web site at *www.medschool.ucsf.edu/admissions/apply/index.aspx.*

Financial Aid

Scholarships are awarded to entering students on the basis of scholarship and/or need. General financial support is awarded through the Student Financial Services Office. Aid packages consist of a combination of loans, grants-in-aid, and scholarships. Financial aid is only available to U.S. citizens or permanent residents. For detailed information, please visit *http://saawww.ucsf.edu/financial/welcome.htm.*

Information about Diversity Programs

The School of Medicine welcomes applicants from all ethnic, economic, and cultural

backgrounds without discrimination, and has a long-standing commitment to increasing the number of physicians who come from communities that are underserved and/or underrepresented in medicine. As a result, over the last 30 years, UCSF has had one of the highest minority enrollment and graduation rates of any continental U.S. medical school. The curriculum includes both coursework and practical opportunities focused on narrowing health care disparities.

Campus Information

Setting

The main UCSF campus is located in the center of San Francisco, a short walk from Golden Gate Park and no more than 10 minutes from the Pacific Ocean. Downtown San Francisco, easily accessible by car or public transportation, is located approximately two miles from the main campus. Other major UCSF teaching sites include San Francisco General Hospital, the VA Medical Center, the Cancer Center, and the new Mission Bay campus. The surrounding area of northern California provides a natural backdrop and opportunities for recreation that are hard to match.

Enrollment

For 2007, total enrollment was: 595

Special Features

Please visit the UCSF Web site for the latest facts and figures unique to the campus: *www.ucsf.edu/about_ucsf/profile.html.*

Housing

For detailed information about housing, please visit the UCSF Housing Services Web site at *www.cas.ucsf.edu/cho/default.html.*

Satellite Campuses/Facilities

Student rotations may be conducted at the UCSF Parnassus Campus, San Francisco General Hospital, UCSF/Mt Zion, SF VA Medical Center, and the UCSF Fresno Medical Education Program, as well as at several other Bay Area affiliated hospitals and clinics.

Application Process and Requirements 2009–2010

Primary Application Service: AMCAS
Earliest filing date: June 1, 2008
Latest filing date: October 15, 2008

Secondary Application Required?: Yes
Sent to: Screened applicants
after preliminary review
Contact: UCSF School of Medicine Admissions
(415) 476-4044, admissions@medsch.ucsf.edu
Fee: Yes, $60
Fee waiver available: Yes
Earliest filing date: August 1, 2008
Latest filing date: January 12, 2009

Latest MCAT® considered: September 2008
Oldest MCAT® considered: August 2006

Early Decision Program
School does not have EDP
Applicants notified: n/a
EDP available for: n/a

Regular Acceptance Notice
Earliest date: December 15, 2008
Latest date: Until class is full

Applicant's Response to Acceptance
Offer – Maximum Time: Two weeks

Requests for Deferred
Entrance Considered: Yes

Deposit to Hold Place in Class: No
Deposit (Resident): n/a
Deposit (Non-Resident): n/a
Deposit due: n/a
Applied to tuition: n/a
Deposit refundable: n/a
Refundable by: n/a

Estimated number of new entrants: 168
EDP: n/a, special program: n/a

Start Month/Year: June 2009 (UCB/UCSF
Joint Medical Program); September 2009 (UCSF)

Interview Format: Required to interview
at UCSF, if invited. Two interviews, 40 minutes
to one hour each. Regional interviews are
not available.

Other Programs

PREPARATORY PROGRAMS
Postbaccalaureate Program: Yes,
www.medschool.ucsf.edu/outreach
Summer Program: No

COMBINED DEGREE PROGRAMS
Baccalaureate/MD: No
MD/MPH: Yes,
www.medschool.ucsf.edu/admissions/degrees/
Curriculum.aspx
MD/MBA: No
MD/JD: No
MD/PhD: Yes,
http://medschool.ucsf.edu/mstp
Joint Medical Program: Yes,
http://jmp.berkeley.edu/

Premedical Coursework

Course	Req.	Rec.	Lab.	Hrs.
Inorganic Chemistry	•		•	12
Behavioral Sciences				
Biochemistry				
Biology				
Biology/Zoology	•		•	12
Calculus				
College English				
College Mathematics				

Course	Req.	Rec.	Lab.	Hrs.
Computer Science				
Genetics				
Humanities				
Organic Chemistry	•			8
Physics	•		•	12
Psychology				
Social Sciences				
Other				

Selection Factors: 2007 Accepted Applicants

Proportion of Accepted Applicants with Relevant Experience (Data Self-Reported to AMCAS®)		
Community Service/Volunteer		69%
Medically-Related Work		89%
Research		91%

Shaded bar represents accepted scores ranging from the 10th percentile to the 90th percentile. School Median ● National Median ●

Overall GPA	2.0	2.1	2.2	2.3	2.4	2.5	2.6	2.7	2.8	2.9	3.0	3.1	3.2	3.3	3.4	3.5	3.6	3.7	(3.8)	3.9	4.0
Science GPA	2.0	2.1	2.2	2.3	2.4	2.5	2.6	2.7	2.8	2.9	3.0	3.1	3.2	3.3	3.4	3.5	3.6	3.7	(3.8)	3.9	4.0

MCAT® required: Yes, 100% of 2007 accepted applicants took MCAT®

Verbal Reasoning	3	4	5	6	7	8	9	(10)	(11)	12	13	14	15
Physical Sciences	3	4	5	6	7	8	9	10	(11)	(12)	13	14	15
Biological Sciences	3	4	5	6	7	8	9	10	(11)	(12)	13	14	15
Writing Sample			J	K	L	M	N	O	P	(Q)	R	S	T

Acceptance & Matriculation Data for 2007–2008 First Year Class

	Resident	Non-Resident	International	Total
Applied	3305	2839	159	6303
Interviewed	0	0	0	0
Deferred	3	0	0	3
Matriculants				
Early Assurance Program	n/a	n/a	n/a	n/a
Early Decision Program	0	0	0	0
Baccalaureate/MD	n/a	n/a	n/a	n/a
MD/PhD	3	9	0	12
Matriculated	129	34	0	**163**

Applications accepted from International Applicants: Yes

Matriculant Demographics: 2007–2008 First Year Class

Men: 67   **Women:** 96

Matriculants' Self-Reported Race/Ethnicity

Mexican American	19	Korean	6
Cuban	1	Vietnamese	3
Puerto Rican	3	Other Asian	4
Other Hispanic	7	**Total Asian**	53
Total Hispanic	29	Native American	4
Chinese	19	Black	22
Asian Indian	7	Native Hawaiian	1
Pakistani	3	White	90
Filipino	7	**Unduplicated Number**	
Japanese	6	**of Matriculants**	163

Science and Math Majors: 67%
Matriculants with:
    Baccalaureate degree: 100%
    Graduate degree(s): 10%

Specialty Choice

2003, 2004, 2005 Graduates, Specialty Choice (As reported by program directors to GME Track™)	
Anesthesiology	7%
Emergency Medicine	11%
Family Practice	5%
Internal Medicine	15%
Obstetrics/Gynecology	5%
Orthopaedic Surgery	2%
Pediatrics	9%
Psychiatry	8%
Radiology	4%
Surgery	5%

Financial Information

Source: 2006–2007 LCME I-B survey
and 2007–2008 AAMC TSF questionnaire

	Residents	Non-Residents
Total Cost of Attendance	$44,063	$56,308
Tuition and Fees	$21,218	$33,463
Other (includes living expenses)	$20,625	$20,625
Health Insurance (cannot be waived)	$2,220	$2,220

Average 2007 Graduate Indebtedness: $85,020
% of Enrolled Students Receiving Aid: 80%

Criminal Background Check

This Medical school requires a criminal background check prior to matriculation.

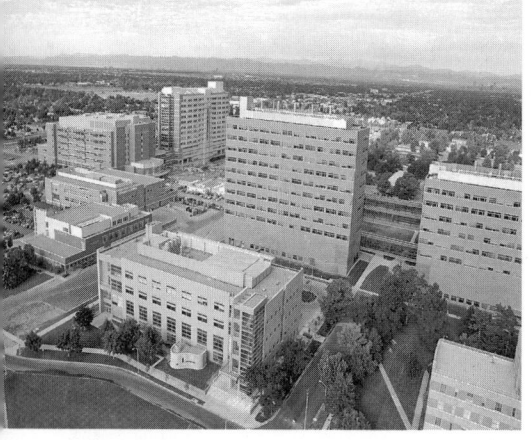

University Colorado Denver School of Medicine

Denver, Colorado

Medical School Admissions
University of Colorado Denver School of Medicine
Anschutz Medical Campus, Mail Stop 297
P.O. Box 6508
Aurora, Colorado 80045
T 303 724 8025   **F** 303 724 8028

Admissions www.uchsc.edu/som/admissions/
Main www.uchsc.edu/som
Financial www.uchsc.edu/finaid/
Email SOMadmin@uchsc.edu

Public Institution

Dr. Richard D. Krugman, Dean

Dominic Martinez, Coordinator of Student Outreach and Support

General Information

The University of Colorado Denver School of Medicine (UCDSOM) is a part of the University of Colorado Denver located in Denver and Aurora, Colorado. The Anshutz Medical Campus in Aurora includes the schools of dentistry, nursing, and pharmacy and the graduate school as well as the SOM. Clinical opportunities for medical students are located throughout the Denver metropolitan area and Colorado. The UCDSOM is home to 1,927 full-time and 2,956 volunteer faculty. In addition to educating students and participating in research, the faculty assumes considerable responsibility for patient care. Student research opportunities and a variety of extracurricular activities are available. The UCDSOM moved to the new 217-acre Anschutz Medical Campus in Aurora in January 2008.

Mission Statement

The mission of the University of Colorado School of Medicine is to provide Colorado, the nation, and the world with programs of excellence in: Education – through the provision of educational programs to medical students, allied health students, graduate students and house staff, practicing health professionals, and the public at large; Research – through the development of new knowledge in the basic and clinical sciences, as well as in health policy and health care education; Clinical Care – through state-of-the-art clinical programs, which reflect the unique educational environment of the university, as well as the needs of the patients it serves; and Community Service – through sharing the School's expertise and knowledge to enhance the broader community, including our affiliated institutions, other health care professionals, alumni and other colleagues, and citizens of the state.

Curricular Highlights

Community Service Requirement: Optional. Many community service electives are available.

Research/Thesis Requirement: Required. A scholarly project is required for graduation.

The curriculum is designed to provide the scientific and clinical background to prepare graduates for the practice of medicine. A systems-based curriculum was introduced in 2005. The Essentials block runs for 18 months. The core clinical year runs through April of year 3. The elective year allows students time to do sub-internships, critical care rotations and other courses essential to their career choices. A capstone science course occurs in the spring of year 4. The Foundations of Doctoring curriculum begins in the first week of medical school and continues through year 3. Standardized patients are widely used in Foundations.

USMLE

Step 1: Required. Students must record a passing score for promotion.
Step 2: Clinical Skills (CS): Required. Students must record a passing score to graduate.
Step 2: Clinical Knowledge (CK): Required. Students must record a passing total score to graduate.

Selection Factors

Places are offered to the applicants who are most highly qualified in terms of intelligence, achievement, character, motivation, and maturity. Grades, MCAT® scores, recommendations, and personal interviews are assessed. Humanistic qualities, indications of peer collaboration, and professionalism are characteristics of our students. Approximately 75 percent of the class is comprised of Colorado residents. Applicants from rural areas and from groups underrepresented in medicine are encouraged to apply. Wyoming and Montana (WICHE) applicants are treated as in-state. All undergraduate majors are considered acceptable. Excellent performance in the required science courses is essential. The medical school has an active MD/PhD program for those who wish to combine medical school with intensive laboratory research. The UCDSOM does not discriminate on the basis of race, sex, creed, national origin, age, or disability. Financial status is not a factor in the selection of applicants.

Financial Aid

The UCSOM participates in federal aid programs and has a number of scholarships which are merit-based. Colorado student grant funds are available for Colorado residents. Financial aid questions should be directed to (303) 556-2886.

Information about Diversity Programs

The UCSOM encourages applications from qualified students from groups underrepresented in American medicine. Detailed information may be obtained from the Office of Diversity at (303) 724-8005.

Campus Information

Setting

The UCDSOM is an urban campus in Aurora, Colorado. In addition to the schools on the campus, the University of Colorado Hospital, The Children's Hospital, the Barbara Davis Center for Childhood Diabetes, and the Ben Nighthorse Campbell Center for Native American Studies are on the Anschutz Medical Campus. The Veterans Affairs Medical Center will move to the campus in 2010.

Enrollment

For 2007, total enrollment was: 586

Special Features

In 2006, the total research budget of UCSOM was in excess of $374 million/year.

Housing

Rental property and roommate information are available in the Student Assistance Office. Call (303) 724-7684 or visit *www.uchsc.edu/ studentassistance.*

Satellite Campuses/Facilities

Besides the hospitals on the Anschutz campus, students rotate through Denver Health Medical Center, National Jewish Hospital, and multiple hospitals throughout Denver and Colorado.

Application Process and Requirements 2009–2010

Primary Application Service: AMCAS
Earliest filing date: June 1, 2008
Latest filing date: November 1, 2008

Secondary Application Required?: Yes
Sent to: All applicants
Sean Spellman, (303) 724-8025
sean.spellman@uchsc.edu
URL: n/a
Fee: Yes, $100
Fee waiver available: Yes
Earliest filing date: August 1, 2008
Latest filing date: December 31, 2008

Latest MCAT® considered: September 2008
Oldest MCAT® considered: 2006

Early Decision Program
School does not have EDP
Applicants notified: n/a
EDP available for: n/a

Regular Acceptance Notice
Earliest date: October 16, 2008
Latest date: Until class is full

Applicant's Response to Acceptance
Offer – Maximum Time: Two weeks

Requests for Deferred
Entrance Considered: Yes

Deposit to Hold Place in Class: Yes
Deposit (Resident): $200
Deposit (Non-Resident): $200
Deposit due: Upon acceptance
Applied to tuition: Yes
Deposit refundable: Yes
Refundable by: July 1, 2009

Estimated number of new entrants: 158
EDP: n/a, special program: n/a

Start Month/Year: August 2009

Interview Format: Two one-on-one academically blind interviews. Regional interviews are not available.

Other Programs

PREPARATORY PROGRAMS
Postbaccalaureate Program: Yes
By invitation only
Summer Program: No

COMBINED DEGREE PROGRAMS
Baccalaureate/MD: No
MD/MPH: No
MD/MBA: Yes,
www.uchsc.edu/sm/sm/mdmbadegree.htm
MD/JD: No
MD/PhD: Yes, www.uchsc.edu/sm/mstp/

Premedical Coursework

Course	Req.	Rec.	Lab.	Hrs.	Course	Req.	Rec.	Lab.	Hrs.
Inorganic Chemistry	•		•	8	Computer Science		•		
Behavioral Sciences					Genetics		•		
Biochemistry		•			Humanities		•		
Biology	•		•	8	Organic Chemistry	•		•	8
Biology/Zoology					Physics	•		•	8
Calculus	•				Psychology				
College English	•			9	Social Sciences		•		
College Mathematics	•			6	Other		•		

Selection Factors: 2007 Accepted Applicants

Proportion of Accepted Applicants with Relevant Experience (Data Self-Reported to AMCAS")		Community Service/Volunteer	71%
		Medically-Related Work	81%
		Research	77%

Shaded bar represents accepted scores ranging from the 10th percentile to the 90th percentile ▪   School Median ● National Median ●

Overall GPA	2.0	2.1	2.2	2.3	2.4	2.5	2.6	2.7	2.8	2.9	3.0	3.1	3.2	3.3	3.4	3.5	3.6	3.7	③.8	3.9	4.0
Science GPA	2.0	2.1	2.2	2.3	2.4	2.5	2.6	2.7	2.8	2.9	3.0	3.1	3.2	3.3	3.4	3.5	3.6	3.7	③.8	3.9	4.0

MCAT® required: Yes, 100% of 2007 accepted applicants took MCAT®

Verbal Reasoning	3	4	5	6	7	8	9	⑩	⑪	12	13	14	15
Physical Sciences	3	4	5	6	7	8	9	10	⑪	12	13	14	15
Biological Sciences	3	4	5	6	7	8	9	10	⑪	12	13	14	15
Writing Sample				J	K	L	M	N	O	P	⑫	R	S	T

Acceptance & Matriculation Data for 2007–2008 First Year Class

	Resident	Non-Resident	International	Total
Applied	606	2292	55	2953
Interviewed	326	243	0	569
Deferred	11	2	0	13
Matriculants				
Early Assurance Program	0	0	0	0
Early Decision Program	0	0	0	0
Baccalaureate/MD	n/a	n/a	n/a	n/a
MD/PhD	2	5	0	7
Matriculated	126	31	0	**157**

Applications accepted from International Applicants: Yes

Specialty Choice

2003, 2004, 2005 Graduates, Specialty Choice (As reported by program directors to GME Track™)

Anesthesiology	9%
Emergency Medicine	7%
Family Practice	15%
Internal Medicine	17%
Obstetrics/Gynecology	3%
Orthopaedic Surgery	4%
Pediatrics	8%
Psychiatry	3%
Radiology	3%
Surgery	9%

Matriculant Demographics: 2007–2008 First Year Class

Men: 83   **Women:** 74

Matriculants' Self-Reported Race/Ethnicity

Mexican American	4	Korean	1
Cuban	0	Vietnamese	2
Puerto Rican	1	Other Asian	1
Other Hispanic	3	Total Asian	11
Total Hispanic	8	Native American	4
Chinese	5	Black	5
Asian Indian	2	Native Hawaiian	0
Pakistani	0	White	138
Filipino	0	Unduplicated Number	
Japanese	1	of Matriculants	157

Science and Math Majors: 76%
Matriculants with:
Baccalaureate degree: 99%
Graduate degree(s): 11%

Financial Information

Source: 2006–2007 LCME I-B survey and 2007–2008 AAMC TSF questionnaire

	Residents	Non-Residents
Total Cost of Attendance	$44,221	$67,423
Tuition and Fees	$24,828	$48,030
Other (includes living expenses)	$17,210	$17,210
Health Insurance (can be waived)	$2,183	$2,183

Average 2007 Graduate Indebtedness: $121,987
% of Enrolled Students Receiving Aid: 93%

Criminal Background Check

This medical school requires a criminal background check prior to matriculation.

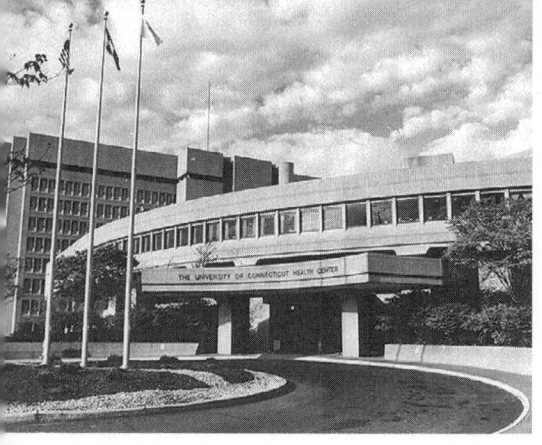

University of Connecticut School of Medicine

Farmington, Connecticut

Admissions Center
University of Connecticut
School of Medicine
263 Farmington Avenue, Rm. AG-062
Farmington, Connecticut 06030-3906
T 860 679 4306   **F** 860 679 1282

Admissions http://medicine.uchc.edu/prospective/admissions/
Main http://medicine.uchc.edu
Financial http://medicine.uchc.edu/prospective/financialaid/
Email fox@nso1.uchc.edu, sanford@nso1.uchc.edu

Public Institution

Dr. Peter J. Deckers, Dean

Dr. Keat Sanford, Assistant Dean for Admissions and Medical Student Affairs

Dr. Marja Hurley, Associate Dean of Minority Affairs

Andrea Devereux, Director of Financial Assistance

Lisa Francini, Administrative Coordinator

Lynda Fox, Administrative Coordinator

General Information

The School of Medicine occupies the University of Connecticut Health Center complex in Farmington. The Health Center also includes the School of Dental Medicine, graduate programs in Biomedical Sciences and Public Health, the University Hospital and Ambulatory Unit, Research buildings, and Stowe Library. Students receive clinical training in Hartford area-affiliated hospitals.

Mission Statement

The School of Medicine's curriculum is designed to prepare professional men and women to practice medicine in a health care system that is evolving at an accelerated rate. The curriculum will equip students to formulate creative and courageous solutions to health care problems and issues. The primary goal is to develop in all students a fund of knowledge, skills, and attitudes that will enable them to pursue the postgraduate training necessary for their chosen career.

Curricular Highlights

Community Service Requirement: Required. Numerous opportunities available.
Research/Thesis Requirement: Optional. Numerous opportunities available.

The curriculum is based on a multi-departmental, organ-system approach. Normal structure/function is presented first, followed by pathophysiology and therapeutic approaches. Students learn medical history-taking, physical diagnosis, and other aspects of the physician-patient relationship. They participate in longitudinal ambulatory clinical experience all four years. Students rotate through major clinical disciplines in the third year. Students complete a sub-internship, courses in emergent and urgent care, a selective experience, and five elective months in the fourth year. The grading system is pass/fail; grading in year three is honors and pass/fail; no class rank or class standing scales are used.

USMLE

Step 1: Required. Students must record a passing score for promotion.
Step 2: Clinical Skills (CS): Required. Students must record a passing total score to graduate.
Step 2: Clinical Knowledge (CK): Required. Students must record a passing total score to graduate.

Selection Factors

The University of Connecticut accepts highly qualified Connecticut residents, with special effort to include those who are disadvantaged. Highly qualified out-of-state residents are considered to achieve a diverse class. The Admissions Committee considers the applicant's interests, achievements, abilities, motivation, and character. GPA and MCAT scores are considered, along with academic program difficulty, academic achievement beyond regular coursework, intellectual growth and development, nonacademic activities, and recommendations. UCSOM policy prohibits discrimination in education, in employment, and in the provision of services on account of race, religion, sex, age, marital status, national origin, ancestry, sexual orientation, disabled veteran status, physical or mental disability, mental retardation, other specifically covered mental disabilities, and criminal records that are not job-related, in accordance with provisions of the Civil Rights Act of 1964, Title IX Education Amendments of 1972, the Rehabilitation Act of 1973, the Americans with Disabilities Act, and other existing federal and state laws and executive orders pertaining to equal rights.

Financial Aid

Educational costs are modest and the financial assistance program is strong. Financial need is not considered relevant to the admissions process. Every effort is made to meet each student's financial requirements through scholarships and loans. Entrance, exit, and debt counseling are provided.

Information about Diversity Programs

The UCSOM recruits disadvantaged applicants and applicants from groups underrepresented in medicine through the Admissions Office and the Department of Health Careers Opportunity Programs (HCOP). The Admissions Committee reviews applications from these candidates in the same manner as those of all other candidates. Candidates receive a full and sensitive review and are selected on a competitive basis. Candidates invited for an interview meet with HCOP staff. Summer enrichment programs are available for high school and college students from groups traditionally underrepresented in American medicine. the HCOP Department's telephone number is (860) 679-3483.

Campus Information

Setting

The 162 acre Health Science Complex is seven miles west of Hartford, with panoramic views of rural hills and the Hartord skyline. The John Dempsey University Hospital is onsite. A major research university, extensive research facilities are an integral part of the Health Center's lifeblood.

Enrollment

For 2007, total enrollment was: 320

Special Features

Signature programs include The Pat and Jim Calhoun Cardiology Center, The Carole and Ray Neag Comprehensive Cancer Center, and The Musculoskeletal Institute. Research centers include: International Community Health Studies, Microbial Pathogenesis, Molecular Medicine, Immunotherapy of Cancer and Infectious Diseases, and Women's Health Research.

Housing

The School of Medicine helps students identify housing in the local community.

Satellite Campuses/Facilities

Students rotate through clinical sites to insure a mix of inpatient and ambulatory experiences. Students complete a Continuity Practice experience with a physician in the community.

Application Process and Requirements 2009–2010

Primary Application Service: AMCAS
Earliest filing date: June 1, 2008
Latest filing date: December 15, 2008

Secondary Application Required?: Yes
Sent to: All applicants
Contact: Lynda Fox, (860) 679-4306
fox@nso1.uchc.edu
Fee: Yes, $85
Fee waiver available: Yes
Earliest filing date: June 1, 2008
Latest filing date: January 30, 2009

Latest MCAT® considered: 2008
Oldest MCAT® considered: 2005

Early Decision Program
School does have EDP
Applicants notified: October 1, 2008
EDP available for: Both Residents
and Non-Residents

Regular Acceptance Notice
Earliest date: October 15, 2008
Latest date: Until class is full

Applicant's Response to Acceptance Offer – Maximum Time: Two weeks

Requests for Deferred Entrance Considered: Yes

Deposit to Hold Place in Class: Yes
Deposit (Resident): $100
Deposit (Non-Resident): $100
Deposit due: with response to acceptance offer
Applied to tuition: Yes
Deposit refundable: Yes
Refundable by: May 15, 2009

Estimated number of new entrants: 85
EDP: 8, special program: n/a

Start Month/Year: August 2009

Interview Format: Three one-on-one interviews. Some regional interviews are done.

Other Programs

PREPARATORY PROGRAMS
Postbaccalaureate Program: Yes,
http://medicine.uchc.edu/prospective/postbac
Summer Research Fellowships Program:
Keat Sanford, (860)679-3874
sanford@nso1.uchc.edu
Medical/Dental Preparatory Program:
http://medicine.uchc.edu/prospective/enrichment/
collegefellow
COMBINED DEGREE PROGRAMS
Baccalaureate/MD: http://medicine.uchc.edu/
prospective/admissions/babs_md.html
MD/MPH: Yes, http://publichealth.uconn.edu/
acprgms_mph_combined.php
MD/MBA: Yes, Keat Sanford, http://medicine.
uchc.edu/prospective/admissions/mba_md.html
MD/JD: No
MD/PhD: No

Premedical Coursework

Course	Req.	Rec.	Lab.	Hrs.	Course	Req.	Rec.	Lab.	Hrs.
Inorganic Chemistry	•		•	8	Computer Science				
Behavioral Sciences					Genetics		•		
Biochemistry		•			Humanities		•		
Biology		•			Organic Chemistry	•		•	8
Biology/Zoology	•		•	8	Physics	•		•	8
Calculus		•			Psychology		•		
College English		•			Social Sciences		•		
College Mathematics		•			Physiology		•		

Selection Factors: 2007 Accepted Applicants

Proportion of Accepted Applicants with Relevant Experience (Data Self-Reported to AMCAS®)		
Community Service/Volunteer		68%
Medically-Related Work		80%
Research		88%

Shaded bar represents accepted scores ranging from the 10th percentile to the 90th percentile. **School Median** ● **National Median** ●

Overall GPA	2.0	2.1	2.2	2.3	2.4	2.5	2.6	2.7	2.8	2.9	3.0	3.1	3.2	3.3	3.4	3.5	3.6	⊙3.7	3.8	3.9	4.0
Science GPA	2.0	2.1	2.2	2.3	2.4	2.5	2.6	2.7	2.8	2.9	3.0	3.1	3.2	3.3	3.4	3.5	3.6	⊙3.7	3.8	3.9	4.0

MCAT® required: Yes, 99% of 2007 accepted applicants took MCAT®

Verbal Reasoning	3	4	5	6	7	8	9	⑩	11	12	13	14	15
Physical Sciences	3	4	5	6	7	8	9	10	⑪	12	13	14	15
Biological Sciences	3	4	5	6	7	8	9	10	⑪	12	13	14	15
Writing Sample			J	K	L	M	N	O	P	ⓠ	R	S	T

Acceptance & Matriculation Data for 2007–2008 First Year Class

	Resident	Non-Resident	International	Total
Applied	404	2294	278	2976
Interviewed	225	150	10	385
Deferred	5	0	1	6
Matriculants				
Early Assurance Program	4	0	0	4
Early Decision Program	1	0	0	1
Baccalaureate/MD	3	0	0	3
MD/PhD	1	1	0	2
Matriculated	70	9	2	**81**

Applications accepted from International Applicants: Yes

Specialty Choice

2003, 2004, 2005 Graduates, Specialty Choice (As reported by program directors to GME Track™)	
Anesthesiology	5%
Emergency Medicine	8%
Family Practice	5%
Internal Medicine	26%
Obstetrics/Gynecology	7%
Orthopaedic Surgery	2%
Pediatrics	14%
Psychiatry	5%
Radiology	2%
Surgery	9%

Matriculant Demographics: 2007–2008 First Year Class

Men: 33 **Women:** 48

Matriculants' Self-Reported Race/Ethnicity

Mexican American	2	**Korean**	1
Cuban	0	**Vietnamese**	1
Puerto Rican	0	**Other Asian**	4
Other Hispanic	4	**Total Asian**	14
Total Hispanic	6	**Native American**	1
Chinese	2	**Black**	8
Asian Indian	6	**Native Hawaiian**	0
Pakistani	0	**White**	56
Filipino	0	**Unduplicated Number**	
Japanese	0	**of Matriculants**	81

Science and Math Majors: 67%
Matriculants with:
Baccalaureate degree: 98%
Graduate degree(s): 6%

Financial Information

Source: 2006–2007 LCME I-B survey
and 2007–2008 AAMC TSF questionnaire

	Residents	Non-Residents
Total Cost of Attendance	$26,827	$49,463
Tuition and Fees	$24,142	$46,778
Other (includes living expenses)	$0	$0
Health Insurance (can not be waived)	$2,685	$2,685

Average 2007 Graduate Indebtedness: $118,839
% of Enrolled Students Receiving Aid: 86%

Criminal Background Check

This medical school does not require a criminal background check prior to matriculation.

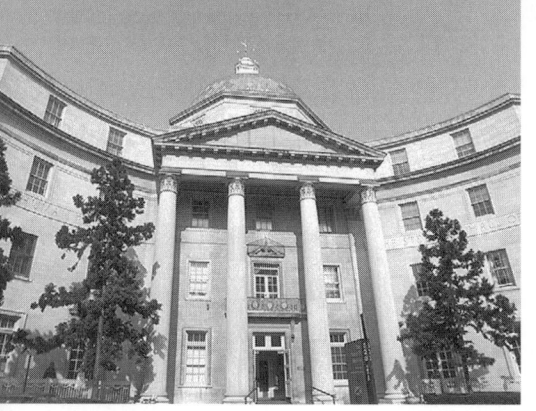

Yale University School of Medicine

New Haven, Connecticut

Richard A. Silverman, Director of Admissions
Yale University School of Medicine
Edward S. Harkness Hall, 367 Cedar Street
New Haven, Connecticut 06510
T 203 785 2696 **F** 203 785 3234

Admissions
http://info.med.yale.edu/education/admissions/
Main http://info.med.yale.edu/ysm/
Financial www.med.yale.edu/education/finaid/index.html
Email medical.admissions@yale.edu

Private Institution

Dr. Robert J. Alpern, Dean

*Dr. Laura R. Ment, Associate Dean
for Admissions*

*Dr. Forrester A. Lee, Assistant Dean for
Multicultural Affairs*

Pamela J. Nyiri, Director of Financial Aid

*Dr. Richard Belitsky, Deputy Dean
for Education*

*Dr. Nancy R. Angoff, Associate Dean
for Student Affairs*

General Information

The Yale University School of Medicine was established in 1810 as the Medical Institution of Yale College. The present-day Yale-New Haven Medical Center includes the School of Medicine, the School of Nursing, and Yale-New Haven Hospital.

Mission Statement

The mission of the Yale University School of Medicine is to educate and inspire scholars and future leaders who will advance the practice of medicine and the biomedical sciences.

Curricular Highlights

Community Service Requirement: Optional. Extensive community service opportunities.
Research/Thesis Requirement: Required. Original thesis required since 1839.

The Yale System of Medical Education is founded on a belief in the maturity and responsibility of students. Highlights of the program are anonymous examinations, the absence of competitive grades, and a required thesis. The ideal Yale physician is schooled in the current state of knowledge of both medical biology and patient care, with a lifelong commitment to learning. The first two years of the curriculum focus on the basic and clinical sciences. The first year emphasizes normal biological form and function, the second year the study of disease. Throughout both years, a pre-clinical clerkship course provides instruction in history, physical examination, and the art of communicating with patients. The third year is largely devoted to clinical clerkships.

In the fourth year, students take electives and a primary care clerkship, and complete their thesis. Required since 1839, the thesis is designed to develop critical thinking, habits of self-education, and application of the scientific method to medicine. Thesis work also gives students an opportunity to work closely with Yale faculty members.

USMLE

Step 1: Required. Students must record a passing score for promotion.
Step 2: Clinical Skills (CS): Required. Students must record a passing total score to graduate.
Step 2: Clinical Knowledge (CK): Required. Students must record a passing total score to graduate.

Selection Factors

The Admissions Committee seeks exceptional students who best suit the educational philosophy of the school. Because of the importance of diversity, applications are encouraged from women and persons from groups underrepresented in medicine. The committee considers each applicant's academic record, MCAT® scores, premedical committee evaluations, letters of recommendation, extracurricular and community activities, and personal qualities. In general, the school strives to admit students with the ability to make significant contributions in medicine and a demonstrated capacity for leadership. Interviews are arranged only by invitation of the Admissions Committee. The class of 100 students that enrolled in 2007 includes graduates of 48 undergraduate colleges. The diversity of the student body is also reflected in a wide variety of academic, professional, and personal interests. The Yale School of Medicine does not discriminate on the basis of sex, race, color, religion, age, disability, national or ethnic origin, sexual orientation, or gender identity or expression.

Financial Aid

Financial aid is based on need and is intended to enable any accepted student to attend without unreasonable hardship. All financial aid applicants must submit the FAFSA and the Yale financial aid application, which will be available (online only) on January 1. In addition, those applying for Yale scholarship funds must submit a supplemental needs analysis, which requires student, spouse, and family financial statements.

Information about Diversity Programs

Diversity is important in Yale's interactive, collaborative learning environment, and applications are encouraged from individuals from groups underrepresented in medicine. Several student organizations sponsor a range of activities throughout the year, all supported by the Office of Multicultural Affairs.

Campus Information

Setting

In completing their studies near the heart of the Yale University campus, medical students benefit from academic and extracurricular opportunities provided by other Yale schools and by the city of New Haven, a culturally diverse city located 75 miles east of New York.

Enrollment

For 2007, total enrollment was: 395

Special Features

The Anlyan Center for Medical Research and Education is an immense structure for disease-based research, with state-of-the-art teaching space for anatomy and histology. Construction of an enlarged Yale Cancer Center will be completed in 2009. Yale was recently honored with a Clinical and Translational Science Award from NIH, reflecting the school's strong commitment to clinical research. A Master of Health Science degree is now available as a joint degree option for MD students who choose to take a tuition-free fifth year. These and other new facilities and programs are part of an unprecedented period of growth at Yale.

Housing

On-campus housing is available for single and married students, and the Yale Housing Office provides access to off-campus apartments in the area.

Satellite Campuses/Facilities

Clinical training occurs at Yale-New Haven Hospital and other nearby hospitals and clinics. In addition, training sites have been established elsewhere in the United States and abroad. International research and community service opportunities are also available.

Application Process and Requirements 2009–2010

Primary Application Service: AMCAS
Earliest filing date: June 1, 2008
Latest filing date: October 15, 2008

Secondary Application Required?: Yes
Sent to: All applicants
URL: http://info.med.yale.edu/education/admissions/
Fee: Yes, $85
Fee waiver available: Yes
Earliest filing date: June 1, 2008
Latest filing date: November 15, 2008

Latest MCAT® considered: September 2008
Oldest MCAT® considered: 2005

Early Decision Program
School does have EDP
Applicants notified: October 1, 2008
EDP available for: Both Residents and Non-Residents

Regular Acceptance Notice
Earliest date: March 15, 2009
Latest date: Until class is full

Applicant's Response to Acceptance Offer – Maximum Time: Three weeks

Requests for Deferred Entrance Considered: Yes

Deposit to Hold Place in Class: Yes
Deposit (Resident): $100
Deposit (Non-Resident): $100
Deposit due: With response to acceptance offer
Applied to tuition: Yes
Deposit refundable: Yes
Refundable by: May 15, 2009

Estimated number of new entrants: 100
EDP: 2, special program: n/a

Start Month/Year: August 2009

Interview Format: One-on-one, open-file interviews. Regional interviews only available if applicant is unable to come to campus.

Other Programs

PREPARATORY PROGRAMS
Postbaccalaureate Program: No
Summer Program: Yes,
http://info.med.yale.edu/omca/programs/mmep.htm
Yale Summer Medical and Dental Education Program:
http://info.med.yale.edu/omca/programs/mmep.htm
Biomedical Science Training & Enrichment Program:
http://info.med.yale.edu/omca/programs/biostep.htm

COMBINED DEGREE PROGRAMS
Baccalaureate/MD: No
MD/MPH: Yes, http://info.med.yale.edu/
ysm/admissions/index.html
MD/MBA: Yes, http://mba.yale.edu/MBA/
curriculum/md_mba/index.shtml
MD/JD: Yes, http://www.law.yale.edu/
academics/jointdegrees.asp
MD/PhD: Yes, http://info.med.yale.edu/mdphd/
Additional Program: Yes,
http://info.med.yale.edu/ysm/admissions/index.html

Premedical Coursework

Course	Req.	Rec.	Lab.	Hrs.	Course	Req.	Rec.	Lab.	Hrs.
Inorganic Chemistry	•		•	6-8	Computer Science				
Behavioral Sciences					Genetics				
Biochemistry					Humanities				
Biology					Organic Chemistry	•		•	6-8
Biology/Zoology	•		•	6-8	Physics	•		•	6-8
Calculus					Psychology				
College English					Social Sciences				
College Mathematics					Other				

Selection Factors: 2007 Accepted Applicants

Proportion of Accepted Applicants with Relevant Experience (Data Self-Reported to AMCAS®)		
Community Service/Volunteer		72%
Medically-Related Work		86%
Research		93%

Shaded bar represents accepted scores ranging from the 10th percentile to the 90th percentile. **School Median** ● **National Median** ●

Overall GPA	2.0	2.1	2.2	2.3	2.4	2.5	2.6	2.7	2.8	2.9	3.0	3.1	3.2	3.3	3.4	3.5	3.6	3.7	(3.8)	3.9	4.0
Science GPA	2.0	2.1	2.2	2.3	2.4	2.5	2.6	2.7	2.8	2.9	3.0	3.1	3.2	3.3	3.4	3.5	3.6	3.7	(3.8)	3.9	4.0

MCAT® required: Yes, 100% of 2007 accepted applicants took MCAT®

Verbal Reasoning	3	4	5	6	7	8	9	(10)	(11)	12	13	14	15
Physical Sciences	3	4	5	6	7	8	9	10	(11)	(12)	13	14	15
Biological Sciences	3	4	5	6	7	8	9	10	(11)	(12)	13	14	15
Writing Sample			J	K	L	M	N	O	P	(Q)	R	S	T

Acceptance & Matriculation Data for 2007–2008 First Year Class

	Resident	Non-Resident	International	Total
Applied	198	4441	382	5021
Interviewed	68	852	78	998
Deferred	0	5	1	6
Matriculants				
Early Assurance Program	n/a	n/a	n/a	n/a
Early Decision Program	0	0	1	1
Baccalaureate/MD	n/a	n/a	n/a	n/a
MD/PhD	1	9	0	10
Matriculated	11	75	14	**100**

Applications accepted from International Applicants: Yes

Specialty Choice

2003, 2004, 2005 Graduates, Specialty Choice (As reported by program directors to GME Track™)	
Anesthesiology	1%
Emergency Medicine	5%
Family Practice	2%
Internal Medicine	21%
Obstetrics/Gynecology	4%
Orthopaedic Surgery	4%
Pediatrics	8%
Psychiatry	5%
Radiology	5%
Surgery	8%

Matriculant Demographics: 2007–2008 First Year Class

Men: 53 **Women:** 47

Matriculants' Self-Reported Race/Ethnicity

Mexican American	2	Korean	3
Cuban	2	Vietnamese	2
Puerto Rican	1	Other Asian	3
Other Hispanic	2	Total Asian	25
Total Hispanic	7	Native American	0
Chinese	10	Black	13
Asian Indian	7	Native Hawaiian	0
Pakistani	0	White	47
Filipino	0	Unduplicated Number	
Japanese	0	of Matriculants	100

Science and Math Majors: 68%
Matriculants with:
Baccalaureate degree: 100%
Graduate degree(s): 10%

Financial Information

Source: 2006–2007 LCME I-B survey and 2007–2008 AAMC TSF questionnaire

	Residents	Non-Residents
Total Cost of Attendance	$59,910	$59,910
Tuition and Fees	$41,220	$41,220
Other (includes living expenses)	$16,850	$16,850
Health Insurance (can be waived)	$1,840	$1,840

Average 2007 Graduate Indebtedness: $115,385
% of Enrolled Students Receiving Aid: 87%

Criminal Background Check

This medical school does not require a criminal background check prior to matriculation.

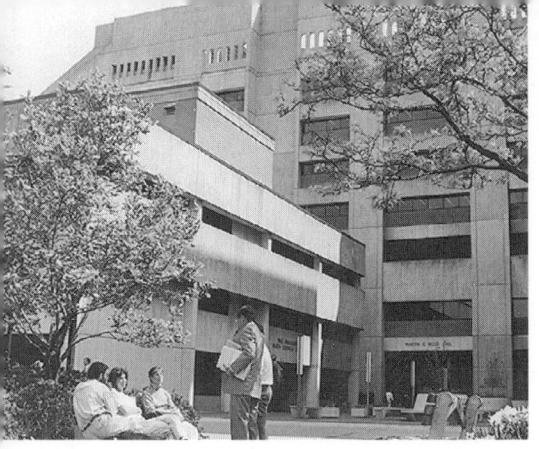

The George Washington University
School of Medicine and Health Sciences
Washington, D.C.

The George Washington University
School of Medicine and Health Sciences
Office of MD Admissions
2300 I Street, N.W., Ross Hall 716
Washington, District of Columbia 20037
T 202 994 3506 F 202 994 1753

Admissions www.gwumc.edu/edu/admis
Main www.gwumc.edu/smhs
Financial www.gwumc.edu/smhs/Fin-Aid
Email medadmit@gwu.edu

Private Institution

*Dr. John F. Williams, Provost and
Vice President for Health Affairs*

*Dr. James L. Scott, Dean,
School of Medicine and Health Sciences*

Diane P. McQuail, Assistant Dean of Admissions

Charles W. Carpenter, Director of Financial Aid

General Information

Founded in 1825, the School of Medicine and Health Sciences is the 11th oldest medical school in the country. The school is housed in Ross Hall, a research, educational and administrative facility located in the nation's capital. Located adjacent to Ross Hall, the new, state-of-the-art GW Hospital opened in August 2002. The facility boasts an Educational Center consisting of a clinical simulation facility, a standardized patient examination facility, a computer resource center, and lounge/conference areas.

Mission Statement

With a vision to be a pre-eminent health institution in the Washington area, GW is committed to providing the highest quality of care and health services to the public; excellence and innovation in education; and research that expands the frontiers of science and knowledge.

Curricular Highlights

Community Service Requirement: Required.
Research/Thesis Requirement: Optional.

The curriculum contains a course entitled "The Practice of Medicine" (POM). This course spans all four years, allowing students to begin clinical training during the first two years while studying the basic sciences. Each first-year student has a physician mentor. Clinical clerkships begin in the third year, and opportunities for international clinical experiences are available during the fourth year. An Honors/Pass/Conditional/Fail system is used for grading. Early Selection Programs are available to sophomores in the spring semester at GW, the University of Maryland-College Park, St. Bonaventure, and George Mason Universities, and Franklin & Marshall, Claremont McKenna, Scripps, Rowan, Knox, Colgate, Lyon, Rhodes,

and Hampden-Sydney Colleges. In addition, linkage agreements exist with postbaccalaureate programs at Goucher College, the University of Pennsylvania, Brandeis University, New York University, Scripps College, Johns Hopkins University, and Bryn Mawr College. Transfer information for the second- and third-year classes is available at *www.gwumc.edu/edu/admis/html/admissions/transfer.html.*

USMLE

Step 1: Required. Students must record a passing score for promotion.
Step 2: Clinical Skills (CS): Required. Students must record a passing total score to graduate.
Step 2: Clinical Knowledge (CK): Required. Students must record a passing total score to graduate.

Selection Factors

The initial evaluation is based on data in the AMCAS and GW applications. This evaluation reviews academic performance; MCAT® scores; extracurricular, health-related, research, and work experiences; and evidence of non-scholastic accomplishments. The next phase of the selection procedure is based on examination of personal comments and letters of recommendation. The most promising applicants are invited for interview. The last phase includes the review by the Committee on Admissions of the entire dossier. This phase selects academically prepared students with motivational and personal characteristics the Committee considers important in future physicians.

Financial Aid

Information is available at *www.gwumc.edu/smhs/Fin-Aid/.* Merit-based admissions scholarships are available.

Information about Diversity Programs

The School of Medicine is committed to providing an education to students from groups underrepresented in medicine. Applicants are encouraged to meet with students and faculty from groups underrepresented in medicine. There are focused student organizations such as NBLHO and SNMA.

Campus Information

Setting

The Medical Center is on the Foggy Bottom campus of The George Washington University in Washington, DC. A subway stop sits immediately outside the medical school. The campus is within walking distance of the White House and the National Mall.

Enrollment

For 2007, total enrollment was: 700

Special Features

Students study histology and pathology in a state-of-the-art laboratory, reviewing digital slides on computer monitors. The newly created Office of Student Opportunities serves as a clearinghouse for various research, scholarships, awards, conferences, and study abroad opportunities. The Track Program offers students an opportunity to choose a program of study outside the standard curriculum, *www.gwumc.edu/smhs/students/opportunities.* Humanities in medicine electives are available. GW operates a Mobile Mammography Program (GW Mammovan), which provides screening mammograms to women in the DC area. The Interdisci-plinary Student Community-Oriented Prevention Enhancement Service (ISCOPES) is an interdisciplinary team service-learning experience providing a wide range of health-related services. The student-run Healing Clinic also provides health care to DC underserved.

Housing

Some graduate student housing is available. The Washington, DC area has abundant off-campus housing options. For information, visit *www.gwumc.edu/smhs/students/Housing2.htm.*

Satellite Campuses/Facilities

In addition to the GW Hospital, the teaching services of the Children's National Medical Center, Inova Fairfax Hospital, Holy Cross Hospital, National Naval Medical Center, St. Elizabeth's Hospital, Veterans Administration Hospital, and Washington Hospital Center are also available to students. A variety of ambulatory sites in the DC area are also utilized, including neighborhood clinics that serve indigent patients.

Application Process and Requirements 2009–2010

Primary Application Service: AMCAS
Earliest filing date: June 1, 2008
Latest filing date: December 1, 2008

Secondary Application Required?: Yes
Sent to: All applicants
URL: n/a
Fee: Yes, $125
Fee waiver available: Yes
Earliest filing date: June 1, 2008
Latest filing date: January 1, 2009

Latest MCAT® considered: September 2008
Oldest MCAT® considered: April 2006

Early Decision Program
School does have EDP
Applicants notified: October 1, 2008
EDP available for: Both Residents and Non-Residents

Regular Acceptance Notice
Earliest date: October 15, 2008
Latest date: Until class is full

Applicant's Response to Acceptance
Offer – Maximum Time: Two weeks

Requests for Deferred
Entrance Considered: Yes

Deposit to Hold Place in Class: Yes
Deposit (Resident): $100
Deposit (Non-Resident): $100
Deposit due: May 15, 2009
Applied to tuition: Yes
Deposit refundable: Yes
Refundable by: May 15, 2009

Estimated number of new entrants: 177
EDP: 5, special program: 40

Start Month/Year: August 2009

Interview Format: Two blind interviews with a faculty member and a student. All interviews take place at GW.

Other Programs
PREPARATORY PROGRAMS
Postbaccalaureate Program: No
Summer Program: No

COMBINED DEGREE PROGRAMS
Baccalaureate/MD: Yes, 7 year program with George Washington University, http://gwired.gwu.edu/adm/apply/special_prog.html, 8 year program with St. Bonaventure University, www.sbu.edu and www.gwumc.edu
MD/MPH: Yes, www.gwumc.edu/edu/admis/html/academics/specialprog.html
MD/MBA: No
MD/JD: No
MD/PhD: Yes, www.gwumc.edu/edu/admis/html/academics/specialprog.html

Premedical Coursework

Course	Req.	Rec.	Lab.	Hrs.	Course	Req.	Rec.	Lab.	Hrs.
Inorganic Chemistry	•		•	8	Computer Science				
Behavioral Sciences					Genetics				
Biochemistry					Humanities				
Biology					Organic Chemistry	•		•	8
Biology/Zoology	•		•	8	Physics	•		•	8
Calculus					Psychology				
College English	•			6	Social Sciences				
College Mathematics					Other				

Selection Factors: 2007 Accepted Applicants

Proportion of Accepted Applicants with Relevant Experience (Data Self-Reported to AMCAS)		
Community Service/Volunteer		73%
Medically-Related Work		88%
Research		77%

Shaded bar represents accepted scores ranging from the 10th percentile to the 90th percentile. School Median ● National Median ●

Overall GPA	2.0	2.1	2.2	2.3	2.4	2.5	2.6	2.7	2.8	2.9	3.0	3.1	3.2	3.3	3.4	3.5	(3.6)	3.7	3.8	3.9	4.0
Science GPA	2.0	2.1	2.2	2.3	2.4	2.5	2.6	2.7	2.8	2.9	3.0	3.1	3.2	3.3	3.4	(3.5)	3.6	3.7	3.8	3.9	4.0

MCAT® required: Yes, 83% of 2007 accepted applicants took MCAT®

Verbal Reasoning	3	4	5	6	7	8	9	(10)	11	12	13	14	15
Physical Sciences	3	4	5	6	7	8	9	(10)	(11)	12	13	14	15
Biological Sciences	3	4	5	6	7	8	9	(10)	(11)	12	13	14	15
Writing Sample				J	K	L	M	N	O	P	(Q)	R	S	T

Acceptance & Matriculation Data for 2007–2008 First Year Class

	Resident	Non-Resident	International	Total
Applied	57	12572	453	13082
Interviewed	19	923	n/a	942
Deferred	0	5	0	5
Matriculants				
Early Assurance Program	0	30	n/a	30
Early Decision Program	0	10	1	11
Baccalaureate/MD	1	17	n/a	18
MD/PhD	n/a	1	n/a	1
Matriculated	6	168	3	**177**

Applications accepted from International Applicants: Yes

Specialty Choice

2003, 2004, 2005 Graduates, Specialty Choice (As reported by program directors to GME Track™)	
Anesthesiology	8%
Emergency Medicine	7%
Family Practice	5%
Internal Medicine	19%
Obstetrics/Gynecology	4%
Orthopaedic Surgery	5%
Pediatrics	12%
Psychiatry	5%
Radiology	5%
Surgery	8%

Matriculant Demographics: 2007–2008 First Year Class

Men: 70   **Women:** 107

Matriculants' Self-Reported Race/Ethnicity

Mexican American	0	Korean	4
Cuban	1	Vietnamese	0
Puerto Rican	1	Other Asian	7
Other Hispanic	2	Total Asian	46
Total Hispanic	4	Native American	2
Chinese	8	Black	23
Asian Indian	25	Native Hawaiian	2
Pakistani	3	White	100
Filipino	2	Unduplicated Number	
Japanese	0	of Matriculants	177

Science and Math Majors: 52%
Matriculants with:
Baccalaureate degree: 100%
Graduate degree(s): 18%

Financial Information

Source: 2006–2007 LCME I-B survey and 2007–2008 AAMC TSF questionnaire

	Residents	Non-Residents
Total Cost of Attendance	$44,915	$44,915
Tuition and Fees	$44,915	$44,915
Other (includes living expenses)	$0	$0
Health Insurance (can not be waived)	$0	$0

Average 2007 Graduate Indebtedness: $172,978
% of Enrolled Students Receiving Aid: 82%

Criminal Background Check

This school currently requires a criminal background check prior to matriculation.

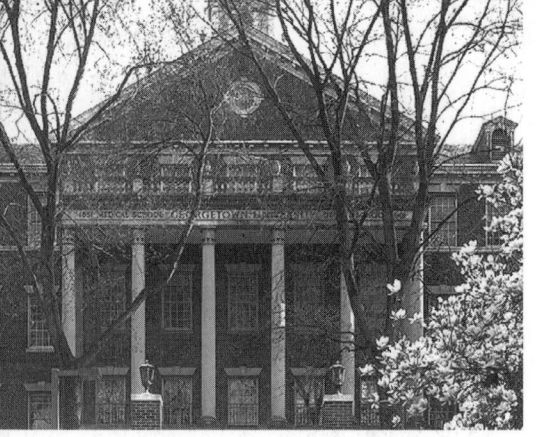

Georgetown University School of Medicine
Washington, D.C.

Office of Admissions
Georgetown University School of Medicine
Box 571421
Washington, District of Columbia 20057-1421
T 202 687 1154   F 202 687 3079

Admissions http://som.georgetown.edu/admissions
Main http://som.georgetown.edu
Financial http://som.georgetown.edu/finaid
Email medicaladmissions@georgetown.edu

Private Institution

Dr. S. Ray Mitchell, Dean for Medical Education

Brandon C. Schneider, Director of Admissions

Joy P. Williams, Associate Dean for Students and Special Programs

David J. Pollock, Assistant Dean for Student Financial Planning

Dr. Russell T. Wall III, Associate Dean for Admissions and Student Services

General Information
The School of Medicine works in association with the 535-bed Georgetown University Hospital, part of the MedStar not-for-profit health care system. The school has affiliations with eight federal and community hospitals in the Washington, DC area. The campus contains a health science library and an integrated learning center with 10 clinical examination rooms. Adjacent to the hospital is the Lombardi Cancer Research Center, which provides both research and clinical care. The school is near the NIH and other internationally prominent health care and research facilities. The Yates Field House offers swimming, jogging tracks, and other athletic programs. The Leavey Center hosts dining establishments and guest quarters.

Mission Statement
Guided by the University's Jesuit tradition of 'cura personalis,' caring for the whole person, Georgetown University School of Medicine will educate, in an integrated way, knowledgeable, skillful, ethical, and compassionate physicians and biomedical scientists, dedicated to the care of others and the health needs of our society. Our educational approach involves excellent basic science and clinical faculty who are committed to providing first-rate scientific information in an environment conducive to learning and application. All of our students participate in small-group and independent learning. Students also serve on educational and student affairs committees.

Curricular Highlights
Community Service Requirement: Required.
Research/Thesis Requirement: Research project required.

Georgetown's curriculum in the first two years emphasizes the body's normal and altered structure and functions reinforced with clinically oriented educational experiences, early introduction to patients, the art of advocacy, and the ethical/cultural dimensions of medicine. Small-group teaching in labs, seminars, and at the bedside begins early in the first year. The third year provides comprehensive clinical training to care of patients through clerkships in the major medical specialties. The fourth year gives each student substantial responsibility for the management of patient care through acting internships, elective study, and research. The grading system consists of Honors, High Pass, Pass, and Fail.

USMLE
Step 1: Required. Students must record a passing score for promotion.
Step 2: Clinical Skills (CS): Required. Students must record a passing total score to graduate.
Step 2: Clinical Knowledge (CK): Required. Students must record a passing total score to graduate.

Selection Factors
The Committee on Admissions selects students on the basis of academic achievement, character, maturity, and motivation. The committee evaluates the applicant's entire academic record, performance on the MCAT®, college premedical committee evaluations or letters of recommendation, personal essays, and personal interviews. Personal interviews are required and conducted on the medical center campus. Applicants may be invited to interview once all credentials have been reviewed by the committee. A secondary application and essay are required for all applicants. Applicants are urged to submit their applications and supporting credentials early. The School of Medicine does not discriminate on the basis of race, sex, creed, age, disability, sexual orientation, or national or ethnic origin. The School of Medicine has an Early Assurance Program with its undergraduate institution. Applicants for transfer are only considered from LCME-accredited medical schools.

Financial Aid
The school participates in federal financial aid programs and awards school-administered scholarships and low-interest loans to students on the basis of financial need. Parents' financial information is required for students seeking school-administered aid. Loan indebtedness counseling is an important function of the Office of Student Financial Planning, as a majority of students incur substantial educational debt. Candidates for admission are strongly encouraged to contact the office with questions.

Information about Diversity Programs
The School of Medicine has a diverse student body, with students from groups underrepresented in medicine. Questions about programs may be addressed to the director, Office of Programs for Minority Student Development. The Georgetown Experimental Medical Studies (GEMS) Program is a one-year postbaccalaureate program for qualified disadvantaged students and those from groups underrepresented in medicine. Priority consideration is given to residents of the District of Columbia. For more information, please telephone the GEMS program coordinator at (202) 687-1406.

Campus Information

Setting
On the university campus, in an urban setting.

Enrollment
For 2007, total enrollment was: 755

Special Features
Special features include Georgetown's state-of-the-art Clinical Skills Center, the Lombardi Cancer Center, opportunities for international clerkships following the first year and in the fourth year, and several community outreach programs.

Housing
No on-campus housing is available. The Office of Admissions attempts to assist students in finding housing.

Satellite Campuses/Facilities
Rotations are divided among the university hospital and other hospitals in the metro area. Ambulatory care experiences are within the area.

Application Process and Requirements 2009–2010

Primary Application Service: AMCAS
Earliest filing date: June 1, 2008
Latest filing date: October 31, 2008

Secondary Application Required?: Yes
Sent To: All applicants
URL: http://som.georgetown.edu/admissions
Fee: $130
Fee Waiver Available: Yes
Earliest filing date: June 15, 2008
Latest filing date: January 5, 2009

Latest MCAT® considered: September 2008
Oldest MCAT® considered: 2006

Early Decision Program
School does not have EDP
Applicants notified: n/a
EDP available for: n/a

Regular Acceptance Notice
Earliest date: October 15, 2008
Latest date: Until class is full

Applicant's Response to Acceptance
Offer – Maximum Time: Three weeks

Requests for Deferred
Entrance Considered: Yes

Deposit to Hold Place in Class: Yes
Deposit (Resident): $100
Deposit (Non-Resident): $100
Deposit due: March 15, 2009. Partial tuition prepayment due June 1, 2009
Applied to tuition: Yes
Deposit refundable: Yes
Refundable by: May 15, 2009

Estimated number of new entrants: 190
EDP: n/a, special program: n/a

Start Month/Year: August 2009

Interview Format: Interviews are one-on-one. Regional interviews are not available.

Other Programs

PREPARATORY PROGRAMS
Postbaccalaureate Program: Yes
http://www3.georgetown.edu/som/student/gems.html
Summer Program: Yes
http://gsmi.georgetown.edu

COMBINED DEGREE PROGRAMS
Baccalaureate/MD: No
MD/MPH: No
MD/MBA: Yes,
http://www3.georgetown.edu/som/curriculum/infosheet4.pdf
MD/JD: No
MD/PhD: Yes, http://biomedgrad.georgetown.edu/MDPhD/index.html

Premedical Coursework

Course	Req.	Rec.	Lab.	Sems.	Course	Req.	Rec.	Lab.	Sems.
Inorganic Chemistry	•		•	2	Computer Science		•		
Behavioral Sciences					Genetics		•		
Biochemistry		•			Humanities		•		
Biology	•		•	2	Organic Chemistry	•		•	2
Biology/Zoology					Physics	•		•	2
Calculus					Psychology				
College English	•			2	Social Sciences				
College Mathematics	•			1	Other				

Selection Factors: 2007 Accepted Applicants

Proportion of Accepted Applicants with Relevant Experience (Data Self-Reported to AMCAS)		
Community Service/Volunteer	66%	
Medically-Related Work	86%	
Research	81%	

Shaded bar represents accepted scores ranging from the 10th percentile to the 90th percentile. School Median ● National Median ●

Overall GPA	2.0	2.1	2.2	2.3	2.4	2.5	2.6	2.7	2.8	2.9	3.0	3.1	3.2	3.3	3.4	3.5	3.6	(3.7)	3.8	3.9	4.0
Science GPA	2.0	2.1	2.2	2.3	2.4	2.5	2.6	2.7	2.8	2.9	3.0	3.1	3.2	3.3	3.4	3.5	3.6	(3.7)	3.8	3.9	4.0

MCAT® required: Yes, 98% of 2007 accepted applicants took MCAT®

Verbal Reasoning	3	4	5	6	7	8	9	(10)	11	12	13	14	15
Physical Sciences	3	4	5	6	7	8	9	10	(11)	12	13	14	15
Biological Sciences	3	4	5	6	7	8	9	10	(11)	12	13	14	15
Writing Sample			J	K	L	M	N	O	P	(Q)	R	S	T

Acceptance & Matriculation Data for 2007–2008 First Year Class

	Resident	Non-Resident	International	Total
Applied	47	10139	457	10643
Interviewed	14	1281	17	1312
Deferred	0	5	0	5
Matriculants				
Early Assurance Program	0	7	0	7
Early Decision Program	0	0	0	0
Baccalaureate/MD	n/a	n/a	n/a	n/a
MD/PhD	0	2	0	2
Matriculated	8	176	6	**190**

Applications accepted from International Applicants: Yes

Specialty Choice

2003, 2004, 2005 Graduates, Specialty Choice (As reported by program directors to GME Track™)	
Anesthesiology	6%
Emergency Medicine	9%
Family Practice	7%
Internal Medicine	19%
Obstetrics/Gynecology	4%
Orthopaedic Surgery	9%
Pediatrics	7%
Psychiatry	3%
Radiology	4%
Surgery	9%

Matriculant Demographics: 2007–2008 First Year Class

Men: 98   **Women:** 92

Matriculants' Self-Reported Race/Ethnicity

Mexican American	1	**Korean**	4
Cuban	0	**Vietnamese**	4
Puerto Rican	1	**Other Asian**	1
Other Hispanic	4	**Total Asian**	33
Total Hispanic	6	**Native American**	0
Chinese	11	**Black**	16
Asian Indian	10	**Native Hawaiian**	0
Pakistani	2	**White**	135
Filipino	0	**Unduplicated Number**	
Japanese	2	**of Matriculants**	190

Science and Math Majors: 68%
Matriculants with:
   Baccalaureate degree: 99%
   Graduate degree(s): 19%

Financial Information

Source: 2006–2007 LCME I-B survey and 2007–2008 AAMC TSF questionnaire

	Residents	Non-Residents
Total Cost of Attendance	$64,700	$64,700
Tuition and Fees	$42,536	$42,536
Other (includes living expenses)	$20,525	$20,525
Health Insurance (can be waived)	$1,639	$1,639

Average 2007 Graduate Indebtedness: $168,256
% of Enrolled Students Receiving Aid: 90%

Criminal Background Check

This medical school requires a criminal background check prior to matriculation.

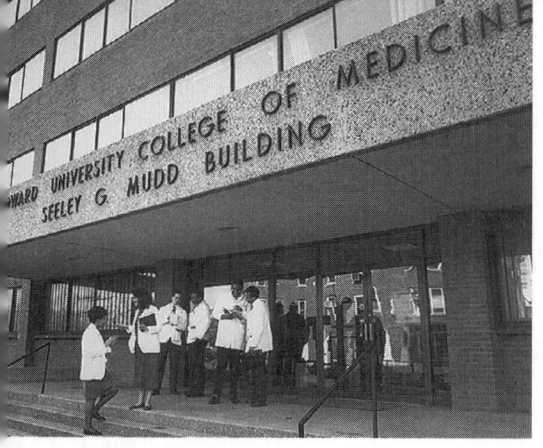

Howard University College of Medicine

Washington, D.C.

Office of Admissions, Office of the Dean
Howard University College of Medicine,
520 W Street, N.W., Room 2310
Washington, District of Columbia 20059
T 202 806 6270 **F** 202 265 0048

Admissions www.med.howard.edu/Admissions
Main www.med.howard.edu
Financial www.med.howard.edu/finaid
Email hucmadmissions@howard.edu

Private Institution

Dr. Robert E. Taylor, Dean

Judith M. Walk, Director of Admissions

Dr. Dawn L. Cannon, Associate Dean for Student Affairs and Admissions

Ann Finney, Admissions Officer

General Information

The Howard University College of Medicine is the oldest and largest historically black medical school in the United States and the 36th oldest of all 129 medical schools in this country. The medical department's primary goal at inception remains the college's goal today: to train students to become competent, compassionate physicians who will provide care in medically underserved communities. The college has more than 4,000 living alumni, including approximately 25 percent of all black practicing physicians in this country. During the first half of this century, the college contributed nearly half of the black physicians in the United States. The 321-bed Howard University Hospital was completed in 1975. It is the college's primary teaching hospital for medical students and is used for postgraduate training in the various specialties of medicine. Medical students also serve clerkships at the Children's National Medical Center, INOVA Fairfax Hospital, St. Elizabeth's Hospital, the Washington Veterans Affairs Medical Center, Providence Hospital, the Washington Hospital Center, and Prince George's Hospital Center.

Mission Statement

Howard University College of Medicine recognizes as its primary obligation the provision of a quality medical education for any student, irrespective of race, creed, sex, or national origin, but with emphasis upon the provision of educational opportunities for those socially, economically and culturally disadvantaged students, who may not otherwise have an opportunity to acquire an education.

Curricular Highlights

Community Service Requirement: Optional.
Research/Thesis Requirement: Optional.

An integrated curriculum was implemented in August 2001. Students in the first year complete curriculum blocks in Molecules and Cells, Structure and Function, and Medicine and Society. In year two, pathophysiology, pathology and pharmacology are integrated according to organ systems. The Medicine and Society block continues throughout the second year, and blocks in Physical Diagnosis and Introduction to Clinical Medicine are also included in year two. The third and fourth years consist of blocks of instruction in a continuum of clerkships and examinations in core clinical disciplines. During the fourth year, opportunity is available for additional clinical or research experience through 24 or 28 weeks of required electives. Grades in the College of Medicine are reported as H (honors), S (satisfactory), or U (unsatisfactory).

USMLE

Step 1: Required. Students must record a passing score for promotion.
Step 2: Clinical Skills (CS): Required. Students must record a passing total score to graduate.
Step 2: Clinical Knowledge (CK): Required. Students must record a passing total score to graduate.

Selection Factors

There are four major criteria used in the selection of applicants for admission to the College of Medicine: (1) character and discernible motivation for a career in medicine, (2) scholastic record, (3) results of the MCAT®, and (4) letters of recommendation from preprofessional advisors and faculty. Candidates for admission and alternates are selected from among those applicants who satisfy the criteria and who are most likely to serve in communities needing physician services. An invitation for an interview may be extended to an applicant after the Committee on Admissions has made a preliminary examination of the applicant's credentials and has decided that an interview is desirable. Although the total student is evaluated, the Committee on Admissions gives strongest consideration to those who have GPAs of 3.0 and above. There are no residence restrictions. All applicants will be evaluated

regardless of the applicants sex, race, religion, national or ethnic origin, age, marital status, or disability. A $100 (refundable) deposit and a $300 (non-refundable) enrollment fee (due with response to acceptance) is required of accepted applicants who have never previously enrolled at Howard University.

Financial Aid

Nearly all of the students enrolled in the College of Medicine receive some sort of financial assistance. Financial aid applicants must submit the FAFSA. Students with demonstrated need may receive school-based scholarships and loans, and those who qualify are recommended for federally guaranteed and private educational loans. Some merit awards are offered to outstanding entering first-year students and for exceptional academic performance in the medical curriculum. Some students receive scholarships funded by the National Health Service Corps or by the military.

Campus Information

Setting

The location of the campus in Washington, D.C., provides a cosmopolitan setting with a diversity of population and activities. The campus is Metrorail and Metrobus-accessible, and within walking distance of the hospital.

Enrollment

For 2007, total enrollment was: 469

Housing

Limited on-campus housing is available for graduate and professional students. Most medical students live off-campus within a short commute to the university.

Satellite Campuses/Facilities

Student rotations are divided between Howard University Hospital and several hospitals, ambulatory centers, and private physicians' offices in the metropolitan area.

Application Process and Requirements 2009–2010

Primary Application Service: AMCAS
Earliest filing date: June 1, 2008
Latest filing date: December 15, 2008

Secondary Application Required?: Yes, www.med.howard.edu/Secondary%20Application%20%20Online.doc
Sent to: All applicants
Contact: Ms. Judith Walk
(202) 806-6279, jwalk@howard.edu
Fee: Yes, $45
Fee waiver available: No
Earliest filing date: August 15, 2008
Latest filing date: January 30, 2009

Latest MCAT® considered: September 2008
Oldest MCAT® considered: 2006

Early Decision Program
School does not have EDP
Applicants notified: n/a
EDP available for: n/a

Regular Acceptance Notice
Earliest date: October 15, 2008
Latest date: Until class is full

Applicant's Response to Acceptance Offer – Maximum Time: Applicant's Response to Acceptance Offer – Maximum Time: 30 days, until April 15, 2009

Requests for Deferred Entrance Considered: Yes

Deposit to Hold Place in Class: Yes
Deposit (Resident): $400
Deposit (Non-Resident): $400
Deposit due: With acceptance offer, accompanied by non-refundable enrollment fee
Applied to tuition: Yes
Deposit refundable: Yes
Refundable by: April 15, 2009

Estimated number of new entrants: 121
EDP: n/a, special program: n/a

Start Month/Year: July 2009

Interview Format: One-on-one interview with admissions committee member. Regional interviews may be arranged upon request.

Other Programs

PREPARATORY PROGRAMS
Postbaccalaureate Program: No
Summer Program: Yes, www.founders.howard.edu/preprof/enrichmentprog.htm
Summer Medical and Dental Education Program (SMDEP) www.med.howard.edu/lloyd/HUCM_Information_06-07.pdf
COMBINED DEGREE PROGRAMS
Baccalaureate/MD: Yes, www.founders.howard.edu/preprof/BSMD-Brochure.pdf
MD/MPH: No
MD/MBA: No
MD/JD: No
MD/PhD: Yes, Dr. Verle Headings
(202) 806-6100, vheadings@howard.edu

Premedical Coursework

Course	Req.	Rec.	Lab.	Hrs.
Inorganic Chemistry	•		•	8
Behavioral Sciences				
Biochemistry		•	•	4
Biology				
Biology/Zoology	•			8
Calculus				
College English	•			6
College Mathematics	•			6

Course	Req.	Rec.	Lab.	Hrs.
Computer Science				
Genetics				
Humanities				
Organic Chemistry	•		•	8
Physics	•		•	8
Psychology				
Social Sciences				
Other				

Selection Factors: 2007 Accepted Applicants

Proportion of Accepted Applicants with Relevant Experience (Data Self-Reported to AMCAS®)		
Community Service/Volunteer		68%
Medically-Related Work		77%
Research		74%

Shaded bar represents accepted scores ranging from the 10th percentile to the 90th percentile ▨   **School Median** ●   **National Median** ●

Overall GPA	2.0	2.1	2.2	2.3	2.4	2.5	2.6	2.7	2.8	2.9	3.0	3.1	3.2	3.3	③.4	3.5	3.6	3.7	3.8	3.9	4.0
Science GPA	2.0	2.1	2.2	2.3	2.4	2.5	2.6	2.7	2.8	2.9	3.0	3.1	3.2	③.3	3.4	3.5	3.6	3.7	3.8	3.9	4.0

MCAT® required: Yes, 100% of 2007 accepted applicants took MCAT®

Verbal Reasoning	3	4	5	6	7	⑧	9	⑩	11	12	13	14	15
Physical Sciences	3	4	5	6	7	⑧	9	10	⑪	12	13	14	15
Biological Sciences	3	4	5	6	7	8	⑨	10	⑪	12	13	14	15
Writing Sample			J	K	L	M	N	ⓞ	P	ⓠ	R	S	T

Acceptance & Matriculation Data for 2007–2008 First Year Class

	Resident	Non-Resident	International	Total
Applied	40	4926	544	5510
Interviewed	30	273	25	328
Deferred	0	3	2	5
Matriculants				
Early Assurance Program	0	0	0	0
Early Decision Program	0	0	0	0
Baccalaureate/MD	0	0	0	8
MD/PhD	0	0	0	0
Matriculated	3	115	12	**130**

Applications accepted from International Applicants: Yes

Matriculant Demographics: 2007–2008 First Year Class

Men: 66   **Women:** 64

Matriculants' Self-Reported Race/Ethnicity

Mexican American	1	Korean		0
Cuban	0	Vietnamese		5
Puerto Rican	2	Other Asian		1
Other Hispanic	7	Total Asian		13
Total Hispanic	10	Native American		1
Chinese	1	Black		96
Asian Indian	4	Native Hawaiian		0
Pakistani	1	White		9
Filipino	1	**Unduplicated Number**		
Japanese	0	**of Matriculants**		130

Science and Math Majors: 78%
Matriculants with:
Baccalaureate degree: 92%
Graduate degree(s): 13%

Specialty Choice

2003, 2004, 2005 Graduates, Specialty Choice (As reported by program directors to GME Track™)	
Anesthesiology	4%
Emergency Medicine	5%
Family Practice	12%
Internal Medicine	18%
Obstetrics/Gynecology	11%
Orthopaedic Surgery	3%
Pediatrics	9%
Psychiatry	2%
Radiology	3%
Surgery	9%

Financial Information

Source: 2006–2007 LCME I-B survey and 2007–2008 AAMC TSF questionnaire

	Residents	Non-Residents
Total Cost of Attendance	$49,458	$49,458
Tuition and Fees	$29,846	$29,846
Other (includes living expenses)	$19,612	$19,612
Health Insurance	$0	$0

Average 2007 Graduate Indebtedness: $145,677
% of Enrolled Students Receiving Aid: 92%

Criminal Background Check

Criminal background check policy was not reported.

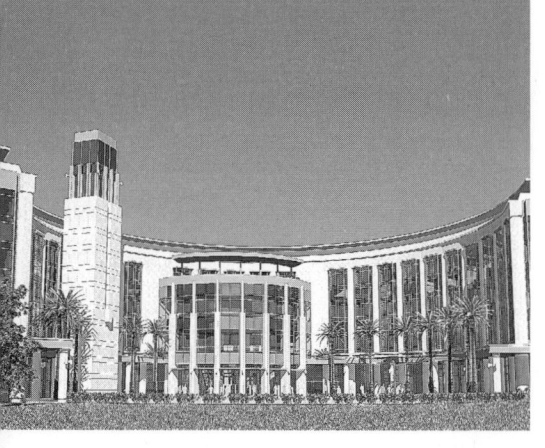

University of Central Florida
College of Medicine

Orlando, Florida

12201 Research Parkway, 3rd Floor
PO Box 160116
Orlando, FL, 32816-0116
T 407 823 4244 **F** 407 823 4048

Admissions www.med.ucf.edu/admissions
Main www.med.ucf.edu
Financial www.med.ucf.edu/financialservices
Email mdadmissions@mail.ucf.edu

Public Institution

Dr. Deborah C. German, Dean

REL Larkin, Director of Admissions

Ruthanne Madsen, Director of Financial Services

Teresa Lyons-Oten, Registrar

General Information

Enrolling our charter class in August 2009, the UCF COM will be fully integrated into Central Florida's healthcare and medical research community. UCF COM will be the premier medical school born in the 21st century. By partnering with Orlando Regional Hospital and Florida Hospital systems, the new Veterans Affairs and Nemours Hospitals, UCF students will have 17 major hospitals available for clinical training in all specialties of medicine. Central Florida has embraced the UCFCOM and each member of our first class should receive a Charter Class Scholarship which will cover tuition, fees, and conservative living expenses valued at $40,000 a year for each year.

Mission Statement

The College of Medicine pursues excellence in education, research, healthcare delivery, and promotion of health for the public good. In an environment of academic scholarship, diversity, partnership, and opportunity, we educate individuals to become exemplary physicians, leaders in medicine, scholars in discovery, and innovators in technology. We conduct basic and applied research to further the understanding and treatment of disease, improve the delivery of healthcare, and enhance the conduct of medical education.

Curricular Highlights

Community Service Requirement: Required.
Research/Thesis Requirement: Required.

The curriculum is a unique and exciting blend of state-of-the-art technology, virtual patients, clinical and laboratory experiences, research, directed small group sessions, and interactive didactic lectures. The first two years of the curriculum are structured into instructional

modules: the first year focuses on how basic science relates to the human body and disease; the second year is an organ system-based approach, applying first-year knowledge to the study of clinical disease, pathological processes, diagnosis, and treatment. Numerous clinical experiences will occur throughout the first two years that also includes a Focused Individualized Study and Research module. Third and fourth year curriculum is devoted to clinical experience through core clerkships and electives in our affiliated hospital facilities.

USMLE

Step 1: Required. Students must record a passing score for graduation, but not promotion.
Step 2: Clinical Skills (CS): Required. Students must only record a score.
Step 2: Clinical Knowledge (CK): Required. Students must only record a score.

Selection Factors

Supplemental applications are available to all qualified U.S. citizens, permanent residents, and those granted asylum who have submit a verified AMCAS application. Applicants chosen for an interview will be highly motivated, capable, passionate, academically proven, and have diverse skills, talents, and life experiences that will benefit the program, community, and fellow classmates.

Financial Aid

The financial status of the applicant is not considered in the admissions process. Student Financial Services staff assist M.D. students in obtaining funding resources and also provide counseling for many financial and debt management topics

Information about Diversity Programs

Increasing diversity and inclusiveness is one of the central goals of UCF. Minorities account for nearly 20 percent of UCF faculty, and an aggressive minority recruitment plan continues to be a priority for the university.

Campus Information

Setting

The College of Medicine will spend its entire first year adjacent to the UCF main campus in Orlando, only a short ride from the Space Coast and Daytona Beach. The COM will move to a new building in the UCF Health Sciences Campus at Lake Nona in the spring of 2010. This phenomenal medical campus will initially include the College of Medicine and the Burnett Bio-medical Research buildings, with additional buildings in the health sciences planned in the future. Adjacent to the campus will be a new Veteran's Hospital, Burnham Institute for Medical Research, Nemours Children's Hospital, and many additional clinical and research facilities in our new medical city at Lake Nona. The rapidly growing complex also includes single and multi-family housing, retail areas, schools, and spacious parks.

Enrollment

For 2007, total enrollment was: n/a

Special Features

All facilities from the classrooms to the numerous study areas are equipped with the latest communication and teaching technologies. Students will enjoy the latest developments in medical simulation and clinical cases. Clinical experiences will be fully integrated into all four years of the program and into the community allowing participation in rural or urban medicine at multiple hospitals and clinics in the Central Florida area.

Housing

On-campus housing is not available. A list of affordable housing near the UCF campus in Orlando as well as the Lake Nona area is available.

Application Process and Requirements 2009–2010

Primary Application Service: AMCAS
Earliest filing date: June 1, 2008
Latest filing date: December 1, 2008

Secondary Application
URL: Provided to qualified applicants via email
Sent to: Screened Applicants
Fee: Yes, $30
Fee Waiver Available: Yes
Earliest filing date: July 1, 2008
Latest filing date: January 15, 2009

Latest MCAT® considered: September 2008
Oldest MCAT® considered: 2006

Early Decision Program
School does have EDP
Applicants notified: October 1, 2008
EDP available for: Both Residents and Non-Residents

Regular Acceptance Notice
Earliest date: October 15, 2008
Latest date: Until Class is Full

Applicant's Response to Acceptance Offer – Maximum Time: 2 weeks
Requests for deferred entrance considered: Yes

Deposit to Hold Place in Class: None
Deposit (Resident): n/a
Deposit (Non-Resident): n/a
Deposit due: n/a
Applied to tuition: n/a
Deposit refundable: n/a
Refundable by: n/a

Estimated number of new entrants: 40
EDP: 4, special program: n/a

Start month/year: August 2009

Interview format: Two closed-file interviews by COM faculty. Regional interviews are not available.

Other Programs

PREPARATORY PROGRAMS
Postbaccalaureate Program: No
Summer Program: No

COMBINED DEGREE PROGRAMS
Baccalaureate/MD: No
MD/MPH: No
MD/MBA: No
MD/JD: No
MD/PhD: No

Premedical Coursework

Course	Req.	Rec.	Lab.	Hrs.
Inorganic Chemistry	•		•	8
Behavioral Sciences				
Biochemistry		•		
Biology	•		•	8
Biology/Zoology				
Calculus/Statistics		•		
College English	•			6
College Mathematics	•			6

Course	Req.	Rec.	Lab.	Hrs.
Computer Science				
Genetics		•		
Humanities		•		
Organic Chemistry	•		•	8
Physics	•		•	8
Psychology				
Social Sciences				
Molecular Biology		•		

Selection Factors: 2007 Accepted Applicants

Proportion of Accepted Applicants with Relevant Experience (Data Self-Reported to AMCAS®)	DATA NOT AVAILABLE

Shaded bar represents accepted scores ranging from the 10th percentile to the 90th percentile ▪   School Median ● National Median ●

Overall GPA Science GPA	DATA NOT AVAILABLE

MCAT® required: Yes, n/a of 2007 accepted applicants took MCAT®

Verbal Reasoning Physical Sciences Biological Sciences Writing Sample	DATA NOT AVAILABLE

Acceptance & Matriculation Data for 2007–2008 First Year Class

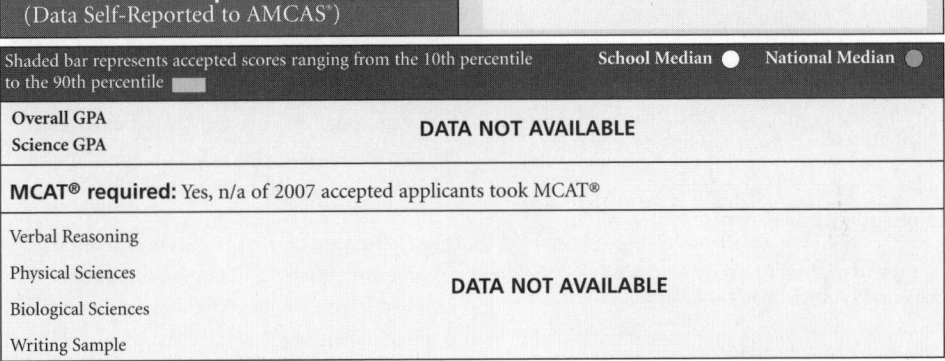

	Resident	Non-Resident	International	Total
Applied				
Interviewed				
Deferred				
Matriculants				
Early Assurance Program				
Early Decision Program	DATA NOT AVAILABLE			
Baccalaureate/MD Program				
MD/PhD Program				
Matriculated				

Applications accepted from International Applicants:

Specialty Choice

2003, 2004, 2005 Graduates, Specialty Choice
(As reported by program directors to GME Track™)

Anesthesiology
Emergency Medicine
Family Practice
Int
Ob   DATA NOT AVAILABLE
Or
Pediatrics
Psychiatry
Radiology
Surgery

Matriculant Demographics: 2007–2008 First Year Class

Men: n/a   **Women:** n/a

Matriculants' Self-Reported Race/Ethnicity

Mexican American   Korean
Cuban   Vietnamese
Puerto Rican   Other Asian
Othe
Total
Chine   DATA NOT AVAILABLE
Asian
Pakis
Filipino   **Unduplicated Number**
Japanese   **of Matriculants**

Science Majors: n/a
Matriculants with:
   Baccalaureate Degree: n/a
   Graduate Degree(s): n/a

Financial Information (Estimated)

Source: 2006–2007 LCME I-B survey and 2007–2008 AAMC TSF questionnaire

	Residents	Non-Residents
Total Cost of Attendance	$40,000	$60,000
Tuition and Fees	$22,500	$42,500
Other (includes living expenses)	$15,700	$15,700
Health Insurance (can be waived)	$1,800	$1,800

Average 2007 Graduate Indebtedness: n/a
% of Enrolled Students Receiving Aid: n/a

Criminal Background Check

This medical school requires a criminal background check prior to matriculation.

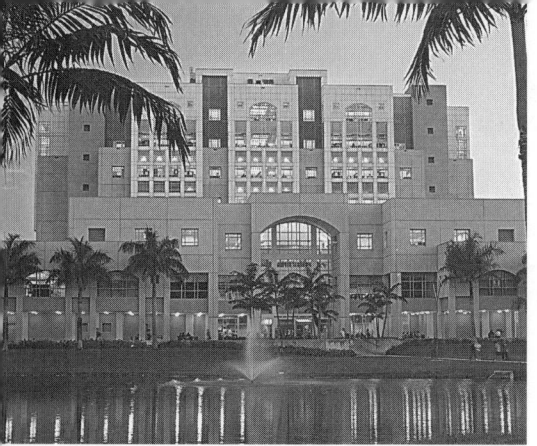

Florida International University College of Medicine

Miami, Florida

Office of Admissions
Florida International University
College of Medicine
11200 S.W 8th Street – HLSII 660 W2
Miami, Florida 33199
T 305 348 0644 **F** 305 348 0650

Admissions http://medicine.fiu.edu/admissions
Main http://medicine.fiu.edu
Email med.admissions@fiu.edu

Public Institution

Dr. John Rock, Founding Dean and Senior VP for Medical Affairs

Dr. Sanford Markham, Executive Associate Dean for Student Affairs

Dr. Robert Dollinger, Assistant Dean, Student Affairs, Counseling and Communities

Dr. Barbra Roller, Assistant Dean, Student Affairs, Admissions and Records

Betty L. Monfort, M.P.H., Director, Admissions and Records

Charlotte Rhine, M.Ed., Associate Director, Admissions and Records

General Information

In August 2009, the College of Medicine will welcome the inaugural class. The four year program, leading to the MD degree, involves in-depth exposure and training in all areas of medical education with specific focus on family and community medicine. Unique to the College is the hands-on experience each student receives in observing and caring for families who have little or no access to medical care. Key in the medical training is the focus on the importance of the doctor-patient relationship in a diverse patient population.

Mission Statement

The Mission of the College of Medicine at Florida International University is to serve as a model for the next generation of medical education and to elevate the level of care available to the Florida community. Our goals are to: (1) Educate culturally competent physicians to serve diverse populations; (2) Provide South Florida students greater access to medical education, admitting a student body that reflects the rich diversity of the region; (3) Develop a curriculum focused on community medicine, elevating the quality of medical care; and (4) Develop basic, translational and clinical research programs that will ensure state of the art care and will substantially expand the economic growth potential of the region.

General Information

Curricular Highlights

Community Service Requirement: Required. Community Service is an integral part of our mission and innovative curriculum.

Research/Thesis Requirement: Optional. The emphasis is community-based, patient-centered learning with the development of an understanding of personal, cultural and social factors affecting health care. Students will develop competencies in a full range of medical specialties.

The College has created a new curriculum that is community based and emphasizes patient-centered learning with a focus on developing an understanding of personal, cultural and social factors in health care. Organized as a four year integration of studies, the curriculum has five strands: Clinical Medicine, Disease, Illness and Injury (pathological approaches), Human Biology (basic medical sciences), Medicine and Society and Professional Development (statistical and evidence based medicine). Curricular innovations include the Medicine and Society strand the goal of which is to enable students to gain an understanding of factors that affect personal and community health care. Students work with individuals, families and communities in interdisciplinary student teams from Public Health, Nursing and Social Work. This strand integrates ethics, public health, cultural competency and sustained community experiences. Cases will be used throughout the curriculum as a context for learning. Small class sizes will provide individualized attention. Small group learning and independent study are emphasized; research is encouraged as an option. The founding faculty has been selected for their excellence in teaching; the learning format is focused on individual student achievement.

USMLE

Step 1: Required. Students must record a passing score for promotion.
Step 2: Clinical Skills (CS): Required. Students must only record a score.
Step 2: Clinical Knowledge (CK): Required. Students must only record a score.

Selection Factors

The Admissions Committee uses AMCAS, a secondary application, Letters of Recommendation and interview feedback to select applicants who have demonstrated a well-rounded, rigorous academic preparation, character and maturity and who best suit our mission. Applicants must show a strong interest in medicine, a record of personal experiences suggesting medical care exposure, research, altruism, integrity, community service, leadership with the ability and desire to pursue lifelong learning and the personal attributes necessary to be a competent, compassionate physician. See *http://medicine.fiu.edu/admissions.*

Financial Aid

Financial aid is awarded on the basis of demonstrated financial need. Scholarships (need-based and merit), low-interest loans and other sources of financial assistance will be available.

Information about Diversity Programs

FIU takes pride in its commitment to diversity as exemplified among our students, faculty and staff.

Campus Information

Setting

Located in Miami, a major international financial and cultural center, FIU is an urban, multi-campus, research university serving South Florida, the state, the nation and the international community. The 344-acre University Park campus, where the College of Medicine is housed, offers a wealth of services and access to many living and learning communities and is only minutes from Miami International Airport, the Port of Miami, cultural centers, and beautiful beaches.

Enrollment

Starting August 2009, the inaugural class will have 40 students.

Housing

The Department of Housing and Residential Life provides state-of-the-art on-campus housing complimented by a supportive Residential Life program. Off-campus housing is also available.

Application Process and Requirements 2009–2010

Primary Application Service: AMCAS
Earliest filing date: June 1, 2008
Latest filing date: December 15, 2008

Secondary Application
URL: n/a
Name: Betty L. Monfort, (305) 348-0644
med.admissions@fiu.edu
Sent to: Screened applicants with minimum required scores
Fee: Yes, $65.00
Fee Waiver Available: Yes, (if waived by AMCAS)
Earliest filing date: June 2008
Latest filing date: January 15, 2009

Latest MCAT® considered: September 2008
Oldest MCAT® considered: 2006

Early Decision Program
School does have EDP
Applicants notified: October 1, 2008
EDP available for: All qualified applicants

Regular Acceptance Notice
Earliest date: October 15, 2008
Latest date: Varies

Applicant's Response to Acceptance Offer – Maximum Time: 4 weeks from date of offer

Requests for deferred entrance considered: No

Deposit to Hold Place in Class: Yes
Deposit (Resident): Yes, $200
Deposit (Non-Resident): Yes, $200
Deposit due: with offer acceptance
Applied to tuition: Yes
Deposit refundable: No
Refundable by: n/a

Estimated number of new entrants: 40
EDP: n/a, special program: n/a

Start month/year: August 2009

Interview format: Two committee members will interview invited applicants. Regional interviews are not available.

Other Programs

PREPARATORY PROGRAMS
Postbaccalaureate Program: No
Summer Program: No

COMBINED DEGREE PROGRAMS
Baccalaureate/MD: No
MD/MPH: No
MD/MBA: No
MD/JD: No
MD/PhD: No

Premedical Coursework

Course	Req.	Rec.	Lab.	Sems.
Inorganic Chemistry	•		•	2
Behavioral Sciences		•		
Biochemistry		•		
Biology	•		•	2
Biology/Zoology				
Calculus and/or Statistics	•			2
College English	•			2
College Mathematics		•		

Course	Req.	Rec.	Lab.	Sems.
Computer Science		•		
Genetics		•		
Humanities		•		
Organic Chemistry	•		•	2
Physics	•		•	2
Psychology				
Social Sciences				
Cell Biology or equivalent	•			1

Selection Factors: 2007 Accepted Applicants

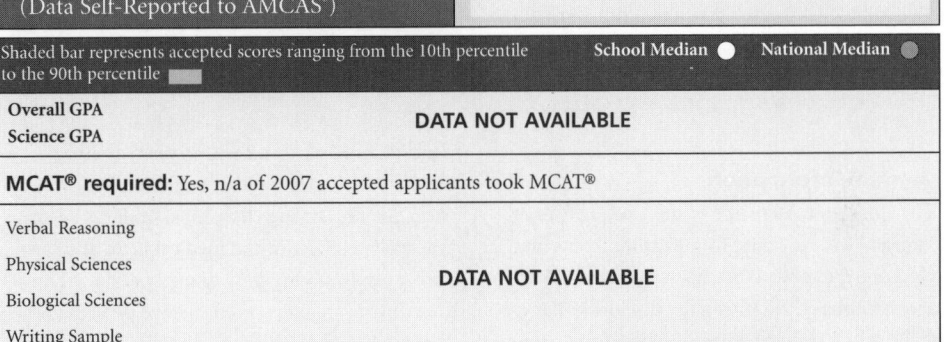

Proportion of Accepted Applicants with Relevant Experience (Data Self-Reported to AMCAS®)	DATA NOT AVAILABLE

Shaded bar represents accepted scores ranging from the 10th percentile to the 90th percentile ▪ School Median ● National Median ●

| Overall GPA | DATA NOT AVAILABLE |
| Science GPA | |

MCAT® required: Yes, n/a of 2007 accepted applicants took MCAT®

Verbal Reasoning	
Physical Sciences	DATA NOT AVAILABLE
Biological Sciences	
Writing Sample	

Acceptance & Matriculation Data for 2007–2008 First Year Class

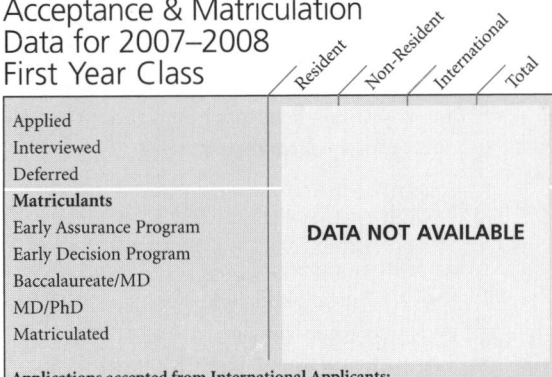

	Resident	Non-Resident	International	Total
Applied				
Interviewed				
Deferred				
Matriculants				
Early Assurance Program		DATA NOT AVAILABLE		
Early Decision Program				
Baccalaureate/MD				
MD/PhD				
Matriculated				

Applications accepted from International Applicants:

Specialty Choice

2003, 2004, 2005 Graduates, Specialty Choice (As reported by program directors to GME Track™)
Anesthesiology
Emergency Medicine
Family Practice
Int...
Ob... DATA NOT AVAILABLE
Or...
Pediatrics
Psychiatry
Radiology
Surgery

Matriculant Demographics: 2007–2008 First Year Class

Men: n/a   **Women:** n/a

Matriculants' Self-Reported Race/Ethnicity

Mexican American	Korean
Cuban	Vietnamese
Puerto Rican	Other Asian
Other	
Total H...	
Chines... DATA NOT AVAILABLE	
Asian I...	
Pakista...	
Filipino	**Unduplicated Number**
Japanese	**of Matriculants**

Science Majors: n/a
Matriculants with:
     Baccalaureate Degree: n/a
     Graduate Degree(s): n/a

Financial Information

Source: 2006–2007 LCME I-B survey and 2007–2008 AAMC TSF questionnaire

	Residents	Non-Residents
Total Cost of Attendance	$41,360	$70,786
Tuition and Fees	$24,500	$53,926
Other (includes living expenses)	$16,860	$16,860
Health Insurance (included in fees)		

Average 2007 Graduate Indebtedness: n/a
% of Enrolled Students Receiving Aid: n/a

Criminal Background Check

This medical school requires a criminal background check prior to matriculation.

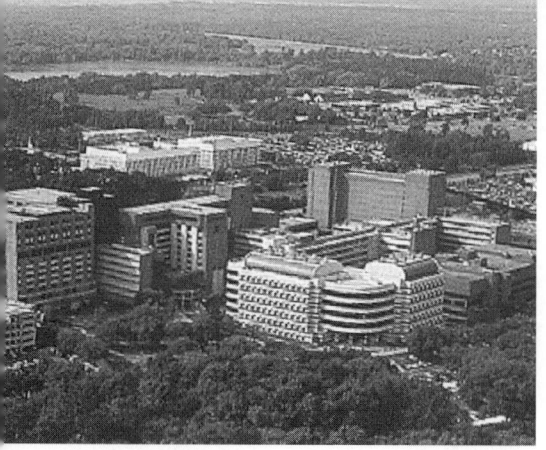

University of Florida College of Medicine
Gainesville, Florida

Director, Office of Admissions
PO Box 100216, UF Health Sciences Center
Univ. of Florida College of Medicine
Gainesville, Florida 32610-0216
T 352 273 7990 **F** 352 392 1307

Admissions www.med.ufl.edu/oea/admiss
Main www.med.ufl.edu
Financial www.med.ufl.edu/oea/finaid
Email robyn@dean.med.ufl.edu

Public Institution

Dr. Bruce C. Kone, Dean

Robyn Sheppard, Director of Admissions

Dr. Donna M. Parker, Assistant Dean for Minority Affairs

Eileen M. Parris, Coordinator of Financial Aid

Denise Chichester, Admissions Program Assistant

General Information
The College of Medicine of the University of Florida Health Science Center admitted its first class in September 1956. Located on the 2,000-acre campus of the University of Florida, the College of Medicine enjoys the benefit of strong ties with other university programs and the other Health Science Center colleges. The HSC complex also includes the Chandler A. Stetson Medical Science Building, the Communicore Building, the Academic Research Building, the Health Professions Building, the Cancer and Genetics Research Building, Shands Hospital, the Brain Institute, and the Veterans Affairs Medical Center, located across the street from the Health Science Center. The UF Health Science Center Jacksonville is our urban campus. The Jacksonville campus is the location of the newest Proton Beam facility in the world. Formal educational affiliations have also been established in Ft. Lauderdale, Miami, Orlando, and Pensacola.

Mission Statement
To educate medical students in humanistic, scientific and practical principles of medicine to become, and remain, exemplary practitioners, academicians and leaders. To educate scientists for research, teaching or industry careers. To provide compassionate, skilled and innovative healthcare. To foster discovery, promote health, prevent disease, and so educate the public. To promote the professional and personal growth of faculty and staff.

Curricular Highlights
Community Service Requirement: Required. Consistent health care experience preferred.
Research/Thesis Requirement: Optional.

The four years are divided into three blocks of time – Preclinical Coursework (2 years), Clinical Clerkships (1 year), and Post-clerkship Electives and Required Courses (1 year). Preclinical coursework provides students with essential basic science and general clinical information necessary for clinical training. The third year is devoted to clinical clerkships. Required clerkships include family medicine, medicine, neurology, pediatrics, psychiatry, obstetrics/gynecology, and surgery. Students spend 10-12 weeks participating in clerkships at UF Health Science Center Jacksonville. During clerkships, students become integral members of the medical team and have direct responsibility for assigned patients. The fourth year includes seven elective periods and three required courses: anesthesiology, emergency medicine, and either senior medicine, community medicine, or pediatrics. An eleventh period is available for accomplishing residency interviews. For students who have already chosen a specialty, fourth-year programs may be designed to provide career choice-related experiences.

USMLE
Step 1: Required. Students must record a passing score for promotion.
Step 2: Clinical Skills (CS): Required. Students must only record a score.
Step 2: Clinical Knowledge (CK): Required. Students must only record a score.

Selection Factors
Applicants will be appraised on the basis of personal attributes, academic record, evaluation of past activities, the MCAT, and letters of recommendation. A personal interview is required to complete the application process and is granted at the discretion of the Medical Selection Committee. The school does not discriminate on the basis of race, sex, age, disability, creed, or national origin. Although Florida residents are given preference in admission, a limited number of non-residents are considered each year. Non-resident applicants must demonstrate superior qualifications. The COM welcomes applications from members of groups

underrepresented in medicine and from persons who demonstrate a clear, long-standing commitment to underserved populations.

Financial Aid
Financial assistance is available to all enrolled students who show need. The college has scholarships and low interest loans available. Applications are mailed to all accepted applicants. Summer and school-year research fellowships are also available.

Information about Diversity Programs
There are summer research programs offered by the Office of Minority Affairs.

Campus Information

Setting
The campus in Gainesville is located midway between the Atlantic Ocean and the Gulf of Mexico in the lush beauty of north central Florida. The surrounding area includes fresh water springs, open wild prairies, and many parks exhibiting a great diversity of wildlife. Arts and culture abound in Gainesville. The Phillips Centers for Performing Arts programs feature world-class entertainers from all areas of performance. The Harn Art Museum houses some of the finest art in the world and includes the new MacQuire Butterfly Rainforest.

Enrollment
For 2007, total enrollment was: 467

Special Features
Several new facilities are under construction, including the Cancer Center, the Nanotechnology Center, and the Trauma I Center.

Housing
On-campus housing is not available.

Satellite Campuses/Facilities
UF Health Sciences Center at Jacksonville, Malcom Randall VA Hospital, Lake City VA Hospital, Shands at Alachua General Hospital, Sacred Heart Hospital in Pensacola, Orlando Regional Medical Center. McKnight Brain Institute, Canter & Genetics Institute, and Proton Beam Facility in Jacksonville.

Application Process and Requirements 2009–2010

Primary Application Service: AMCAS
Earliest filing date: June 1, 2008
Latest filing date: December 1, 2008

Secondary Application Required?: Yes
Sent to: Applicants of interest
URL: n/a
Fee: No
Fee waiver available: n/a
Earliest filing date: July 15, 2008
Latest filing date: January 15, 2009

Latest MCAT® considered: September 2008
Oldest MCAT® considered: August 2006

Early Decision Program
School does not have EDP
Applicants notified: n/a
EDP available for: n/a

Regular Acceptance Notice
Earliest date: October 16, 2008
Latest date: Until class is full

Applicant's Response to Acceptance
Offer – Maximum Time: Two weeks

Requests for Deferred
Entrance Considered: Yes

Deposit to Hold Place in Class: Yes
Deposit (Resident): $200
Deposit (Non-Resident): $200
Deposit due: Two weeks after notice of acceptance
Applied to tuition: Yes
Deposit refundable: Yes
Refundable by: May 15, 2009

Estimated number of new entrants: 135
EDP: n/a, special program: 16

Start Month/Year: August 2009

Interview Format: Two open-file interviews at COM. Regional interviews are not available.

Other Programs

PREPARATORY PROGRAMS
Postbaccalaureate Program: No
Summer Program: Yes,
www.med.ufl.edu/oma/srp.shtml
Office of Minority Affairs, (352) 273-6656

COMBINED DEGREE PROGRAMS
Baccalaureate/MD: Yes,
www.med.ufl.edu/oea/admiss
MD/MPH: Yes,
www.med.ufl.edu/oea/admiss
MD/MBA: Yes, www.med.ufl.edu/oea/admiss
MD/JD: Yes,
www.med.ufl.edu/oea/admiss
MD/PhD: Yes,
www.med.ufl.edu/md-phd/
Additional Program: Yes,
www.msrp.med.ufl.edu

Premedical Coursework

Course	Req.	Rec.	Lab.	Hrs.	Course	Req.	Rec.	Lab.	Hrs.
Inorganic Chemistry	•		•	8	Computer Science				
Behavioral Sciences					Genetics				
Biochemistry	•		•	4	Humanities				
Biology	•				Organic Chemistry	•		•	4
Biology/Zoology	•		•	8	Physics	•		•	8
Calculus					Psychology				
College English					Social Sciences				
College Mathematics					Other				

Selection Factors: 2007 Accepted Applicants

Proportion of Accepted Applicants with Relevant Experience (Data Self-Reported to AMCAS®)		Community Service/Volunteer	67%
		Medically-Related Work	86%
		Research	82%

Shaded bar represents accepted scores ranging from the 10th percentile to the 90th percentile. School Median ● National Median ●

Overall GPA	2.0	2.1	2.2	2.3	2.4	2.5	2.6	2.7	2.8	2.9	3.0	3.1	3.2	3.3	3.4	3.5	3.6	3.7	(3.8)	3.9	4.0
Science GPA	2.0	2.1	2.2	2.3	2.4	2.5	2.6	2.7	2.8	2.9	3.0	3.1	3.2	3.3	3.4	3.5	3.6	3.7	(3.8)	3.9	4.0

MCAT® required: Yes, 95% of 2007 accepted applicants took MCAT®

Verbal Reasoning	3	4	5	6	7	8	9	(10)	(11)	12	13	14	15
Physical Sciences	3	4	5	6	7	8	9	10	(11)	12	13	14	15
Biological Sciences	3	4	5	6	7	8	9	10	(11)	12	13	14	15
Writing Sample			J	K	L	M	N	O	P	(Q)	R	S	T

Acceptance & Matriculation Data for 2007–2008 First Year Class

	Resident	Non-Resident	International	Total
Applied	1429	1079	42	2550
Interviewed	320	26	0	346
Deferred	2	1	0	3
Matriculants				
Early Assurance Program	n/a	n/a	n/a	n/a
Early Decision Program	0	0	0	0
Baccalaureate/MD	12	0	0	12
MD/PhD	0	0	0	0
Matriculated	127	5	0	**132**

Applications accepted from International Applicants: No

Specialty Choice

2003, 2004, 2005 Graduates, Specialty Choice (As reported by program directors to GME Track™)	
Anesthesiology	7%
Emergency Medicine	6%
Family Practice	7%
Internal Medicine	14%
Obstetrics/Gynecology	7%
Orthopaedic Surgery	3%
Pediatrics	11%
Psychiatry	5%
Radiology	6%
Surgery	7%

Matriculant Demographics: 2007–2008 First Year Class

Men: 72   **Women:** 60

Matriculants' Self-Reported Race/Ethnicity

Mexican American	0	Korean	1
Cuban	7	Vietnamese	0
Puerto Rican	0	Other Asian	3
Other Hispanic	6	Total Asian	36
Total Hispanic	12	Native American	0
Chinese	9	Black	7
Asian Indian	20	Native Hawaiian	0
Pakistani	3	White	88
Filipino	2	Unduplicated Number	
Japanese	0	of Matriculants	132

Science and Math Majors: 57%
Matriculants with:
  Baccalaureate degree: 99%
  Graduate degree(s): 11%

Financial Information

Source: 2006–2007 LCME I-B survey and 2007–2008 AAMC TSF questionnaire

	Residents	Non-Residents
Total Cost of Attendance	$40,349	$69,589
Tuition and Fees	$23,170	$52,410
Other (includes living expenses)	$17,179	$17,179
Health Insurance (not applicable)	$0	$0

Average 2007 Graduate Indebtedness: $112,262
% of Enrolled Students Receiving Aid: 89%

Criminal Background Check

This medical school does not require a criminal background check prior to matriculation.

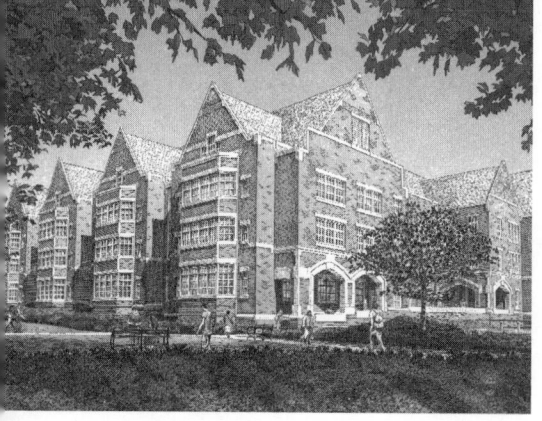

Florida State University College of Medicine

Tallahassee, Florida

Office of Student Affairs and Admissions
Florida State University College of Medicine
Administration Building, Room 1110-F
Tallahassee, Florida 32306-4300
T 850 644 7904   **F** 850 645 2846

Admissions www.med.fsu.edu/StudentAffairs
Main www.med.fsu.edu
Financial www.med.fsu.edu/StudentAffairs/FinAid
Email medadmissions@med.fsu.edu

Public Institution

Dr. J. Ocie Harris, Dean

Dr. Elena Reyes, Associate Dean for Student Affairs, Admissions and Outreach

Thesla Anderson, Director of Outreach Programs

Melinda Oglesby, Enrollment Services Coordinator

Dana Urrutia, Admissions Coordinator

General Information

The Florida State University College of Medicine was created in July 2000 by a legislative act to train physicians with a focus on serving medically underserved populations in rural and inner-city areas and the growing geriatric population in the state. The FSU College of Medicine is located in Tallahassee, with regional medical campuses, where students complete third and fourth-year clerkships, in Pensacola, Orlando, Sarasota, Tallahassee, Daytona Beach, and Fort Pierce.

Mission Statement

The mission of the FSU COM is to educate and develop exemplary physicians who practice patient-centered health care, discover and advance knowledge, and respond to community needs, especially through service to elder, rural, and other medically underserved populations.

Curricular Highlights

Community Service Requirement: Optional.
Research/Thesis Requirement: Optional.

The academic program includes instruction in the biopsychosocial sciences and community-based health care. The first and second-year integrated curriculum uses a combination of lecture and case-based and problem-based learning in small-group discussions and simulated standardized-patient interviews. A three-year doctoring course, composed of lecture, small-group discussion, patient encounters, clinical skills instruction, and preceptorships, provides application models to complement years 1, 2, and 3. The third year and part of the fourth year consist of required rotations in internal medicine, surgery, pediatrics, obstetrics-gynecology, family medicine/rural medicine, geriatrics, emergency medicine, advanced medicine (critical care unit), advanced family practice, and psychiatry. Students may spend up to 24 weeks in electives designed to provide a foundation on which to develop and fulfill personal interests, broaden clinical knowledge, and prepare for postgraduate medical training.

USMLE

Step 1: Required. Students must record a passing score for promotion.
Step 2: Clinical Skills (CS): Required. Students must record a passing total score to graduate.
Step 2: Clinical Knowledge (CK): Required. Students must record a passing total score to graduate.

Selection Factors

Although scholastic aptitude is necessary to complete studies in medical school, neither high GPAs nor high MCAT scores alone or in combination are adequate to obtain admission. Only Florida residents will be considered for admission. International applicants must have a permanent resident visa. Applicants who have grades and test scores predictive of success in medical school, have demonstrated through their experiences a high degree of motivation for medicine and a strong commitment to the service of others, and have a likelihood of practicing medicine with medically underserved populations will be invited to interview. The committee evaluates all aspects of the applicant's academic record, including trends in scholastic performance.

Financial Aid

Scholarships and loan funds from private, state, and federal sources are available to qualified students and are awarded on the basis of need and/or scholarship.

Information about Diversity Programs

Because of the mission of the College of Medicine and the educational value of admitting a diverse class, Florida State University College of Medicine developed a Postbaccalaureate Bridge Program to provide opportunities for applicants from groups underrepresented in medicine. Applicants from these groups who embody the characteristics valued by the college are selected for the Bridge year, which is used to develop and enhance study, time management, and test-taking skills; psychosocial and basic science backgrounds; and clinical experiences. If these students meet all requirements established for the year, they are admitted to the next year's medical school class. Students may contact Eugene Trowers, MD, at (850) 644-4607 for more information.

Campus Information

Setting

The main medical school campus is located on the Florida State University campus in a newly constructed 65 million dollar medical school complex. Each regional campus is located near affiliated hospitals in its respective community and includes study and resource areas. Applicants are invited to take a virtual tour of the campus at *www.med.fsu.edu.*

Enrollment

For 2007, total enrollment was: 358

Special Features

The FSU College of Medicine utilizes a state of the art Clinical Learning Center on the main campus and community resources to ensure that students receive a significant amount of one-on-one training with physician preceptors. The College of Medicine has affiliation agreements with over 30 hospitals across the state of Florida, as well as affiliations with nearby rural community hospitals. A wide range of elective opportunities is available in the fourth year at each of the regional sites, as well as at other accredited institutions both nationally and internationally.

Housing

On-campus housing is available. A list of affordable housing within Tallahassee and at each of the regional campuses is maintained.

Satellite Campuses/Facilities

Student rotations in the third year occur at one of the regional campuses. Rural learning opportunities are also available within driving distance of each site.

Application Process and Requirements 2009–2010

Primary Application Service: AMCAS
Earliest filing date: June 1, 2008
Latest filing date: December 14, 2008

Secondary Application Required?: Yes
Sent to: Screened applicants
Contact: Dana Urrutia, (850) 644-1857,
dana.urrutia@med.fsu.edu

Fee: No
Fee waiver available: No
Earliest filing date: June 1, 2008
Latest filing date: January 7, 2009

Latest MCAT® considered: September 2008
Oldest MCAT® considered: 2004

Early Decision Program
School does have EDP
Applicants notified: October 1, 2008
EDP available for: Both Residents
and Non-Residents

Regular Acceptance Notice
Earliest date: October 15, 2008
Latest date: Until Class is Full

**Applicant's Response to Acceptance
Offer – Maximum Time:** Two weeks

**Requests for Deferred
Entrance Considered:** Yes

Deposit to Hold Place in Class: Yes
Deposit (Resident): $30
Deposit (Non-Resident): n/a
Deposit due: Within two weeks of receipt
of letter of acceptance
Applied to tuition: No
Deposit refundable: No
Refundable by: n/a

Estimated number of new entrants: 120
EDP: 15, special program: 10

Start Month/Year: June 2009

Interview Format: Two committee
members interview invited applicants.
Regional interviews are not available.

Other Programs

PREPARATORY PROGRAMS
Postbaccalaureate Program: Yes,
www.med.fsu.edu/StudentAffairs/admissions/
bridge.asp

COMBINED DEGREE PROGRAMS
Baccalaureate/MD: Yes, http://med.fsu.edu/
news/2005/MedicalScholars.pdf
MD/MPH: No
MD/MBA: No
MD/JD: No
MD/PhD: No

Premedical Coursework

Course	Req.	Rec.	Lab.	Hrs.
Inorganic Chemistry	•		•	8
Behavioral Sciences				
Biochemistry	•		•	4
Biology	•		•	8
Biology/Zoology				
Calculus				
College English	•			6
College Mathematics	•			6

Course	Req.	Rec.	Lab.	Hrs.
Computer Science				
Genetics		•		
Humanities				
Organic Chemistry	•		•	8
Physics	•		•	8
Psychology				3
Social Sciences		•		3
Other				

Selection Factors: 2007 Accepted Applicants

Proportion of Accepted Applicants with Relevant Experience (Data Self-Reported to AMCAS)		
Community Service/Volunteer	65%	
Medically-Related Work	92%	
Research	77%	

Shaded bar represents accepted scores ranging from the 10th percentile to the 90th percentile. **School Median** ● **National Median** ●

Overall GPA	2.0	2.1	2.2	2.3	2.4	2.5	2.6	2.7	2.8	2.9	3.0	3.1	3.2	3.3	3.4	3.5	3.6	(3.7)	3.8	3.9	4.0
Science GPA	2.0	2.1	2.2	2.3	2.4	2.5	2.6	2.7	2.8	2.9	3.0	3.1	3.2	3.3	3.4	3.5	(3.6)	3.7	3.8	3.9	4.0

MCAT® required: Yes, 100% of 2007 accepted applicants took MCAT®

Verbal Reasoning	3	4	5	6	7	8	9	(10)	11	12	13	14	15
Physical Sciences	3	4	5	6	7	8	9	(10)	(11)	12	13	14	15
Biological Sciences	3	4	5	6	7	8	9	(10)	(11)	12	13	14	15
Writing Sample			J	K	L	M	N	O	(P)	(Q)	R	S	T

Acceptance & Matriculation Data for 2007–2008 First Year Class

	Resident	Non-Resident	International	Total
Applied	1501	1	3	1505
Interviewed	372	0	0	372
Deferred	4	0	0	4
Matriculants				
Early Assurance Program	0	0	0	0
Early Decision Program	8	0	0	8
Baccalaureate/MD	n/a	n/a	n/a	n/a
MD/PhD	n/a	n/a	n/a	n/a
Matriculated	119	0	0	**119**

Applications accepted from International Applicants: No

Specialty Choice

2003, 2004, 2005 Graduates, Specialty Choice (As reported by program directors to GME Track™)	
Anesthesiology	0%
Emergency Medicine	10%
Family Practice	6%
Internal Medicine	3%
Obstetrics/Gynecology	1%
Orthopaedic Surgery	3%
Pediatrics	3%
Psychiatry	1%
Radiology	0%
Surgery	4%

Matriculant Demographics: 2007–2008 First Year Class

Men: 52   **Women:** 67

Matriculants' Self-Reported Race/Ethnicity

Mexican American	0	Korean	0
Cuban	3	Vietnamese	1
Puerto Rican	0	Other Asian	1
Other Hispanic	4	Total Asian	14
Total Hispanic	7	Native American	0
Chinese	2	Black	11
Asian Indian	8	Native Hawaiian	2
Pakistani	1	White	95
Filipino	2	Unduplicated Number	
Japanese	0	of Matriculants	119

Science and Math Majors: 60%
Matriculants with:
    Baccalaureate degree: 98%
    Graduate degree(s): 8%

Financial Information

Source: 2006–2007 LCME I-B survey
and 2007–2008 AAMC TSF questionnaire

	Residents	Non-Residents
Total Cost of Attendance	$45,591	$0
Tuition and Fees	$18,447	$0
Other (includes living expenses)	$27,144	$0
Health Insurance (can be waived)	$0	$0

Average 2007 Graduate Indebtedness: $123,277
% of Enrolled Students Receiving Aid: 89%

Criminal Background Check

This medical school requires a criminal background check prior to matriculation.

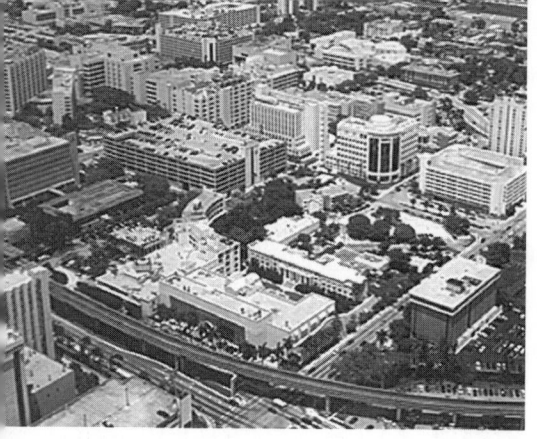

University of Miami
Miller School of Medicine
Miami, Florida

Office of Admissions
University of Miami Miller School of Medicine
P.O. Box 016159
Miami, Florida 33101
T 305 243 6791   **F** 305 243 6548

Admissions www.miami.edu/medical-admissions
Main www.med.miami.edu
Financial www.mededu.miami.edu/OSFA
Email med.admissions@miami.edu

Private Institution

Dr. Pascal Goldschmidt, Dean

Dr. R.E. Hinkley, Associate Dean for Admissions and Enrollment Management

Dr. Astrid Mack, Associate Dean for Minority Affairs

Laura L. Kasperski, Assistant Dean for Student Financial Assistance

General Information

The University of Miami Miller School of Medicine is the largest and oldest medical school in the state of Florida. Six hospitals containing nearly 3,000 beds are located on the medical campus and provide a complete spectrum of clinical experiences. Specialty centers at the Miller School of Medicine include The Bascom Palmer Eye Institute and Anne Bates Leach Eye Hospital, the Ambulatory Care Center, the Diabetes Research Institute, the Lois Pope Life Center (which houses The Miami Project to Cure Spinal Cord Paralysis), the Bachelor Children's Research Institute, the Ryder Trauma Center, and the Sylvester Comprehensive Cancer Center.

Mission Statement

The Miller School of Medicine has four interrelated missions: patient care, teaching, research, and community service.

Curricular Highlights

Community Service Requirement: Required.
Research/Thesis Requirement: Optional.

The curriculum is an integrated program that requires students to be active and responsible learners. It emphasizes faculty and student-led small-group experiences wherein basic science concepts are introduced and assimilated in light of common disease states and clinical relevance. It also includes material not traditionally emphasized: professionalism, humanism and ethics, population medicine, prevention and screening, quality and outcome assessment, medical informatics, geriatrics, alternative medicine, nutrition, medical economics, and

end-of-life care. An over-arching theme throughout all four years is the continuous acquisition and refinement of clinical skills through expert teaching and patient encounters, starting in the first weeks of the first year of the curriculum.

USMLE

Step 1: Required. Students must record a passing score for promotion.
Step 2: Clinical Skills (CS): Required. Students must only record a score.
Step 2: Clinical Knowledge (CK): Required. Students must only record a score.

Selection Factors

Secondary applications are sent to all U.S. citizens and permanent residents who submit a verified AMCAS application. In deciding whether to return secondary materials, applicants are reminded that the last entering class had an average undergraduate cumulative GPA of 3.7 and an average composite MCAT® score of 31. Factors assessed by the committee to rate all completed applications include: preparedness to study medicine, diversity of life experiences, meaningfulness of direct patient contact experiences, and quality of letters of recommendation. Applicants with the highest ratings are invited for an interview. Applicants' files are reviewed without regard to race, creed, sex, national origin, age, or handicap.

Financial Aid

In 2007-2008, the amount of financial aid awarded totaled about $22 million. The school participates in all major federal and state programs. A number of scholarships are awarded each year for merit and for life diversity and financial need. Information concerning financial assistance and student budgets may be obtained on the Office of Financial Assistance web site at *www.mededu.miami.edu/OSFA* or by calling 305-243-6211.

Information about Diversity Programs

The school sponsors a special seven-week summer program that provides pre-medical undergraduates with opportunities to gain

first-hand knowledge of the requirements of a medical education. Applications and information may be obtained by calling 305-243-5998.

Campus Information

Setting

The School of Medicine is located in the Civic Center area of Miami, about midway between Miami International Airport and downtown Miami. The regional medical campus is located in Boca Raton, Florida, on the campus of Florida Atlantic University, about 50 miles north of the parent campus.

Enrollment

For 2007, total enrollment was: 655

Special Features

The entire medical campus is completely "wireless," and lectures are now podcasted, both in audio and in video formats. Numerous opportunities exist for students to participate in community medicine, outreach programs, and international medicine to study the root causes of medical inequalities at multiple sites in the Caribbean, Russia, Central America, and Africa.

Housing

Many medical students live in two apartment buildings adjacent to campus. The Medical Campus is served by Metro Rail, an elevated light railway, which has made large areas of Miami accessible to medical students.

Satellite Campuses/Facilities

The School of Medicine has a regional medical campus in Boca Raton on the campus of Florida Atlantic University. Thirty-two students each year will start and complete their medical educations at the regional campus. While the Medical Campus and regional campus curricula are identical in their missions, they have different emphases. Students at the regional campus gain their clinical training at Boca Raton Community Hospital and other local hospitals and clinics in a patient-centered environment.

Application Process and Requirements 2009–2010

Primary Application Service: AMCAS
Earliest filing date: June 1, 2008
Latest filing date: December 1, 2008

Secondary Application Required?: Yes
Sent to: All U.S. citizens and permanent residents
Contact: R. E. Hinkley, (305) 243-6791
med.admissions@miami.edu
Fee: Yes, $65
Fee waiver available: No
Earliest filing date: June 15, 2008
Latest filing date: January 31, 2009

Latest MCAT® considered: September 2008
Oldest MCAT® considered: 2006

Early Decision Program
School does not have EDP
Applicants notified: n/a
EDP available for: n/a

Regular Acceptance Notice
Earliest date: October 15, 2008
Latest date: Until class is full

Applicant's Response to Acceptance
Offer – Maximum Time: Two weeks

Requests for Deferred
Entrance Considered: Yes

Deposit to Hold Place in Class: Yes
Deposit (Resident): $100
Deposit (Non-Resident): $100
Deposit due: response to acceptance letter
Applied to tuition: Yes
Deposit refundable: No
Refundable by: May 15, 2009

Estimated number of new entrants: 182
EDP: 0, special program: 25

Start Month/Year: August 2009

Interview Format: Open file, structured, one hour interviews. Regional interviews are not available.

Other Programs

PREPARATORY PROGRAMS
Postbaccalaureate Program: Yes
www.miami.edu
Linette Aguiar, (305) 284-5176
Summer Program: Yes
www.miami.edu/medical-admissions
Astrid Mack, Ph.D. , (305) 284-5998

COMBINED DEGREE PROGRAMS
Baccalaureate/MD: Yes
www.miami.edu/medical-admissions
MD/MPH: Yes
http://spider.med.miami.edu/grad/phd.html
Dr. Jay Wilkinson, (305) 243-2209
MD/MBA: Yes
MD/JD: No
MD/PhD: Yes, http://chroma.med.miami.edu/mdphd
Dr. Sandra Lemmon, (305) 243-1094

Premedical Coursework

Course	Req.	Rec.	Lab.	Hrs.
Inorganic Chemistry	•		•	8
Behavioral Sciences				
Biochemistry		•		
Biology				
Biology/Zoology	•			6
Calculus				
College English	•			6
College Mathematics				

Course	Req.	Rec.	Lab.	Hrs.
Computer Science				
Genetics		•		
Humanities				
Organic Chemistry	•		•	8
Physics	•		•	8
Psychology				
Social Sciences				
Additional Sciences		•		6

Selection Factors: 2007 Accepted Applicants

Proportion of Accepted Applicants with Relevant Experience (Data Self-Reported to AMCAS®)		
Community Service/Volunteer		66%
Medically-Related Work		92%
Research		80%

Shaded bar represents accepted scores ranging from the 10th percentile to the 90th percentile   School Median ●   National Median ●

	2.0	2.1	2.2	2.3	2.4	2.5	2.6	2.7	2.8	2.9	3.0	3.1	3.2	3.3	3.4	3.5	3.6	3.7	3.8	3.9	4.0
Overall GPA	2.0	2.1	2.2	2.3	2.4	2.5	2.6	2.7	2.8	2.9	3.0	3.1	3.2	3.3	3.4	3.5	3.6	3.7	(3.8)	3.9	4.0
Science GPA	2.0	2.1	2.2	2.3	2.4	2.5	2.6	2.7	2.8	2.9	3.0	3.1	3.2	3.3	3.4	3.5	3.6	(3.7)	3.8	3.9	4.0

MCAT® required: Yes, 100% of 2007 accepted applicants took MCAT®

Verbal Reasoning	3	4	5	6	7	8	9	(10)	11	12	13	14	15
Physical Sciences	3	4	5	6	7	8	9	10	(11)	12	13	14	15
Biological Sciences	3	4	5	6	7	8	9	10	(11)	12	13	14	15
Writing Sample				J	K	L	M	N	O	(P)	(Q)	R	S	T

Acceptance & Matriculation Data for 2007–2008 First Year Class

	Resident	Non-Resident	International	Total
Applied	1472	2901	53	4426
Interviewed	313	180	1	494
Deferred	6	0	0	6
Matriculants				
Early Assurance Program	0	0	0	0
Early Decision Program	0	0	0	0
Baccalaureate/MD	21	1	0	22
MD/PhD	6	1	0	7
Matriculated	124	52	0	**176**

Applications accepted from International Applicants: No

Specialty Choice

2003, 2004, 2005 Graduates, Specialty Choice (As reported by program directors to GME Track™)	
Anesthesiology	10%
Emergency Medicine	5%
Family Practice	5%
Internal Medicine	22%
Obstetrics/Gynecology	6%
Orthopaedic Surgery	2%
Pediatrics	8%
Psychiatry	3%
Radiology	4%
Surgery	5%

Matriculant Demographics: 2007–2008 First Year Class

Men: 101   **Women:** 75

Matriculants' Self-Reported Race/Ethnicity

Mexican American	1	Korean	3
Cuban	10	Vietnamese	1
Puerto Rican	2	Other Asian	2
Other Hispanic	10	Total Asian	38
Total Hispanic	23	Native American	1
Chinese	11	Black	11
Asian Indian	16	Native Hawaiian	0
Pakistani	2	White	130
Filipino	3	Unduplicated Number	
Japanese	4	of Matriculants	176

Science and Math Majors: 70%
Matriculants with:
Baccalaureate degree: 99%
Graduate degree(s): 12%

Financial Information

Source: 2006–2007 LCME I-B survey and 2007–2008 AAMC TSF questionnaire

	Residents	Non-Residents
Total Cost of Attendance	$54,818	$64,524
Tuition and Fees	$30,048	$39,254
Other (includes living expenses)	$22,955	$23,455
Health Insurance (can be waived)	$1,815	$1,815

Average 2007 Graduate Indebtedness: $143,783
% of Enrolled Students Receiving Aid: 87%

Criminal Background Check

This medical school does not require a criminal background check prior to matriculation.

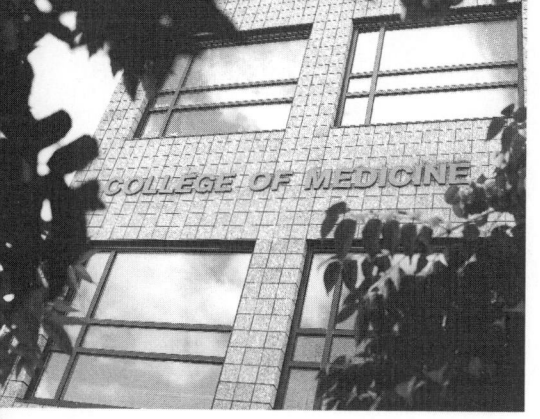

University of South Florida College of Medicine
Tampa, Florida

Office of Admissions/MDC-3
University of South Florida College of Medicine
12901 Bruce B. Downs Boulevard
Tampa, Florida 33612-4799
T 813 974 2229   **F** 813-974-4990

Admissions www.hsc.usf.edu/medicine/mdadmissions/index.htm
Main http://health.usf.edu/medicine/home.html
Financial http://hsc.usf.edu/medicine/studentaffairs/financial_aid/index.htm
Email md-admissions@lyris.health.usf.edu

Public Institution

Dr. Steven S. Klasko, Dean College of Medicine and VP for USF Health

Dr. Gretchen Koehler, Assistant Dean for Recruitment and Admissions

Suzanne Jackson, Director of Student Diversity and Enrichment

Michelle Williamson, Director of Financial Aid

General Information

The College of Medicine, along with the Colleges of Public Health and Nursing and the School of Physical Therapy compose USF Health and offers students unique opportunities for inter-professional relationships and experiences. The College of Medicine admitted the first class of medical students in 1971. The MD curriculum carefully integrates basic science learning with early clincial training. Located in Tampa, the College offers medical students a rich and diverse set of patients in nationally-ranked clinical sites.

Mission Statement

The mission of the College of Medicine is to provide for the education of students and professionals of the health and biomedical sciences through the creation of a scholarly environment that fosters excellence in the lifelong goals of education, research, and compassionate care.

Curricular Highlights

Community Service Requirement: Required.
Research/Thesis Requirement: Optional.

The faculty at the COM strive to create a four-year curriculum that is dynamic and forward-looking, reflecting a health care system that is ever-changing and increasingly global in its scope. It is designed to permit the student to learn the fundamental principles of medicine, to acquire skills of critical judgment based on evidence and experience, and to develop an ability to use principles and skills wisely in solving problems of health and disease. Areas of study include the sciences basic to medicine, the major clinical disciplines, and other significant elements such as behavioral science, medical ethics, and human values. The preclinical curriculum (years 1 and 2) utilizes an integrated, systems-based approach with an emphasis on early clinical experiences. In the major clinical years (years 3 and 4), student participate in direct patient care using both ambulatory and hospital settings across a number of excellent clinical facilities, gaining exposure to a vast array of patient populations. Required clerkships emphasize a patient-centered, interdisciplinary approach to care. Students are given increasing responsibility for patient care in preparation for graduate medical education residencies.

USMLE

Step 1: Required. Students must record a passing score for promotion.
Step 2: Clinical Skills (CS): Required. Students must record a passing total score to graduate.
Step 2: Clinical Knowledge (CK): Required. Students must record a passing total score to graduate.

Selection Factors

Applicants are selected for interviews based on academic achievement, demonstrated motivation to practice medicine and humanism, and leadership. The Admissions Committee reviews all materials including evaluation of the interviews and letters of recommendation, course load and types of courses taken. The majority of the matriculating class are Florida residents, but highly qualified non-Florida residents are also considered. Applicants are encouraged to apply early and complete their applications as soon as possible.

Financial Aid

The financial status of applicants does not affect their acceptance. Limited funds are available for loans and scholarships. First-year students are not permitted to engage in outside employment. There are employment opportunities in Tampa and the surrounding area for spouses. Contact our Office of Financial Aid at (813) 974-2068.

Information about Diversity Programs

The Office of Student Diversity and Enrichment (OSDE) works closely with the Office of MD Admissions and the rest of USF Health to recruit and support a diverse student body. Events, activities, programs, and facilities of the University of South Florida are available to all. For specific infomration about specific programs and services offered call (813) 974-4707 or visit *http://health.usf.edu/medicine/osde/index.htm.*

Campus Information

Setting
The USF MD Program is located in the nation's fifth most diverse large city area and is partners with an array of medical training hospitals in the Tampa Bay and central Florida area. The diversity of the patient population and medical training facilities contribute to an extraordinary clinical training program.

Enrollment
For 2007, total enrollment was: 480

Special Features
The College of Medicine's community training partners include the nation's 12th busiest transplant hospital and Level 1 Trauma/Burn Centers at Tampa General Hospital, All Children's Hospital (ranked among the top 10 children's hospitals), the Moffitt Cancer Center (3rd busiest outpatient cancer hospital in the nation and Florida's only NCI-accredited comprehensive cancer hospital and research center), two very large Veterans Affairs hospitals (the J.A. Haley VA is the busiest outpatient VA facility in the nation), and Florida's only Shriner's Hospital, as well as many other large local hospitals and rural clinics.

Housing
While on-campus student housing is limited, there are many student-centered complexes within close proximity. In addition, the MD Student Peer Advisory Council provides an unofficial housing directory to new students in the spring of their matriculation year.

Satellite Campuses/Facilities
Since clinical training at USF is integrated into the entire Tampa Bay medical community, students may rotate through a vast array of excellent hospitals and clinics in both city and rural environments.

Application Process and Requirements 2009–2010

Primary Application Service: AMCAS
Earliest filing date: June 1, 2008
Latest filing date: December 1, 2008

Secondary Application Required?: Yes
Sent to: Screened applicants
URL: Admissions office, (813) 974-2299, md-admissions@lyris.health.usf.edu
Fee: Yes, $30
Fee waiver available: Yes
Earliest filing date: June 1, 2008
Latest filing date: January 15, 2009

Latest MCAT® considered: October 2008
Oldest MCAT® considered: 2006

Early Decision Program
School does have EDP
Applicants notified: October 1, 2008
EDP available for: Both Residents and Non-Residents

Regular Acceptance Notice
Earliest date: October 15, 2008
Latest date: Until class is full

Applicant's Response to Acceptance Offer – Maximum Time: Two weeks

Requests for Deferred Entrance Considered: Yes

Deposit to Hold Place in Class: Yes
Deposit (Resident): $100
Deposit (Non-Resident): $100
Deposit due: Within two weeks of acceptance.
Applied to tuition: Yes
Deposit refundable: Yes
Refundable by: May 15, 2009

Estimated number of new entrants: 120
EDP: 15, special program: 15

Start Month/Year: August 2009

Interview Format: Closed file.
Regional interviews are not available.

Other Programs

PREPARATORY PROGRAMS
Postbaccalaureate Program: No
Summer Program: Yes,
http://health.usf.edu/medicine/osde/programs.htm
Pre-Matriculation Program: Yes,
http://health.usf.edu/medicine/osde/programs.htm
COMBINED DEGREE PROGRAMS
Baccalaureate/MD: Yes, www.hsc.usf.edu/medicine/mdadmissions/special_programs.htm
MD/MPH: Yes, www.hsc.usf.edu/medicine/mdadmissions/special_programs.html
MD/MBA: Yes, www.hsc.usf.edu/medicine/mdadmissions/special_programs.html
MD/JD: Yes, www.hsc.usf.edu/medicine/mdadmissions/special_programs.html
MD/PhD: Yes, www.hsc.usf.edu/medicine/mdadmissions/special_programs.html

Premedical Coursework

Course	Req.	Rec.	Lab.	Sems.	Course	Req.	Rec.	Lab.	Sems.
Inorganic Chemistry	•		•	2	Computer Science				
Behavioral Sciences					Genetics				
Biochemistry		•			Humanities		•		
Biology	•		•	2	Organic Chemistry	•		•	2
Biology/Zoology					Physics	•		•	2
Calculus					Psychology		•		
College English	•			2	Social Sciences		•		
College Mathematics	•			2	Other				

Selection Factors: 2007 Accepted Applicants

Proportion of Accepted Applicants with Relevant Experience (Data Self-Reported to AMCAS®)		
Community Service/Volunteer		71%
Medically-Related Work		94%
Research		79%

Shaded bar represents accepted scores ranging from the 10th percentile to the 90th percentile. School Median ● National Median ●

Overall GPA	2.0	2.1	2.2	2.3	2.4	2.5	2.6	2.7	2.8	2.9	3.0	3.1	3.2	3.3	3.4	3.5	3.6	3.7	(3.8)	3.9	4.0
Science GPA	2.0	2.1	2.2	2.3	2.4	2.5	2.6	2.7	2.8	2.9	3.0	3.1	3.2	3.3	3.4	3.5	3.6	3.7	(3.8)	3.9	4.0

MCAT® required: Yes, 100% of 2007 accepted applicants took MCAT®

Verbal Reasoning	3	4	5	6	7	8	9	(10)	11	12	13	14	15
Physical Sciences	3	4	5	6	7	8	9	(10)	(11)	12	13	14	15
Biological Sciences	3	4	5	6	7	8	9	(10)	(11)	12	13	14	15
Writing Sample				J	K	L	M	N	O	(P)	(Q)	R	S	T

Acceptance & Matriculation Data for 2007–2008 First Year Class

	Resident	Non-Resident	International	Total
Applied	1624	968	30	2622
Interviewed	381	38	0	419
Deferred	2	1	0	3
Matriculants				
Early Assurance Program	n/a	n/a	n/a	n/a
Early Decision Program	6	0	0	6
Baccalaureate/MD	13	0	0	13
MD/PhD	0	0	0	0
Matriculated	109	11	0	**120**

Applications accepted from International Applicants: No

Specialty Choice

2003, 2004, 2005 Graduates, Specialty Choice (As reported by program directors to GME Track™)	
Anesthesiology	4%
Emergency Medicine	7%
Family Practice	10%
Internal Medicine	17%
Obstetrics/Gynecology	6%
Orthopaedic Surgery	3%
Pediatrics	11%
Psychiatry	6%
Radiology	8%
Surgery	7%

Matriculant Demographics: 2007–2008 First Year Class

Men: 63   **Women:** 57

Matriculants' Self-Reported Race/Ethnicity

Mexican American	4	Korean	2
Cuban	6	Vietnamese	3
Puerto Rican	2	Other Asian	5
Other Hispanic	4	Total Asian	32
Total Hispanic	15	Native American	1
Chinese	2	Black	8
Asian Indian	16	Native Hawaiian	0
Pakistani	3	White	81
Filipino	2	Unduplicated Number	
Japanese	0	of Matriculants	120

Science and Math Majors: 69%
Matriculants with:
Baccalaureate degree: 99%
Graduate degree(s): 23%

Financial Information

Source: 2006–2007 LCME I-B survey and 2007–2008 AAMC TSF questionnaire

	Residents	Non-Residents
Total Cost of Attendance	$42,234	$74,108
Tuition and Fees	$21,192	$53,066
Other (includes living expenses)	$19,842	$19,842
Health Insurance (can be waived)	$1,200	$1,200

Average 2007 Graduate Indebtedness: $113,568
% of Enrolled Students Receiving Aid: 88%

Criminal Background Check

This medical school requires a criminal background check prior to matriculation.

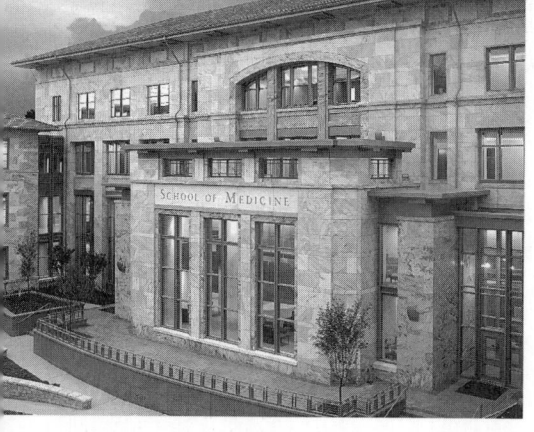

Emory University School of Medicine

Atlanta, Georgia

Emory University School of Medicine
Office of Admissions
1648 Pierce Drive NE, Suite 231
Atlanta, Georgia 30322-4510
T 404 727 5660   F 404 727 5456

Admissions www.med.emory.edu
Main www.med.emory.edu
Financial www.emory.edu/FINANCIAL_AID
Email medadmiss@emory.edu

Private Institution

Dr. Thomas J. Lawley, Dean

Dr. Ira K. Schwartz, Associate Dean for Medical Education/Student Affairs, Director of Admissions

Dr. Robert Lee, Associate Dean and Director, Office of Multicultural Affairs

Michael Behler, Associate Director of Financial Aid

Dr. J. William Eley, Executive Associate Dean for Medical Education/Student Affairs

General Information

Located six miles east of Atlanta, the Emory University School of Medicine was founded in 1915, resulting from several reorganizations dating from 1854 when the Atlanta Medical College was founded. Student clinical experiences are in numerous teaching hospitals, which provide more than 3,000 beds and large outpatient clinics. The university has close ties with Grady Memorial Hospital, the Centers for Disease Control and Prevention, the Carter Center of Emory University, and other affiliated institutions.

Mission Statement

Emory University School of Medicine is committed to providing leadership in medicine and science through the development of recognized programs of excellence and innovation in medical education, biomedical research, and patient care.

Curricular Highlights

Community Service Requirement: Optional.
Research/Thesis Requirement: Optional.

In 2007, EUSM implemented a progressive new curriculum which coincided with the opening of our new state-of-the-art medical education building. The new curriculum features a hybrid of lectures, small groups, and enhanced clinical exposure throughout the first 18 months of training. Students begin 12 months of clinical rotations midway through the second year, followed by a 5 month Discovery Phase which allows time for clinical or bench research, international experience, or other academic inquiry. The curriculum offers flexibility to allow students to take advantage of all of Emory's diverse opportunities. The fourth year is highlighted by a capstone experience which helps further prepare students for entering residency.

USMLE

Step 1: Required. Students must record a passing score for promotion.
Step 2: Clinical Skills (CS): Required. Students must only record a score.
Step 2: Clinical Knowledge (CK): Required. Students must record a passing total score to graduate.

Selection Factors

Students are selected on the basis of scholastic achievement and personal qualifications, without regard to race, sex, sexual orientation, age, disability, creed, veteran status, or national origin. In addition to the AMCAS application, all applicants must (a) present a very high level of scholarship; (b) take the MCAT® within four years of the matriculating year; (c) complete the Emory supplemental application form and fee (available on-line upon Emory's receipt of the AMCAS application); (d) have the required evaluation(s) submitted; and (e) appear for a personal interview, if invited. Students from foreign schools must have completed at least one year of academic work in an accredited U.S. or Canadian institution. Anyone enrolled in a graduate degree program should complete all required work for the degree by the date of matriculation. Only students enrolled in U.S. LCME-accredited medical schools with a similar curriculum are eligible to apply for transfer. Advanced standing is not given for work completed in other professional or graduate schools.

Financial Aid

Those who show documented need are eligible to receive funding in the form of scholarships and loans. Parental financial information is necessary to determine need-based funding. Each year, Emory awards 5 entering students merit-based Woodruff Fellowships, which provide full tuition and stipend for all four years.

Information about Diversity Programs

EUSM is strongly committed to increasing diversity in medicine. The Office of Multicultural Affairs works in conjunction with the Admission Committee and the Office of Student Affairs in the recruitment, selection, and retention of qualified students from groups underrepresented in medicine.

Campus Information

Setting

EUSM is located on the main university campus, situated on 631 acres of land in the historic neighborhood of Druid Hills. Emory is positioned along the Clifton Corridor, which also includes the U.S. Centers for Disease Control and Prevention.

Enrollment

For 2007, total enrollment was: 480

Special Features

Emory's clinical facilities provide for an extraordinary variety of training opportunities with diverse patient populations. Students are trained at the Emory University Hospital, Emory Crawford Long Hospital, Wesley Woods Geriatric Center, Children's Healthcare of Atlanta at Egleston and at Hughes Spalding, The Emory Clinic, Winship Cancer Center, Atlanta VA Medical Center, Grady Memorial Hospital, and numerous out-patient clinical sites. Grady Memorial Hospital is one of the largest hospitals in the U.S. Students have opportunities to volunteer in clinics, conduct research, and spend elective time abroad.

Housing

Off-campus apartments and houses are plentiful and affordable. New graduate housing will open in August 2009, offering all the modern amenities of luxury apartment complexes.

Application Process and Requirements 2009–2010

Primary Application Service: AMCAS
Earliest filing date: June 1, 2008
Latest filing date: October 15, 2008

Secondary Application Required?: Yes
Sent to: All applicants
Contact: Medical School Admissions
(404) 727-5660, medadmiss@emory.edu
Fee: Yes, $90
Fee waiver available: Yes
Earliest filing date: August 1, 2008
Latest filing date: December 1, 2008

Latest MCAT® considered: September 2008
Oldest MCAT® considered: 2005

Early Decision Program
School does not have EDP
Applicants notified: n/a
EDP available for: n/a

Regular Acceptance Notice
Earliest date: October 28, 2008
Latest date: Until class is full

Applicant's Response to Acceptance
Offer – Maximum Time: Two weeks

Requests for Deferred
Entrance Considered: Yes

Deposit to Hold Place in Class: No
Deposit (Resident): n/a
Deposit (Non-Resident): n/a
Deposit due: n/a
Applied to tuition: n/a
Deposit refundable: n/a
Refundable by: n/a

Estimated number of new entrants: 132
EDP: n/a, special program: n/a

Start Month/Year: August 2009

Interview Format: Group interview and individual interview. Regional interviews are not available.

Other Programs

PREPARATORY PROGRAMS
Postbaccalaureate Program: No
Summer Program: No

COMBINED DEGREE PROGRAMS
Baccalaureate/MD: No
MD/MPH: Yes, www.med.emory.edu
John E. McGowan, Jr., MD
jmcgowa@sph.emory.edu
MD/MBA: No
MD/JD: No
MD/PhD: Yes, www.med.emory.edu
Mary Horton, MPH, MA
(404) 727-6977, mdphd@emory.edu

Premedical Coursework

Course	Req.	Rec.	Lab.	Hrs.
Inorganic Chemistry	•	•		8
Behavioral Sciences	•			
Biochemistry		•		
Biology	•		•	8
Biology/Zoology				
Calculus				
College English	•			6
College Mathematics				

Course	Req.	Rec.	Lab.	Hrs.
Computer Science				
Genetics				
Humanities	•			18
Organic Chemistry	•		•	8
Physics	•		•	8
Psychology				
Social Sciences	•			
Other				

Selection Factors: 2007 Accepted Applicants

Proportion of Accepted Applicants with Relevant Experience (Data Self-Reported to AMCAS®)		Community Service/Volunteer	69%
		Medically-Related Work	86%
		Research	88%

Shaded bar represents accepted scores ranging from the 10th percentile to the 90th percentile   School Median ●   National Median ●

Overall GPA	2.0	2.1	2.2	2.3	2.4	2.5	2.6	2.7	2.8	2.9	3.0	3.1	3.2	3.3	3.4	3.5	3.6	3.7	(3.8)	3.9	4.0
Science GPA	2.0	2.1	2.2	2.3	2.4	2.5	2.6	2.7	2.8	2.9	3.0	3.1	3.2	3.3	3.4	3.5	3.6	3.7	(3.8)	3.9	4.0

MCAT® required: Yes, 100% of 2007 accepted applicants took MCAT®

Verbal Reasoning	3	4	5	6	7	8	9	(10)	(11)	12	13	14	15
Physical Sciences	3	4	5	6	7	8	9	10	(11)	(12)	13	14	15
Biological Sciences	3	4	5	6	7	8	9	10	(11)	(12)	13	14	15
Writing Sample			J	K	L	M	N	O	P	(Q)	R	S	T

Acceptance & Matriculation Data for 2007–2008 First Year Class

	Resident	Non-Resident	International	Total
Applied	544	4908	284	5736
Interviewed	142	570	22	734
Deferred	6	1	0	7
Matriculants				
Early Assurance Program	n/a	n/a	n/a	n/a
Early Decision Program	0	0	0	0
Baccalaureate/MD	n/a	n/a	n/a	n/a
MD/PhD	1	6	2	9
Matriculated	42	85	3	130

Applications accepted from International Applicants: Yes

Specialty Choice

2003, 2004, 2005 Graduates, Specialty Choice (As reported by program directors to GME Track™)	
Anesthesiology	5%
Emergency Medicine	5%
Family Practice	5%
Internal Medicine	23%
Obstetrics/Gynecology	3%
Orthopaedic Surgery	3%
Pediatrics	9%
Psychiatry	3%
Radiology	7%
Surgery	7%

Matriculant Demographics: 2007–2008 First Year Class

Men: 64   **Women:** 66

Matriculants' Self-Reported Race/Ethnicity

Mexican American	1	Korean	1
Cuban	0	Vietnamese	1
Puerto Rican	2	Other Asian	4
Other Hispanic	5	Total Asian	33
Total Hispanic	7	Native American	0
Chinese	11	Black	5
Asian Indian	13	Native Hawaiian	0
Pakistani	3	White	89
Filipino	0	**Unduplicated Number**	
Japanese	1	**of Matriculants**	130

Science and Math Majors: 62%
Matriculants with:
Baccalaureate degree: 100%
Graduate degree(s): 8%

Financial Information

Source: 2006–2007 LCME I-B survey and 2007–2008 AAMC TSF questionnaire

	Residents	Non-Residents
Total Cost of Attendance	$67,576	$67,576
Tuition and Fees	$39,976	$39,976
Other (includes living expenses)	$25,704	$25,704
Health Insurance (can be waived)	$1,896	$1,896

Average 2007 Graduate Indebtedness: $120,321
% of Enrolled Students Receiving Aid: 88%

Criminal Background Check

This medical school requires a criminal background check prior to matriculation.

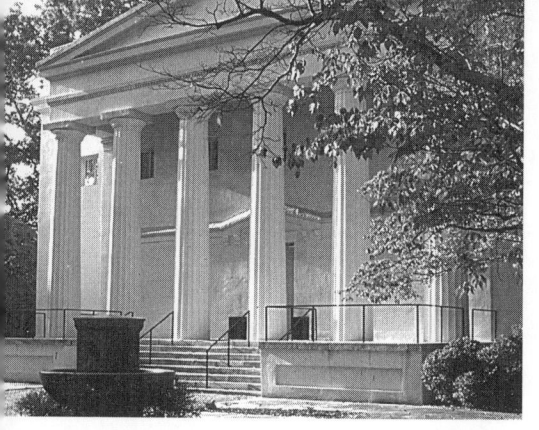

Medical College of Georgia
School of Medicine

Augusta, Georgia

Dr. Geoffrey H. Young
Associate Dean for Admissions
School of Medicine Medical College of Georgia
Augusta, Georgia 30912-4760
T 706 721 3186   F 706 721 0959

Admissions www.mcg.edu/careers/medicine.htm
Main www.mcg.edu
Financial www.mcg.edu/students/finaid
Email stdadmin@mail.mcg.edu

Public Institution

Dr. D. Douglas Miller, Dean

Dr. Geoffrey H. Young, Associate Dean for Admissions

Wilma A. Sykes-Brown, M.A., Assistant Dean for Educational Outreach and Partnerships

Dr. Beverly Ann Boggs, Director of Student Financial Aid

Linda R. DeVaughn, Director of Admissions

General Information

The School of Medicine of the Medical College of Georgia was founded in 1828 and is the nation's 13th oldest medical school. The institution is a separate university under the University System of Georgia. It consists of five schools: medicine, allied health, dentistry, graduate studies, and nursing.

Mission Statement

The Medical College of Georgia is committed to a supportive campus climate, necessary services, and leadership and development opportunities, all to educate the whole person and meet the needs of students, faculty, and staff; cultural, ethnic, racial, and gender diversity supported by practices that embody the ideals of an open democratic and global society; technology to advance education; collaborative relationships with other System institutions, state agencies, local schools and technical institutes, and industry, sharing physical, human, and information resources to enhance services available to the citizens of Georgia.

Curricular Highlights

Community Service Requirement: Optional.
Research/Thesis Requirement: Optional.

Basic Sciences: During the two pre-clinical years, students acquire the building blocks that underlie medical practice. The modular content of the curriculum is taught in lectures and labs with integrated clinical conferences and small-group activities. In the first semester, the Cellular and Systems Structures module introduces students to Gross Anatomy, Histology, and Development. In the

second semester, Biochemistry, Genetics, and Physiology are taught, while the Brain and Behavior module covers Psychiatry and Neuroscience. The Essentials of Clinical Medicine (ECM) is a two-year sequence emphasizing patient care skills, including interviewing and physical examination, information retrieval/analysis, ethics, and health promotion/disease prevention. In year two, the year-long Cellular and Systems Disease States module exposes students to Microbiology, Pathology, and Pharmacology in the context of clinical medicine. Clinical Training: Patient contact begins in year one in the ECM course that extends through year two. Year three consists of required core clerkships in Family Medicine, Internal Medicine, Neurology, OB/Gyn, Pediatrics, Psychiatry, and Surgery. During year four, students complete rotations in Emergency Medicine, Critical Care, Ambulatory Medicine, and an acting internship, with the remainder of the year for electives that can include research.

USMLE

Step 1: Required. Students must record a passing score for promotion.
Step 2: Clinical Skills (CS): Required. Students must record a passing total score to graduate.
Step 2: Clinical Knowledge (CK): Required. Students must record a passing total score to graduate.

Selection Factors

Applicants for admission are evaluated on a competitive basis. Information used includes, but is not limited to, the applicant's responsibilities prior to application; activities; shadowing physicians; ethnic, socioeconomic, and cultural background; region of residence with respect to its health professional needs; commitment to practice in an underserved area; references; motivation and potential for serving as a physician; interviews; MCAT® performance; and grades. In addition, students must meet specified technical standards to participate effectively in the medical education program and in the practice of medicine. Preference is given to Georgia residents. See *www.mcg.edu/SOM/admit/* for more information.

Financial Aid

The Office of Financial Aid coordinates programs

of assistance available to students. Information may be obtained at *www.mcg.edu/students/finaid*.

Information about Diversity Programs

The Medical College of Georgia seeks to encourage applications from qualified students from groups underrepresented in medicine. A summer program is designed for disadvantaged college students who show academic promise and who desire to practice medicine. Students may apply by writing to: Wilma A. Sykes-Brown, M.A., Assistant Dean for Educational Outreach and Partnerships, CB-1801, Medical College of Georgia, Augusta, GA 30912-1900.

Campus Information

Setting

The medical school is located in Augusta, GA, the second-largest city in Georgia, which is located on the south bank of the Savannah River, midway between the Great Smokey Mountains and the Atlantic Ocean. Augusta is a thriving city and a leading health care center, with nine area hospitals.

Enrollment

For 2007, total enrollment was: 739

Special Features

MCG Children's Medical Center is dedicated to serving the health care needs of children, from newborns to teenagers. The 149-bed modern center recognizes the importance of family involvement in a child's healing process and embraces the philosophy of family-centered care. A new $54 million Cancer Research Center opened in 2006. A new student Wellness Center features impact-absorbing treadmills, step and rowing machines, many computerized fitness tools, an indoor track, basketball courts, and a group exercise studio.

Housing

A variety of on-campus living environments are available.

Satellite Campuses/Facilities

Core clerkships take place at the MCG Hospitals and Clinics, the Children's Medical Center, and affiliated hospitals and community-based teaching sites throughout Georgia.

Application Process and Requirements 2009–2010

Primary Application Service: AMCAS
Earliest filing date: June 1, 2008
Latest filing date: November 1, 2008

Secondary Application Required?: Yes
Sent to: All Georgia residents; others are screened
URL: Provided by school
Fee: No
Fee waiver available: n/a
Earliest filing date: n/a
Latest filing date: January 7, 2009

Latest MCAT® considered: September 2008
Oldest MCAT® considered: 2006

Early Decision Program
School does have EDP
Applicants notified: October 1, 2008
EDP available for: Residents only

Regular Acceptance Notice
Earliest date: October 23, 2008
Latest date: Until class is full

Applicant's Response to Acceptance Offer – Maximum Time: Two weeks

Requests for Deferred Entrance Considered: Yes

Deposit to Hold Place in Class: Yes
Deposit (Resident): $100
Deposit (Non-Resident): $100
Deposit due: With response to acceptance offer
Applied to tuition: Yes
Deposit refundable: Yes
Refundable by: May 15, 2009

Estimated number of new entrants: 190
EDP: 60, special program: 6

Start Month/Year: August 2009

Interview Format: Two individual interviews with faculty. Regional interviews are not available.

Other Programs

PREPARATORY PROGRAMS
Postbaccalaureate Program: No
Summer Program: Yes,
mcg.edu/careers/specop/
Wilma A. Sykes-Brown, MA, 706-721-2522,
wsykes@mail.mcg.edu
Summer Student Training and Research (STAR) Program: www.mcg.edu/star

COMBINED DEGREE PROGRAMS
Baccalaureate/MD: No
MD/MPH: No
MD/MBA: No
MD/JD: No
MD/PhD: Yes,
www.mcg.edu/som/mdphd/geninfo.htm
Edward Inscho, PhD, 706-721-5615,
einscho@mcg.edu

Premedical Coursework

Course	Req.	Rec.	Lab.	Sems.	Course	Req.	Rec.	Lab.	Sems.
Inorganic Chemistry	•		•	2	Genetics				
Behavioral Sciences					Humanities				
Biochemistry		•			Organic Chemistry	•		•	1
Biology					Physics	•		•	2
Biology/Zoology	•		•	2	Psychology				
Calculus					Social Sciences				
College English	•			2	Advanced Chemistry	•			1
College Mathematics					Cellular Biology			•	
Computer Science					Statistics			•	

Selection Factors: 2007 Accepted Applicants

Proportion of Accepted Applicants with Relevant Experience (Data Self-Reported to AMCAS®)		Community Service/Volunteer	70%
		Medically-Related Work	84%
		Research	73%

Shaded bar represents accepted scores ranging from the 10th percentile to the 90th percentile. School Median ● National Median ●

Overall GPA	2.0	2.1	2.2	2.3	2.4	2.5	2.6	2.7	2.8	2.9	3.0	3.1	3.2	3.3	3.4	3.5	3.6	3.7	(3.8)	3.9	4.0
Science GPA	2.0	2.1	2.2	2.3	2.4	2.5	2.6	2.7	2.8	2.9	3.0	3.1	3.2	3.3	3.4	3.5	3.6	(3.7)	3.8	3.9	4.0

MCAT® required: Yes, 100% of 2007 accepted applicants took MCAT®

Verbal Reasoning	3	4	5	6	7	8	9	(10)	11	12	13	14	15
Physical Sciences	3	4	5	6	7	8	9	(10)	(11)	12	13	14	15
Biological Sciences	3	4	5	6	7	8	9	10	(11)	12	13	14	15
Writing Sample						J	K	L	M	N	(O)	P	(Q)	R	S	T

Acceptance & Matriculation Data for 2007–2008 First Year Class

	Resident	Non-Resident	International	Total
Applied	933	945	72	1950
Interviewed	453	29	0	482
Deferred	3	0	0	3
Matriculants				
Early Assurance Program	0	0	0	0
Early Decision Program	70	0	0	70
Baccalaureate/MD	n/a	n/a	n/a	n/a
MD/PhD	4	0	0	4
Matriculated	183	6	1	**190**

Applications accepted from International Applicants: Only Canadian

Matriculant Demographics: 2007–2008 First Year Class

Men: 110   **Women:** 80

Matriculants' Self-Reported Race/Ethnicity

Mexican American	1	Korean	5
Cuban	1	Vietnamese	3
Puerto Rican	1	Other Asian	1
Other Hispanic	5	**Total Asian**	36
Total Hispanic	7	Native American	0
Chinese	5	Black	11
Asian Indian	22	Native Hawaiian	0
Pakistani	2	White	139
Filipino	0	**Unduplicated Number**	
Japanese	0	**of Matriculants**	190

Science and Math Majors: 84%
Matriculants with:
    Baccalaureate degree: 99%
    Graduate degree(s): 7%

Specialty Choice

2003, 2004, 2005 Graduates, Specialty Choice (As reported by program directors to GME Track™)	
Anesthesiology	9%
Emergency Medicine	5%
Family Practice	9%
Internal Medicine	18%
Obstetrics/Gynecology	5%
Orthopaedic Surgery	5%
Pediatrics	18%
Psychiatry	1%
Radiology	4%
Surgery	6%

Financial Information

Source: 2006–2007 LCME I-B survey and 2007–2008 AAMC TSF questionnaire

	Residents	Non-Residents
Total Cost of Attendance	$35,124	$52,550
Tuition and Fees	$14,237	$31,663
Other (includes living expenses)	$19,762	$19,762
Health Insurance (can be waived)	$1,125	$1,125

Average 2007 Graduate Indebtedness: $105,086
% of Enrolled Students Receiving Aid: 78%

Criminal Background Check

This medical school does not require a criminal background check prior to matriculation.

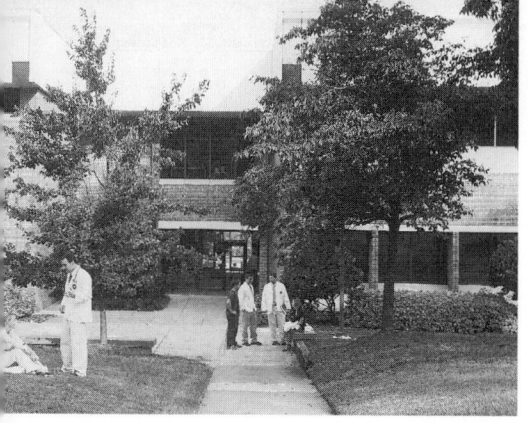

Mercer University School of Medicine
Macon, Georgia

Office of Admissions and Student Affairs
Mercer University School of Medicine
1550 College Street
Macon, Georgia 31207
T 478 301 2542   **F** 478 301 2547

Admissions http://medicine.mercer.edu/admissions_main
Main http://medicine.mercer.edu
Financial http://medicine.mercer.edu/Admissions/admissions_financial
Email admissions@med.mercer.edu

Private Institution

Dr. Martin L. Dalton, Dean

Dr. Maurice S. Clifton, Associate Dean for Admissions and Student Affairs

Dr. Youvette D. Hudson, Director for Financial Aid

General Information

Mercer University School of Medicine was founded in 1982 to improve health care access to the residents of Georgia. A private institution with strong state support, MUSM has been a leader in educating physicians who practice in the state after their training. In addition to the medical school, MUSM offers multiple graduate degrees including a Masters in Public Health.

Mission Statement

The mission of Mercer University School of Medicine (MUSM) is to educate physicians and health professionals to meet the primary care and health care needs of rural and medically underserved areas of Georgia.

Curricular Highlights

Community Service Requirement: Required. Numerous volunteer opportunities are available
Research/Thesis Requirement: Optional.

One of the first schools to adopt an all Problem-Based-Learning curriculum, there are no lectures and students take responsibility for their own learning. This open-ended nature requires and generates maturity and confidence not seen in traditional curricula. Learning must go well beyond the basic facts in that students are called upon to integrate and demonstrate verbally their basic science knowledge base to explain clinical findings. In addition, students are evaluated in areas related to group and interpersonal, problem-solving, information-gathering and evaluation skills. Students interview and examine actual and standardized patients early in the first year. The Community Medicine program provides a continuity experience in the clinical aspects of a community-oriented primary care medical practice during the first, second and fourth years. The third year consists of

required clinical rotations in internal medicine, surgery, pediatrics, obstetrics-gynecology, family medicine, and psychiatry. The fourth year includes required clerkships in acute and critical care and community medicine.

USMLE

Step 1: Required. Students must record a passing score for promotion.
Step 2: Clinical Skills (CS): Required. Students must only record a score.
Step 2: Clinical Knowledge (CK): Required. Students must record a passing total score to graduate.

Selection Factors

The Admissions Committee has accepted only applicants who are legal residents of Georgia. Each applicant must show promise of learning effectively in Mercer's curriculum and strong potential for practice in a medical specialty commensurate with the health care needs of rural and other underserved areas of Georgia. Most counties in Georgia have underserved status by the Federal Government, and the specialties that are needed include the primary care specialties of Internal Medicine, Pediatrics and Family Medicine, but also Surgery, and Obstetrics and Gynecology. Interviews are by invitation only and are held in Macon. In making the final decisions for acceptance or rejection, the Admissions Committee considers all criteria, but emphasizes strongly an applicant's demonstrated desire to fulfill the mission of the institution. The committee does not discriminate on the basis of race, sex, creed, national origin, age, or handicap. The average age of entering students was 23 years in 2007.

Financial Aid

Financial aid in the form of loans and scholarships is available to incoming accepted students. Financial need is determined by a federally approved need analysis and awards are made on the basis of need and merit. Most scholarships are based on need and mission compliance. The Office of Student Financial Planning provides easy access to information about all financial aid programs available and financial planning and debt

management thru financial management conferences and workshops.

Information about Diversity Programs

MUSM embraces the position that promoting and supporting diversity among the student body is central to the mission of the School. A diverse student body enriches professional education by providing a multiplicity of views and prospective that enhances learning within this highly interactive, student centered curriculum. For additional information and opportunities, please contact diversity@med.mercer.edu.

Special Features

The assessment system includes oral exams which foster integration of basic science knowledge base to explain clinical findings. Our students participate in a wide variety of leadership and community service programs, and many in international outreach programs in Africa, Central and South America.

Campus Information

Setting

There are two branch campuses, the Macon campus at Mercer University and at the Medical Center of Central Georgia, and the Savannah campus at the Memorial Health University Medical Center. Clinical teaching is also provided at several rural hospitals and clinics throughout Georgia.

Enrollment

For 2007, total enrollment was: 245

Housing

The Office of Student Affairs maintains a housing list of available apartments/houses and a list of those students who wish to secure roommates.

Satellite Campuses/Facilities

Students may study all four years on either the Macon or Savannah campus with a limited number of spaces for students to complete the first two years in Macon, and the clinical years in Savannah. There are many sites available for the Community Medicine program, and most students are able to return to a location near their home.

Application Process and Requirements 2009–2010

Primary Application Service: AMCAS
Earliest filing date: June 1, 2008
Latest filing date: November 1, 2008

Secondary Application Required?: Yes
Sent to: Screened applicants
Contact: Mary Putnam, (478) 301-2542, admissions@mercer.edu
Fee: Yes, $50
Fee waiver available: Yes
Earliest filing date: June 2008
Latest filing date: January 15, 2009

Latest MCAT® considered: September 2008
Oldest MCAT® considered: 2006

Early Decision Program
School does have EDP
Applicants notified: October 1, 2008
EDP available for: Residents only

Regular Acceptance Notice
Earliest date: November 2008
Latest date: Until class is full

Applicant's Response to Acceptance
Offer – Maximum Time: Two weeks

Requests for Deferred
Entrance Considered: Yes

Deposit to Hold Place in Class: Yes
Deposit (Resident): $100
Deposit (Non-Resident): n/a
Deposit due: With response to acceptance offer
Applied to tuition: Yes
Deposit refundable: Yes
Refundable by: May 15, 2009

Estimated number of new entrants: 70
EDP: 20, special program: n/a

Start Month/Year: August 2009

Interview Format: Two, one-hour interviews, open file.

Other Programs

PREPARATORY PROGRAMS
Postbaccalaureate Program: No
Summer Program: Yes, Admissions@med.mercer.edu

COMBINED DEGREE PROGRAMS
Baccalaureate/MD: No
MD/MPH: No
MD/MBA: No
MD/JD: No
MD/PhD: No

Premedical Coursework

Course	Req.	Rec.	Lab.	Hrs.	Course	Req.	Rec.	Lab.	Hrs.
Inorganic Chemistry	•		•	2	Computer Science				
Behavioral Sciences					Genetics				
Biochemistry		•			Humanities				
Biology	•		•	2	Organic Chemistry	•		•	2
Biology/Zoology					Physics	•		•	2
Calculus					Psychology				
College English					Social Sciences				
College Mathematics					Other				

Selection Factors: 2007 Accepted Applicants

Proportion of Accepted Applicants with Relevant Experience (Data Self-Reported to AMCAS®)		
Community Service/Volunteer		74%
Medically-Related Work		82%
Research		58%

Shaded bar represents accepted scores ranging from the 10th percentile to the 90th percentile — **School Median** ● **National Median** ●

Overall GPA	2.0	2.1	2.2	2.3	2.4	2.5	2.6	2.7	2.8	2.9	3.0	3.1	3.2	3.3	3.4	3.5	(3.6)	3.7	3.8	3.9	4.0
Science GPA	2.0	2.1	2.2	2.3	2.4	2.5	2.6	2.7	2.8	2.9	3.0	3.1	3.2	3.3	3.4	(3.5)	3.6	3.7	3.8	3.9	4.0

MCAT® required: Yes, 100% of 2007 accepted applicants took MCAT®

Verbal Reasoning	3	4	5	6	7	8	(9)	(10)	11	12	13	14	15
Physical Sciences	3	4	5	6	7	8	(9)	10	(11)	12	13	14	15
Biological Sciences	3	4	5	6	7	8	(9)	10	(11)	12	13	14	15
Writing Sample				J	K	L	M	N	(O)	P	(Q)	R	S	T

Acceptance & Matriculation Data for 2007–2008 First Year Class

	Resident	Non-Resident	International	Total
Applied	709	0	4	713
Interviewed	261	0	0	261
Deferred	0	0	0	0
Matriculants				
Early Assurance Program	n/a	n/a	n/a	n/a
Early Decision Program	25	0	0	25
Baccalaureate/MD	n/a	n/a	n/a	n/a
MD/PhD	n/a	n/a	n/a	n/a
Matriculated	62	0	1	**63**

Applications accepted from International Applicants: No

Specialty Choice

2003, 2004, 2005 Graduates, Specialty Choice (As reported by program directors to GME Track™)	
Anesthesiology	4%
Emergency Medicine	6%
Family Practice	9%
Internal Medicine	23%
Obstetrics/Gynecology	8%
Orthopaedic Surgery	3%
Pediatrics	16%
Psychiatry	0%
Radiology	8%
Surgery	12%

Matriculant Demographics: 2007–2008 First Year Class

Men: 37   **Women:** 26

Matriculants' Self-Reported Race/Ethnicity

Mexican American	0	Korean	0
Cuban	0	Vietnamese	0
Puerto Rican	0	Other Asian	0
Other Hispanic	1	Total Asian	8
Total Hispanic	1	Native American	0
Chinese	1	Black	1
Asian Indian	7	Native Hawaiian	0
Pakistani	0	White	54
Filipino	1	Unduplicated Number	
Japanese	0	of Matriculants	63

Science and Math Majors: 81%
Matriculants with:
Baccalaureate degree: 100%
Graduate degree(s): 3%

Financial Information

Source: 2006–2007 LCME I-B survey and 2007–2008 AAMC TSF questionnaire

	Residents	Non-Residents
Total Cost of Attendance	$58,932	$0
Tuition and Fees	$35,132	$0
Other (includes living expenses)	$23,090	$0
Health Insurance (can be waived)	$710	$0

Average 2007 Graduate Indebtedness: $158,908
% of Enrolled Students Receiving Aid: 93%

Criminal Background Check

This medical school does not require a criminal background check prior to matriculation.

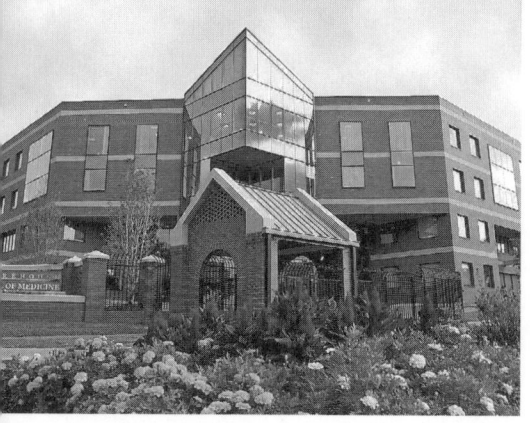

Morehouse School of Medicine
Atlanta, Georgia

Admissions and Student Affairs
Morehouse School of Medicine
720 Westview Drive, S.W.
Atlanta, Georgia 30310-1495
T 404 752 1650   F 404 752 1512

Admissions www.msm.edu/educational/mdprogram.htm
Main www.msm.edu/
Financial www.msm.edu/admissions/
fa/financial_aid.htm
Email mdadmissions@msm.edu

Private Institution

Dr. Ngozi Anachebe, Interim Assistant Dean for Student Affairs

Dr. Sterling Roaf, Director of Admissions

Cynthia Handy, Director of Student Fiscal Affairs

General Information

Morehouse School of Medicine is one of three medical schools in the nation founded by historically black institutions and was the first such medical school begun in the 20th century. In 2002 the new National Center for Primary Care opened. This facility features a 570-seat auditorium, cafeteria services, as well as additional office and teaching space. Clinical instruction takes place in affiliated hospitals and clinics, including Grady Memorial Hospital and South Fulton Medical Center.

Mission Statement

Morehouse School of Medicine is dedicated to improving the health and well-being of individuals and communities; increasing the diversity of the health professional and scientific workforce; and addressing primary health-care needs through programs in education, research, and service, with emphasis on people of color and the underserved urban and rural populations in Georgia and the nation.

Curricular Highlights

Community Service Requirement: Optional.
Research/Thesis Requirement: Optional.

The first two years of the curriculum emphasize an understanding of the principles, concepts, and major factual background of the basic medical sciences. Exposure to clinical medicine begins in the first year through assignment to a preceptor and increases in the second year with introduction to clinical medicine. Clinical education is continued through core clerkships during the third and fourth years, with 20 weeks of electives in the senior year. Student performance is evaluated primarily by letter grades. Learning resources and other support services are available to all students throughout their four years.

USMLE

Step 1: Required. Students must record a passing score for promotion.
Step 2: Clinical Skills (CS): Required. Students must record a passing total score to graduate.
Step 2: Clinical Knowledge (CK): Required. Students must record a passing total score to graduate.

Selection Factors

Selection of students for admission is made after careful consideration of many factors. These include MCAT® scores, the academic record, the extent of academic improvement, balance and depth of academic program, difficulty of courses taken, and other indicators of maturation of learning ability. Additional factors considered are extracurricular activities, hobbies, the need to work, research projects and experiences, evidence of activities that indicate concurrence with the school's mission, and evidence of pursuing interests and talents in depth. Finally, the committee looks for evidence of those traits of personality and character essential to success in medicine: compassion, integrity, motivation, and perseverance. All information available about each applicant is considered without assigning priority to any single factor. Students are admitted on the basis of individual qualifications regardless of sex, age, race, creed, national origin, or handicap. Preferential consideration is given to qualified applicants who are residents of the state of Georgia. Foreign applicants must have a permanent resident visa. Technical standards have been established as a prerequisite for admission and graduation from the MSM. A candidate for the M.D. degree must have aptitude, abilities, and skills in five areas: observation, communication, motor, conceptual integrative and quantitative, and behavioral and social. Applicants are not considered for admission who have been dismissed from another medical school for academic or disciplinary reasons. Transfer applications are considered only from students in good standing at an LCME-accredited U.S. or Canadian medical school; transfers from foreign medical schools or osteopathic, veterinary, or dental schools are not accepted. Transfers are accepted into the second year only on a space-available basis. The transfer application deadline is May 1.

Financial Aid

In addition to federal loan programs, a number of scholarships and grants are available.

Campus Information

Setting

Morehouse School of Medicine is situated five minutes from downtown Atlanta within the Atlanta University Center (AUC) in the historic West End. The AUC is a consortium of six independent institutions that constitute the largest predominately African American educational complex in the world. Atlanta is also home to the Centers for Disease Control and Prevention (CDC), over 20 major medical centers, the Carter Presidential Library, the Martin Luther King Center for Nonviolent Social Change, and a plethora of educational, entertainment, and cultural opportunities. Atlanta's sports teams, led by the Atlanta Braves, Atlanta Falcons, and Atlanta Hawks, are consistently competitive in their respective divisions. Home to one of the busiest airports in the world, Hartsfield-Jackson Atlanta International Airport, the city is a major international transportation hub. A premier city for the 21st century, Atlanta is a bustling, progressive metropolis with an energy all its own.

Enrollment

For 2007, total enrollment was: 210

Housing

On-campus housing is not available. Students seeking assistance in their relocation can access the school's very useful Web site at *http://web. msm.edu/relocation_guide/housing.htm*.

Application Process and Requirements 2009–2010

Primary Application Service: AMCAS
Earliest filing date: June 1, 2008
Latest filing date: December 1, 2008

Secondary Application Required?: Yes
Sent to: All eligible applicants after preliminary screening
URL: URL given to invited applicants only
Fee: Yes, $50
Fee waiver available: Yes
Earliest filing date: July 15, 2008
Latest filing date: January 9, 2009

Latest MCAT® considered: September 2008
Oldest MCAT® considered: 2006

Early Decision Program
School does have EDP
Applicants notified: October 1, 2008
EDP available for: Residents only

Regular Acceptance Notice
Earliest date: November 2008
Latest date: Until class is full

Applicant's Response to Acceptance
Offer – Maximum Time: 14 days

Requests for Deferred
Entrance Considered: Yes

Deposit to Hold Place in Class: Yes
Deposit (Resident): $100
Deposit (Non-Resident): $100
Deposit due: 14 days from acceptance offer
Applied to tuition: Yes
Deposit refundable: Yes
Refundable by: May 15, 2009

Estimated number of new entrants: 52
EDP: 1, special program: n/a

Start Month/Year: July 2009

Interview Format: One one-on-one Interview. Regional interviews are not available.

Other Programs

PREPARATORY PROGRAMS
Postbaccalaureate Program: No
Summer Program: Yes
www.applyweb.com/apply/mhsum/index.html

COMBINED DEGREE PROGRAMS
Baccalaureate/MD: No
MD/MPH: Yes, Sterling Roaf, M.D.
(404) 752-1650, sroaf@msm.edu
MD/MBA: No
MD/JD: No
MD/PhD: Yes

Premedical Coursework

Course	Req.	Rec.	Lab.	Sems.	Course	Req.	Rec.	Lab.	Sems.
Inorganic Chemistry	•		•	2	Computer Science				
Behavioral Sciences		•		1	Genetics		•	•	1
Biochemistry		•	•	1	Humanities				
Biology	•		•	2	Organic Chemistry	•		•	2
Biology/Zoology					Physics	•		•	2
Calculus					Psychology				
College English	•			2	Social Sciences				
College Mathematics	•			2	Other				

Selection Factors: 2007 Accepted Applicants

Proportion of Accepted Applicants with Relevant Experience (Data Self-Reported to AMCAS®)		
Community Service/Volunteer		71%
Medically-Related Work		82%
Research		74%

Shaded bar represents accepted scores ranging from the 10th percentile to the 90th percentile · · · School Median ● · · National Median ●

Overall GPA 2.0 2.1 2.2 2.3 2.4 2.5 2.6 2.7 2.8 2.9 3.0 3.1 3.2 3.3 ③.④ 3.5 3.6 3.7 3.8 3.9 4.0
Science GPA 2.0 2.1 2.2 2.3 2.4 2.5 2.6 2.7 2.8 2.9 3.0 3.1 3.2 ③.③ 3.4 3.5 3.6 3.7 3.8 3.9 4.0

MCAT® required: Yes, 100% of 2007 accepted applicants took MCAT®

Verbal Reasoning	3	4	5	6	7	8	⑨	⑩	11	12	13	14	15
Physical Sciences	3	4	5	6	7	8	⑨	10	⑪	12	13	14	15
Biological Sciences	3	4	5	6	7	8	⑨	10	⑪	12	13	14	15
Writing Sample			J	K	L	M	N	ⓞ	P	ⓠ	R	S	T

Acceptance & Matriculation Data for 2007–2008 First Year Class

	Resident	Non-Resident	International	Total
Applied	421	3093	109	3623
Interviewed	113	135	0	248
Deferred	1	0	0	1
Matriculants				
Early Assurance Program	0	0	0	0
Early Decision Program	1	0	0	1
Baccalaureate/MD	n/a	n/a	n/a	n/a
MD/PhD	n/a	n/a	n/a	n/a
Matriculated	32	20	0	**52**

Applications accepted from International Applicants: No

Specialty Choice

2003, 2004, 2005 Graduates, Specialty Choice (As reported by program directors to GME Track™)	
Anesthesiology	2%
Emergency Medicine	7%
Family Practice	12%
Internal Medicine	15%
Obstetrics/Gynecology	11%
Orthopaedic Surgery	1%
Pediatrics	20%
Psychiatry	4%
Radiology	2%
Surgery	5%

Matriculant Demographics: 2007–2008 First Year Class

Men: 21   **Women:** 31

Matriculants' Self-Reported Race/Ethnicity

Mexican American	0	Korean	2
Cuban	0	Vietnamese	0
Puerto Rican	1	Other Asian	2
Other Hispanic	0	Total Asian	9
Total Hispanic	1	Native American	1
Chinese	0	Black	39
Asian Indian	5	Native Hawaiian	0
Pakistani	0	White	4
Filipino	0	Unduplicated Number	
Japanese	0	of Matriculants	52

Science and Math Majors: 67%
Matriculants with:
Baccalaureate degree: 98%
Graduate degree(s): 12%

Financial Information

Source: 2006–2007 LCME I-B survey and 2007–2008 AAMC TSF questionnaire

	Residents	Non-Residents
Total Cost of Attendance	$58,102	$58,102
Tuition and Fees	$29,248	$29,248
Other (includes living expenses)	$26,771	$26,771
Health Insurance (can be waived)	$2,083	$2,083

Average 2007 Graduate Indebtedness: $136,118
% of Enrolled Students Receiving Aid: 94%

Criminal Background Check

This medical school requires a criminal background check prior to matriculation.

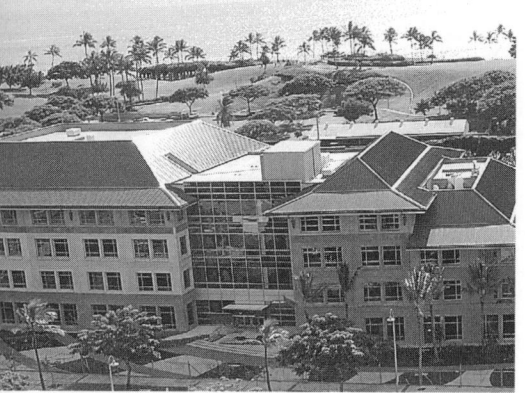

University of Hawai'i
John A. Burns School of Medicine

Honolulu, Hawaii

Office of Student Affairs/Admissions
Medical Education Building
University of Hawai'i, John A. Burns
School of Medicine
651 Ilalo Street
Honolulu, Hawaii 96813-5534
T 808 692 1000   **F** 808 692 1251

Admissions http://jabsom.hawaii.edu/
Main http://jabsom.hawaii.edu
Financial http://jabsom.hawaii.edu/
Email mnishiki@hawaii.edu

Public Institution

Dr. Gary K. Ostrander, Interim Dean

Dr. Satoru Izutsu, Senior Associate Dean

*Gail C. Koki, Student Liaison, Financial
Aid and Scholarships*

*Marilyn M. Nishiki,
Admissions Officer & Registrar*

General Information
The University of Hawai'i at Manoa John A.
Burns School of Medicine is in the College of
Health Sciences and Social Welfare. The School
of Medicine is located at the Kaka'ako campus.
It also has teaching facilities in affiliated com-
munity hospitals and primary care clinics
throughout the state.

Mission Statement
John A. Burns School of Medicine's mission is to
teach and train high quality physicians, biomedical students, and allied health professionals for
Hawai'i and the Pacific, and to conduct both clinical and basic research in areas of specific interest
to the community and region. JABSOM is the
most culturally and ethnically diverse medical
school in the country. Its student body mirrors
the rich diversity of the state's population.

Curricular Highlights
Community Service Requirement: Optional.
Research/Thesis Requirement: Optional.

The school utilizes a problem-based learning
curriculum (PBL), in which basic sciences are
learned in the context of the study of health care
problems. These activities are supplemented by
selected lecture and laboratory sessions. Clinical
skills and community health activities are
prominent, and begin in the first year of the
curriculum. Special features include an emphasis
on PBL as the primary instructional method in
the pre-clinical years; early introduction of clinical training, community service, and research
experiences; rural health training opportunities;
a longitudinal, interdisciplinary clerkship
opportunity in the third-year; and opportunities

for training experiences in various communities
throughout Hawaii, the Pacific, and Asia.

USMLE
Step 1: Required. Students must record a passing
score for promotion.
Step 2: Clinical Skills (CS): Required. Students
must record a passing total score to graduate.
Step 2: Clinical Knowledge (CK): Required. Students must record a passing total score to graduate.

Selection Factors
Applicants are considered without discrimination as to age, sex, race, creed, national origin,
religion, or handicap. The school admits 62 students to its regular first-year class. A priority is to
admit applicants with strong ties to the state of
Hawaii. Applications go through two screens.
The first screen determines an applicant's ties to
the State of Hawaii. This screen reviews an applicant's state or country of legal residence, birth-
place, high school graduated, college attended,
parents' legal residence, and legacy. An applicant
who meets three of the six categories is considered a resident of the state for application purposes. The second screen is the academic screen.
The following characteristics are examined:
GPAs, MCAT® scores, graduate/other professional degrees, academic honors, participation
in extracurricular activities and employment in
areas of human services, and research. Interviews
are conducted in Hawaii for those passing the
second screen. Acceptance, alternate, and rejection letters are mailed in April.

Financial Aid
Financial status is not a factor in considering
applicants for acceptance. Although financial aid is
limited, efforts are made to assist medical students
in obtaining loans and scholarships, wherever possible. Loan funds from federal sources are available only to U.S. citizens and permanent residents.
In general, students are discouraged from engag-
ing in outside employment.

Information about Diversity Programs
The student body and faculty are culturally
diverse. The school is actively involved in the

recruitment, admission, and retention of students from disadvantaged backgrounds who
have potential and are interested in pursuing
an M.D. degree. The school provides a range of
student services. The Imi Ho'ola Post-Baccalaureate Program is for students from disadvantaged
backgrounds. Interested persons are encouraged
to contact Dr. Nanette L.K. Judd, Program Director, Imi Ho'ola Post-Baccalaureate Program, at
judd@hawaii.edu or 808-692-1030.

Campus Information

Setting
The School of Medicine is located at a 10.5-
acre state-owned parcel in Kaka'ako, on the
water's edge, between Waikiki and downtown
Honolulu. It is an environment conducive to the
school's goal of becoming a top-ranked research-
intensive medical school with the opportunity to
attract world-class research scientists to join the
school's faculty.

Enrollment
For 2007, total enrollment was: 257

Special Features
The school's problem-based learning curriculum has been in place since 1989. For the past
several years, emphasis has been placed on promoting biomedical research. Recruitment of
world-class scientists has resulted in an increase
of research funding. It is envisioned that these
research areas will be further developed at the
new quarters in Kaka'ako.

Housing
Medical students and candidates for graduate
degrees in the medical school are expected to
make their own living arrangements. The
University provides limited dormitory and
apartment facilities.

Satellite Campuses/Facilities
Clinical activities of the school's curriculum
are conducted in affiliated community hospitals
and clinics. There is no university hospital
connected to the school of medicine.

Application Process and Requirements 2009–2010

Primary Application Service: AMCAS
Earliest filing date: June 1, 2008
Latest filing date: November 1, 2008

Secondary Application Required?: Yes
Sent to: Screened applicants who minimally achieve the required cut-off scores.
Contact: Marilyn Nishiki
(808) 692-1000, mnishiki@hawaii.edu
Fee: Yes, $50
Fee waiver available: No
Earliest filing date: School-specific deadlines
Latest filing date: School-specific deadlines

Latest MCAT® considered: September 2008
Oldest MCAT® considered: 2006

Early Decision Program
School does have EDP
Applicants notified: October 1, 2008
EDP available for: Residents only

Regular Acceptance Notice
Earliest date: October 15, 2008
Latest date: Until class is full

Applicant's Response to Acceptance Offer – Maximum Time: Two weeks

Requests for Deferred Entrance Considered: Yes

Deposit to Hold Place in Class: No
Deposit (Resident): n/a
Deposit (Non-Resident): n/a
Deposit due: n/a
Applied to tuition: n/a
Deposit refundable: n/a
Refundable by: n/a

Estimated number of new entrants: 62
EDP: 1, special program: n/a

Start Month/Year: July 2009

Interview Format: One-on-one interviews. Regional interviews are not available.

Other Programs

PREPARATORY PROGRAMS
Postbaccalaureate Program: Yes
http://jabsom.hawaii.edu
Nanette K. Judd, PhD, MPH, RN
(808) 692-1030, judd@hawaii.edu
Summer Program: No

COMBINED DEGREE PROGRAMS
Baccalaureate/MD: No
MD/MPH: No
MD/MBA: No
MD/JD: No
MD/PhD: No

Premedical Coursework

Course	Req.	Rec.	Lab.	Hrs.	Course	Req.	Rec.	Lab.	Hrs.
Inorganic Chemistry	•		•	8	Computer Science				
Behavioral Sciences					Genetics		•		
Biochemistry	•			3	Humanities				
Biology	•		•	8	Organic Chemistry	•		•	8
Biology/Zoology					Physics	•		•	8
Calculus					Psychology		•		
College English		•			Social Science		•		
College Mathematics		•			Cell & Molecular Biology		•		3

Selection Factors: 2007 Accepted Applicants

Proportion of Accepted Applicants with Relevant Experience (Data Self-Reported to AMCAS®)		
Community Service/Volunteer		64%
Medically-Related Work		92%
Research		83%

Shaded bar represents accepted scores ranging from the 10th percentile to the 90th percentile ▭   School Median ● National Median ●

Overall GPA	2.0	2.1	2.2	2.3	2.4	2.5	2.6	2.7	2.8	2.9	3.0	3.1	3.2	3.3	3.4	3.5	3.6	3.7	(3.8)	3.9	4.0
Science GPA	2.0	2.1	2.2	2.3	2.4	2.5	2.6	2.7	2.8	2.9	3.0	3.1	3.2	3.3	3.4	3.5	3.6	(3.7)	3.8	3.9	4.0

MCAT® required: Yes, 100% of 2007 accepted applicants took MCAT®

Verbal Reasoning	3	4	5	6	7	8	9	(10)	11	12	13	14	15
Physical Sciences	3	4	5	6	7	8	9	10	(11)	12	13	14	15
Biological Sciences	3	4	5	6	7	8	9	10	(11)	12	13	14	15
Writing Sample				J	K	L	M	N	O	P	(Q)	R	S	T

Acceptance & Matriculation Data for 2007–2008 First Year Class

	Resident	Non-Resident	International	Total
Applied	191	1597	113	1901
Interviewed	174	57	9	240
Deferred	2	0	0	2
Matriculants				
Early Assurance Program	0	0	0	0
Early Decision Program	0	0	0	0
Baccalaureate/MD	n/a	n/a	n/a	n/a
MD/PhD	n/a	n/a	n/a	n/a
Matriculated	48	12	2	**62**

Applications accepted from International Applicants: Yes

Specialty Choice

2003, 2004, 2005 Graduates, Specialty Choice (As reported by program directors to GME Track™)	
Anesthesiology	6%
Emergency Medicine	5%
Family Practice	8%
Internal Medicine	25%
Obstetrics/Gynecology	5%
Orthopaedic Surgery	2%
Pediatrics	6%
Psychiatry	4%
Radiology Diagnostic	2%
Surgery General	7%

Matriculant Demographics: 2007–2008 First Year Class

Men: 25   **Women:** 37

Matriculants' Self-Reported Race/Ethnicity

Mexican American	0	**Korean**	5
Cuban	0	**Vietnamese**	4
Puerto Rican	0	**Other Asian**	1
Other Hispanic	0	**Total Asian**	47
Total Hispanic	0	**Native American**	1
Chinese	23	**Black**	0
Asian Indian	0	**Native Hawaiian**	11
Pakistani	0	**White**	19
Filipino	0	**Unduplicated Number**	
Japanese	29	**of Matriculants**	62

Science and Math Majors: 74%
Matriculants with:
  Baccalaureate degree: 100%
  Graduate degree(s): 15%

Financial Information

Source: 2006–2007 LCME I-B survey and 2007–2008 AAMC TSF questionnaire

	Residents	Non-Residents
Total Cost of Attendance	$48,530	$68,426
Tuition and Fees	$20,692	$40,588
Other (includes living expenses)	$27,838	$27,838
Health Insurance (can be waived)	$0	$0

Average 2007 Graduate Indebtedness: $26,223
% of Enrolled Students Receiving Aid: 86%

Criminal Background Check

This medical school requires a criminal background check prior to matriculation.

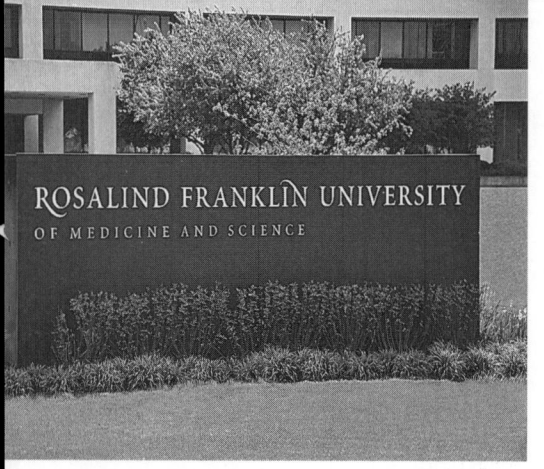

Rosalind Franklin University of Medicine and Science Chicago Medical School

North Chicago, Illinois

Rosalind Franklin University of Medicine and Science
Office of Medical School Admissions
3333 Green Bay Road
North Chicago, Illinois 60064
T 847 578 3204

Admissions www.rosalindfranklin.edu/admissions
Main www.rosalindfranklin.edu/cms
Financial www.rosalindfranklin.edu/osa/financialaid
Email cms.admissions@rosalindfranklin.edu

Private Institution

Arthur J. Ross III, M.D., M.B.A., Dean

Maryann DeCaire, Associate Vice President of Enrollment Services

Cathy Lazarus, M.D., Senior Associate Dean for Student Affairs and Medical Education

Rebecca Durkin, Associate Vice President, Office of Student Development

General Information

Founded in 1912, The Chicago Medical School has been dedicated to excellence in medical education for nearly a century. The Chicago Medical School has educated thousands of professionals with recognized innovation in health education, excellence in the creation of knowledge and scientific discovery focused on prediction and prevention of disease, outstanding clinical programs, and compassionate community service. Major hospital affiliates include: Advocate Lutheran General Hospital, John H. Stroger, Jr., Hospital of Cook County, Mount Sinai Hospital and Medical Center, and the North Chicago Veterans Affairs Medical Center (NCVAMC). The University's clinical campus consists of the NCVAMC and The Clinics at Rosalind Franklin University, and the Rosalind Franklin University.

Mission Statement

The Chicago Medical School educates physicians and scientists dedicated to providing exemplary, compassionate patient care and excellence in scientific discovery within an inter-professional environment.

Curricular Highlights

Community Service Requirement: Optional.
Research/Thesis Requirement: Optional.

The Chicago Medical School's curriculum offers a strong grounding in the sciences basic to medicine along with assuring competency in skills necessary for the practice of medicine. The CMS curriculum features a unique interprofessional approach, with interaction among a broad range of health professional students and practitioners. The curriculum is a mix of lectures, labs, small-group discussions, team-based learning, and

opportunities for peer-to-peer learning. The educational information system, Desire to Learn (D2L), provides 24-hour-a-day access to learning materials. Students have early clinical experiences in the state-of-the-art evaluation and education center, as well as opportunities to connect with physician preceptors. The required junior clinical clerkships include medicine, ambulatory care, surgery, family medicine, obstetrics/gynecology, psychiatry, medCore, pediatrics, neurology, and emergency medicine. The senior requirements include four weeks in a medicine or pediatrics subinternship, plus 32 weeks of approved electives (14 of which must be completed at one of the school's primary affiliated sites). The elective period gives students an opportunity, through both intramural and extramural experiences, to explore and strengthen their personal career interests.

USMLE

Step 1: Required. Students must record a passing score for promotion.
Step 2: Clinical Skills (CS): Required. Students must record a passing total score to graduate.
Step 2: Clinical Knowledge (CK): Required. Students must record a passing total score to graduate.

Selection Factors

Students are selected on the basis of various criteria, including scholarship, character, motivation, and educational background. A student's potential for the study and practice of medicine will be evaluated on the basis of academic achievement, MCAT® results, appraisals by a preprofessional advisory committee or individual instructors, and a personal interview, if requested by the Student Admissions Committee. To fulfill the mission of The Chicago Medical School, admissions policies are designed to ensure that the selection process matriculates a class made up of individuals capable of meeting the needs of current and future patients. Applicants will be evaluated not only for educational potential, but with the aim of providing diverse educational experience for other members of the class.

Financial Aid

The Financial Aid Office is committed to helping students secure the funding needed to pursue their educational endeavors. Financial Aid is available in the form of loans, scholarships, and work-study. For more information, contact the Financial Aid Office at (847) 578-3217.

Information about Diversity Programs

The school maintains an extensive recruitment and retention program for students from groups underrepresented in medicine.

Campus Information

Setting

Rosalind Franklin University of Medicine and Science is situated in the northern suburbs of Chicago, with easy access to downtown Chicago and the surrounding areas by car or public transportation. State-of-the-art facilities include a recently completed $10 million research wing expansion; multimedia classrooms and gross anatomy laboratory; and an Education and Evaluation Center for physical examination skills training. Recreational facilities include an exercise room, game room, and the Student Union (home to the University Bookstore, Union Café, and dedicated e-mail stations).

Enrollment

For 2007, total enrollment was: 758

Housing

On-campus housing is available at Rosalind Franklin University. Each of the University's three apartment buildings has five floors and consists of 60 one and two-bedroom apartments. Individual apartments feature a variety of amenities, such as kitchen appliances (range, refrigerator, dishwasher, and microwave), fully networked Internet connectivity, and washer/dryer hookups. Each apartment building also includes study and lounge areas, shared laundry facilities on every floor, and individual storage units. For more information about student housing, contact the Office of Student Housing at (847) 578-8350 or campus.housing@rosalindfranklin.edu.

Application Process and Requirements 2009–2010

Primary Application Service: AMCAS
Earliest filing date: June 1, 2008
Latest filing date: November 1, 2008

Secondary Application Required?: Yes
Sent to: All applicants
URL: n/a
Fee: Yes, $100
Fee waiver available: Yes
Earliest filing date: July 1, 2008
Latest filing date: December 15, 2008

Latest MCAT® considered: September 2008
Oldest MCAT® considered: 2006

Early Decision Program
School does have EDP
Applicants notified: October 1, 2008
EDP available for: Both Residents and Non-Residents

Regular Acceptance Notice
Earliest date: October 15, 2008
Latest date: Until class is full

Applicant's Response to Acceptance Offer – Maximum Time: Two weeks

Requests for Deferred Entrance Considered: Yes

Deposit to Hold Place in Class: Yes
Deposit (Resident): $100
Deposit (Non-Resident): $100
Deposit due: With acceptance offer
Applied to tuition: Yes
Deposit refundable: Yes
Refundable by: May 15, 2009

Estimated number of new entrants: 185
EDP: 3, special program: n/a

Start Month/Year: August 2009

Interview Format: Two open-file interviews with committee members, faculty, staff, and/or fourth-year students. Regional interviews are not available.

Other Programs

PREPARATORY PROGRAMS
Postbaccalaureate Program: No
Summer Program: No

COMBINED DEGREE PROGRAMS
Baccalaureate/MD: No
MD/MPH: No
MD/MBA: No
MD/JD: No
MD/PhD: Yes,
www.rosalindfranklin.edu/sgpds/mdphd

Premedical Coursework

Course	Req.	Rec.	Lab.	Sems.	Course	Req.	Rec.	Lab.	Sems.
Inorganic Chemistry	•		•	2	Computer Science				
Behavioral Sciences					Genetics				
Biochemistry					Humanities				
Biology					Organic Chemistry	•		•	2
Biology/Zoology	•		•	2	Physics	•		•	2
Calculus					Psychology				
College English					Social Sciences				
College Mathematics					Other				

Selection Factors: 2007 Accepted Applicants

Proportion of Accepted Applicants with Relevant Experience (Data Self-Reported to AMCAS)		
Community Service/Volunteer		66%
Medically-Related Work		88%
Research		79%

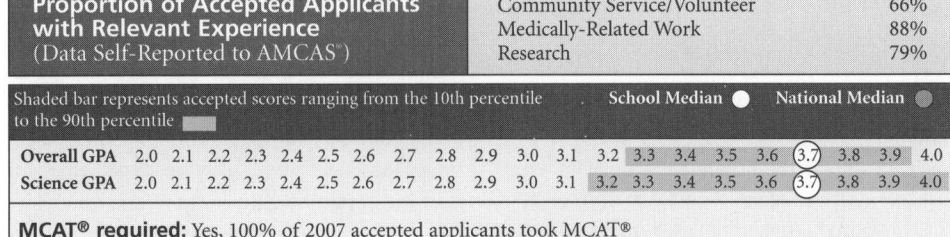

Shaded bar represents accepted scores ranging from the 10th percentile to the 90th percentile   School Median ●   National Median ●

	2.0	2.1	2.2	2.3	2.4	2.5	2.6	2.7	2.8	2.9	3.0	3.1	3.2	3.3	3.4	3.5	3.6	3.7	3.8	3.9	4.0
Overall GPA	2.0	2.1	2.2	2.3	2.4	2.5	2.6	2.7	2.8	2.9	3.0	3.1	3.2	3.3	3.4	3.5	3.6	⦿3.7	3.8	3.9	4.0
Science GPA	2.0	2.1	2.2	2.3	2.4	2.5	2.6	2.7	2.8	2.9	3.0	3.1	3.2	3.3	3.4	3.5	3.6	⦿3.7	3.8	3.9	4.0

MCAT® required: Yes, 100% of 2007 accepted applicants took MCAT®

Verbal Reasoning	3	4	5	6	7	8	9	⑩	11	12	13	14	15
Physical Sciences	3	4	5	6	7	8	9	⑩	⑪	12	13	14	15
Biological Sciences	3	4	5	6	7	8	9	10	⑪	12	13	14	15
Writing Sample			J	K	L	M	N	O	Ⓟ	Ⓠ	R	S	T

Acceptance & Matriculation Data for 2007–2008 First Year Class

	Resident	Non-Resident	International	Total
Applied	1151	7993	691	9835
Interviewed	250	480	53	783
Deferred	1	2	0	3
Matriculants				
Early Assurance Program	0	0	0	0
Early Decision Program	0	0	0	0
Baccalaureate/MD	n/a	n/a	n/a	n/a
MD/PhD	0	0	3	3
Matriculated	71	102	17	**190**

Applications accepted from International Applicants: Yes

Specialty Choice

2003, 2004, 2005 Graduates, Specialty Choice (As reported by program directors to GME Track™)	
Anesthesiology	6%
Emergency Medicine	10%
Family Practice	8%
Internal Medicine	21%
Obstetrics/Gynecology	4%
Orthopaedic Surgery	4%
Pediatrics	11%
Psychiatry	4%
Radiology	5%
Surgery	6%

Matriculant Demographics: 2007–2008 First Year Class

Men: 100   **Women:** 90

Matriculants' Self-Reported Race/Ethnicity

Mexican American	0	Korean	6
Cuban	0	Vietnamese	3
Puerto Rican	1	Other Asian	4
Other Hispanic	2	Total Asian	63
Total Hispanic	2	Native American	0
Chinese	17	Black	10
Asian Indian	25	Native Hawaiian	0
Pakistani	4	White	101
Filipino	3	Unduplicated Number	
Japanese	3	of Matriculants	190

Science and Math Majors: 70%
Matriculants with:
    Baccalaureate degree: 98%
    Graduate degree(s): 20%

Financial Information

Source: 2006–2007 LCME I-B survey and 2007–2008 AAMC TSF questionnaire

	Residents	Non-Residents
Total Cost of Attendance	$57,727	$57,727
Tuition and Fees	$39,472	$39,472
Other (includes living expenses)	$16,380	$16,380
Health Insurance (can be waived)	$1,875	$1,875

Average 2007 Graduate Indebtedness: $159,444
% of Enrolled Students Receiving Aid: 79%

Criminal Background Check

This medical school requires a criminal background check prior to matriculation.

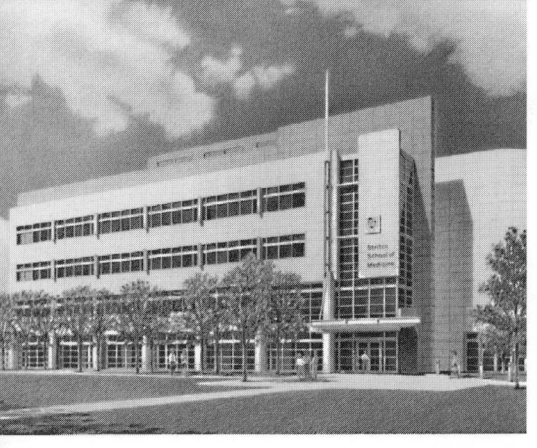

Loyola University Chicago
Stritch School of Medicine
Maywood, Illinois

Loyola University Chicago Stritch School of Medicine
Office of Admissions
2160 South First Avenue
Maywood, Illinois 60153
T 708-216-3229

Admissions www.meddean.luc.edu/admissions/
admissions.htm
Main www.meddean.luc.edu
Financial www.meddean.luc.edu\financialaid
Email n/a

Private Institution

Dr. John M. Lee, Dean

Teresa Wronski, Associate Dean for Student Affairs and Interim Dean for Admissions

Donna J. Sobie, Director, Financial Aid

General Information

Loyola University Chicago, founded in 1870 by the Jesuits, is one of the largest Catholic universities in the United States. By 1909, the university had organized several small medical colleges into a new medical school and, in 1948, the school was named in honor of Samuel Cardinal Stritch, Archbishop of Chicago. In 1969 the university opened the Loyola University Medical Center, built on land given by the Veterans Administration, in Maywood, a suburban community located 12 miles west of downtown Chicago. The medical center is home to the Stritch School of Medicine, Loyola University Hospital, Cardinal Bernardin Cancer Center, and Loyola Outpatient Center. Students receive their clinical training at the 570-bed Loyola University Hospital, 248-bed Hines Veterans Affairs Hospital, and other affiliated hospitals in the Chicago area.

Curricular Highlights

Community Service Requirement: Optional. Highly desirable.
Research/Thesis Requirement: Optional.

The primary purpose of the Stritch School of Medicine is to train physicians who will care for their patients with skill, respect, and compassion. The personal and intellectual development of each student is promoted through close contact with faculty members and the administration. Students are exposed to the operation of a large academic medical center, as well as to VA and community offices and hospitals, where they learn in an atmosphere of cooperation and mutual assistance. The first year of the curriculum concentrates on the basic principles and processes related to the normal structure, function, and regulation of the human body. In addition, the first year includes instruction in health promotion/disease prevention, health care finance and access, medical ethics, medical/legal issues, and the doctor/patient relationship. Students also have the opportunity to visit ambulatory care sites to experience the delivery of medical care in the ambulatory setting. The second year of the curriculum focuses on basic science principles related to the mechanisms of human disease, neuroscience, and the therapeutic approach to disease. Additionally, students have the opportunity to continue to develop their knowledge about human behavioral science, physical examination skills, basic clinical skills, evidence-based clinical decision-making, and medical ethics and humanities. The third and fourth years are organized into clinical clerkships which include up to 34 weeks of elective time during the fourth year. Special curricular features include an emphasis on bioethics and professionalism and intensive training in history-taking, physical examination, and communication skills using the extensive Clinical Skills Center, which combines the latest in educational technology and patient simulation activities.

USMLE

Step 1: Required. Students must record a passing score for graduation, but not promotion.
Step 2: Clinical Skills (CS): Required. Students must record a passing total score to graduate.
Step 2: Clinical Knowledge (CK): Required. Students must record a passing total score to graduate.

Selection Factors

A bachelor's degree and the MCAT®, preferably taken in the Spring, but no later than September of the year of application, are required. Any undergraduate major is acceptable. Applicants must be U.S. citizens or hold a permanent resident visa. As a rule, applicants are limited to applying no more than twice. Applicants enrolled in advanced degree programs must expect to complete their degrees prior to matriculation. Applicants who present academic credentials that indicate they are capable of succeeding in the rigorous medical education program will be evaluated for evidence of the personal qualifications they can bring to the medical profession. Essential characteristics include an interest in learning, integrity, compassion, and the ability to assume responsibility. Of particular concern will be an applicant's exploration of the field of medicine and the nature of the motivation to enter this profession. Early submission of the AMCAS application and prompt return of all supporting material will enhance an applicant's chance of being offered a place in the class. Loyola University does not discriminate on the basis of race, religion, national origin, sex, age, or disability.

Financial Aid

Financial aid is primarily in the form of loans, but limited scholarship and grant money is also available. Applicants should receive a preliminary financial aid award approximately two months after submitting financial aid forms.

Information about Diversity Programs

The Summer Enrichment Program (SEP) at Loyola University Chicago Stritch School of Medicine is a four-week experience for premedical students. The program offers students a variety of educational experiences and service activities to enhance their preparation for a career in medicine. The program targets students who have the potential to enrich the diversity of the medical student community.

Campus Information

Enrollment
For 2007, total enrollment was: 552

Application Process and Requirements 2009–2010

Primary Application Service: AMCAS
Earliest filing date: June 1, 2008
Latest filing date: November 15, 2008

Secondary Application Required?: Yes
Sent to: Screened applicants
URL: n/a
Fee: Yes, $70
Fee waiver available: Yes
Earliest filing date: June 2008
Latest filing date: February 2009

Latest MCAT® considered: September 2008
Oldest MCAT® considered: 2005

Early Decision Program
School does not have EDP
Applicants notified: n/a
EDP available for: n/a

Regular Acceptance Notice
Earliest date: October 15, 2008
Latest date: Until class is full

Applicant's Response to Acceptance
Offer – Maximum Time: Two weeks

Requests for Deferred
Entrance Considered: Yes

Deposit to Hold Place in Class: No
Deposit (Resident): n/a
Deposit (Non-Resident): n/a
Deposit due: n/a
Applied to tuition: n/a
Deposit refundable: n/a
Refundable by: n/a

Estimated number of new entrants: 145
EDP: n/a, special program: n/a

Start Month/Year: July 2009

Interview Format: Semi-open file with admission committee members. Regional interviews are not available.

Other Programs

PREPARATORY PROGRAMS
Postbaccalaureate Program: No
Summer Program: Yes, Office of Student Affairs, (708) 216-3220, kcalhoun@lumc.edu

COMBINED DEGREE PROGRAMS
Baccalaureate/MD: No
MD/MPH: No
MD/MBA: No
MD/JD: No
MD/PhD: Yes, www.meddean.luc.edu/prospective/mdphd/index.htm
Additional Program: Yes, http://bioethics.lumc.edu/education/MD_MA_Program.html

Premedical Coursework

Course	Req.	Rec.	Lab.	Sems.
Inorganic Chemistry	•		•	2
Behavioral Sciences				
Biochemistry		•		
Biology				
Biology/Zoology	•		•	2
Calculus				
College English				
College Mathematics				

Course	Req.	Rec.	Lab.	Sems.
Computer Science				
Genetics		•		
Humanities				
Organic Chemistry	•		•	2
Physics	•		•	2
Psychology				
Social Sciences				
Molecular Biology		•		

Selection Factors: 2007 Accepted Applicants

Proportion of Accepted Applicants with Relevant Experience (Data Self-Reported to AMCAS®)		
Community Service/Volunteer		70%
Medically-Related Work		86%
Research		76%

Shaded bar represents accepted scores ranging from the 10th percentile to the 90th percentile ▪   **School Median** ●   **National Median** ●

Overall GPA	2.0	2.1	2.2	2.3	2.4	2.5	2.6	2.7	2.8	2.9	3.0	3.1	3.2	3.3	3.4	3.5	3.6	(3.7)	3.8	3.9	4.0
Science GPA	2.0	2.1	2.2	2.3	2.4	2.5	2.6	2.7	2.8	2.9	3.0	3.1	3.2	3.3	3.4	3.5	(3.6)	3.7	3.8	3.9	4.0

MCAT® required: Yes, 100% of 2007 accepted applicants took MCAT®

Verbal Reasoning	3	4	5	6	7	8	9	(10)	11	12	13	14	15
Physical Sciences	3	4	5	6	7	8	9	(10)	(11)	12	13	14	15
Biological Sciences	3	4	5	6	7	8	9	10	(11)	12	13	14	15
Writing Sample				J	K	L	M	N	O	P	(Q)	R	S	T

Acceptance & Matriculation Data for 2007–2008 First Year Class

	Resident	Non-Resident	International	Total
Applied	1463	7999	25	9487
Interviewed	186	342	0	528
Deferred	0	0	0	0
Matriculants				
Early Assurance Program	n/a	n/a	n/a	n/a
Early Decision Program	0	0	0	0
Baccalaureate/MD	n/a	n/a	n/a	n/a
MD/PhD	1	2	0	3
Matriculated	70	76	0	**146**

Applications accepted from International Applicants: No

Specialty Choice

2003, 2004, 2005 Graduates, Specialty Choice (As reported by program directors to GME Track™)	
Anesthesiology	5%
Emergency Medicine	8%
Family Practice	11%
Internal Medicine	20%
Obstetrics/Gynecology	5%
Orthopaedic Surgery	5%
Pediatrics	9%
Psychiatry	2%
Radiology	2%
Surgery	8%

Matriculant Demographics: 2007–2008 First Year Class

Men: 70   **Women:** 76

Matriculants' Self-Reported Race/Ethnicity

Mexican American	7	**Korean**	4
Cuban	0	**Vietnamese**	0
Puerto Rican	4	**Other Asian**	3
Other Hispanic	0	**Total Asian**	19
Total Hispanic	10	**Native American**	0
Chinese	3	**Black**	5
Asian Indian	7	**Native Hawaiian**	0
Pakistani	2	**White**	117
Filipino	0	**Unduplicated Number**	
Japanese	1	**of Matriculants**	146

Science and Math Majors: 65%
Matriculants with:
      Baccalaureate degree: 100%
      Graduate degree(s): 7%

Financial Information

Source: 2006–2007 LCME I-B survey and 2007–2008 AAMC TSF questionnaire

	Residents	Non-Residents
Total Cost of Attendance	$54,940	$55,440
Tuition and Fees	$37,620	$37,620
Other (includes living expenses)	$15,725	$16,225
Health Insurance (can be waived)	$1,595	$1,595

Average 2007 Graduate Indebtedness: $157,299
% of Enrolled Students Receiving Aid: 89%

Criminal Background Check

This medical school requires a criminal background check prior to matriculation.

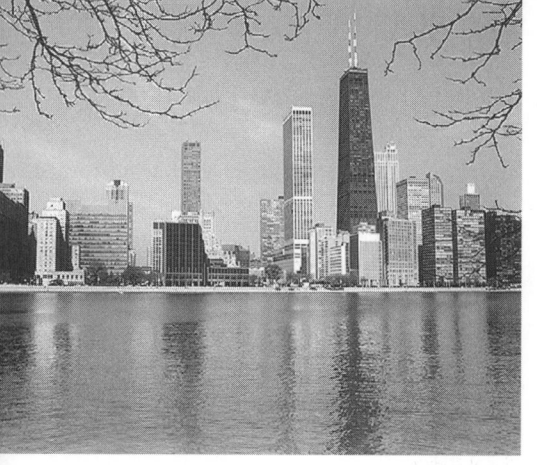

Northwestern University Feinberg School of Medicine

Chicago, Illinois

Office of Admissions
Northwestern University
Feinberg School of Medicine
303 East Chicago Avenue, Morton I-606
Chicago, Illinois 60611-3008
T 312 503 8206   F 312 503 0550

Admissions www.feinberg.northwestern.edu/admissions/md/index.html
Main www.feinberg.northwestern.edu
Financial http://chicagofinancialaid.northwestern.edu
Email med-admissions@northwestern.edu

Private Institution

Dr. Larry Jameson, Dean

Dr. Warren H. Wallace, Associate Dean for Admissions

Dr. John E. Franklin, Associate Dean for Minority and Cultural Affairs

Diann R. Lapin, Assistant Dean for Admissions

General Information

The Feinberg School was founded in 1859. Close to 4,000 faculty members offer instruction in the basic sciences and clinical medicine. Students gain clinical experience at the McGaw affiliated group of hospitals, which include Northwestern Memorial, Children's Memorial, Evanston Northwestern Health Care, the Rehabilitation Institute of Chicago, and the Jesse Brown VA Medical Center.

Mission Statement

Students who graduate from Northwestern University's Feinberg School of Medicine are well-grounded scientifically and clinically. Committed to the ethical and humane practice of medicine, they learn how to approach patients, perform physical examinations, and formulate a plan of investigation for optimal health management. Beyond diagnosis and treatment, they appreciate the importance of disease prevention, utilizing the skills of allied health professionals and ascertaining the role of the patient's relationships with family, friends, and the community in producing and alleviating symptoms. Students become lifelong learners, understanding that knowledge at any time is only a prologue to new facts and concepts. They are well-prepared for their choice of careers in either the practice of medicine or a research-oriented career in academic medicine.

Curricular Highlights

Community Service Requirement: Optional.
Research/Thesis Requirement: Optional.

Students are trained through an integrated, organ system-based curriculum that contains the essential basic science and the biopsychosocial foundations of medicine. The first and second years integrate traditional medical school coursework (see the Web site for specific detail). In addition, three short blocks of time are devoted to medical decision-making, which develops a student's abilities in analyzing and managing information and clinical decision-making. During the first two years, students take Patient, Physician, and Society (PPS). Periodic PPS sessions are part of the third and fourth-year curricula, in which students learn from attending physicians and residents during clinical clerkships. A subinternship and electives round out the curriculum.

USMLE

Step 1: Required. Students must record a passing score for graduation but not for promotion.
Step 2: Clinical Skills (CS): Required. Students must record a passing score in each section to graduate.
Step 2: Clinical Knowledge (CK): Required. Students must record a passing score in each section to graduate.

Selection Factors

All applicants are required to take the MCAT®. The latest MCAT® considered is September 2008. The Committee on Admissions looks for evidence of emotional maturity, motivation, achievement, character, and academic excellence. A premium is placed on the breadth and depth of the academic program, life experiences, and clinical/research exposure. Applicants should be liberally educated men and women who have studied in some depth subjects beyond the conventional premedical sciences. The faculty has established technical performance standards. Candidates should demonstrate the mental capability, moral integrity, and physical skills required to function effectively in a variety of clinical situations. The Illinois Medical School Matriculant Criminal History Records Act requires each medical student to submit to a criminal history records check before official matriculation. Northwestern University does not discriminate on the basis of race, religion, national origin, gender, sexual orientation, age, or handicap in its educational programs or activities.

Financial Aid

Financial considerations do not influence admissions decisions. Feinberg makes every attempt to ensure that accepted students receive a competitive financial aid package that includes support through national and local loan programs, scholarships, and grants. Feinberg students also receive financial management counseling. Feinberg offers a loan program to international students who have a credit-worthy U.S. loan co-signer.

Information about Diversity Programs

The school is committed to diversity in the student body, and it makes a concerted effort to recruit, admit, and graduate students from groups underrepresented in medicine. Faculty and staff are comprised of diverse members.

Campus Information

Setting

The School of Medicine is located in the Streeterville neighborhood of downtown Chicago, adjacent to Lake Michigan and within walking distance of apartments, museums, restaurants, athletic facilities, and retailers. Public and university transportation is available.

Enrollment

For 2007, total enrollment was: 700

Special Features

The School of Medicine administers numerous research programs, including centers for comprehensive cancer research, genetic medicine, cardiovascular medicine and bionanotechnology. The campus includes Northwestern Memorial Hospital (a Level I trauma center), the new Prentice Women's Hospital(the largest birthing center in the Midwest), and the world-renowned Rehabilitation Institute of Chicago.

Housing

Most students live in high rise apartments in the surrounding neighborhood.

Satellite Campuses/Facilities

Clinical rotations occur at the McGaw Medical Center hospitals and clinics and at other affiliated urban and suburban facilities.

Application Process and Requirements 2009–2010

Primary Application Service: AMCAS
Earliest filing date: June 1, 2008
Latest filing date: October 15, 2008

Secondary Application Required?: Yes
Sent to: All AMCAS applicants
URL: https://medicalapp.northwestern.edu
Fee: Yes, $75
Fee waiver available: Yes
Earliest filing date: July 15, 2008
Latest filing date: Varies

Latest MCAT® considered: September 2008
Oldest MCAT® considered: 2006

Early Decision Program
School does not have EDP
Applicants notified: n/a
EDP available for: n/a

Regular Acceptance Notice
Earliest date: November 2008
Latest date: Varies
Applicant's Response to Acceptance
Offer – Maximum Time: Two weeks

Requests for Deferred
Entrance Considered: Yes

Deposit to Hold Place in Class: No
Deposit (Resident): n/a
Deposit (Non-Resident): n/a
Deposit due: n/a
Applied to tuition: n/a
Deposit refundable: n/a
Refundable by: n/a

Estimated number of new entrants: 170
EDP: n/a, special program: n/a

Start Month/Year: August 2009

Interview Format: Individual and panel interviews. Regional interviews are not available.

Other Programs

PREPARATORY PROGRAMS
Postbaccalaureate Program: No
Summer Program: No

COMBINED DEGREE PROGRAMS
Baccalaureate/MD: Yes,
www.feinberg.northwestern.edu/hpme/index.html
MD/MPH: Yes, www.publichealth.
northwestern.edu/admissions_mdmph.htm
MD/MBA: No
MD/JD: No
MD/PhD: Yes,
www.mstp.northwestern.edu/index.htm
MD/MA-Medical Humanities & Bioethics: Yes,
www.bioethics.northwestern.edu/masters/
feinbergma.html

Premedical Coursework

Course	Req.	Rec.	Lab.	Sems.	Course	Req.	Rec.	Lab.	Sems.
Inorganic Chemistry	•		•	2	Computer Science				
Behavioral Sciences					Genetics				
Biochemistry					Humanities		•		2
Biology	•		•	2	Organic Chemistry	•		•	2
Biology/Zoology					Physics	•		•	2
Calculus					Psychology		•		
College English		•		2	Social Sciences				
College Mathematics					Statistics		•		2

Selection Factors: 2007 Accepted Applicants

Proportion of Accepted Applicants with Relevant Experience (Data Self-Reported to AMCAS*)		
Community Service/Volunteer		66%
Medically-Related Work		80%
Research		87%

Shaded bar represents accepted scores ranging from the 10th percentile to the 90th percentile ▪   School Median ●   National Median ●

Overall GPA	2.0	2.1	2.2	2.3	2.4	2.5	2.6	2.7	2.8	2.9	3.0	3.1	3.2	3.3	3.4	3.5	3.6	3.7	(3.8)	3.9	4.0
Science GPA	2.0	2.1	2.2	2.3	2.4	2.5	2.6	2.7	2.8	2.9	3.0	3.1	3.2	3.3	3.4	3.5	3.6	3.7	(3.8)	3.9	4.0

MCAT® required: Yes, 100% of 2007 accepted applicants took MCAT®

Verbal Reasoning	3	4	5	6	7	8	9	(10)	(11)	12	13	14	15
Physical Sciences	3	4	5	6	7	8	9	10	(11)	12	(13)	14	15
Biological Sciences	3	4	5	6	7	8	9	10	(11)	12	(13)	14	15
Writing Sample			J	K	L	M	N	O	P	(Q)	R	S	T

Acceptance & Matriculation Data for 2007–2008 First Year Class

	Resident	Non-Resident	International	Total
Applied	1003	6106	418	7527
Interviewed	130	693	40	863
Deferred	3	8	0	11
Matriculants				
Early Assurance Program	4	1	0	5
Early Decision Program	0	0	0	0
Baccalaureate/MD	9	27	0	36
MD/PhD	4	11	0	15
Matriculated	38	121	10	**169**

Applications accepted from International Applicants: Yes

Specialty Choice

2003, 2004, 2005 Graduates, Specialty Choice (As reported by program directors to GME Track™)	
Anesthesiology	5%
Emergency Medicine	7%
Family Practice	2%
Internal Medicine	26%
Obstetrics/Gynecology	3%
Orthopaedic Surgery	6%
Pediatrics	10%
Psychiatry	3%
Radiology	5%
Surgery	7%

Matriculant Demographics: 2007–2008 First Year Class

Men: 85   **Women:** 84

Matriculants' Self-Reported Race/Ethnicity

Mexican American	5	**Korean**	2
Cuban	0	**Vietnamese**	1
Puerto Rican	0	**Other Asian**	0
Other Hispanic	6	**Total Asian**	54
Total Hispanic	10	**Native American**	2
Chinese	26	**Black**	8
Asian Indian	23	**Native Hawaiian**	1
Pakistani	1	**White**	94
Filipino	0	**Unduplicated Number**	
Japanese	2	**of Matriculants**	169

Science and Math Majors: 69%
Matriculants with:
    Baccalaureate degree: 100%
    Graduate degree(s): 11%

Financial Information

Source: 2006–2007 LCME I-B survey and 2007–2008 AAMC TSF questionnaire

	Residents	Non-Residents
Total Cost of Attendance	$66,606	$66,606
Tuition and Fees	$40,313	$40,313
Other (includes living expenses)	$24,205	$24,205
Health Insurance (can be waived)	$2,088	$2,088

Average 2007 Graduate Indebtedness: $170,368
% of Enrolled Students Receiving Aid: 77%

Criminal Background Check

This medical school requires a criminal background check prior to matriculation.

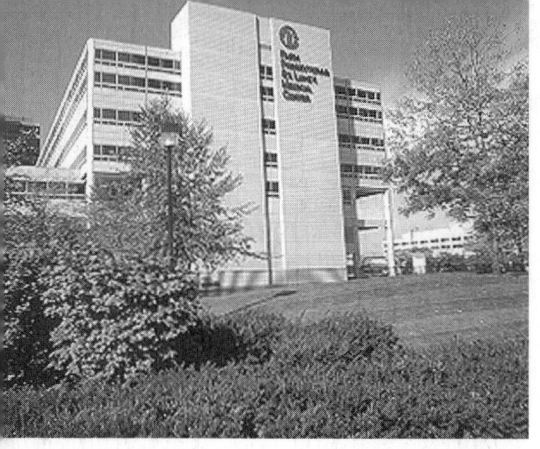

Rush Medical College of Rush University

Chicago, Illinois

Rush Medical College of Rush University
Office of Admissions, Suite 524
600 South Paulina Street
Chicago, Illinois 60612
T 312 942 6915 F 312 942 2333

Admissions www.rushu.rush.edu/
medcol/admissions.html
Main www.rushu.rush.edu/medcol
Financial www.rushu.rush.edu/finaid
Email RMC_Admissions@rush.edu

Private Institution

Dr. Thomas A. Deutsch, Dean

Dr. Cynthia Boyd, Recruitment Team Leader

David Nelson, Acting Director of Student Financial Aid

Dr. Susan K. Jacob, Associate Dean

Jill M. Volk-Porter, Director of Recruitment and Special Programs

General Information

Rush Medical College, founded in 1837, is the oldest component of Rush University. Through an academic and health care network of more than a dozen affiliated hospitals and a neighborhood health center, Rush University Medical Center serves 1.5 to 2 million people annually. Thus, students train in urban and suburban areas in a variety of socioeconomic and ethnic settings.

Mission Statement

Rush educates students as practitioners, scientists, and teachers who will become leaders in advancing health care and furthering the advancement of knowledge through research. The university integrates patient care, education, and research through the practitioner-teacher model. Rush encourages the growth of its students by committing itself to the pursuit of excellence, dedication to community service, free inquiry, and the highest intellectual and ethical standards.

Curricular Highlights

Community Service Requirement: Optional.
Research/Thesis Requirement: Optional.

Rush provides a firm background in the science of medicine and a balanced introduction to the practice of clinical medicine in a four-year curriculum designed to provide educational flexibility. The faculty have created an environment that fosters commitments to competent and compassionate patient care and to attitudes of inquiry and life-long learning. Preclinical Curriculum – The first year exposes students to the vocabulary and fundamental concepts upon which clinical medicine is based. The courses utilize lecture, lab, small groups and case study workshops. The second year centers on the causes and effects of disease and therapeutics and utilizes a case-based approach. Students also participate in clinical skills courses and see patients. Clinical Curriculum – The third and fourth years provide students with training in clinical skills, diagnosis and patient management in a variety of clinical settings. The third year is comprised of required core clerkships, while the fourth year provides students with the opportunity to pursue areas of special interest. Students complete the majority of their required clinical rotations at Rush University Medical Center or the John H. Stroger, Jr. Hospital.

USMLE

Step 1: Required. Students must record a passing score for promotion.
Step 2: Clinical Skills (CS): Required. Students must only record a score.
Step 2: Clinical Knowledge (CK): Required. Students must only record a score.

Selection Factors

The Committee on Admissions considers both the academic and non-academic qualifications of applicants in making its decisions and places strong emphasis on the applicant's humanistic concerns, unique experiences and demonstrated motivation for a career in medicine. All applicants are invited to complete the supplemental application and submit letters of recommendation. The Committee looks for objective evidence that the applicant will be able to handle the academic demands of the curriculum. Health-care-related experiences and social service activities are measures of how an applicant pursues their values, engages in activities that move them outside of their usual boundaries and expands their horizons. Academic achievement, letters of recommendation, MCAT® performance, health care experience and interviews are considered in the final evaluation of all applicants. Only U.S. citizens or permanent residents are considered for admission.

Financial Aid

Financial aid awards are made after acceptance into medical school. Rush University grant eligibility is based on both student and parent resources, regardless of the student's age or status. Students are awarded financial aid packages, grants, scholarships and loans to meet 100 percent of the demonstrated financial need during each year of their medical education.

Information about Diversity Programs

Rush seeks to attract applicants who will promote an environment of tolerance, respect and compassion, and who will make the student body more representative of the national population and more informed about the social problems affecting the delivery of health care.

Campus Information

Setting

Rush Medical College is located on the near west side of Chicago; the John H. Stroger, Jr. Hospital of Cook County, a major teaching affiliate, is two blocks away. The community is thriving and culturally diverse, with easy access by public transportation.

Enrollment

For 2007, total enrollment was: 536

Special Features

The Rush Community Service Initiatives Program creates a network of community programs that matches students' interest and initiative with the social and healthcare needs of Chicago's underserved population. Students have the opportunity to participate in clinical and non-clinical programs.

Application Process and Requirements 2009–2010

Primary Application Service: AMCAS
Earliest filing date: June 1, 2008
Latest filing date: November 1, 2008

Secondary Application Required?: Yes
Sent to: All applicants
URL: http://rush.infostatz.com
Contact: RMC_Admissions@rush.edu
Fee: Yes, $75
Fee waiver available: Yes
Earliest filing date: July 31, 2008
Latest filing date: December 31, 2008

Latest MCAT® considered: November 2008
Oldest MCAT® considered: January 2007

Early Decision Program
School does not have EDP
Applicants notified: n/a
EDP available for: n/a

Regular Acceptance Notice
Earliest date: November 2008
Latest date: Varies

Applicant's Response to Acceptance
Offer – Maximum Time: Six week

Requests for Deferred
Entrance Considered: Yes

Deposit to Hold Place in Class: Yes
Deposit (Resident): $100
Deposit (Non-Resident): $100
Deposit due: With acceptance offer
Applied to tuition: Yes
Deposit refundable: Yes
Refundable by: May 15, 2009

Estimated number of new entrants: 128
EDP: n/a, special program: n/a

Start Month/Year: August/September 2009

Interview Format: Two individual interviews with faculty. Regional interviews are not available.

Other Programs

PREPARATORY PROGRAMS
Postbaccalaureate Program: No
Summer Program: No

COMBINED DEGREE PROGRAMS
Baccalaureate/MD: No
MD/MPH: No
MD/MBA: No
MD/JD: No
MD/PhD: Yes,
RMC_Admissions@rush.edu

Premedical Coursework

Course	Req.	Rec.	Lab.	Hrs.	Course	Req.	Rec.	Lab.	Hrs.
Inorganic Chemistry	•			8	Computer Science				
Behavioral Sciences					Genetics				
Biochemistry					Humanities				
Biology	•			8	Organic Chemistry	•			8
Biology/Zoology					Physics	•			8
Calculus					Psychology				
College English					Social Sciences				
College Mathematics					Other				

Selection Factors: 2007 Accepted Applicants

Proportion of Accepted Applicants with Relevant Experience (Data Self-Reported to AMCAS®)		
Community Service/Volunteer		69%
Medically-Related Work		83%
Research		83%

Shaded bar represents accepted scores ranging from the 10th percentile to the 90th percentile ▬   School Median ●   National Median ●

Overall GPA	2.0	2.1	2.2	2.3	2.4	2.5	2.6	2.7	2.8	2.9	3.0	3.1	3.2	3.3	3.4	3.5	(3.6)	3.7	3.8	3.9	4.0
Science GPA	2.0	2.1	2.2	2.3	2.4	2.5	2.6	2.7	2.8	2.9	3.0	3.1	3.2	3.3	3.4	3.5	(3.6)	3.7	3.8	3.9	4.0

MCAT® required: Yes, 100% of 2007 accepted applicants took MCAT®

Verbal Reasoning	3	4	5	6	7	8	9	(10)	11	12	13	14	15
Physical Sciences	3	4	5	6	7	8	9	(10)	(11)	12	13	14	15
Biological Sciences	3	4	5	6	7	8	9	10	(11)	12	13	14	15
Writing Sample			J	K	L	M	N	O	P	(Q)	R	S	T

Acceptance & Matriculation Data for 2007–2008 First Year Class

	Resident	Non-Resident	International	Total
Applied	1458	3959	40	5457
Interviewed	285	107	0	392
Deferred	3	1	0	4
Matriculants				
Early Assurance Program	n/a	n/a	n/a	n/a
Early Decision Program	0	0	0	0
Baccalaureate/MD	n/a	n/a	n/a	n/a
MD/PhD	0	0	0	0
Matriculated	107	21	0	**128**

Applications accepted from International Applicants: No

Matriculant Demographics: 2007–2008 First Year Class

Men: 71   **Women:** 57

Matriculants' Self-Reported Race/Ethnicity

Mexican American	6	**Korean**	6
Cuban	1	**Vietnamese**	1
Puerto Rican	1	**Other Asian**	3
Other Hispanic	3	**Total Asian**	40
Total Hispanic	10	**Native American**	0
Chinese	8	**Black**	1
Asian Indian	22	**Native Hawaiian**	0
Pakistani	2	**White**	88
Filipino	1	**Unduplicated Number**	
Japanese	0	**of Matriculants**	128

Science and Math Majors: 65%
Matriculants with:
    Baccalaureate degree: 100%
    Graduate degree(s): 9%

Specialty Choice

2003, 2004, 2005 Graduates, Specialty Choice (As reported by program directors to GME Track™)	
Anesthesiology	7%
Emergency Medicine	7%
Family Practice	7%
Internal Medicine	20%
Obstetrics/Gynecology	5%
Orthopaedic Surgery	4%
Pediatrics	11%
Psychiatry	3%
Radiology	4%
Surgery	7%

Financial Information

Source: 2006–2007 LCME I-B survey and 2007–2008 AAMC TSF questionnaire

	Residents	Non-Residents
Total Cost of Attendance	$61,820	$61,820
Tuition and Fees	$43,680	$43,680
Other (includes living expenses)	$18,140	$18,140
Health Insurance (not applicable)	$0	$0

Average 2007 Graduate Indebtedness: $159,701
% of Enrolled Students Receiving Aid: 89%

Criminal Background Check

This medical school requires a criminal background check prior to matriculation.

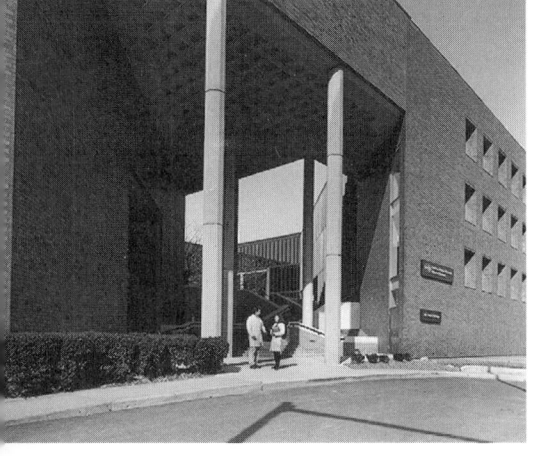

Southern Illinois University School of Medicine
Springfield, Illinois

Office of Admissions
Southern Illinois University
School of Medicine, P.O. Box 19624
Springfield, Illinois 62794-9624
T 217 545 6013   **F** 217 545 5538

Admissions www.siumed.edu/studentaffairs
Main www.siumed.edu
Financial www.siumed.edu/studentaffairs
Email admissions@siumed.edu

Public Institution

Dr. J. Kevin Dorsey, Dean and Provost

*Dr. Erik J. Constance,
Associate Dean for Student Affairs*

*Dr. Wesley Robinson-McNeese, Executive
Assistant to the Dean for Diversity*

Nancy Calvert, Director of Financial Aid

Evan Wilson, Director of Admissions

General Information
Southern Illinois University School of Medicine
was established in 1969 and graduated its first
class in 1975. Students spend the first 12 months
of the program at the medical education facilities
on the Carbondale campus and the remaining
three years at the Medical Center in Springfield.

Mission Statement
SIU School of Medicine is guided by a clear
mandate to assist the people of central and
southern Illinois in meeting their present and
future health care needs through education,
research and service.

Curricular Highlights
Community Service Requirement: Optional.
Highly recommended.
Research/Thesis Requirement: Optional.

The overall focus of the first two years of the
curriculum is on case-based, student-directed
learning in a small-group setting supported by
lectures/resource sessions. Close integration of
basic science and clinical information takes place
throughout the four-year course of study. Clinical training begins in the first year with simulated patients and real patients. An increased
emphasis on issues such as community health
care and the psychosocial issues of medicine
continues SIU School of Medicine's emphasis
on caring while curing and treating patients as
people rather than medical conditions. The third
year consists of a series of multidisciplinary clinical rotations, with emphasis on both hospital-
based and ambulatory practice. The fourth year
comprises a series of electives designed to help
students with final preparations for residency

and offers opportunities for off-campus training.
The grading system is honors/pass/fail. The
school also offers a six-year M.D.-J.D. program.

USMLE
Step 1: Required. Students must record a passing
score for graduation, but not promotion.
Step 2: Clinical Skills (CS): Required. Students
must only record a score.
Step 2: Clinical Knowledge (CK): Required.
Students must only record a score.

Selection Factors
Applications for the M.D. program are accepted
from Illinois residents who are U.S. citizens or
possess a permanent resident visa. Completion of
a minimum of 90 semester hours of undergraduate work in an accredited degree-granting college
or university is required. Foreign students are
advised to have completed at least 60 semester
hours of coursework in the United States. The
M.D.-J.D. program is open to non-Illinois residents. All applicants are expected to have a
strong foundation in the natural sciences, social
sciences, and humanities; they must demonstrate
facility in writing and speaking the English language, as well as achieve competitive MCAT®
scores. Preference is given to those with sufficient
recent academic activity to demonstrate the
potential for successful completion of the rigorous educational program and to those who
demonstrate the necessary noncognitive characteristics of a successful medical student and
physician. Applicants are invited for interviews
according to their strengths in academics,
extracurricular activities, employment and volunteer experiences, and area of residence, with
preference given to central and southern Illinois
residents. The School of Medicine does not discriminate on the basis of race, religion, age, sex,
handicap, or national or ethnic origin in administration of its education policies, admissions
policies, scholarship and loan programs, or other
school-administered programs.

Financial Aid
The School participates in all major federal
student aid programs. Students receive aid on
the basis of need as calculated on the FAFSA.

Scholarship and grant aid are generally limited
to students who demonstrate exceptional need.

Information about Diversity Programs
An effort is made to recruit qualified applicants
from groups that have been underrepresented
in the medical profession. The school has several active minority student organizations.
For more information, contact the Office of
Diversity at 217-545-7334. The School of
Medicine also sponsors the Medical/Dental
Education Preparatory Program (MEDPREP),
a non-degree granting program in Carbondale
for disadvantaged undergraduate or postbaccalaureate students, as well as underrepresented, rural, or low-income students
(*www.siumed.edu/medprep/*).

Campus Information

Setting
SIU School of Medicine holds the first year of
medical school in a small-town, collegiate environment on the main quad at SIU-Carbondale,
an institution serving over 20,000 undergraduate,
graduate, and professional students. The remaining three years take place at the SIU medical campus in the north central residential/commercial
region of Springfield (pop. 115,000), the state capital. The facilities in Springfield are located in one
of downstate Illinois' largest and fastest growing
medical districts. The main medical instructional
buildings are adjacent to Memorial Medical Center.
A second affiliated hospital, St. John's, and additional clinics are situated within blocks of the
main campus.

Enrollment
For 2007, total enrollment was: 291

Housing
Carbondale and Springfield: off-campus
housing. Monthly rates for apartments in
both locations: $300 to $550 per month.

Satellite Campuses/Facilities
Students receive training in affiliated clinical locations throughout central and southern Illinois.

Application Process and Requirements 2009–2010

Primary Application Service: AMCAS
Earliest filing date: June 1, 2008
Latest filing date: November 15, 2008
Secondary Application Required?: Yes
Sent to: Selected applicants
Name: Denise Thomas, (217)-545-6013
dthomas@siumed.edu
Fee: Yes, $50
Fee waiver available: Yes
Earliest filing date: July 1, 2008
Latest filing date: February 1, 2009

Latest MCAT® considered: September 2008
Oldest MCAT® considered: August 2006

Early Decision Program
School does not have EDP
Applicants notified: n/a
EDP available for: n/a

Regular Acceptance Notice
Earliest date: October 16, 2008
Latest date: Until class is full

Applicant's Response to Acceptance
Offer – Maximum Time: Two weeks

Requests for Deferred
Entrance Considered: Yes

Deposit to Hold Place in Class: Yes
Deposit (Resident): $100
Deposit (Non-Resident): $100
Deposit due: With receipt of acceptance offer
Applied to tuition: Yes
Deposit refundable: Yes
Refundable by: May 15, 2009

Estimated number of new entrants: 72
EDP: n/a, special program: 2

Start Month/Year: August 2009

Interview Format: MD two one-on-one interviews; MD/JD three one-on-one. Regional interviews are not available.

Other Programs

PREPARATORY PROGRAMS
Postbaccalaureate Program: Yes,
www.siumed.edu/medprep/
Summer Program: No

COMBINED DEGREE PROGRAMS
Baccalaureate/MD: No
MD/MPH: No
MD/MBA: No
MD/JD: Yes,
www.siumed.edu/medhum/mdjdprog.htm
MD/PhD: No

Premedical Coursework

Course	Req.	Rec.	Lab.	Sems.	Course	Req.	Rec.	Lab.	Sems.
Inorganic Chemistry		•	•	2	Computer Science				
Behavioral Sciences					Humanities		•		
Biochemistry		•		1	Organic Chemistry		•	•	2
Biology		•	•	2	Physics		•	•	2
Biology/Zoology					Psychology		•		
Calculus					Social Sciences		•		
College English		•		2	Cell/Molecular Biology		•		1
College Mathematics		•		2	Physiology & Microbiology		•	•	1

Selection Factors: 2007 Accepted Applicants

Proportion of Accepted Applicants with Relevant Experience (Data Self-Reported to AMCAS®)		
Community Service/Volunteer		69%
Medically-Related Work		84%
Research		72%

Shaded bar represents accepted scores ranging from the 10th percentile to the 90th percentile.   School Median ●   National Median ●

Overall GPA	2.0	2.1	2.2	2.3	2.4	2.5	2.6	2.7	2.8	2.9	3.0	3.1	3.2	3.3	3.4	3.5	3.6	(3.7)	3.8	3.9	4.0
Science GPA	2.0	2.1	2.2	2.3	2.4	2.5	2.6	2.7	2.8	2.9	3.0	3.1	3.2	3.3	3.4	3.5	(3.6)	3.7	3.8	3.9	4.0

MCAT® required: Yes, 100% of 2007 accepted applicants took MCAT®

Verbal Reasoning	3	4	5	6	7	8	9	(10)	11	12	13	14	15
Physical Sciences	3	4	5	6	7	8	(9)	10	(11)	12	13	14	15
Biological Sciences	3	4	5	6	7	8	9	(10)	(11)	12	13	14	15
Writing Sample				J	K	L	M	N	O	(P)	(Q)	R	S	T

Acceptance & Matriculation Data for 2007–2008 First Year Class

	Resident	Non-Resident	International	Total
Applied	1133	239	8	1380
Interviewed	268	2	0	270
Deferred	3	2	0	5
Matriculants				
Early Assurance Program	0	0	0	0
Early Decision Program	0	0	0	0
Baccalaureate/MD	n/a	n/a	n/a	n/a
MD/PhD	n/a	n/a	n/a	n/a
Matriculated	72	0	0	**72**

Applications accepted from International Applicants: No

Specialty Choice

2003, 2004, 2005 Graduates, Specialty Choice (As reported by program directors to GME Track™)	
Anesthesiology	4%
Emergency Medicine	9%
Family Practice	10%
Internal Medicine	16%
Obstetrics/Gynecology	10%
Orthopaedic Surgery	6%
Pediatrics	13%
Psychiatry	1%
Radiology Diagnostic	5%
Surgery General	7%

Matriculant Demographics: 2007–2008 First Year Class

Men: 35   **Women:** 37

Matriculants' Self-Reported Race/Ethnicity

Mexican American	2	Korean	1
Cuban	0	Vietnamese	1
Puerto Rican	1	Other Asian	2
Other Hispanic	1	Total Asian	10
Total Hispanic	4	Native American	1
Chinese	2	Black	8
Asian Indian	4	Native Hawaiian	0
Pakistani	0	White	55
Filipino	2	**Unduplicated Number**	
Japanese	0	**of Matriculants**	72

Science and Math Majors: 86%
Matriculants with:
    Baccalaureate degree: 100%
    Graduate degree(s): 13%

Financial Information

Source: 2006–2007 LCME I-B survey and 2007–2008 AAMC TSF questionnaire

	Residents	Non-Residents
Total Cost of Attendance	$37,126	$79,430
Tuition and Fees	$23,370	$65,674
Other (includes living expenses)	$13,270	$13,270
Health Insurance (can be waived)	$486	$486

Average 2007 Graduate Indebtedness: $119,121
% of Enrolled Students Receiving Aid: 93%

Criminal Background Check

This medical school requires a criminal background check prior to matriculation.

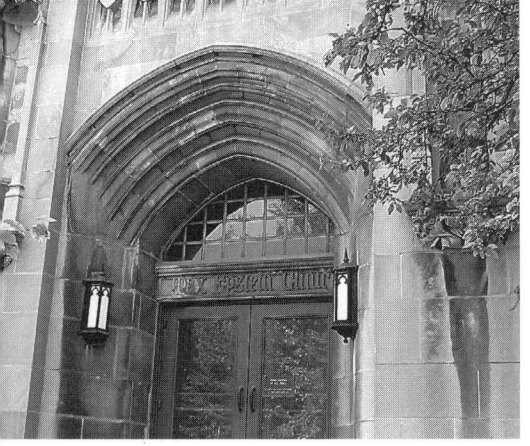

University of Chicago Division of the Biological Sciences, The Pritzker School of Medicine

Chicago, Illinois

Office of Admissions, University of Chicago
Pritzker School of Medicine
924 E. 57th Street, BSLC 104W
Chicago, Illinois 60637-5416
T 773 702 1937   **F** 773 834 5412

Admissions http://pritzker.bsd.uchicago.edu
Main http://pritzker.bsd.uchicago.edu
Financial http://pritzker.bsd.uchicago.edu
Email pritzkeradmissions@bsd.uchicago.edu

Private Institution

Dr. Holly J. Humphrey,
Dean for Medical Education

Sylvia Robertson, Assistant Dean
for Admissions and Financial Aid

Dr. William McDade, Associate Dean
for Multicultural Affairs

Dr. Herbert Abelson, Associate Dean
for Admissions

General Information

The Pritzker School of Medicine is unique among medical schools in that it is a part of the academic Division of the Biological Sciences. As an integral part of a world-class university, it offers medical students opportunities for interdisciplinary learning, clinical training, and research in a setting where recognized experts from all disciplines contribute to the development of physicians-in-training.

Mission Statement

At the University of Chicago, in an atmosphere of interdisciplinary scholarship and discovery, the Pritzker School of Medicine is dedicated to inspiring diverse students of exceptional promise to become leaders and innovators in science and medicine for the betterment of humanity.

Curricular Highlights

Community Service Requirement: Optional. Students have an impressive record of service.
Research/Thesis Requirement: Optional. Research is encouraged and supported.

The basic competencies which underlie the curriculum at Pritzker are grouped into four areas: the scientific basis of medicine; the scientific basis of diagnosis, prevention, and treatment of disease; interpersonal communication and teaching; and professional growth and development. Significant programs are devoted to helping students excel in these educational objectives. The library provides a comprehensive set of on-line medical and scientific materials with off-site access by students and faculty. This complements a Web-based curriculum that includes

multimedia presentations and searchable text. A Clinical Performance Center uses standardized patients and videotaped performance to educate students in taking a history, performing a physical examination, and clinical decision-making. The scientific foundation of medicine is achieved through lectures, labs, case-based problem-solving, and computer-based guided self-study and assessment. The clinical biennium consists of eight clinical clerkships and electives taught entirely by full-time clinical faculty and by selected residents who are trained in the humanistic teaching of medical students.

USMLE

Step 1: Required. Students must only record a score.
Step 2: Clinical Skills (CS): Required. Students must only record a score.
Step 2: Clinical Knowledge (CK): Required. Students must only record a score.

Selection Factors

A supplementary application is made available to everyone who submits an AMCAS application to the Pritzker School of Medicine. The Committee on Admissions reviews an application once the supplementary application is returned and the required letters of evaluation are received. About 600 applicants are invited to interview on the university campus from September through February. Offers of admission are extended on a rolling basis from October through April. Offers of admission are made solely on the basis of ability, achievement, motivation, and humanistic qualities. Outstanding personal characteristics and a strong career commitment are as important as excellence in academics.

Financial Aid

Scholarships and low-interest loans are made available to all students who have demonstrated need. There are both federally subsidized loans and low-interest loans from the university. Merit scholarships are available for a limited number of exceptionally well-qualified students. Individual counseling and debt management programs are available to all students. Financial aid packets are

mailed to all accepted applicants after January 1. Financial aid resources for international applicants are extremely limited.

Information about Diversity Programs

Pritzker is particularly interested in providing a diverse educational experience for its students. Medical students from groups underrepresented in medicine who have attended Pritzker often assume strong leadership roles, both within their class and at the national level.

Campus Information

Setting

The University of Chicago is located on the south side of Chicago in the ethnically diverse community of Hyde Park, just minutes by train from downtown Chicago. The resources of this world-class city and its extraordinary lake-front are at the campus doorstep. The University of Chicago Medical Center campus, including its 21 buildings with 22 acres of space for research, teaching, and patient care, are within easy walking distance of Pritzker's libraries, classrooms, and labs.

Enrollment

For 2007, total enrollment was: 440

Special Features

The University of Chicago is made up predominantly of graduate and professional students participating in four major academic divisions and six professional schools, all sharing one campus. In this environment, graduates acquire superb skills in medical reasoning, problem-solving, team-building, and life-long learning, which help them assume leadership roles in residency training programs and as faculty in academic medicine. Over 90 percent of Pritzker students engage in some form of scholarly activity prior to completing their M.D. degree, and approximately 20 percent pursue combined degrees.

Housing

As a part of an extensive orientation program, students are guided in their housing search. Rents average $800/month.

Application Process and Requirements 2009–2010

Primary Application Service: AMCAS
Earliest filing date: June 1, 2008
Latest filing date: October 15, 2008

Secondary Application Required?: Yes
Sent to: All applicants
Contact: Sylvia Robertson, (773) 702-1937, pritzkeradmissions@bsd.uchicago.edu
Fee: Yes, $75
Fee waiver available: Yes
Earliest filing date: July 1, 2008
Latest filing date: December 1, 2008

Latest MCAT® considered: September 2008
Oldest MCAT® considered: 2006

Early Decision Program
School does have EDP
Applicants notified: October 1, 2008
EDP available for: Both Residents and Non-Residents

Regular Acceptance Notice
Earliest date: October 15, 2008
Latest date: Until class is full

Applicant's Response to Acceptance Offer – Maximum Time: On or before May 15, 2009

Requests for Deferred Entrance Considered: Yes

Deposit to Hold Place in Class: No
Deposit (Resident): n/a
Deposit (Non-Resident): n/a
Deposit due: n/a
Applied to tuition: n/a
Deposit refundable: n/a
Refundable by: n/a

Estimated number of new entrants: 112
EDP: 2, special program: n/a

Start Month/Year: August 2009

Interview Format: Three individual interviews. On-campus interviews only.

Other Programs

PREPARATORY PROGRAMS
Postbaccalaureate Program: No
Summer Program: Yes,
http://pritzker.bsd.uchicago.edu/about/diversity/pipeline/psomer.shtml

COMBINED DEGREE PROGRAMS
Baccalaureate/MD: No
MD/MPH: No
MD/MBA: Yes,
http://pritzker@.bsd.uchicago.edu/jointdegrees/
MD/JD: Yes,
http://pritzker@.bsd.uchicago.edu/jointdegrees/
MD/PhD: Yes,
http://pritzker@.bsd.uchicago.edu/jointdegrees/

Premedical Coursework

Course	Req.	Rec.	Lab.	Sems.	Course	Req.	Rec.	Lab.	Sems.
Inorganic Chemistry	•		•	2	Computer Science				
Behavioral Sciences					Genetics		•		
Biochemistry		•	•		Humanities		•		
Biology	•		•	2	Organic Chemistry	•		•	2
Biology/Zoology					Physics	•		•	2
Calculus		•			Psychology				
College English		•			Social Sciences				
College Mathematics					Other				

Selection Factors: 2007 Accepted Applicants

Proportion of Accepted Applicants with Relevant Experience (Data Self-Reported to AMCAS®)		
Community Service/Volunteer		74%
Medically-Related Work		90%
Research		92%

Shaded bar represents accepted scores ranging from the 10th percentile to the 90th percentile. School Median ● National Median ●

Overall GPA	2.0	2.1	2.2	2.3	2.4	2.5	2.6	2.7	2.8	2.9	3.0	3.1	3.2	3.3	3.4	3.5	3.6	3.7	(3.8)	3.9	4.0
Science GPA	2.0	2.1	2.2	2.3	2.4	2.5	2.6	2.7	2.8	2.9	3.0	3.1	3.2	3.3	3.4	3.5	3.6	3.7	(3.8)	3.9	4.0

MCAT® required: Yes, 99% of 2007 accepted applicants took MCAT®

Verbal Reasoning	3	4	5	6	7	8	9	(10)	(11)	12	13	14	15
Physical Sciences	3	4	5	6	7	8	9	10	(11)	(12)	13	14	15
Biological Sciences	3	4	5	6	7	8	9	10	(11)	(12)	13	14	15
Writing Sample			J	K	L	M	N	O	P	(Q)	R	S	T

Acceptance & Matriculation Data for 2007–2008 First Year Class

	Resident	Non-Resident	International	Total
Applied	994	6346	447	7787
Interviewed	118	559	72	749
Deferred	2	3	2	7
Matriculants				
Early Assurance Program	n/a	n/a	n/a	n/a
Early Decision Program	0	0	0	0
Baccalaureate/MD	n/a	n/a	n/a	n/a
MD/PhD	4	5	0	9
Matriculated	31	77	4	**112**

Applications accepted from International Applicants: Yes

Matriculant Demographics: 2007–2008 First Year Class

Men: 53   **Women:** 59

Matriculants' Self-Reported Race/Ethnicity

Mexican American	5	Korean	5
Cuban	0	Vietnamese	0
Puerto Rican	4	Other Asian	5
Other Hispanic	2	Total Asian	30
Total Hispanic	11	Native American	2
Chinese	10	Black	13
Asian Indian	9	Native Hawaiian	2
Pakistani	1	White	63
Filipino	0	Unduplicated Number	
Japanese	0	of Matriculants	112

Science and Math Majors: 71%
Matriculants with:
   Baccalaureate degree: 100%
   Graduate degree(s): 3%

Specialty Choice

2003, 2004, 2005 Graduates, Specialty Choice (As reported by program directors to GME Track™)	
Anesthesiology	6%
Emergency Medicine	4%
Family Practice	2%
Internal Medicine	24%
Obstetrics/Gynecology	3%
Orthopaedic Surgery	6%
Pediatrics	13%
Psychiatry	3%
Radiology	5%
Surgery	7%

Financial Information

Source: 2006–2007 LCME I-B survey and 2007–2008 AAMC TSF questionnaire

	Residents	Non-Residents
Total Cost of Attendance	$57,926	$57,926
Tuition and Fees	$35,985	$35,985
Other (includes living expenses)	$20,168	$20,168
Health Insurance (can be waived)	$1,773	$1,773

Average 2007 Graduate Indebtedness: $162,859
% of Enrolled Students Receiving Aid: 87%

Criminal Background Check

This medical school requires a criminal background check prior to matriculation.

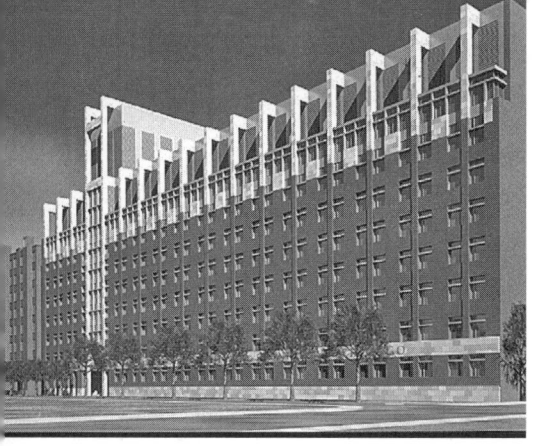

University of Illinois at Chicago
College of Medicine
Chicago, Peoria, Rockford, and Urbana, Illinois

Medical College Admissions
University of Illinois College of Medicine
808 South Wood St., Room 165 CME M/C 783
Chicago, Illinois 60612-7302
T 312 996 5635   **F** 312 996 6693

Admissions www.uic.edu/depts/mcam/admissions
Main www.medicine.uic.edu
Financial www.uic.edu/depts/mcam/finaid
Email medadmit@uic.edu

Public Institution

Dr. Joseph A. Flaherty, Dean

Dr. Jorge A. Girotti, Associate Dean and Director

Dr. Javette Orgain, Assistant Dean Urban Health Program

Carmelita Gee, Director of Financial Aid

Linda Singleton, Associate Director of Admissions

General Information
The college opened in 1882 as a private institution and joined the University of Illinois in 1913. Since 1982, the programs leading to the M.D. degree are conducted at four geographic sites. The Chicago site is located in the Medical Center of the university. The Urbana-Champaign site offers a four-year curriculum integrated with the programs of a comprehensive campus. The Peoria site includes facilities in each of the hospitals in that community and a modern downtown campus. The Rockford site has a centrally located campus and conducts programs in each of the Rockford hospitals and in several nearby smaller communities.

Mission Statement
The mission of the UIC College of Medicine is to enhance the health of the citizens of Illinois through the education of physicians and biomedical scientists, the advancement of our understanding and knowledge of health and disease, and the provision of health care in a setting of education and research. In pursuit of this mission, the college is committed to the goal of achieving excellence in teaching, research, and service in the science, art, and practice of medicine. This goal is best attained by applying valid educational principles, demonstrating high-quality patient care, and establishing a spirit of inquiry leading to scholarly achievement in basic and clinical research.

Curricular Highlights
Community Service Requirement: Optional.
Research/Thesis Requirement: Optional.

The college offers a generalist curriculum whose goal is to graduate physicians who are well grounded in basic and clinical sciences, oriented and competent as beginning general physicians, capable of entering graduate training in either generalist specialties or subspecialties, and able to function in an ever changing health care environment. We offer several special programs that allow students to combine medicine with doctoral degrees, business and public health, and independent study options to carry out in-depth studies of topics of their choosing.

USMLE
Step 1: Required. Students must record a passing score for promotion.
Step 2: Clinical Skills (CS): Required. Students must only record a score.
Step 2: Clinical Knowledge (CK): Required. Students must record a passing total score to graduate.

Selection Factors
The college selects applicants with the best combination of academic and extracurricular achievement, maturity, integrity, and motivation. Selection of students is based on an individualized evaluation of all available data and a personal interview. We consider the quality of work in all subject areas, breadth of education, and experiences that demonstrate initiative and creativity. The college gives preference to Illinois residents and does not discriminate on the basis of race, creed, sex, religion, national origin, age, disability, or status as a disabled veteran.

Financial Aid
Students are encouraged to apply early for loans and scholarships. Financial aid information is available by calling (312) 413-0127.

Information about Diversity Programs
The College has programs to encourage applicants from medically underserved areas of Illinois, and has staff to provide guidance to students from groups underrepresented in medicine and in-state candidates interested in a rural Illinois practice. The college accepts students on the basis of their potential for successfully meeting all standards leading to the M.D. degree.

Campus Information

Setting
UIC offers high-quality education to medical and graduate students at four sites across Illinois. Chicago is the largest of the college's four programs, and is located in the heart of the Illinois Medical District, about two miles west of downtown Chicago. The Urbana/Champaign campus is a complete four-year program leading to the M.D., located 130 miles south of Chicago. The first-year basic science program at Urbana also serves students who will complete their last three years of medical school at Peoria or Rockford. Peoria is located about 60 miles west of Urbana. With a greater metropolitan population of over 356,000, Peoria offers the best of both urban and country living. Rockford is the third largest city in Illinois, located just an hour's drive from Chicago and offers the appeal of a small town with the advantages of a large city.

Enrollment
For 2007, total enrollment was: 1,443

Special Features
As a research-oriented institution, UIC offers first-rate research facilities and resources. For instance, the Molecular Biology Research Building (MBRB), which opened in 1995, is a 230,000 square feet state-of-the-art research facility. The building houses 56 Principal Investigators and 108 laboratories. Researchers from both basic and clinical science departments conduct individual and collaborative research at the MBRB. The campus houses a 9.4 Tesla magnet, which is the world's strongest magnetic field for human imaging. Finally, a new 300,000 square feet Research Building opened in summer 2005. The building will be one of the most modern, architecturally innovative facilities in the country, with laboratory space for over 100 investigators.

Housing
On-campus housing is available at Chicago and Urbana. All campuses have private housing available nearby.

Application Process and Requirements 2009–2010

Primary Application Service: AMCAS
Earliest filing date: June 1, 2008
Latest filing date: November 15, 2008

Secondary Application Required?: Yes
Sent to: UIC College of Medicine – Admissions
Contact: Admissions Office, (312) 996-5635
medadmit@uic.edu
Fee: Yes, $70
Fee waiver available: Yes
Earliest filing date: June 15, 2008
Latest filing date: January 15, 2009

Latest MCAT® considered: September 2008
Oldest MCAT® considered: 2006

Early Decision Program
School does have EDP
Applicants notified: October 1, 2008
EDP available for: Both Residents
and Non-Resident

Regular Acceptance Notice
Earliest date: October 14, 2008
Latest date: Until class is full

Applicant's Response to Acceptance
Offer – Maximum Time: Two weeks

Requests for Deferred
Entrance Considered: Yes

Deposit to Hold Place in Class: Yes
Deposit (Resident): $100
Deposit (Non-Resident): $100
Deposit due: With response to acceptance offer
Applied to tuition: Yes
Deposit refundable: Yes
Refundable by: May 15, 2009

Estimated number of new entrants: 300
EDP: 6-10, special program: n/a

Start Month/Year: August 2009

Interview Format: Individual or panel.
Regional interviews in Peoria and Rockford are offered.

Other Programs

PREPARATORY PROGRAMS
Postbaccalaureate Program: Yes,
Dr. Javette Orgain (312)996-6491, uhpcom@uic.edu

Summer Program: Yes,
Dr. Javette Orgain, (312)996-6491, uhpcom@uic.edu
COMBINED DEGREE PROGRAMS
Baccalaureate/MD: Yes,
www.iuic.edu/depts/oaa/spec_prog/gppa
Josephine Volpe, (312) 355-2477, gppa@uic.edu
MD/MPH: Yes, www.uic.edu/sph, Susan S. O'Keefe,
(312) 996-6920, sokeefe@uic.edu
MD/MBA: Yes, www.lgsb.uic.edu,
Susan S. O'Keefe, (312)996-6920, sokeefe@uic.edu
MD/JD: Yes, www.med.uiuc.edu/msp/mdjd.asp
Amanda Cuevas, (217) 244-7800, acuevas@uiuc.edu
MD/PhD: Yes, www.uic.edu/com/mdphd
Roberta Bernstein, (312) 996-7473, roberta@uic.edu
MCAT Program Yes, Dr. Javette Orgain,
(312) 996-6491, uhpcom@uic.edu

Premedical Coursework

Course	Req.	Rec.	Lab.	Sems.	Course	Req.	Rec.	Lab.	Sems.
Inorganic Chemistry	•		•	2	Genetics		•		
Behavioral Sciences					Humanities				
Biochemistry					Organic Chemistry	•		•	2
Biology	•		•	2	Physics	•		•	2
Biology/Zoology					Psychology	•			2
Calculus					Social Sciences				
College English					Anthropology or Sociology	•			1
College Mathematics					Advanced Level Biology	•			1
Computer Science									

Selection Factors: 2007 Accepted Applicants

Proportion of Accepted Applicants with Relevant Experience (Data Self-Reported to AMCAS®)		
Community Service/Volunteer	67%
Medically-Related Work	86%
Research	80%

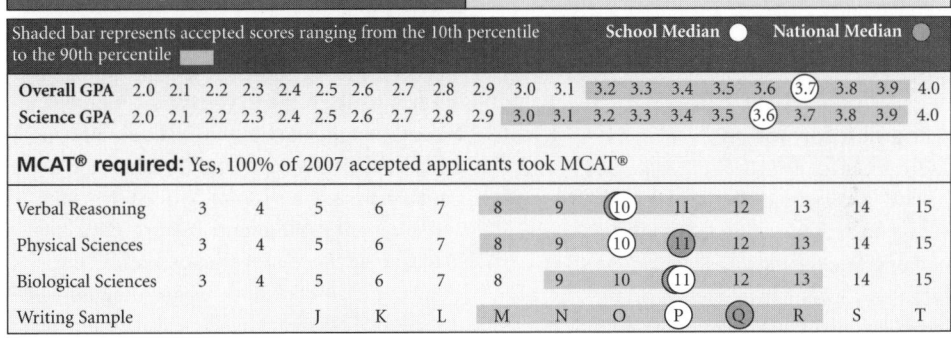

Shaded bar represents accepted scores ranging from the 10th percentile to the 90th percentile.   School Median ●   National Median ●

Overall GPA	2.0	2.1	2.2	2.3	2.4	2.5	2.6	2.7	2.8	2.9	3.0	3.1	3.2	3.3	3.4	3.5	3.6	(3.7)	3.8	3.9	4.0
Science GPA	2.0	2.1	2.2	2.3	2.4	2.5	2.6	2.7	2.8	2.9	3.0	3.1	3.2	3.3	3.4	3.5	(3.6)	3.7	3.8	3.9	4.0

MCAT® required: Yes, 100% of 2007 accepted applicants took MCAT®

Verbal Reasoning	3	4	5	6	7	8	9	(10)	11	12	13	14	15
Physical Sciences	3	4	5	6	7	8	9	(10)	(11)	12	13	14	15
Biological Sciences	3	4	5	6	7	8	9	10	(11)	12	13	14	15
Writing Sample				J	K	L	M	N	O	(P)	Q	R	S	T

Acceptance & Matriculation Data for 2007–2008 First Year Class

	Resident	Non-Resident	International	Total
Applied	1787	5296	10	7093
Interviewed	547	300	0	874
Deferred	2	1	0	3
Matriculants				
Early Assurance Program	0	0	0	0
Early Decision Program	2	0	0	2
Baccalaureate/MD	24	0	0	24
MD/PhD	8	12	0	20
Matriculated	239	68	0	**307**
Applications accepted from International Applicants: No				

Specialty Choice

2003, 2004, 2005 Graduates, Specialty Choice (As reported by program directors to GME Track™)	
Anesthesiology	9%
Emergency Medicine	8%
Family Practice	8%
Internal Medicine	16%
Obstetrics/Gynecology	3%
Orthopaedic Surgery	4%
Pediatrics	9%
Psychiatry	6%
Radiology	7%
Surgery	8%

Matriculant Demographics: 2007–2008 First Year Class

Men: 170   **Women:** 137

Matriculants' Self-Reported Race/Ethnicity

Mexican American	22	**Korean**	18
Cuban	2	**Vietnamese**	1
Puerto Rican	3	**Other Asian**	5
Other Hispanic	14	**Total Asian**	97
Total Hispanic	41	**Native American**	4
Chinese	25	**Black**	26
Asian Indian	42	**Native Hawaiian**	0
Pakistani	5	**White**	167
Filipino	4	**Unduplicated Number**	
Japanese	2	**of Matriculants**	307

Science and Math Majors: 69%
Matriculants with:
   Baccalaureate degree: 100%
   Graduate degree(s): 13%

Financial Information

Source: 2006–2007 LCME I-B survey
and 2007–2008 AAMC TSF questionnaire

	Residents	Non-Residents
Total Cost of Attendance	$42,986	$71,882
Tuition and Fees	$27,828	$56,724
Other (includes living expenses)	$14,356	$14,356
Health Insurance (can be waived)	$802	$802

Average 2007 Graduate Indebtedness: $143,533
% of Enrolled Students Receiving Aid: 89%

Criminal Background Check

This medical school requires a criminal background check prior to matriculation.

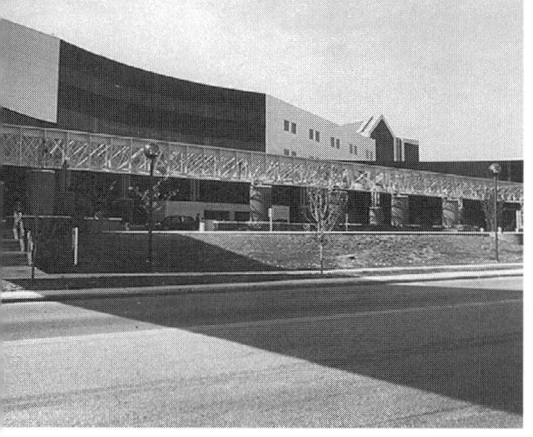

Indiana University School of Medicine
Indianapolis, Indiana

Medical School Admissions Office,
Indiana University School of Medicine
1120 South Drive, Fesler Hall 213
Indianapolis, Indiana 46202-5113
T 317 274 3772

Admissions www.medicine.iu.edu/body.cfm?id=166
Main www.medicine.iu.edu
Financial http://msaa.iusm.iu.edu/FinancialAid/
finaidtxt.html
Email inmedadm@iupui.edu

Public Institution

Dr. D. Craig Brater, Dean

Robert M. Stump Jr., Director of Admissions

Jose Espada, Director, Student Financial Services

Karen Smartt, Associate Director of Admissions

Dr. Stephen B. Leapman, Executive Associate Dean and Chair, Admissions Committee

General Information
Indiana University School of Medicine, founded in 1903, is the sole institution responsible for providing medical education in the state of Indiana and operates the Indiana Statewide Medical Education System. In addition to its responsibilities in teaching, patient care, and service, Indiana University School of Medicine is a major academic research center. In conducting its medical educational programs, Indiana University School of Medicine utilizes six teaching hospitals on or near the medical center campus, as well as other affiliated hospitals in Indianapolis and throughout the state.

Mission Statement
The goal of the Indiana University School of Medicine is the education of physicians, scientists, and other health professionals in an intellectually rich environment with research as its scientific base. In education, we are committed to imparting a fundamental understanding of both clinical practice and the basic scientific knowledge upon which it rests, to provide a firm foundation for lifelong learning. In research, we are committed to the advancement of knowledge. In patient care, we are committed to the highest standards of medical practice in an atmosphere of respect and empathy for our patients. Education, research, and delivery of health care are inseparable components of our mission. Excellence can only be achieved when all components are of highest quality, well integrated, and mutually supportive.

Curricular Highlights
Community Service Requirement: Optional, but expected.
Research/Thesis Requirement: Optional.

The School of Medicine's faculty have adopted a competency-based curriculum which equips students with excellent clinical skills balanced by the development of interpersonal and professional skills. The basic medical sciences are presented in the first two years. In addition, an intensive multidisciplinary course, Introduction to Clinical Medicine, spans both years. The faculty utilizes small problem-based learning groups throughout the first two years. A 12-month clinical clerkship program at the medical center in Indianapolis occupies the third year. In the fourth year, students complete three clerkships, and select seven one-month electives. Students may arrange elective experiences around the country and abroad. Students pursuing the M.D. degree may simultaneously pursue graduate degrees in a variety of disciplines, or elect to participate in the five-year Physician Scholar Program which incorporates a year of research into the M.D. degree program.

USMLE
Step 1: Required. Students must record a passing score for graduation, but not promotion.
Step 2: Clinical Skills (CS): Required. Students must record a passing total score to graduate.
Step 2: Clinical Knowledge (CK): Required. Students must record a passing total score to graduate.

Selection Factors
Students are offered places in the class on the basis of scholarship, character, personality, references, residence, interview, and performance on the MCAT®. In addition, the medical school faculty has specified non-academic criteria (technical standards), which all applicants must meet in order to participate effectively in the medical education program and the practice of medicine. The School of Medicine is state-assisted, and the Admissions Committee shows preference to Indiana residents. Nevertheless, a number of non-residents are offered acceptances each year (e.g., 163 for 2007). The applications of non-residents who have significant ties to the state of Indiana may be given greater consideration. The School of Medicine does not discriminate on the basis of age, color, disability, ethnicity, gender, marital status, national origin, race, religion, sexual orientation, or veteran status.

Financial Aid
Both merit and need-based scholarships are available, as are need-based loans. There are scholarships for Indiana residents who commit to practicing primary care medicine in a medically underserved location in Indiana.

Information about Diversity Programs
Indiana University School of Medicine is committed to diversity in its student body, faculty, and staff.

Campus Information

Setting
The Indiana University Medical Center campus covers some 85 acres within one mile of the center of Indianapolis and is part of the 30,000 student Indiana University-Purdue University at Indianapolis. The medical center is also host to outstanding schools of dentistry and nursing.

Enrollment
For 2007, total enrollment was: 1,173

Special Features
A Physician Scholars Program permits students to take up to a year off to pursue research or other medically-related interests. The Kenya Program allows students to work with IU faculty at Moi University to provide medical care for Kenyans. Similar programs in Latin America are under development.

Housing
On-campus housing is limited, but there is an abundance of available housing within 5-20 minutes of campus.

Satellite Campuses/Facilities
First- and second-year students may be enrolled at host higher education campuses in Bloomington, Evansville, Fort Wayne, Gary, Lafayette, Muncie, South Bend, and Terre Haute, in addition to Indianapolis. A new Rural Health Program was implemented at Terre Haute in 2008.

Application Process and Requirements 2009–2010

Primary Application Service: AMCAS
Earliest filing date: June 1, 2008
Latest filing date: December 15, 2008

Secondary Application Required?: Yes
Sent to: Only applicants to be interviewed
Contact: Admissions Office, (317) 274-3772, inmedadm@iupui.edu
URL: n/a
Fee: Yes, $50
Fee waiver available: No
Earliest filing date: June 1, 2008
Latest filing date: Varies

Latest MCAT® considered: September 2008
Oldest MCAT® considered: 2005

Early Decision Program
School does have EDP
Applicants notified: October 1, 2008
EDP available for: Both Residents and Non-Residents

Regular Acceptance Notice
Earliest date: October 15, 2008
Latest date: Until class is full

Applicant's Response to Acceptance Offer – Maximum Time: Three weeks

Requests for Deferred Entrance Considered: Yes

Deposit to Hold Place in Class: No
Deposit (Resident): n/a
Deposit (Non-Resident): n/a
Deposit due: n/a
Applied to tuition: n/a
Deposit refundable: n/a
Refundable by: n/a

Estimated number of new entrants: 308
EDP: 25, special program: n/a

Start Month/Year: August 2009

Interview Format: Individual interviews. Regional interviews are not available.

Other Programs

PREPARATORY PROGRAMS
Postbaccalaureate Program: No
Summer Program: No
COMBINED DEGREE PROGRAMS
Baccalaureate/MD: No
MD/MPH: Yes, www.medicine.iu.edu/body.cfm?id=1853
MD/MBA: Yes, www.medicine.iu.edu/body.cfm?id=1852
MD/JD: No
MD/PhD: www.medicine.iu.edu/body.cfm?id=1851
Additional Program: www.medicine.iu.edu/body.cfm?id=1854

Premedical Coursework

Course	Req.	Rec.	Lab.	Sems.
Inorganic Chemistry				
Behavioral Sciences				
Biochemistry				
Biology	•		•	2
Biology/Zoology				
Calculus				
College English				
College Mathematics				

Course	Req.	Rec.	Lab.	Sems.
Computer Science				
Genetics				
Humanities				
Organic Chemistry	•		•	2
Physics	•		•	2
Psychology				
Social Sciences				
General Chemistry	•		•	2

Selection Factors: 2007 Accepted Applicants

Proportion of Accepted Applicants with Relevant Experience (Data Self-Reported to AMCAS®)		
Community Service/Volunteer		73%
Medically-Related Work		76%
Research		71%

Shaded bar represents accepted scores ranging from the 10th percentile to the 90th percentile ▬   **School Median** ●   **National Median** ●

Overall GPA	2.0	2.1	2.2	2.3	2.4	2.5	2.6	2.7	2.8	2.9	3.0	3.1	3.2	3.3	3.4	3.5	3.6	3.7	(3.8)	3.9	4.0
Science GPA	2.0	2.1	2.2	2.3	2.4	2.5	2.6	2.7	2.8	2.9	3.0	3.1	3.2	3.3	3.4	3.5	3.6	3.7	(3.8)	3.9	4.0

MCAT® required: Yes, 100% of 2007 accepted applicants took MCAT®

Verbal Reasoning	3	4	5	6	7	8	9	(10)	11	12	13	14	15
Physical Sciences	3	4	5	6	7	8	9	(10)	(11)	12	13	14	15
Biological Sciences	3	4	5	6	7	8	9	10	(11)	12	13	14	15
Writing Sample				J	K	L	M	N	O	(P)	(Q)	R	S	T

Acceptance & Matriculation Data for 2007–2008 First Year Class

	Resident	Non-Resident	International	Total
Applied	689	2551	250	3490
Interviewed	572	391	40	1003
Deferred	3	1	1	5
Matriculants				
Early Assurance Program	0	0	0	0
Early Decision Program	17	1	0	18
Baccalaureate/MD	n/a	n/a	n/a	n/a
MD/PhD	4	1	0	5
Matriculated	251	39	4	**294**

Applications accepted from International Applicants: Yes

Matriculant Demographics: 2007–2008 First Year Class

Men: 161   **Women:** 133

Matriculants' Self-Reported Race/Ethnicity

Mexican American	10	**Korean**	9
Cuban	1	**Vietnamese**	2
Puerto Rican	0	**Other Asian**	4
Other Hispanic	4	**Total Asian**	52
Total Hispanic	15	**Native American**	3
Chinese	9	**Black**	14
Asian Indian	24	**Native Hawaiian**	0
Pakistani	5	**White**	224
Filipino	3	**Unduplicated Number**	
Japanese	1	**of Matriculants**	294

Science and Math Majors: 72%
Matriculants with:
  Baccalaureate degree: 100%
  Graduate degree(s): 12%

Specialty Choice

2003, 2004, 2005 Graduates, Specialty Choice (As reported by program directors to GME Track™)	
Anesthesiology	11%
Emergency Medicine	8%
Family Practice	10%
Internal Medicine	14%
Obstetrics/Gynecology	4%
Orthopaedic Surgery	5%
Pediatrics	10%
Psychiatry	3%
Radiology	6%
Surgery	6%

Financial Information

Source: 2006–2007 LCME I-B survey and 2007–2008 AAMC TSF questionnaire

	Residents	Non-Residents
Total Cost of Attendance	$51,437	$68,427
Tuition and Fees	$26,207	$43,197
Other (includes living expenses)	$22,654	$22,654
Health Insurance (can be waived)	$2,576	$2,576

Average 2007 Graduate Indebtedness: $163,007
% of Enrolled Students Receiving Aid: 84%

Criminal Background Check

This medical school requires a criminal background check prior to matriculation.

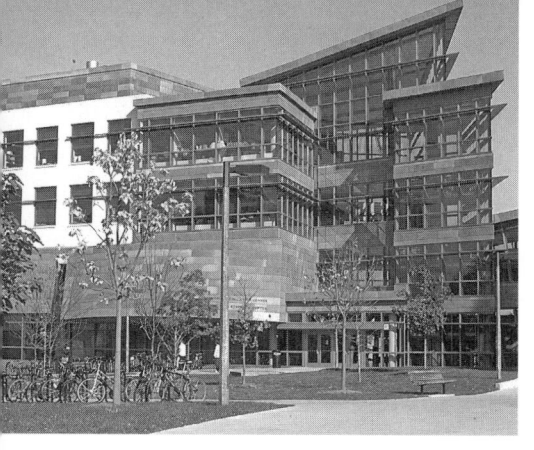

University of Iowa Roy J. and Lucille A. Carver College of Medicine

Iowa City, Iowa

Medical Student Admissions, University of Iowa
Roy J. & Lucille A. Carver College of Medicine
1213 Medical Education and Research Facility
Iowa City, Iowa 52242-1101
T 319 335 8052   F 319 335 8049

Admissions www.medicine.uiowa.edu/osac/admissions
Main www.medicine.uiowa.edu
Financial www.medicine.uiowa.edu/osac/
financial/index.htm
Email medical-admissions@uiowa.edu

Public Institution

Dr. Jean Robillard, Vice President of Medical Affairs & Dean

Catherine M. Solow,
Assistant Dean of Student Affairs

Barbara E. Barlow, Recruitment Coordinator and Minority Affairs Coordinator

Linda G. Bissell, Director of Financial Services

Judith D. Lehman,
Admissions Process Coordinator

General Information

The college is part of a major health center serving the state and region. The health sciences campus includes the University of Iowa Hospitals and Clinics; Veterans Affairs Hospital; Hardin Health Sciences Library; and medical college, basic sciences, dental, nursing, and pharmacy buildings. The Medical Education and Research Facility opened in 2001.

Mission Statement

The Carver College of Medicine has three inextricably linked missions: education, research, and service. The college aspires to be responsive to the needs of society, and in particular the citizens of Iowa, through the excellence of its educational programs in the health professions and biomedical sciences, by the outstanding quality of its research, and through the provision of innovative and comprehensive health care and other services.

Curricular Highlights

Community Service Requirement: Optional.
Research/Thesis Requirement: Optional.

Case-based and self-directed learning, clinical correlation, computer-based learning, small-group activities, and vertical integration of material are emphasized in the curriculum. Year 1: investigation of the normal structure and function of the human body. Year 2: investigation of abnormal structure and function. Patient contact, introduction to medical history-taking and physical diagnosis, and coverage of emerging topic areas are presented in Foundations of Clinical Practice, a course that runs the first two years of the

curriculum. In the fourth semester, this course provides students with a foundation in clinical medicine that will prepare them to perform in the clinical arena. The two clinical years of the curriculum afford a broad base of training to provide the student with the essential skills and knowledge required to enter residency training. A generalist core is a feature of the clinical years. Ample time for electives is provided.

USMLE

Step 1: Required. Students must record a passing score for promotion.
Step 2: Clinical Skills (CS): Required. Students must record a passing score in each section to graduate.
Step 2: Clinical Knowledge (CK): Required. Students must record a passing score in each section to graduate.

Selection Factors

The Admissions Committee selects applicants best qualified for the study and practice of medicine. To be eligible for admission, the applicant must attain at least a 2.5 GPA (based on a 4.0 scale) for all college work undertaken. Factors considered: 1. Overall undergraduate academic record. 2. Science GPA. 3. MCAT Scores. 4. Residence: Preference given to Iowa residents with high scholastic standing. Consideration also given to outstanding non-residents. 5. Personal characteristics: Evaluated through letters of recommendation, information on the AMCAS application, and information on the supplemental form. 6. On-site personal interview. Applications for transfer are not considered.

Financial Aid

Applicants are selected without consideration of their ability to meet the cost of medical school. Students receive financial aid on the basis of need as calculated using the FAFSA. Scholarship assistance is available. Students are responsible for their own financial support, but the college provides information on locating funding sources. Loan and grant funds from private, state, collegiate, and federal sources are available.

Information about Diversity Programs

The college is committed to the recruitment, selection, and retention of a diverse student body. Financial and academic assistance is provided to disadvantaged students and those from groups underrepresented in American medicine. Financial aid packages are designed on the basis of need, and grant assistance is available. The application fee and admission deposit may be waived for financially disadvantaged students upon request.

Campus Information

Setting

The college is on the 1,900-acre campus of a major research institution, the University of Iowa, and is located in a community of 60,000. University Hospitals and Clinics, one of the largest university-owned teaching hospitals, is adjacent. Cultural activities, Big 10 sports, shopping and nearby parks provide outlets for recreation and services.

Enrollment

For 2007, total enrollment was: 576

Special Features

The college provides opportunities in international and domestic cross-cultural sites. Courses are offered in global health and U.S. health policy issues. The writing program provides consultation on personal statements, CVs, and creative writing. The program coordinates activities for medical students involving literature, music, and the visual and performing arts.

Housing

On-campus housing is generally not available. The university offers a clearinghouse to help students find housing. Rents range from $350-1,600/month. There are two coed medical fraternities with rents ranging from $295-$450/month.

Satellite Campuses/Facilities

The major satellite campus is the Des Moines Medical Education Consortium, a cooperative venture of several Des Moines hospitals, where some students complete required clerkships. Some ambulatory care clerkships are completed with adjunct faculty across the state.

Application Process and Requirements 2009–2010

Primary Application Service: AMCAS
Earliest filing date: June 1, 2008
Latest filing date: November 1, 2008

Secondary Application Required?: Yes
Sent to: Screened applicants
URL: www.medicine.uiowa.edu/osac/admissions
Fee: Yes, $60
Fee waiver available: Yes
Earliest filing date: July 1, 2008
Latest filing date: December 15, 2008

Latest MCAT® considered: September 2008
Oldest MCAT® considered: 2003

Early Decision Program
School does have EDP
Applicants notified: October 1, 2008
EDP available for: Both Residents and Non-Residents

Regular Acceptance Notice
Earliest date: October 15, 2008
Latest date: Until class is full

Applicant's Response to Acceptance Offer – Maximum Time: Two weeks from date of letter

Requests for Deferred Entrance Considered: Yes

Deposit to Hold Place in Class: Yes
Deposit (Resident): $50
Deposit (Non-Resident): $50
Deposit due: March 1, 2009, or within 3 weeks after acceptance offer if after March 1, 2009
Applied to tuition: Yes
Deposit refundable: Yes
Refundable by: June 15, 2009

Estimated number of new entrants: 148
EDP: 5, special program: n/a

Start Month/Year: August 20, 2009
(first day of orientation)

Interview Format: Candidates interviewed by two faculty members in one room. Regional interviews are not available.

Other Programs

PREPARATORY PROGRAMS
Postbaccalaureate Program: No
Summer Program: No
Prematriculation Summer Program (for admitted candidates): Yes, www.medicine.uiowa.edu/osac/imei.htm

COMBINED DEGREE PROGRAMS
Baccalaureate/MD: No
MD/MPH: Yes, www.public-health.uiowa.edu/mph/about/combined_degrees/md_mph.html
MD/MBA: Yes, www.medicine.uiowa.edu/osac/programsrecords/CombinedDegrees.htm
MD/JD: Yes, www.medicine.uiowa.edu/osac/programsrecords/CombinedDegrees.htm
MD/PhD: Yes, www.medicine.uiowa.edu/mstp

Premedical Coursework

Course	Req.	Rec.	Lab.	Sems.	Course	Req.	Rec.	Lab.	Sems.
Inorganic Chemistry	•		•	2	Genetics		•		
Behavioral Sciences					Humanities				
Biochemistry		•			Organic Chemistry	•		•	2
Biology	•		•	2	Physics	•		•	2
Biology/Zoology					Psychology				
Calculus					Social Sciences				
College English	•			2	Advanced Biology				1
College Mathematics	•			1	Social, Behavioral	•			4
Computer Science					Sciences/Humanities				

Selection Factors: 2007 Accepted Applicants

Proportion of Accepted Applicants with Relevant Experience (Data Self-Reported to AMCAS®)		
Community Service/Volunteer		70%
Medically-Related Work		91%
Research		83%

Shaded bar represents accepted scores ranging from the 10th percentile to the 90th percentile. **School Median** ● **National Median** ●

Overall GPA	2.0	2.1	2.2	2.3	2.4	2.5	2.6	2.7	2.8	2.9	3.0	3.1	3.2	3.3	3.4	3.5	3.6	3.7	(3.8)	3.9	4.0
Science GPA	2.0	2.1	2.2	2.3	2.4	2.5	2.6	2.7	2.8	2.9	3.0	3.1	3.2	3.3	3.4	3.5	3.6	3.7	(3.8)	3.9	4.0

MCAT® required: Yes, 100% of 2007 accepted applicants took MCAT®

Verbal Reasoning	3	4	5	6	7	8	9	(10)	11	12	13	14	15
Physical Sciences	3	4	5	6	7	8	9	10	(11)	12	13	14	15
Biological Sciences	3	4	5	6	7	8	9	10	(11)	12	13	14	15
Writing Sample			J	K	L	M	N	O	(P)	(Q)	R	S	T

Acceptance & Matriculation Data for 2007–2008 First Year Class

	Resident	Non-Resident	International	Total
Applied	321	2625	10	2956
Interviewed	260	419	0	679
Deferred	9	6	0	15
Matriculants				
Early Assurance Program	0	0	0	0
Early Decision Program	5	0	0	5
Baccalaureate/MD	n/a	n/a	n/a	n/a
MD/PhD	0	10	0	10
Matriculated	99	49	0	**148**

Applications accepted from International Applicants: No

Matriculant Demographics: 2007–2008 First Year Class

Men: 82   **Women:** 66

Matriculants' Self-Reported Race/Ethnicity

Mexican American	6	Korean	2
Cuban	0	Vietnamese	1
Puerto Rican	0	Other Asian	1
Other Hispanic	0	Total Asian	7
Total Hispanic	6	Native American	3
Chinese	3	Black	8
Asian Indian	1	Native Hawaiian	1
Pakistani	0	White	131
Filipino	0	**Unduplicated Number**	
Japanese	0	**of Matriculants**	**148**

Science and Math Majors: 76%
Matriculants with:
　　Baccalaureate degree: 100%
　　Graduate degree(s): 9%

Specialty Choice

2003, 2004, 2005 Graduates, Specialty Choice
(As reported by program directors to GME Track™)

Anesthesiology	7%
Emergency Medicine	6%
Family Practice	13%
Internal Medicine	13%
Obstetrics/Gynecology	5%
Orthopaedic Surgery	5%
Pediatrics	11%
Psychiatry	4%
Radiology	8%
Surgery	6%

Financial Information

Source: 2006–2007 LCME I-B survey and 2007–2008 AAMC TSF questionnaire

	Residents	Non-Residents
Total Cost of Attendance	$41,975	$58,005
Tuition and Fees	$25,689	$41,719
Other (includes living expenses)	$15,476	$15,476
Health Insurance (can be waived)	$810	$810

Average 2007 Graduate Indebtedness: $120,171
% of Enrolled Students Receiving Aid: 95%

Criminal Background Check

This medical school requires a criminal background check prior to matriculation.

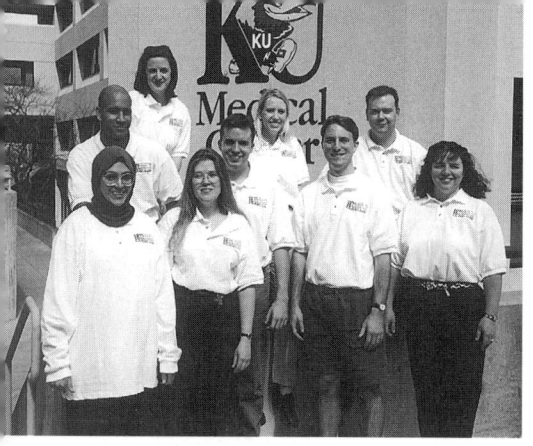

University of Kansas School of Medicine
Kansas City, Kansas

Associate Dean for Admissions
University of Kansas School of Medicine
Mail Stop 1049, 3901 Rainbow Boulevard
Kansas City, Kansas 66160
T 913 588 5245 **F** 913 588 5259

Admissions www.kumc.edu/som/prospectivestudents.html
Main www.kumc.edu/som/
Financial www.kumc.edu/studentcenter/
financialaid.html
Email premedinfo@kumc.edu

Public Institution

Dr. Barbara F. Atkinson, Executive Vice Chancellor and Executive Dean

Sandra J. McCurdy, Associate Dean for Admissions

Dr. Patricia A. Thomas, Associate Dean for Cultural Enhancement and Diversity

Sara Honeck, Director of Student Financial Aid

General Information

Since the establishment of the University of Kansas School of Medicine in 1905, its students and faculty have built upon a tradition of excellence. Through exceptional medical education, patient care, service, and research, the medical faculty and staff are dedicated to preparing students for the future of medicine by providing the innovative education and training needed to practice in today's ever-changing health care delivery system.

Mission Statement

The School of Medicine commits to enhance the quality of life and to serve our community through the discovery of knowledge, the education of health professionals, and improving the health of the public.

Curricular Highlights

Community Service Requirement: Optional.
Research/Thesis Requirement: Optional.

The interdisciplinary curriculum promotes self-directed, active learning to facilitate students' mastery of the knowledge, skills, attitudes, and behaviors required to become highly competent and compassionate healers. In preparation for lifelong acquisition and synthesis of new discoveries and knowledge, students become critical thinkers who can analyze difficult problems, formulate effective action plans, and provide optimal clinical care. Years one and two consist of 13 sequential modules organized around central themes or organ systems, with didactic instruction and self-directed learning balanced between lectures and small-group activities. Each student uses a tablet computer to access

course management, learning, and research systems. Beginning in the first semester, each student is paired with a mentoring physician in a longitudinal ambulatory clinical experience. Several summer programs are offered for clinical credit to students who have completed their first year. For core clinical rotations, students rotate through hospitals and community-based clinics located in Kansas City, Wichita, or select sites throughout the state. Students may also choose the Rural Track, a multidisciplinary clinical training program. Clinical electives may be taken locally, across the country, or at more than 20 approved international locations.

USMLE

Step 1: Required. Students must record a passing score for promotion.
Step 2: Clinical Skills (CS) Required. Students must record a passing total score to graduate.
Step 2: Clinical Knowledge (CK): Required. Students must record a passing total score to graduate.

Selection Factors

Applicants are encouraged to submit their AMCAS applications by September 1. Qualified Kansas residents receive strong first preference for secondary applications, interviews, and admission; successful nonresident applicants will have significant Kansas ties and/or add breadth to the class. Academic performance, MCAT® scores, application materials, letters of recommendation, impressions gained from interviews, and nonacademic activities are assessed throughout the admissions process. Transfer applications are considered only if a position is available in the third-year class; Kansas residents with a compelling need to transfer receive priority.

Financial Aid

Loans and scholarships are available, with the FAFSA used to determine recipients of need-based aid. A major source of assistance for selected students is the Kansas Medical Loan Program, which provides payment of tuition and a stipend of up to $2,000 per month. Recipients receive loan forgiveness by practicing primary care or emergency medicine in an underserved county in Kansas.

Information about Diversity Programs

The University of Kansas and the School of Medicine believe the intentional creation of a diverse learning environment is essential to achieving their educational missions. Diversity and quality in medical education and health care delivery are ensured through programs that recruit, enroll, and graduate a diverse population of students; train culturally competent physicians; recruit a diverse faculty; institutionalize measures that develop and retain minority academic physicians; and expand research on health care issues affecting disadvantaged and underserved populations.

Campus Information

Setting
The School of Medicine is located at the tip of the popular 39th Street West district and just north of historic Westport and the Country Club Plaza. The metropolitan area is well-known for its award-winning parks system and an abundance of venues for athletic events and the visual and performance arts.

Enrollment
For 2007, total enrollment was: 703

Special Features
Student educational resources include a high-tech clinical skills teaching laboratory, a computer testing center, and a newly renovated medical library. A new heart hospital and biomedical research center opened in 2006. Medical students provide medical care to uninsured patients through student-operated JayDoc Clinics in Kansas City and Wichita.

Housing
All housing is off-campus, with affordable housing readily available in the two-county area.

Satellite Campuses/Facilities
Approximately one-third of each class completes clinical training on the KU School of Medicine-Wichita campus. This premier community-based program of medical education, patient care, and research is centered upon a partnership with four hospitals that offer a total capacity of more than 3,000 licensed beds.

Application Process and Requirements 2009–2010

Primary Application Service: AMCAS
Earliest filing date: June 1, 2008
Latest filing date: October 15, 2008

Secondary Application Required?: Yes
Sent to: All Residents and selected Non-Resident applicants
URL: www2.kumc.edu/som/aissupapp/default.asp
Fee: Yes, $50
Fee waiver available: Yes
Earliest filing date: July 1, 2008
Latest filing date: November 15, 2008

Latest MCAT® considered: September, 2008
Oldest MCAT® considered: August, 2006

Early Decision Program
School does have EDP
Applicants notified: October 1, 2008
EDP available for: Both Residents and Non-Residents

Regular Acceptance Notice
Earliest date: November 15, 2008
Latest date: Varies

Applicant's Response to Acceptance Offer – Maximum Time: Two weeks

Requests for Deferred Entrance Considered: Yes

Deposit to Hold Place in Class: Yes
Deposit (Resident): $50
Deposit (Non-Resident): $50
Deposit due: With response to acceptance offer
Applied to tuition: Yes
Deposit refundable: Yes
Refundable by: May 15, 2009

Estimated number of new entrants: 175
EDP: 45, special program: 25

Start Month/Year: July 2009

Interview Format: Two individual interviews, one open-file with a committee member. Regional interviews are not available.

Other Programs

PREPARATORY PROGRAMS
Postbaccalaureate Program: Yes, www2.kumc.edu/oced/hcpp.htm
Summer Program: Yes, www2.kumc.edu/oced/hcpp.htm
Primary Care Workshops: www.kumc.edu/som/primarycareworkshop.html
Premedical Student Conference: www.kumc.edu/som/psc.html

COMBINED DEGREE PROGRAMS
Baccalaureate/MD: No
MD/MPH: Yes, http://mph.kumc.edu/
MD/MBA: No
MD/JD: No
MD/PhD: Yes, www3.kumc.edu/mdphd/
Additional Program: Yes, www.kumc.edu/hpm

Premedical Coursework

Course	Req.	Rec.	Lab.	Sems.
Inorganic Chemistry	•		•	2
Behavioral Sciences		•		
Biochemistry		•		
Biology	•		•	2
Biology/Zoology				
Calculus				
College English	•			2
College Mathematics	•			1

Course	Req.	Rec.	Lab.	Sems.
Computer Science				
Genetics		•		
Humanities		•		
Organic Chemistry	•		•	2
Physics	•		•	2
Psychology				
Social Sciences				
Other				

Selection Factors: 2007 Accepted Applicants

Proportion of Accepted Applicants with Relevant Experience (Data Self-Reported to AMCAS®)		
Community Service/Volunteer		73%
Medically-Related Work		77%
Research		60%

Shaded bar represents accepted scores ranging from the 10th percentile to the 90th percentile | School Median ● | National Median ●

Overall GPA	2.0	2.1	2.2	2.3	2.4	2.5	2.6	2.7	2.8	2.9	3.0	3.1	3.2	3.3	3.4	3.5	3.6	(3.7)	3.8	3.9	4.0
Science GPA	2.0	2.1	2.2	2.3	2.4	2.5	2.6	2.7	2.8	2.9	3.0	3.1	3.2	3.3	3.4	3.5	3.6	(3.7)	3.8	3.9	4.0

MCAT® required: Yes, 100% of 2007 accepted applicants took MCAT®

Verbal Reasoning	3	4	5	6	7	8	9	(10)	11	12	13	14	15
Physical Sciences	3	4	5	6	7	8	(9)	10	(11)	12	13	14	15
Biological Sciences	3	4	5	6	7	8	9	(10)	(11)	12	13	14	15
Writing Sample			J	K	L	M	N	(O)	P	(Q)	R	S	T

Acceptance & Matriculation Data for 2007–2008 First Year Class

	Resident	Non-Resident	International	Total
Applied	423	1481	14	1918
Interviewed	321	144	0	465
Deferred	3	1	0	4
Matriculants				
Early Assurance Program	6	0	0	6
Early Decision Program	60	3	0	63
Baccalaureate/MD	n/a	n/a	n/a	n/a
MD/PhD	3	2	0	5
Matriculated	153	23	0	**176**

Applications accepted from International Applicants: No

Matriculant Demographics: 2007–2008 First Year Class

Men: 83 **Women:** 93

Matriculants' Self-Reported Race/Ethnicity

Mexican American	9	Korean	2
Cuban	0	Vietnamese	5
Puerto Rican	0	Other Asian	0
Other Hispanic	2	Total Asian	16
Total Hispanic	11	Native American	2
Chinese	4	Black	14
Asian Indian	3	Native Hawaiian	0
Pakistani	1	White	142
Filipino	1	Unduplicated Number	
Japanese	0	of Matriculants	176

Science and Math Majors: 75%
Matriculants with:
Baccalaureate degree: 100%
Graduate degree(s): 5%

Specialty Choice

2003, 2004, 2005 Graduates, Specialty Choice (As reported by program directors to GME Track™)	
Anesthesiology	8%
Emergency Medicine	8%
Family Practice	20%
Internal Medicine	13%
Obstetrics/Gynecology	8%
Orthopaedic Surgery	4%
Pediatrics	7%
Psychiatry	2%
Radiology	4%
Surgery	7%

Financial Information

Source: 2006–2007 LCME I-B survey and 2007–2008 AAMC TSF questionnaire

	Residents	Non-Residents
Total Cost of Attendance	$46,165	$63,556
Tuition and Fees	$22,976	$40,367
Other (includes living expenses)	$22,269	$22,269
Health Insurance (can be waived)	$920	$920

Average 2007 Graduate Indebtedness: $115,660
% of Enrolled Students Receiving Aid: 93%

Criminal Background Check

This medical school requires a criminal background check prior to matriculation.

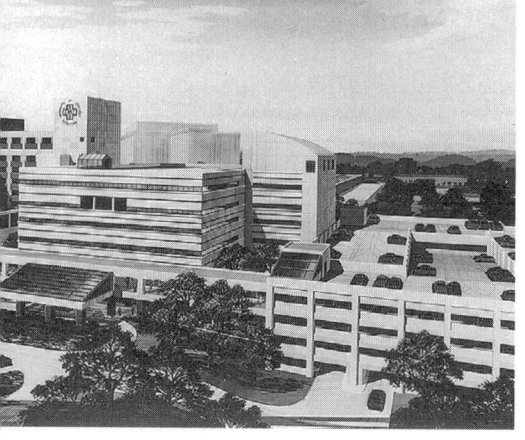

University of Kentucky College of Medicine

Lexington, Kentucky

University of Kentucky College of Medicine
Office of Admissions
138 Leader Avenue
Lexington, Kentucky 40507
T 859 323 6161   F 859 257 3633

Admissions www.mc.uky.edu/meded/admissions/index.asp
Main www.mc.uky.edu/medicine
Financial www.mc.uky.edu/meded/financialaid/index.asp
Email kymedap@uky.edu

Public Institution

Dr. Jay Perman, Dean

*Dr. Carol L. Elam,
Assistant Dean for Admissions
and Institutional Advancement*

Linda A. Gilbert, Financial Aid Coordinator

General Information

The University of Kentucky College of Medicine admitted its first class in 1960. The College of Medicine is part of the University of Kentucky Academic Medical Center located on the university campus in Lexington. The medical center comprises six colleges: medicine, nursing, pharmacy, dentistry, health sciences, and public health. The majority of on-site clinical teaching occurs at the University of Kentucky Chandler Hospital, the Veterans Affairs Medical Center, and the Kentucky Clinic. Hospitals in Lexington and across the Commonwealth hold affiliation agreements with the college for clinical teaching and patient service. Basic science teaching areas for lecture, laboratory, and small-group instruction, and the Medical Center Library, are located in the Willard Medical Sciences Building.

Mission Statement

Our mission is to assume a leadership role in addressing the health care needs of the Commonwealth of Kentucky and to be preeminent among medical schools in selected areas of education, research, and service.

Curricular Highlights

Community Service Requirement: Required. Interprofessional & underserved exposure required.
Research/Thesis Requirement: Optional.

In a curriculum that integrates basic and clinical sciences, students are taught fundamental problems of human biology, how to recognize causes of these problems, and how to prevent disease and treat patients. Year 1 of the curriculum focuses on normal function of the human body (human structure, cellular structure and function, neurosciences, and human function). First-year students receive early exposure and experience in patient care through the study of interviewing, history-taking, physical exam skills, and clinical decision-making using both standardized and real patients in a longitudinal care experience. In the first two years, students explore principles of prevention and assess the impact of social, ethical, legal, economic, and psychological factors using case study discussions. Year 2 exposes students to abnormal functions of the human body. Coursework is designed to integrate studies of infectious disease, immunology, pathology, pharmacology, and psychiatry. Computer-based instruction and simulation reinforce basic science studies and provide linkages to clinical applications. Clinical students work with patients in both inpatient and outpatient settings and are required to take medical histories, perform physical exams, and monitor laboratory tests. Year 3 includes integrated women's maternal and child health clerkships, along with internal medicine and emergency care, neurosciences, family and community medicine, and surgery. Year 4 includes clinical pharmacology, rural medicine experiences, 2 acting internships, and a 4-month elective period. The Rural Track provides clinical education at rural sites.

USMLE

Step 1: Required. Students must record a passing score for promotion.
Step 2: Clinical Skills (CS): Required. Students must record a passing total score to graduate.
Step 2: Clinical Knowledge (CK): Required. Students must record a passing total score to graduate.

Selection Factors

The UKCOM gives preference to qualified applicants who are Kentucky residents. Determination of state residence is made by the registrar's office. Secondary applications are sent to all Kentucky residents and to nonresidents with competitive undergraduate GPAs and MCAT® scores. Selected candidates are invited for interviews conducted at the UKCOM. Necessary personal attributes of applicants include time management abilities, interpersonal skills, leadership, and demonstrated service to others. Admission decisions are based upon review of academic and nonacademic factors, including scholastic excellence, MCAT® performance, personal attributes, exposure to the profession, premedical recommendations, and admission interviews. Transfers from LCME-accredited schools are considered on a space-available basis. The UKCOM does not discriminate on the basis of race, sex, creed, national origin, age, or handicap.

Financial Aid

A limited number of scholarships are awarded to selected students with exceptional achievement. Institutional loan/scholarship assistance is available for eligible resident and nonresident students. The Financial Aid Office provides counseling and assists students in applying for aid. A guaranteed tuition plan locks tuition and fees for each entering class.

Information about Diversity Programs

The UKCOM is committed to the recruitment and retention of disadvantaged students and students from groups underrepresented in medicine. Interested applicants are encouraged to contact the admissions office.

Campus Information

Setting

The UKCOM is located on the University campus in Lexington.

Enrollment

For 2007, total enrollment was: 413

Special Features

Adjacent to UKCOM are biomedical research centers, Markey Cancer Center, Sanders-Brown Center on Aging, University Health Service, Chandler Hospital, UK Children's Hospital, VA Hospital, and the Gill Heart Institute. A new bed tower is under construction.

Housing

Housing is available close to campus. Rents average $600 to $800 per month.

Satellite Campuses/Facilities

Students participate in rural health electives throughout Kentucky through the Area Health Education Centers.

Application Process and Requirements 2009–2010

Primary Application Service: AMCAS
Earliest filing date: June 1, 2008
Latest filing date: November 1, 2008

Secondary Application Required?: Yes
Sent to: Screened applicants
Contact: Kim Scott, (859) 323-6161
kstahlma@email.uky.edu
Fee: Yes, $50
Fee waiver available: Yes
Earliest filing date: July 1, 2008
Latest filing date: January 15, 2009

Latest MCAT® Considered: September 2008
Oldest MCAT® considered: August 2006

Early Decision Program
School does have EDP
Applicants notified: October 1, 2008
EDP available for: Both Residents
and Non-Residents

Regular Acceptance Notice
Earliest date: October 15, 2008
Latest date: Until class is full

Applicant's Response to Acceptance
Offer – Maximum Time: Two weeks

Requests for Deferred
Entrance Considered: Yes

Deposit to Hold Place in Class: Yes
Deposit (Resident): $100
Deposit (Non-Resident): $100
Deposit due: With response to acceptance offer
Applied to tuition: Yes
Deposit refundable: Yes
Refundable by: May 15, 2009

Estimated number of new entrants: 113
EDP: 20, special program: n/a

Start Month/Year: August 2009

Interview Format: Two individual interviews.
Regional interviews are not available.

Other Programs

PREPARATORY PROGRAMS
Postbaccalaureate Program: No
Summer Program: No

COMBINED DEGREE PROGRAMS
Baccalaureate/MD: Yes, www.mc.uky.edu/
meded/bsmd/index.asp
Marlene Sauer, (859) 323-1780,
msauer1@email.uky.edu
MD/MPH: Yes, Kim Scott
(859) 323-6161, kstahlma@email.uky.edu
MD/MBA: No
MD/JD: No
MD/PhD: Yes, www.mc.uky.edu/mdphd/
Marlene Sauer, (859) 323-1780,
msauer1@email.uky.edu

Premedical Coursework

Course	Req.	Rec.	Lab.	Sems.
Inorganic Chemistry	•	•		2
Behavioral Sciences				
Biochemistry		•		
Biology	•	•		2
Biology/Zoology				
Calculus				
College English	•			2
College Mathematics				

Course	Req.	Rec.	Lab.	Sems.
Computer Science				
Genetics				
Humanities		•		
Organic Chemistry	•		•	2
Physics	•		•	2
Psychology				
Social Sciences		•		
Other				

Selection Factors: 2007 Accepted Applicants

Proportion of Accepted Applicants with Relevant Experience (Data Self-Reported to AMCAS®)		
Community Service/Volunteer		72%
Medically-Related Work		82%
Research		73%

Shaded bar represents accepted scores ranging from the 10th percentile to the 90th percentile   **School Median** ●   **National Median** ●

Overall GPA	2.0	2.1	2.2	2.3	2.4	2.5	2.6	2.7	2.8	2.9	3.0	3.1	3.2	3.3	3.4	3.5	3.6	(3.7)	3.8	3.9	4.0
Science GPA	2.0	2.1	2.2	2.3	2.4	2.5	2.6	2.7	2.8	2.9	3.0	3.1	3.2	3.3	3.4	3.5	3.6	(3.7)	3.8	3.9	4.0

MCAT® required: Yes, 100% of 2007 accepted applicants took MCAT®

Verbal Reasoning	3	4	5	6	7	8	9	(10)	11	12	13	14	15
Physical Sciences	3	4	5	6	7	8	9	(10)	11	12	13	14	15
Biological Sciences	3	4	5	6	7	8	9	(10)	(11)	12	13	14	15
Writing Sample			J	K	L	M	N	O	(P)	(Q)	R	S	T

Acceptance & Matriculation Data for 2007–2008 First Year Class

	Resident	Non-Resident	International	Total
Applied	424	1551	107	2082
Interviewed	241	117	9	367
Deferred	2	0	1	3
Matriculants				
Early Assurance Program	n/a	n/a	n/a	n/a
Early Decision Program	18	3	0	21
Baccalaureate/MD	n/a	n/a	n/a	n/a
MD/PhD	1	2	0	3
Matriculated	77	22	4	**103**

Applications accepted from International Applicants: Yes

Specialty Choice

2003, 2004, 2005 Graduates, Specialty Choice (As reported by program directors to GME Track™)	
Anesthesiology	3%
Emergency Medicine	6%
Family Practice	9%
Internal Medicine	17%
Obstetrics/Gynecology	6%
Orthopaedic Surgery	2%
Pediatrics	11%
Psychiatry	6%
Radiology	4%
Surgery	5%

Matriculant Demographics: 2007–2008 First Year Class

Men: 60   **Women:** 43

Matriculants' Self-Reported Race/Ethnicity

Mexican American	0	Korean	0
Cuban	0	Vietnamese	0
Puerto Rican	0	Other Asian	2
Other Hispanic	0	Total Asian	13
Total Hispanic	0	Native American	0
Chinese	4	Black	3
Asian Indian	6	Native Hawaiian	0
Pakistani	0	White	85
Filipino	1	**Unduplicated Number**	
Japanese	0	**of Matriculants**	103

Science and Math Majors: 78%
Matriculants with:
    Baccalaureate degree: 99%
    Graduate degree(s): 9%

Financial Information

Source: 2006–2007 LCME I-B survey
and 2007–2008 AAMC TSF questionnaire

	Residents	Non-Residents
Total Cost of Attendance	$44,500	$65,900
Tuition and Fees	$24,010	$45,413
Other (includes living expenses)	$19,630	$19,627
Health Insurance (can be waived)	$860	$860

Average 2007 Graduate Indebtedness: $115,974
% of Enrolled Students Receiving Aid: 91%

Criminal Background Check

This medical school requires a criminal background check prior to matriculation.

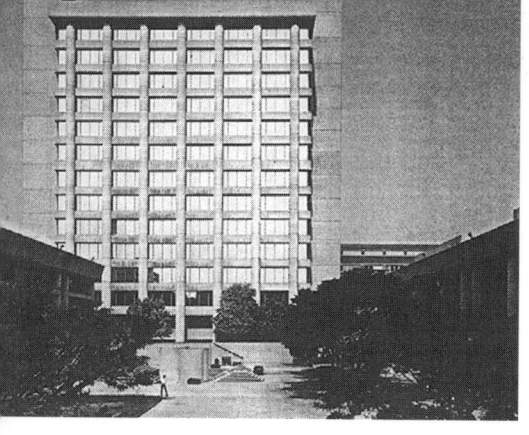

University of Louisville School of Medicine
Louisville, Kentucky

Office of Admissions, School of Medicine
Abell Administration Center
323 East Chestnut, University of Louisville
Louisville, Kentucky 40202-3866
T 502 852 5193   **F** 502 852 0302

Admissions www.louisville.edu/medschool/admissions
Main www.louisville.edu/medschool
Financial www.louisville.edu/medschool/finaid
Email medadm@louisville.edu

Public Institution

Dr. Edward C. Halperin, Dean

*Pamela D. Osborne, Director,
Medical School Admissions*

*Mary Joshua, Associate Director, Office
of Minority and Rural Affairs*

Leslie Kaelin, Director, Financial Aid

*Dr. Stephen F. Wheeler, Associate Dean,
Medical School Admissions*

*Dr. V. Faye Jones, Associate Dean, Office of
Minority and Rural Affairs*

General Information
The School of Medicine was established at the
Louisville Medical Institute in 1833 and became
affiliated with the University of Louisville in
1846. In 1970 the university became a member
of the state system of higher education.

Mission Statement
The University of Louisville School of Medicine's
mission is to excel in the education of physicians
and scientists for careers in teaching, research,
patient care and service, to bring our fundamental discoveries to the bedside, and to be a vital
component in the University's quest to become
a premier, nationally recognized metropolitan
research university.

Curricular Highlights
Community Service Requirement: Optional.
Research/Thesis Requirement: Optional.

The University of Louisville School of Medicine
is committed to training physicians who are
humanistically oriented and patient-centered
and who will meet the diverse health care needs
of Kentucky's citizens. The curriculum is focused
on providing comprehensive exposure to the
fundamental aspects of medicine while retaining
sufficient flexibility for effective development of
an individual student's abilities and interests. It
emphasizes a learning environment that enables
students to maximize their success and prepares
them to achieve their professional goals. Four
goals drive the design, development, implementation and evaluation of our curriculum:

Integration of basic and clinical sciences, within
courses and clinical rotations; Expanded use of
non-lecture teaching and learning modalities
such as directed self-learning, small-group activities, and case-based learning; Expanded use of
technology to support teaching and learning
such as course and clerkship Web sites and
patient simulations; and Development of course
and clerkship learning objectives that support the
overall goals of the Educational Objectives for
the Undergraduate Medical Education Program.

USMLE
Step 1: Required. Students must record a passing
score for promotion.
Step 2: Clinical Skills (CS): Required. Students
must only record a score.
Step 2: Clinical Knowledge (CK): Required.
Students must only record a score.

Selection Factors
The ULSOM is a state institution which gives
preference to residents of Kentucky. International
applicants are only considered if they have both
strong Kentucky ties and a pending permanent
residency application. Applicants are selected
on the basis of their individual merits without
bias concerning sex, race, creed, national origin,
age, or handicap. Applicants are chosen on the
basis of intellect, integrity, maturity, and interpersonal sensitivity. Consideration is given to the
past academic record, college pre-professional
committee evaluations/faculty letters of recommendations, extracurricular activities, and personal interviews held at the medical school and
the Trover Campus.

Financial Aid
Financial needs of the applicant are not a consideration in the selection process. Scholarships
are available on a limited basis and are granted
according to demonstrated financial need, and
scholastic and professional promise.

Information about Diversity Programs
Applications from disadvantaged individuals
and members of groups underrepresented
in medicine are encouraged. Applicants are
reviewed by the full Admissions Committee,

which accepts students on an individual basis.
Selected admitted students have the option to
participate in a summer pre-matriculation program offered through the Office of Minority &
Rural Affairs.

Campus Information

Setting
The ULSOM is located in the heart of downtown
Louisville's medical center. The major acute and
trauma care clinical teaching activities take place
in the 404-bed University Hospital. Within two
blocks are three formally affiliated hospitals:
Kosair Children's Hospital, the only full-service
children's hospital in the state of Kentucky; Jewish
Hospital; and Norton Hospital. Other facilities
include the world-renowned Kentucky Lions Eye
Research Institute; James Graham Brown Cancer
Center; the Veterans Affairs Medical Center; the
Child Evaluation Center; Amelia Brown Frazier
Rehabilitation Center; and the ULSOM Trover
Campus, located in Madisonville, Kentucky.

Enrollment
For 2007, total enrollment was: 600

Special Features
The ULSOM patient simulation center provides students hands-on, risk free learning,
realistic patient encounters and inter-active
self-directed learning. Large portions of the
campus are WI-FI. Additionally, we offer students the opportunity to complete clinical
training in a rural setting at the ULSOM
Trover Campus in Madisonville, Kentucky.

Housing
The U of L medical-dental dormitory/apartment
building is on campus. Non-university housing
listings are available from the Office of Faculty
and Student Advocacy, 502-852-6185.

Satellite Campuses/Facilities
Students rotate at five primary hospital sites; four
sites are within walking distance of the Health
Science Center campus. Interested candidates
may apply for dedicated admission to complete
clinical training at the ULSOM Trover Campus
in Madisonville, Kentucky.

Application Process and Requirements 2009–2010

Primary Application Service: AMCAS
Earliest filing date: June 1, 2008
Latest filing date: October 15, 2008

Secondary Application Required?: Yes
Sent to: Screened applicants
Contact: medadm@louisville.edu
Fee: Yes, $75
Fee waiver available: Yes
Earliest filing date: July 1, 2008
Latest filing date: December 31, 2008

Latest MCAT® considered: 2008
Oldest MCAT® considered: 2006

Early Decision Program
School does have EDP
Applicants notified: October 1, 2008
EDP available for: Both Residents and Non-Residents

Regular Acceptance Notice
Earliest date: October 16, 2008
Latest date: Varies

Applicant's Response to Acceptance Offer – Maximum Time: Two weeks

Requests for Deferred Entrance Considered: Yes

Deposit to Hold Place in Class: Yes
Deposit (Resident): $100
Deposit (Non-Resident): $100
Deposit due: With acceptance letter.
Applied to tuition: Yes
Deposit refundable: Yes
Refundable by: May 15, 2009

Estimated number of new entrants: 155
EDP: 4, special program: 10

Start Month/Year: August 2009

Interview Format: Academically blind interview with two committee members. Regional interviews are not available.

Other Programs

PREPARATORY PROGRAMS
Postbaccalaureate Program: No
Summer Program: Yes, www.louisville.edu/medschool/ahec/special.programs/ Mary Joshua, (502) 852-7159, specprog@louisville.edu

COMBINED DEGREE PROGRAMS
Baccalaureate/MD: No
MD/MPH: Yes, www.louisville.edu/medschool/curr/md_combined.htm
MD/MBA: Yes, Toni Ganzel, M.D., M.B.A., (502) 852-5192, medstuaf@gwise.louisville.edu
MD/JD: No
MD/PhD: Yes, www.louisville.edu/medschool/curr/md_combined.htm
Additional Program: Yes, www.louisville.edu/bioethicsma

Premedical Coursework

Course	Req.	Rec.	Lab.	Sems.
Inorganic Chemistry	•	•		2
Behavioral Sciences				
Biochemistry		•		1
Biology	•	•		2
Biology/Zoology				
Calculus	•			1
College English	•			2
College Mathematics		•		2

Course	Req.	Rec.	Lab.	Sems.
Computer Science				
Genetics		•		1
Humanities				
Organic Chemistry	•	•	•	2
Physics	•	•	•	2
Psychology				
Social Sciences				
Physiology		•		1
Statistics		•		1

Selection Factors: 2007 Accepted Applicants

Proportion of Accepted Applicants with Relevant Experience (Data Self-Reported to AMCAS®)		
Community Service/Volunteer		67%
Medically-Related Work		76%
Research		69%

Shaded bar represents accepted scores ranging from the 10th percentile to the 90th percentile. School Median ● National Median ●

Overall GPA	2.0	2.1	2.2	2.3	2.4	2.5	2.6	2.7	2.8	2.9	3.0	3.1	3.2	3.3	3.4	3.5	3.6	(3.7)	3.8	3.9	4.0
Science GPA	2.0	2.1	2.2	2.3	2.4	2.5	2.6	2.7	2.8	2.9	3.0	3.1	3.2	3.3	3.4	3.5	3.6	(3.7)	3.8	3.9	4.0

MCAT® required: Yes, 100% of 2007 accepted applicants took MCAT®

Verbal Reasoning	3	4	5	6	7	8	9	(10)	11	12	13	14	15
Physical Sciences	3	4	5	6	7	8	9	(10)	(11)	12	13	14	15
Biological Sciences	3	4	5	6	7	8	9	(10)	(11)	12	13	14	15
Writing Sample			J	K	L	M	N	O	(P)	(Q)	R	S	T

Acceptance & Matriculation Data for 2007–2008 First Year Class

	Resident	Non-Resident	International	Total
Applied	411	1763	20	2194
Interviewed	276	93	0	369
Deferred	1	1	0	2
Matriculants				
Early Assurance Program	4	0	0	4
Early Decision Program	0	0	0	0
Baccalaureate/MD	n/a	n/a	n/a	n/a
MD/PhD	2	0	0	2
Matriculated	119	29	0	**148**

Applications accepted from International Applicants: No

Specialty Choice

2003, 2004, 2005 Graduates, Specialty Choice (As reported by program directors to GME Track™)

Anesthesiology	7%
Emergency Medicine	5%
Family Practice	7%
Internal Medicine	17%
Obstetrics/Gynecology	5%
Orthopaedic Surgery	4%
Pediatrics	12%
Psychiatry	5%
Radiology	6%
Surgery	7%

Matriculant Demographics: 2007–2008 First Year Class

Men: 81   **Women:** 67

Matriculants' Self-Reported Race/Ethnicity

Mexican American	0	Korean	1
Cuban	0	Vietnamese	2
Puerto Rican	0	Other Asian	1
Other Hispanic	1	Total Asian	17
Total Hispanic	1	Native American	0
Chinese	0	Black	10
Asian Indian	13	Native Hawaiian	1
Pakistani	0	White	123
Filipino	0	Unduplicated Number	
Japanese	0	of Matriculants	148

Science and Math Majors: 76%
Matriculants with:
Baccalaureate degree: 99%
Graduate degree(s): 9%

Financial Information

Source: 2006–2007 LCME I-B survey and 2007–2008 AAMC TSF questionnaire

	Residents	Non-Residents
Total Cost of Attendance	$42,058	$62,404
Tuition and Fees	$23,079	$43,425
Other (includes living expenses)	$17,359	$17,359
Health Insurance (can be waived)	$1,620	$1,620

Average 2007 Graduate Indebtedness: $124,604
% of Enrolled Students Receiving Aid: 92%

Criminal Background Check

This medical school requires a criminal background check prior to matriculation.

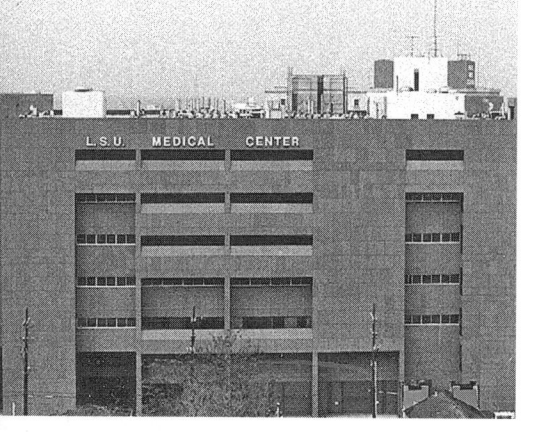

Louisiana State University
School of Medicine in New Orleans

New Orleans, Louisiana

Admissions Office, Louisiana State University
School of Medicine in New Orleans
1901 Perdido Street, Box P3-4
New Orleans, Louisiana 70112-1393
T 504 568 6262   F 504 568 7701

Admissions www.medschool.lsuhsc.edu/admissions
Main www.medschool.lsuhsc.edu
Financial www.medschool.lsuhsc.edu/
admissions/aid.asp
Email ms-admissions@lsuhsc.edu

Public Institution

Dr. Steve Nelson, Dean

*Dr. Sam G. McClugage Jr.,
Associate Dean for Admissions*

*Dr. Edward Helm, Associate Dean, Office of
Community and Minority Health Education*

*Patrick Gorman, Director of
Student Financial Aid*

General Information

LSU School of Medicine in New Orleans was established in 1931 in downtown New Orleans. During the past two decades, several new buildings have been erected, including a state-of-the-art Student Learning Center which includes procedural and simulation labs, a computer lounge, and large and small-group meeting rooms. A new residence facility, Stanislaus Hall, containing a comprehensive fitness center, is among the more recent additions to the campus.

Mission Statement

The LSUSOM is dedicated to providing the opportunity for an excellent medical education to all Louisiana applicants who are prepared to benefit from its curriculum and instruction. To this end, the Admissions Committee will strive to recruit and admit residents from Louisiana from every geographic, economic, social, and cultural dimension of the state of Louisiana.

Curricular Highlights

Community Service Requirement: Required.
Research/Thesis Requirement: Optional.

The first two years of the medical school curriculum emphasize several basic sciences and their relevance to clinical medicine. Clinical experiences begin in the first year in courses such as Science and Practice of Medicine. The second year of medical school utilizes an integrated approach to the teaching of basic science and pre-clinical courses within an environment that fosters an early exposure to patient care. Clerkships begin in the third year where students rotate through the various clinical disciplines. In the fourth year, students are given several months for electives in addition to required rotations in Ambulatory Medicine, Acting Internships, etc. Some of these rotations can be completed at the institutions associated with the LSU School of Medicine throughout the state or at other approved institutions outside the state or country. Computer-assisted instruction is an important component of the curriculum. Entering students are required to purchase laptop computers.

USMLE

Step 1: Required. Students must record a passing score for promotion.
Step 2: Clinical Skills (CS): Required. Students must only record a score.
Step 2: Clinical Knowledge (CK): Required. Students must record a passing total score to graduate.

Selection Factors

Candidates are encouraged to contact the Office of Admissions for a brochure which summarizes the selection process for LSU School of Medicine in New Orleans.

Financial Aid

Financial assistance is available for students through several different methods. There are direct scholarship programs, scholarships for disadvantaged students, state and federal loan programs, work-study programs, and employment opportunities in the New Orleans area for students in their third and fourth years. Financial assistance information is available from the Student Financial Aid Office at (504) 568-4820.

Information about Diversity Programs

Members of groups underrepresented in medicine are encouraged to apply. The School of Medicine's Office of Community and Minority Health Education actively recruits students from groups underrepresented in medicine and provides counseling for high school and college students. Further information may be obtained by contacting Dr. Edward Helm, Associate Dean for Community and Minority Health Education, at (504) 568-8501.

Campus Information

Setting

LSU School of Medicine is located in downtown New Orleans in a medical corridor which is within walking distance of the historic French Quarter, museums, shopping districts, and two sports arenas for professional football and basketball teams.

Enrollment

For 2007, total enrollment was: 697

Special Features

The interdisciplinary Science and Practice of Medicine course and the Isidore Cohn Learning Center were both created to provide a more innovative way for the clinical teaching of students beginning in the first year. The Learning Center includes over 14,000 square feet of space, small-group teaching rooms, simulation laboratories, a computer center, and meeting rooms. More information is available at *www.medschool.lsuhsc.edu/learning_center/*.

Housing

Two recently renovated student housing facilities are available. Furnished and unfurnished apartments are available for married (with or without children) and single students. Many students choose to rent apartments in New Orleans or the surrounding metropolitan area. Lists of available apartments are supplied upon request.

Satellite Campuses/Facilities

LSU School of Medicine rotates its students among one of several public hospitals, mainly in New Orleans, Baton Rouge, or Lafayette, LA, as well as several private hospitals such as Children's Hospital in the city of New Orleans. The LSU Health Care Services Division has oversight for eight public teaching hospitals in the State of Louisiana in which many LSUSOM medical students, residents and fellows receive training. Several clinics in the metropolitan area and around the state are also similarly used for the training of health care professionals.

Application Process and Requirements 2009–2010

Primary Application Service: AMCAS
Earliest filing date: June 1, 2008
Latest filing date: November 30, 2008

Secondary Application Required?: Yes
Sent to: All applicants
URL: www.medschool.lsuhsc.edu/admissions/secondary_application
Fee: Yes, $50
Fee waiver available: Yes
Earliest filing date: June 15, 2008
Latest filing date: January 15, 2009

Latest MCAT® considered: September 2008
Oldest MCAT® considered: August 2005

Early Decision Program
School does have EDP
Applicants notified: October 1, 2008
EDP available for: Both Residents and Non-Residents

Regular Acceptance Notice
Earliest date: October 15, 2008
Latest date: Varies

Applicant's Response to Acceptance Offer – Maximum Time: Two weeks

Requests for Deferred Entrance Considered: Yes

Deposit to Hold Place in Class: Yes
Deposit (Resident): $100
Deposit (Non-Resident): $100
Deposit due: due with acceptance offer
Applied to tuition: Yes
Deposit refundable: Yes
Refundable by: May 15, 2009

Estimated number of new entrants: 180
EDP: 10, special program: n/a

Start Month/Year: August 2009

Interview Format: Three one-on-one interviews. Regional interviews are not available.

Other Programs

PREPARATORY PROGRAMS
Postbaccalaureate Program: Yes
http://graduatestudies.lsuhsc.edu/
Summer Program: No

COMBINED DEGREE PROGRAMS
Baccalaureate/MD: No
MD/MPH: Yes, http://publichealth.lsuhsc.edu/
MD/MBA: No
MD/JD: No
MD/PhD: Yes, http://graduatestudies.lsuhsc.edu/
Additional Program: Yes, Rural Scholars' Track
Cathie Stuckey, (504) 568-6262
ms-admissions@lsuhsc.edu

Premedical Coursework

Course	Req.	Rec.	Lab.	Hrs.
Inorganic Chemistry	•		•	8
Behavioral Sciences		•		
Biochemistry		•		
Biology		•		
Biology/Zoology	•		•	8
Calculus				
College English	•			6
College Mathematics		•		

Course	Req.	Rec.	Lab.	Hrs.
Computer Science		•		
Genetics		•		
Humanities		•		
Organic Chemistry	•		•	8
Physics	•		•	8
Psychology				
Social Sciences				
Other				

Selection Factors: 2007 Accepted Applicants

Proportion of Accepted Applicants with Relevant Experience (Data Self-Reported to AMCAS®)		
Community Service/Volunteer		70%
Medically-Related Work		79%
Research		62%

Shaded bar represents accepted scores ranging from the 10th percentile to the 90th percentile. **School Median** ● **National Median** ●

Overall GPA	2.0	2.1	2.2	2.3	2.4	2.5	2.6	2.7	2.8	2.9	3.0	3.1	3.2	3.3	3.4	3.5	3.6	(3.7)	3.8	3.9	4.0
Science GPA	2.0	2.1	2.2	2.3	2.4	2.5	2.6	2.7	2.8	2.9	3.0	3.1	3.2	3.3	3.4	3.5	3.6	(3.7)	3.8	3.9	4.0

MCAT® required: Yes, 100% of 2007 accepted applicants took MCAT®

Verbal Reasoning	3	4	5	6	7	8	(9)	(10)	11	12	13	14	15
Physical Sciences	3	4	5	6	7	8	(9)	10	(11)	12	13	14	15
Biological Sciences	3	4	5	6	7	8	9	(10)	(11)	12	13	14	15
Writing Sample				J	K	L	M	N	(O)	P	(Q)	R	S	T

Acceptance & Matriculation Data for 2007–2008 First Year Class

	Resident	Non-Resident	International	Total
Applied	638	727	49	1414
Interviewed	387	14	2	403
Deferred	3	0	0	3
Matriculants				
Early Assurance Program	0	0	0	0
Early Decision Program	9	0	0	9
Baccalaureate/MD	n/a	n/a	n/a	n/a
MD/PhD	3	4	0	7
Matriculated	170	9	0	**179**

Applications accepted from International Applicants: Yes

Specialty Choice

2003, 2004, 2005 Graduates, Specialty Choice (As reported by program directors to GME Track™)	
Anesthesiology	6%
Emergency Medicine	5%
Family Practice	7%
Internal Medicine	15%
Obstetrics/Gynecology	6%
Orthopaedic Surgery	5%
Pediatrics	7%
Psychiatry	2%
Radiology	7%
Surgery	8%

Matriculant Demographics: 2007–2008 First Year Class

Men: 98   **Women:** 81

Matriculants' Self-Reported Race/Ethnicity

Mexican American	3	Korean	1
Cuban	0	Vietnamese	3
Puerto Rican	0	Other Asian	2
Other Hispanic	3	Total Asian	17
Total Hispanic	6	Native American	1
Chinese	2	Black	11
Asian Indian	8	Native Hawaiian	3
Pakistani	1	White	153
Filipino	0	Unduplicated Number	
Japanese	0	of Matriculants	179

Science and Math Majors: 78%
Matriculants with:
    Baccalaureate degree: 99%
    Graduate degree(s): 12%

Financial Information

Source: 2006–2007 LCME I-B survey and 2007–2008 AAMC TSF questionnaire

	Residents	Non-Residents
Total Cost of Attendance	$37,431	$51,579
Tuition and Fees	$12,866	$27,014
Other (includes living expenses)	$23,305	$23,305
Health Insurance (can be waived)	$1,260	$1,260

Average 2007 Graduate Indebtedness: $121,509
% of Enrolled Students Receiving Aid: 89%

Criminal Background Check

This medical school does not require a criminal background check prior to matriculation.

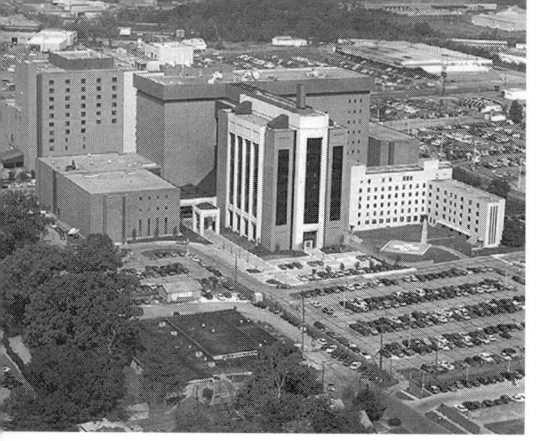

Louisiana State University Health Sciences Center School of Medicine in Shreveport

Shreveport, Louisiana

Office of Student Admissions
Louisiana State University Health Sciences Center
LSU School of Medicine, Office of Student Admissions
P.O. Box 33932, Shreveport, Louisiana 71130-3932
T 318 675 5190 **F** 318 675 8690

Admissions www.admissions.lsuhsc.edu
Main www.sh.lsuhsc.edu/index.html
Financial http://sh-aux.lsuhsc.edu/financialaid/Home2.htm
Email shvadm@lsuhsc.edu

Public Institution

Dr. John C. McDonald, Chancellor and Dean

Dr. F. Scott Kennedy, Assistant Dean for Student Admissions

Shirley Roberson, Director for Multicultural Affairs

Sherry Gladney, Director of Student Financial Aid

Warren E. Cockerham, Registrar

Jacquline Hatcher, Coordinator of Student Admissions

General Information

The LSU Health Sciences Center in Shreveport (LSUHSC-S) provides education, research, patient care services, and community outreach. Educating health professionals and scientists at all levels, its major responsibility includes the advancement and dissemination of knowledge in medicine and the basic sciences. It also provides vital public service through its hospital and clinics.

Mission Statement

LSUHSC-S has a dual mission: to assure the availability of acute and primary health care services to the uninsured, to the underinsured, and to others with problems of access to medical care, and to serve as the principal site for the clinical education of future doctors and other health care professionals.

Curricular Highlights

Community Service Requirement: Optional. Community service is highly desirable.
Research/Thesis Requirement: Optional. Desirable, but not required.

The modern curriculum thoroughly integrates medical issues and applications in the first two years, during which the basic sciences are emphasized. Recently, didactic lecture hours were cut dramatically, and small-group, active-learning experiences were dramatically increased. The overall effect was decreased contact hours and increased self-directed learning. All essential basic-science concepts traditionally taught in the first two years are now integrated with clinical examples, clinical cases and standardized patient experiences. The required clerkships occur in the third year, and the fourth year is devoted to electives.

USMLE

Step 1: Required. Students must record a passing score for promotion.
Step 2: Clinical Skills (CS): Required. Students must only record a score.
Step 2: Clinical Knowledge (CK): Required. Students must only record a score.

Selection Factors

Admission is based upon character, motivation, intellectual ability, and achievement as judged by recommendations of premedical advisors, personal interviews with members of the faculty at the School of Medicine, college grades, and MCAT® scores. In recent years, the number of applications filed by well-qualified residents of Louisiana has exceeded the number of places available. For this reason, places have not been offered to nonresidents. Determination of state residence is determined by LSU system regulations. Twenty-four colleges are represented in the 2007 entering class. The School of Medicine in Shreveport does not discriminate in applicant selection on the basis of race, sex, creed, national origin, age, or handicap.

Financial Aid

Scholarships and long-term, low-interest loan funds are available to students with financial need. In the past, no accepted students have been unable to meet their financial needs. Scholarships and loans are available to students in all four years and are based on applicants' showing verified need. Certain awards are given in recognition primarily of academic accomplishment and promise. The school offers summer employment to many students, but does not advise employment during school sessions, which would interfere with academic performance. Financial need has no bearing on an applicant's acceptance. Applications for financial assistance are furnished by the Financial Aid Office after applicants have been accepted.

Information about Diversity Programs

Applications from students from groups underrepresented in medicine are encouraged and will be given every consideration. All students are encouraged to take advantage of the services provided by the Office of Multicultural Affairs. They include a pre-matriculation program, an MCAT® preparation course, and a summer research program for high school students, as well as informal counseling for medical students and applicants.

Campus Information

Setting
The medical school is located near the intersection of I-49 and I-20, in a peaceful neighborhood near the geographic center of Shreveport. Thus, affordable housing is available within a short commute.

Enrollment
For 2007, total enrollment was: 444

Special Features
The hospital includes an Adult Level-One Trauma Center, a Level-One Pediatric Trauma Center and a Pediatric ICU, as well as all features of a tertiary care hospital.

Satellite Campuses/Facilities
The school is affiliated with other local and regional hospitals.

Application Process and Requirements 2009–2010

Primary Application Service: AMCAS
Earliest filing date: June 1, 2008
Latest filing date: November 1, 2008

Secondary Application Required?: Yes
Sent to: All Louisiana applicants
URL: Provided by school
Student Admissions, (318) 675-5190
shvadm@lsuhsc.edu
Fee: Yes, $50
Fee waiver available: Yes
Earliest filing date: June 1, 2008
Latest filing date: December 15, 2008

Latest MCAT® considered: September 2008
Oldest MCAT® considered: August 2005

Early Decision Program
School does have EDP
Applicants notified: October 1, 2008
EDP available for: Residents only

Regular Acceptance Notice
Earliest date: October 17, 2008
Latest date: Until class is full

Applicant's Response to Acceptance
Offer – Maximum Time: Two weeks

Requests for Deferred
Entrance Considered: Yes

Deposit to Hold Place in Class: Yes
Deposit (Resident): $250
Deposit (Non-Resident): $250
Deposit due: May 15, 2009
Applied to tuition: Yes
Deposit refundable: Yes
Refundable by: May 15, 2009

Estimated number of new entrants: 118
EDP: 12, special program: n/a

Start Month/Year: July 31, 2009

Interview Format: Two closed file and one open file, non-stress interviews. Regional interviews are not available.

Other Programs

PREPARATORY PROGRAMS
Postbaccalaureate Program: No
Summer Program: Yes
Shirley Roberson, (318) 675-5049

COMBINED DEGREE PROGRAMS
Baccalaureate/MD: No
MD/MPH: No
MD/MBA: No
MD/JD: No
MD/PhD: Yes,
www.admissions.lsuhsc.edu

Premedical Coursework

Course	Req.	Rec.	Lab.	Hrs.	Course	Req.	Rec.	Lab.	Hrs.
Inorganic Chemistry	•		•	8	Computer Science				
Behavioral Sciences					Genetics		•		6
Biochemistry		•		6	Humanities				
Biology					Organic Chemistry	•		•	8
Biology/Zoology	•		•	8	Physics	•		•	8
Calculus					Psychology				
College English	•			6	Social Sciences				
College Mathematics					Other Science	•		•	6

Selection Factors: 2007 Accepted Applicants

Proportion of Accepted Applicants with Relevant Experience (Data Self-Reported to AMCAS®)		
Community Service/Volunteer		72%
Medically-Related Work		81%
Research		61%

Shaded bar represents accepted scores ranging from the 10th percentile to the 90th percentile.   School Median ●   National Median ●

Overall GPA	2.0	2.1	2.2	2.3	2.4	2.5	2.6	2.7	2.8	2.9	3.0	3.1	3.2	3.3	3.4	3.5	3.6	3.7	(3.8)	3.9	4.0
Science GPA	2.0	2.1	2.2	2.3	2.4	2.5	2.6	2.7	2.8	2.9	3.0	3.1	3.2	3.3	3.4	3.5	3.6	(3.7)	3.8	3.9	4.0

MCAT® required: Yes, 100% of 2007 accepted applicants took MCAT®

Verbal Reasoning	3	4	5	6	7	8	(9)	(10)	11	12	13	14	15
Physical Sciences	3	4	5	6	7	8	(9)	10	(11)	12	13	14	15
Biological Sciences	3	4	5	6	7	8	9	(10)	(11)	12	13	14	15
Writing Sample			J	K	L	M	N	(O)	P	(Q)	R	S	T

Acceptance & Matriculation Data for 2007–2008 First Year Class

	Resident	Non-Resident	International	Total
Applied	610	383	11	1004
Interviewed	224	1	0	226
Deferred	0	0	0	0
Matriculants				
Early Assurance Program	n/a	n/a	n/a	n/a
Early Decision Program	16	0	0	16
Baccalaureate/MD	n/a	n/a	n/a	n/a
MD/PhD	0	0	0	0
Matriculated	117	0	0	**117**

Applications accepted from International Applicants: No

Specialty Choice

2003, 2004, 2005 Graduates, Specialty Choice (As reported by program directors to GME Track™)	
Anesthesiology	5%
Emergency Medicine	7%
Family Practice	11%
Internal Medicine	14%
Obstetrics/Gynecology	10%
Orthopaedic Surgery	2%
Pediatrics	7%
Psychiatry	2%
Radiology	4%
Surgery	10%

Matriculant Demographics: 2007–2008 First Year Class

Men: 71   **Women:** 46

Matriculants' Self-Reported Race/Ethnicity

Mexican American	1	Korean	1
Cuban	1	Vietnamese	2
Puerto Rican	1	Other Asian	0
Other Hispanic	1	Total Asian	7
Total Hispanic	3	Native American	0
Chinese	0	Black	7
Asian Indian	2	Native Hawaiian	0
Pakistani	1	White	106
Filipino	0	Unduplicated Number	
Japanese	1	of Matriculants	117

Science and Math Majors: 92%
Matriculants with:
Baccalaureate degree: 99%
Graduate degree(s): 6%

Financial Information

Source: 2006–2007 LCME I-B survey
and 2007–2008 AAMC TSF questionnaire

	Residents	Non-Residents
Total Cost of Attendance	$35,339	$49,487
Tuition and Fees	$10,458	$24,606
Other (includes living expenses)	$23,299	$23,299
Health Insurance (can be waived)	$1,582	$1,582

Average 2007 Graduate Indebtedness: $111,605
% of Enrolled Students Receiving Aid: 87%

Criminal Background Check

This medical school requires a criminal background check prior to matriculation.

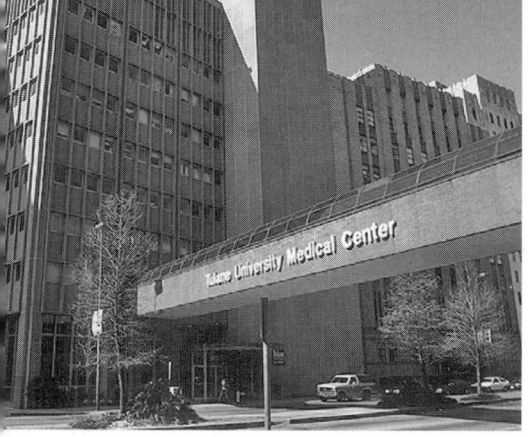

Tulane University School of Medicine

New Orleans, Louisiana

Office of Admissions and Student Affairs
Tulane University School of Medicine
1430 Tulane Avenue, SL67
New Orleans, Louisiana 70112-2699
T 504 988 5187   F 504 988 6735

Admissions www.mcl.tulane.edu/admissions
Main www.mcl.tulane.edu
Financial www.finaidhsc.tulane.edu
Email medsch@tulane.edu

Private Institution

Dr. Benjamin Sachs, Dean

Dr. Marc J. Kahn, Senior Associate Dean for Admissions and Student Affairs

Dr. Ernest Steed, Assistant Dean for Student Affairs

Dr. Barbara S. Beckman, Assistant Dean for Admissions

Michael T. Goodman, Director of Financial Aid

General Information

Tulane University School of Medicine, a private, nonsectarian institution, was founded in 1834. Today it is one of the eleven colleges comprising Tulane University and is the 15th oldest medical school in the U.S.

Mission Statement

Tulane has a rich tradition of education characterized by an environment that is both supportive and enriching in every sense. It strives to present the ideal environment for preparing students to be expert and compassionate clinicians.

Curricular Highlights

Community Service Requirement: Required.
Research/Thesis Requirement: Optional.

Tulane School of Medicine offers a four-year program leading to the M.D. degree. While the emphasis in the first two years is on the principles of the basic medical sciences, the goal of the first two years is helping students develop clinical problem-solving skills instead of emphasizing the transmission of facts devoid of clinical context. The program in Foundations in Medicine, which spans the first two years, is responsible for instructing students in the complex art and science of the patient-doctor interaction. This objective is accomplished through lectures, small-group discussions, clinical demonstrations, visits to community health facilities, and interactions with both real patients and individuals trained as patient instructors. The third and fourth years provide experience in clinical settings where the emphasis is on patient care

and community health. Flexibility is attained throughout the four years by designating approximately one-third of scheduled curriculum time for elective courses and selected advanced studies. The curriculum is under constant review by faculty and students. Tulane offers a wide variety of support systems for medical students, including test-taking skills workshops.

USMLE

Step 1: Required. Students must only record a score.
Step 2: Clinical Skills (CS): Required. Students must record a passing total score to graduate.
Step 2: Clinical Knowledge (CK): Required. Students must record a passing total score to graduate.

Selection Factors

In evaluating applicants, the Committee on Admissions relies on such criteria as grade point averages, MCAT® scores, faculty appraisals from the applicant's college, special accomplishments and talents, and the substance and level of courses taken in a particular college. Tulane has not established mandatory minimal MCAT® or GPA scores, as all components of the application, cognitive and non-cognitive, are taken into account.

Financial Aid

Scholarships and loans (federal, private, and Tulane programs) are available to students based on an analysis of the individual's financial needs. Additionally, each year approximately 25 students are awarded scholarships, which are based exclusively upon academic merit.

Information about Diversity Programs

Tulane encourages qualified disadvantaged students and students from groups underrepresented in medicine to apply. Special activities available for, but not limited to, students from groups underrepresented in medicine include tutorial and counseling services for students in medical school. The diversity in composition of the members of the Committee on Admissions is reflected in the composition of the medical student body.

Campus Information

Setting

Tulane University School of Medicine is located in downtown New Orleans, a few blocks from the New Orleans Superdome and the French Quarter.

Enrollment

For 2007, total enrollment was: 627

Special Features

The School of Medicine and the Tulane University Hospital and Clinic are two components of the Tulane University Health Sciences Center. Other components of the Center include: the School of Public Health and Tropical Medicine, the Tulane/Xavier Center for Bioenvironmental Research, the Tulane National Primate Research Center, and the F. Edward Hebert Research Center. Twelve Centers of Excellence include the Depaul-Tulane Behavioral Health Center, Tulane Cancer Center, Tulane Center for Abdominal Transplant, Tulane Institute of Sports Medicine, Tulane-Xavier National Women's Center, Tulane Center for Gene Therapy, and Tulane Cardio-Vascular Center of Excellence.

Housing

Reasonably priced housing of all kinds is widely available, including the Deming Pavilion student residence, which is adjacent to the Tulane University Hospital and Clinic and across the street from the medical school.

Satellite Campuses/Facilities

Tulane School of Medicine has affiliation agreements with more than 10 hospitals and clinics in New Orleans and other communities; four of its principal clinical teaching facilities are in close proximity to the School of Medicine: the Medical Center of Louisiana in New Orleans (Charity Hospitals), University Hospital (a Charity Hospital), Veterans Affairs Medical Center, and the Tulane University Hospital and Clinic.

Application Process and Requirements 2009–2010

Primary Application Service: AMCAS
Earliest filing date: June 1, 2008
Latest filing date: December 15, 2008

Secondary Application Required?: Yes
Sent to: All applicants
URL: www.som.tulane.edu/departments/admissions/Secondary_App/Tulane_Secondary_App.pdf
Fee: Yes, $95
Fee waiver available: No
Earliest filing date: June 1, 2008
Latest filing date: January 15, 2009

Latest MCAT® considered: August 2008
Oldest MCAT® considered: 2004

Early Decision Program
School does have EDP
Applicants notified: October 15, 2008
EDP available for: Both Residents and Non-Residents

Regular Acceptance Notice
Earliest date: October 16, 2008
Latest date: Until class is full

Applicant's Response to Acceptance Offer – Maximum Time: Two weeks

Requests for Deferred Entrance Considered: Yes

Deposit to Hold Place in Class: Yes
Deposit (Resident): $500
Deposit (Non-Resident): $500
Deposit due: May 15, 2009
Applied to tuition: Yes
Deposit refundable: Yes
Refundable by: May 15, 2009

Estimated number of new entrants: 175
EDP: 10, special program: n/a

Start Month/Year: August 2009

Interview Format: Selected applicants are invited for interviews. Regional interviews are not available.

Other Programs

PREPARATORY PROGRAMS
Postbaccalaureate Program: Yes, www.som/tulane.edu/anatomy/acpinfo.htm
Summer Program: No
Master of Science in Pharmacology: www.pharmacology.tulane.edu
Master of Science in Genetics: www.som.tulane.edu/human_genetics/masters.html
COMBINED DEGREE PROGRAMS
Baccalaureate/MD: No
MD/MPH: Yes, www.mdmph.tulane.edu
MD/MBA: Yes, Marc Kahn, M.D.
(504) 988-5187, mkahn@tulane.edu
MD/JD: No
MD/PhD: Yes, www.som.tulane.edu/psp
Charles Hemenway, M.D., Ph.D.
(504) 988-5412, chemenw@tulane.edu

Premedical Coursework

Course	Req.	Rec.	Lab.	Hrs.	Course	Req.	Rec.	Lab.	Hrs.
Inorganic Chemistry	•		•	6	Computer Science				
Behavioral Sciences					Genetics				
Biochemistry					Humanities				
Biology					Organic Chemistry	•		•	6
Biology/Zoology	•		•	6	Physics	•		•	6
Calculus					Psychology				
College English	•			6	Social Sciences				
College Mathematics					Other				

Selection Factors: 2007 Accepted Applicants

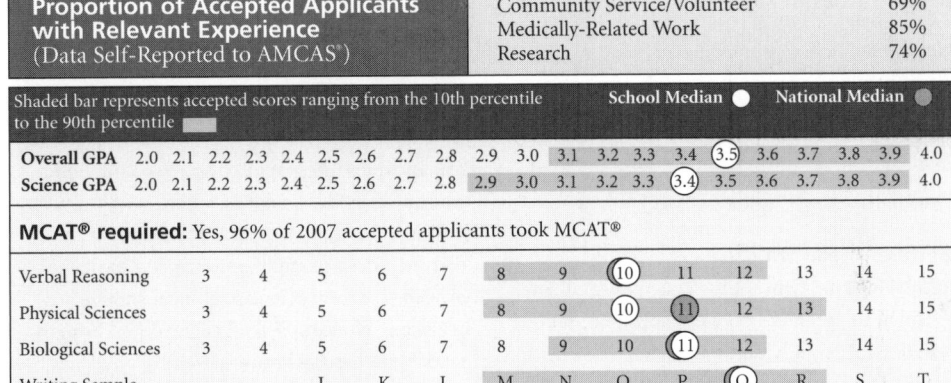

Proportion of Accepted Applicants with Relevant Experience (Data Self-Reported to AMCAS®)		
Community Service/Volunteer		69%
Medically-Related Work		85%
Research		74%

Shaded bar represents accepted scores ranging from the 10th percentile to the 90th percentile. **School Median** ● **National Median** ●

Overall GPA	2.0	2.1	2.2	2.3	2.4	2.5	2.6	2.7	2.8	2.9	3.0	3.1	3.2	3.3	3.4	(3.5)	3.6	3.7	3.8	3.9	4.0
Science GPA	2.0	2.1	2.2	2.3	2.4	2.5	2.6	2.7	2.8	2.9	3.0	3.1	3.2	3.3	(3.4)	3.5	3.6	3.7	3.8	3.9	4.0

MCAT® required: Yes, 96% of 2007 accepted applicants took MCAT®

Verbal Reasoning	3	4	5	6	7	8	9	(10)	11	12	13	14	15
Physical Sciences	3	4	5	6	7	8	9	(10)	(11)	12	13	14	15
Biological Sciences	3	4	5	6	7	8	9	10	(11)	12	13	14	15
Writing Sample				J	K	L	M	N	O	P	(Q)	R	S	T

Acceptance & Matriculation Data for 2007–2008 First Year Class

	Resident	Non-Resident	International	Total
Applied	473	6109	218	6800
Interviewed	141	1023	12	1176
Deferred	0	9	1	10
Matriculants				
Early Assurance Program	11	1	0	12
Early Decision Program	4	4	0	8
Baccalaureate/MD	n/a	n/a	n/a	n/a
MD/PhD	2	7	0	9
Matriculated	36	137	2	**175**

Applications accepted from International Applicants: Yes

Specialty Choice

2003, 2004, 2005 Graduates, Specialty Choice (As reported by program directors to GME Track™)	
Anesthesiology	6%
Emergency Medicine	6%
Family Practice	7%
Internal Medicine	16%
Obstetrics/Gynecology	6%
Orthopaedic Surgery	5%
Pediatrics	8%
Psychiatry	5%
Radiology	6%
Surgery	8%

Matriculant Demographics: 2007–2008 First Year Class

Men: 94　　　　**Women:** 81

Matriculants' Self-Reported Race/Ethnicity

Mexican American	0	Korean	1
Cuban	0	Vietnamese	8
Puerto Rican	0	Other Asian	5
Other Hispanic	2	Total Asian	37
Total Hispanic	2	Native American	0
Chinese	13	Black	6
Asian Indian	7	Native Hawaiian	1
Pakistani	2	White	132
Filipino	2	**Unduplicated Number**	
Japanese	4	**of Matriculants**	175

Science and Math Majors: 63%
Matriculants with:
　Baccalaureate degree: 99%
　Graduate degree(s): 23%

Financial Information

Source: 2006–2007 LCME I-B survey and 2007–2008 AAMC TSF questionnaire

	Residents	Non-Residents
Total Cost of Attendance	$66,160	$66,160
Tuition and Fees	$45,080	$45,080
Other (includes living expenses)	$19,187	$19,187
Health Insurance (can be waived)	$1,893	$1,893

Average 2007 Graduate Indebtedness: $175,598
% of Enrolled Students Receiving Aid: 84%

Criminal Background Check

This medical school does not require a criminal background check prior to matriculation.

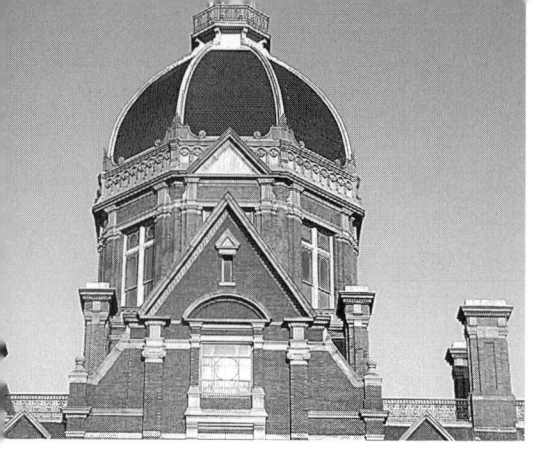

Johns Hopkins University School of Medicine

Baltimore, Maryland

Committee on Admission
Johns Hopkins University School of Medicine
733 North Broadway, Suite G-49
Baltimore, Maryland 21205
T 410 955 3182   **F** 410 955 7494

Admissions www.hopkinsmedicine.org/admissions
Main www.hopkinsmedicine.org/som
Financial www.hopkinsmedicine.org/
admissions/afford.html
Email somadmiss@jhmi.edu

Private Institution

Dr. Edward D. Miller, Dean and Chief Executive

*Dr. James L. Weiss,
Associate Dean for Admissions*

*Hermione Hicks, Assistant Dean
for Admissions*

*Dr. Thomas Koenig, Associate Dean
for Student Affairs*

Terra Jones, Director, Financial Aid

General Information

Johns Hopkins University School of Medicine, founded in 1893, is a private, nondenominational institution which fosters the training of medical practitioners, teachers, and biomedical scientists. The medical center provides library facilities, the Reed Residence Hall, off-campus housing assistance, cafeterias, recreational sports in the Cooley Center, and performing arts programs. Preclinical courses are given in the adjacent basic science complex. Medical care facilities such as the Johns Hopkins Hospital and the Outpatient Center provide an extensive and diverse patient base for the teaching of all clinical subjects. Students also attend educational programs conducted at community hospitals in Baltimore and pursue elective experiences at other medical schools in the U.S. and foreign countries.

Mission Statement

The Johns Hopkins University School of Medicine is dedicated to preparing students to practice compassionate medicine of the highest standards and to contributing to the advancement of medical knowledge.

Curricular Highlights

Community Service Requirement: Optional.
Research/Thesis Requirement: Encouraged. Exceptional research opportunities are available.

The curriculum provides sound foundations in basic sciences and clinical medicine while retaining the flexibility required for students to identify and develop diverse career interests. All students receive honors, high pass, pass or fail grades in lieu of letter grades. The M.D. program includes the integration of basic sciences and clinical experiences and the expanded use of case-based, small-group learning sessions. Students have contact with clinical medicine throughout the first year by working with community physicians. The Physician and Society course spans the four-year program. For more information, see *www.hopkins medicine.org*. First Year includes integrated coverage of introductory basic sciences, neuroscience, epidemiology, and introduction to clinical medicine. Second Year includes the study of advanced basic sciences, behavioral sciences, clinical skills, and beginning clerkships. In the Third and Fourth Years, with the assistance of faculty advisors, students develop individualized programs incorporating required clerkships in major clinical areas and electives. Students may use electives for specialized clerkships, research, and public health experiences.

USMLE

Step 1: Required. Students must only record a score.
Step 2: Clinical Skills (CS): Required. Students must only record a score.
Step 2: Clinical Knowledge (CK): Required. Students must only record a score.

Selection Factors

In addition to proven academic competence, previous achievements and activities help the Committee on Admission to evaluate applicants' suitability for medicine. Applicants who have unusual talents, strong humanistic qualities, demonstrated leadership, and creative abilities are sought. There are no residency·requirements for U.S. citizens; applications are invited from candidates in all sections of the country. Students matriculating at Hopkins are required to undergo a criminal background check. Because of space limitations, Hopkins does not admit transfer students. JHU complies with federal and state laws prohibiting discrimination.

Financial Aid

Financial aid in the form of federal and institutional grants and loans is awarded solely on the basis of need. Financial considerations do not influence admission decisions. Parents' financial information is required of all students requesting institutional aid. Students' aid awards fully meet their demonstrated financial need. The cost for living expenses is based on a 12-month budget. Student fellowship stipends are frequently available for projects carried out in summers. Non-U.S. citizens without permanent resident or immigrant visa status are not eligible to receive financial aid. International students must establish an escrow account currently in the amount of $255,000 and subject to change.

Information about Diversity Programs

Johns Hopkins is committed to the enrollment and education of individuals from all disadvantaged groups. The school values having a diverse student population from all areas of the country. Hopkins has an excellent record of enrolling students from groups underrepresented in medicine. For information, write the assistant dean for student affairs.

Campus Information

Setting

The School of Medicine is located in the eastern part of Baltimore, 20 minutes by car from the undergraduate campus and a short walk from the Inner Harbor. Other institutions on the medical campus include the Schools of Public Health and Nursing and the Johns Hopkins Hospital. The 44-acre campus is accessible to other parts of Baltimore by subway and to other Hopkins divisions by a free shuttle provided to students and faculty.

Enrollment

For 2007, total enrollment was: 475

Housing

Students may live in Reed Hall, the primary residence for the School of Medicine. Many students live throughout Baltimore. Rental costs in Baltimore are relatively low.

Application Process and Requirements 2009–2010

Primary Application Service: AMCAS
Earliest filing date: June 1, 2008
Latest filing date: October 15, 2008

Secondary Application Required?: Yes
Sent to: All applicants
URL: www.hopkinsmedicine.org/admissions
Fee: Yes, $75
Fee waiver available: Yes
Earliest filing date: June 1, 2008
Latest filing date: December 1, 2008

Latest MCAT® considered: September 2008
Oldest MCAT® considered: 2005

Early Decision Program
School does have EDP
Applicants notified: October 1, 2008
EDP available for: Both Residents
and Non-Residents

Regular Acceptance Notice
Earliest date: October 15, 2008
Latest date: Varies

Applicant's Response to Acceptance
Offer – Maximum Time: Three weeks

Requests for Deferred
Entrance Considered: Yes

Deposit to Hold Place in Class: No
Deposit (Resident): n/a
Deposit (Non-Resident): n/a
Deposit due: n/a
Applied to tuition: n/a
Deposit refundable: n/a
Refundable by: n/a

Estimated number of new entrants: 120
EDP: 3, special program: n/a

Start Month/Year: August 2009

Interview Format: Interviews are one-one-one.
Regional interview available in limited areas.

Other Programs

PREPARATORY PROGRAMS
Postbaccalaureate Program: Yes,
www.jhu.edu/postbac/
Summer Program: No

COMBINED DEGREE PROGRAMS
Baccalaureate/MD: No
MD/MPH: No
MD/MBA: No
MD/JD: No
MD/PhD: Yes, www.hopkinsmedicine.org/
admissions/dualdegree.html, Sharon Welling,
(410) 955-8543, swellin1@jhmi.edu

Premedical Coursework

Course	Req.	Rec.	Lab.	Hrs.	Course	Req.	Rec.	Lab.	Hrs.
Inorganic Chemistry	•		•	8	Computer Science		•		
Behavioral Sciences					Genetics				
Biochemistry					Humanities				
Biology	•		•	8	Organic Chemistry	•		•	8
Biology/Zoology					Physics	•		•	8
Calculus	•			6	Psychology				
College English					Social Sciences				
College Mathematics					Humanities or Social and Behavioral Sciences	•			24

Selection Factors: 2007 Accepted Applicants

Proportion of Accepted Applicants with Relevant Experience (Data Self-Reported to AMCAS®)		Community Service/Volunteer	67%
		Medically-Related Work	90%
		Research	92%

Shaded bar represents accepted scores ranging from the 10th percentile to the 90th percentile   School Median ●   National Median ●

Overall GPA	2.0	2.1	2.2	2.3	2.4	2.5	2.6	2.7	2.8	2.9	3.0	3.1	3.2	3.3	3.4	3.5	3.6	3.7	3.8	(3.9)	4.0
Science GPA	2.0	2.1	2.2	2.3	2.4	2.5	2.6	2.7	2.8	2.9	3.0	3.1	3.2	3.3	3.4	3.5	3.6	3.7	3.8	(3.9)	4.0

MCAT® required: Yes, 100% of 2007 accepted applicants took MCAT®

Verbal Reasoning	3	4	5	6	7	8	9	(10)	(11)	12	13	14	15
Physical Sciences	3	4	5	6	7	8	9	10	(11)	12	(13)	14	15
Biological Sciences	3	4	5	6	7	8	9	10	(11)	12	(13)	14	15
Writing Sample			J	K	L	M	N	O	P	(Q)	R	S	T

Acceptance & Matriculation Data for 2007–2008 First Year Class

	Resident	Non-Resident	International	Total
Applied	419	5371	359	6149
Interviewed	91	648	35	774
Deferred	1	10	3	14
Matriculants				
Early Assurance Program	n/a	n/a	n/a	n/a
Early Decision Program	0	0	0	0
Baccalaureate/MD	n/a	n/a	n/a	n/a
MD/PhD	2	9	0	11
Matriculated	22	91	5	**118**

Applications accepted from International Applicants: Yes

Matriculant Demographics: 2007–2008 First Year Class

Men: 59   **Women:** 59

Matriculants' Self-Reported Race/Ethnicity

Mexican American	0	Korean	8
Cuban	0	Vietnamese	2
Puerto Rican	0	Other Asian	1
Other Hispanic	3	Total Asian	42
Total Hispanic	3	Native American	1
Chinese	15	Black	13
Asian Indian	13	Native Hawaiian	0
Pakistani	2	White	62
Filipino	1	Unduplicated Number	
Japanese	0	of Matriculants	118

Science and Math Majors: 78%
Matriculants with:
     Baccalaureate degree: 100%
     Graduate degree(s): 11%

Specialty Choice

2003, 2004, 2005 Graduates, Specialty Choice (As reported by program directors to GME Track™)	
Anesthesiology	5%
Emergency Medicine	6%
Family Practice	1%
Internal Medicine	20%
Obstetrics/Gynecology	1%
Orthopaedic Surgery	5%
Pediatrics	12%
Psychiatry	1%
Radiology	7%
Surgery	6%

Financial Information

Source: 2006–2007 LCME I-B survey
and 2007–2008 AAMC TSF questionnaire

	Residents	Non-Residents
Total Cost of Attendance	$55,575	$55,575
Tuition and Fees	$37,579	$37,579
Other (includes living expenses)	$15,476	$15,476
Health Insurance (can be waived)	$2,520	$2,520

Average 2007 Graduate Indebtedness: $93,753
% of Enrolled Students Receiving Aid: 88%

Criminal Background Check

This medical school requires a criminal background check prior to matriculation.

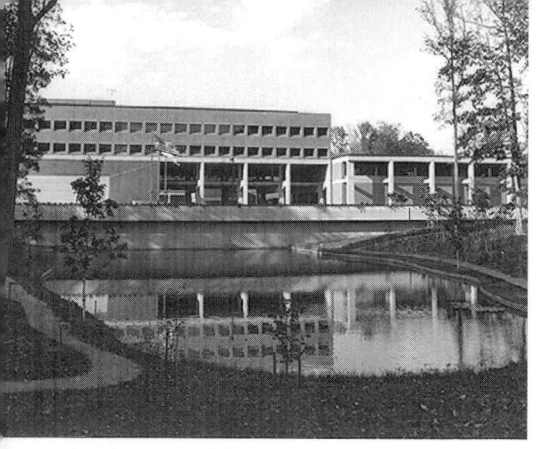

Uniformed Services University of the Health Sciences F. Edward Hébert School of Medicine

Bethesda, Maryland

Admissions Office, Room A-1041
Uniformed Services University of the Health Sciences
F. Edward Hébert School of Medicine
4301 Jones Bridge Road
Bethesda, Maryland 20814-4799
T 301 295 3101   **F** 301 295 3545

Admissions www.usuhs.mil/admissions.html
Main www.usuhs.mil
Financial n/a
Email admissions@usuhs.mil

Public Institution

Dr. Larry W. Laughlin, M.D., Ph.D., Dean

Dr. Margaret Calloway, M.D., CDR, MC, USN, Associate Dean for Recruitment and Admissions

Dr. Cynthia I. Macri, M.D., CAPT, MC, USN, Vice President for Recruitment and Diversity

Joan C. Stearman, M.S.W., Director, Office of Admissions

General Information

Created by public law in 1972, the Uniformed Services University of the Health Sciences (USUHS) was founded to prepare young men and women for careers as health care professionals in the uniformed services. The school's charter is to provide a comprehensive education in medicine and to select individuals who demonstrate potential for and commitment to careers as medical officers in the uniformed services.

Mission Statement

USUHS is the nation's federal health sciences university and is committed to excellence in military medicine and public health during peace and war. Our mission is to provide the nation with health professionals dedicated to career service in the Department of Defense and the United States Public Health Service and with scientists who serve the common good.

Curricular Highlights

Community Service Requirement: Optional.
Research/Thesis Requirement: Optional.

The school has a four-year program culminating in the doctor of medicine degree. Basic science instruction predominates in the initial two academic years, with the final two years devoted to clinical education. Basic science instruction is correlated both interdisciplinarily and clinically. The integration between the clinical and basic sciences is progressive and proceeds with involvement in patient care activities early in the curriculum, starting with the first semester of the first year. The overall

program is designed to educate students to serve as providers of primary health care. The curriculum also includes basic military orientation and concentration on unique aspects of military medicine. A conventional letter grading system is used.

USMLE

Step 1: Required. Students must record a passing score for graduation, but not promotion.
Step 2: Clinical Skills (CS): Required. Students must record a passing total score to graduate.
Step 2: Clinical Knowledge (CK): Required. Students must record a passing total score to graduate.

Selection Factors

The school employs a three-stage, progressive screening process for selecting entrants. The first stage consists of the submission of the AMCAS application; the second, the submission of supplementary materials; and the third, personal interviews, which are conducted at the campus. Advancement in the process is competitive, based on candidates' personal and intellectual characteristics. The Committee on Admissions does not discriminate on the basis of sex, race, religion, marital status, or national origin.

Financial Aid

Upon entering the first-year class of the School of Medicine, the student will be commissioned and will serve on active duty in the grade of second lieutenant in either the Army or Air Force or of ensign in the Navy or Public Health Service, receiving the appropriate pay and benefits of that grade. The time spent in medical school is not creditable toward retirement until retirement eligibility has been established. At graduation, students are promoted to captain in the Air Force or Army or lieutenant in the Navy and PHS upon receipt of the M.D. degree. Graduates are obligated to serve on active duty as medical officers for not less than seven years, as well as six years inactive ready reserve. The period of time spent in internship or residency training is not be acceptable toward satisfying this seven-year obligation. A student

who is dropped from the program for any reason may be required to perform active duty for a period of time equal to the time spent in the program. A disenrolled student may also be required to reimburse the government for tuition and fees. However, one year will be the minimum required active duty for persons separated from the school, regardless of the time spent in the program.

Information about Diversity Programs

The Office of Recruitment and Diversity at USUHS is designed to provide a welcoming environment to all students by promoting and encouraging expression of their diverse ethnic, cultural, economic, and experiential backgrounds. Competitive applicants from groups underrepresented in medicine are actively encouraged to apply. The application and admissions processes are the same for all students. The Vice President and staff seek to support all students throughout the four years of medical school, recognizing that each individual's unique circumstances may require various levels of support and encouragement. The learning environment is enhanced by participation in the Faculty-Student Mentor Program (administered by the Commandant's office) and the three major student-sponsored groups: Women in Medicine and Science, the Asian Pacific American Medical Student Association, and the Student National Medical Association. Administrative and faculty support is provided by the Office of Recruitment and Diversity to advance the community outreach efforts of these student groups.

Campus Information

Enrollment

For 2007, total enrollment was: 670

Housing

Although on-campus housing is not available, students are provided a housing allowance which is non-taxable.

Application Process and Requirements 2009–2010

Primary Application Service: AMCAS
Earliest filing date: June 1, 2008
Latest filing date: November 15, 2008

Secondary Application Required?: Yes
Sent to: All applicants
Contact: (301)-295-3101, admissions@usuhs.mil
Fee: No
Fee waiver available: n/a
Earliest filing date: June 1, 2008
Latest filing date: December 15, 2008

Latest MCAT® considered: 2008
Oldest MCAT® considered: 2006

Early Decision Program
School does not have EDP
Applicants notified: n/a
EDP available for: n/a

Regular Acceptance Notice
Earliest date: October 15, 2008
Latest date: Until class is full

Applicant's Response to Acceptance Offer – Maximum Time: Two weeks

Requests for Deferred Entrance Considered: Yes

Deposit to Hold Place in Class: No
Deposit (Resident): n/a
Deposit (Non-Resident): n/a
Deposit due: n/a
Applied to tuition: n/a
Deposit refundable: n/a
Refundable by: n/a

Estimated number of new entrants: 171
EDP: 0, special program: n/a

Start Month/Year: June 2009

Interview Format: Two thirty-minute interviews with medical corps officers. Regional interviews are not available.

Other Programs

PREPARATORY PROGRAMS
Postbaccalaureate Program: No
Summer Program: No

COMBINED DEGREE PROGRAMS
Baccalaureate/MD: No
MD/MPH: No
MD/MBA: No
MD/JD: No
MD/PhD: Yes,
http://cim.usuhs.mil/geo/mdphd.htm

Premedical Coursework

Course	Req.	Rec.	Lab.	Hrs.	Course	Req.	Rec.	Lab.	Hrs.
Inorganic Chemistry	•		•	8	Computer Science				
Behavioral Sciences					Genetics				
Biochemistry					Humanities				
Biology	•		•	8	Organic Chemistry	•		•	8
Biology/Zoology					Physics	•		•	8
Calculus	•			3	Psychology				
College English	•			6	Social Sciences				
College Mathematics					Other				

Selection Factors: 2007 Accepted Applicants

Proportion of Accepted Applicants with Relevant Experience (Data Self-Reported to AMCAS®)		Community Service/Volunteer	62%
		Medically-Related Work	82%
		Research	69%

Shaded bar represents accepted scores ranging from the 10th percentile to the 90th percentile ▇   School Median ● National Median ●

Overall GPA	2.0	2.1	2.2	2.3	2.4	2.5	2.6	2.7	2.8	2.9	3.0	3.1	3.2	3.3	3.4	3.5	(3.6)	3.7	3.8	3.9	4.0
Science GPA	2.0	2.1	2.2	2.3	2.4	2.5	2.6	2.7	2.8	2.9	3.0	3.1	3.2	3.3	3.4	(3.5)	3.6	3.7	3.8	3.9	4.0

MCAT® required: Yes, 100% of 2007 accepted applicants took MCAT®

Verbal Reasoning	3	4	5	6	7	8	9	(10)	11	12	13	14	15
Physical Sciences	3	4	5	6	7	8	9	(10)	(11)	12	13	14	15
Biological Sciences	3	4	5	6	7	8	9	(10)	(11)	12	13	14	15
Writing Sample				J	K	L	M	N	(O)	P	(Q)	R	S	T

Acceptance & Matriculation Data for 2007–2008 First Year Class

	Resident	Non-Resident	International	Total
Applied	141	1754	13	1908
Interviewed	48	458	0	506
Deferred	1	5	0	6
Matriculants				
Early Assurance Program	n/a	n/a	n/a	n/a
Early Decision Program	0	0	0	0
Baccalaureate/MD	n/a	n/a	n/a	n/a
MD/PhD	0	3	0	3
Matriculated	16	157	0	**173**

Applications accepted from International Applicants: No

Matriculant Demographics: 2007–2008 First Year Class

Men: 114   **Women:** 59

Matriculants' Self-Reported Race/Ethnicity

Mexican American	4	Korean	6
Cuban	0	Vietnamese	2
Puerto Rican	2	Other Asian	4
Other Hispanic	4	Total Asian	33
Total Hispanic	10	Native American	2
Chinese	5	Black	3
Asian Indian	8	Native Hawaiian	0
Pakistani	0	White	141
Filipino	6	Unduplicated Number	
Japanese	2	of Matriculants	173

Science and Math Majors: 74%
Matriculants with:
Baccalaureate degree: 100%
Graduate degree(s): 13%

Specialty Choice

2003, 2004, 2005 Graduates, Specialty Choice (As reported by program directors to GME Track™)	
Anesthesiology	3%
Emergency Medicine	4%
Family Practice	11%
Internal Medicine	8%
Obstetrics/Gynecology	3%
Orthopaedic Surgery	2%
Pediatrics	7%
Psychiatry	3%
Radiology	2%
Surgery	5%

Financial Information

Source: 2006–2007 LCME I-B survey and 2007–2008 AAMC TSF questionnaire

	Residents	Non-Residents
Total Cost of Attendance	n/a	n/a
Tuition and Fees	n/a	n/a
Other (includes living expenses)	n/a	n/a
Health Insurance	n/a	n/a

Average 2007 Graduate Indebtedness: n/a
% of Enrolled Students Receiving Aid: n/a

Criminal Background Check

This medical school requires a criminal background check prior to matriculation.

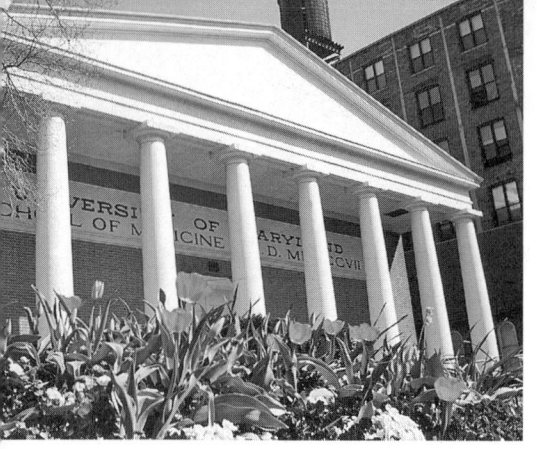

University of Maryland School of Medicine
Baltimore, Maryland

Committee on Admissions, Suite 190
University of Maryland School of Medicine
685 West Baltimore Street
Baltimore, Maryland 21201-1559
T 410 706 7478   F 410 706 0467

Admissions www.medschool.umaryland.edu/admissions
Main www.medschool.umaryland.edu
Financial www.umaryland.edu/fin
Email admissions@som.umaryland.edu

Public Institution

Dr. E. Albert Reece, Dean

*Dr. Milford M. Foxwell Jr.,
Associate Dean for Admissions*

Patricia Scott, Director of Financial Aid

*Dr. Donna L. Parker, Associate Dean
for Student Affairs*

General Information
Organized in 1807, The University of Maryland School of Medicine is the nation's oldest public medical college. The first class was graduated in 1810. Among the first to erect its own hospital for clinical instruction, the university also established the first intramural residency for senior students.

Mission Statement
The University of Maryland School of Medicine is dedicated to providing excellence in biomedical education, basic and clinical research, quality patient care, and service to improve the health of the citizens of Maryland and beyond. The School is committed to the education and training of M.D., M.D./M.P.H., M.D./Ph.D., graduate, physical therapy, and medical research technology students. The school will recruit and develop faculty to serve as exemplary role models for our students.

Curricular Highlights
Community Service Requirement: Optional.
Research/Thesis Requirement: Optional.

During the first two years of medical school the basic sciences are integrated and taught as systems, using interdisciplinary teaching by both basic and clinical science faculty. Mornings include lecture and small group sessions; afternoons are devoted to independent study. Curricular materials are available online and laptop computers are required. "Introduction to Clinical Medicine" begins early in the first year and continues through year two, offering instruction in clinical diagnosis, intimate human behavior, problem-based learning, biomedical ethics and dynamics of ambulatory care. Clinical clerkships

during the last two years include a month in family medicine and an emphasis on ambulatory teaching in other disciplines and two months of subinternship.

USMLE
Step 1: Required. Students must record a passing score for promotion.
Step 2: Clinical Skills (CS): Optional.
Step 2: Clinical Knowledge (CK): Optional.

Selection Factors
Applications are accepted from citizens and permanent residents of the U.S. and citizens of Canada. All AMCAS applicants are invited to submit a Stage II application. Selection of students is based on careful appraisal of character, motivation for medicine, academic achievement, MCAT® scores, letters of reference, extracurricular activities and interviews. The University does not discriminate on the basis of race, creed, sex, national origin, age or handicap.

Financial Aid
Scholarships and loans are available for students with demonstrable need. The amount of the award may vary according to need and the level of funding available.

Information about Diversity Programs
The School of Medicine values diversity very highly in the educational process and is committed to the recruitment and retention of talented students from underrepresented and disadvantaged backgrounds. A major focus of our recruitment efforts is to provide information on admissions requirements and preparation for medical school, the selection process, and educational and research opportunities at the School of Medicine. There are no fixed quotas for any group and the admissions procedures are the same for all applicants. The Office of Admissions will make a special effort to provide information that is relevant to prospective applicants in these groups. Information can be obtained from Ms. Raushanah Kareem, in the Office of Admissions.

Campus Information

Setting
The professional campus is located in downtown Baltimore within easy walking distance of the new Hippodrome Theatre, Inner Harbor, Maryland Science Center, National Aquarium and Pier 6 Pavilion. Oriole Park at Camden Yards and M&T Bank Stadium sit adjacent to campus.

Enrollment
For 2007, total enrollment was: 621

Special Features
Built in 1812, the meticulously restored Davidge Hall is the oldest building in North America in continuous use for medical education. The Health Sciences and Human Services Library is the second largest medical library building on the East Coast. Adjacent to the medical center's new Weinberg and Gudelsky clinical towers are the world-renowned Shock Trauma Center, the Baltimore Veterans Administration Medical Center, the University of Maryland Biotechnology Institute and the new UMB Biopark.

Housing
On-campus housing is available at a cost of about $700-800/month. The new University Suites features furnished apartments plus study lounges, 24-hour security and on-site garage parking. The surrounding neighborhood provides even more choices for students, with both apartments and individual homes (townhomes) available for rent (average $800-1000/month) or purchase. The majority of our students live within walking distance of the campus, particularly during the first two years of medical school.

Satellite Campuses/Facilities
Students complete most of their junior year clinical clerkships at the University of Maryland Medical System and Baltimore Veterans Affairs Medical Center, but do rotate through several of our affiliated community hospitals for selected rotations. During the fourth year of medical school our students will see patients during their ambulatory months at physician's offices in underserved areas of Baltimore City, Western Maryland and the Eastern Shore.

Application Process and Requirements 2009–2010

Primary Application Service: AMCAS
Earliest filing date: June 1, 2008
Latest filing date: November 1, 2008

Secondary Application Required?: Yes
Sent to: All applicants
Contact: Ms. Tawanda Sykes
(410) 706-7478, tsykes@som.umaryland.edu
Fee: Yes, $70
Fee waiver available: No
Earliest filing date: August 1, 2008
Latest filing date: December 15, 2008

Latest MCAT® considered: September 2008
Oldest MCAT® considered: January 2005

Early Decision Program
School does have EDP
Applicants notified: October 1, 2008
EDP available for: Both Residents and Non-Residents

Regular Acceptance Notice
Earliest date: October 15, 2008
Latest date: Until class is full

Applicant's Response to Acceptance Offer – Maximum Time: Three weeks

Requests for Deferred Entrance Considered: Yes

Deposit to Hold Place in Class: No
Deposit (Resident): n/a
Deposit (Non-Resident): n/a
Deposit due: n/a
Applied to tuition: n/a
Deposit refundable: n/a
Refundable by: n/a

Estimated number of new entrants: 160
EDP: 5, special program: n/a

Start Month/Year: August 2009

Interview Format: Two, one-on-one interviews with faculty or student. Regional interviews are not available.

Other Programs

PREPARATORY PROGRAMS
Postbaccalaureate Program: No
Summer Program: Yes, Dr. Sandra Dolan
(410) 706-7669, sdolan@clc.umaryland.edu
COMBINED DEGREE PROGRAMS
Baccalaureate/MD: No
MD/MPH: Yes, www.medschool.umaryland.edu/
MD_MPH/, Dr. Jordan Warnick, (410) 706-3026,
jwarnick@som.umaryland.edu
MD/MBA: No
MD/JD: No
MD/PhD: Yes, Nancy Malson
(410) 706-3990, nmalson@som.umaryland.edu

Premedical Coursework

Course	Req.	Rec.	Lab.	Hrs.
Inorganic Chemistry	•		•	8
Behavioral Sciences				
Biochemistry		•		
Biology				
Biology/Zoology	•		•	8
Calculus				
College English				6
College Mathematics				

Course	Req.	Rec.	Lab.	Hrs.
Computer Science		•		
Genetics				
Humanities		•		
Organic Chemistry	•		•	8
Physics	•		•	8
Psychology				
Social Sciences				
Other				

Selection Factors: 2007 Accepted Applicants

Proportion of Accepted Applicants with Relevant Experience (Data Self-Reported to AMCAS®)		
Community Service/Volunteer		69%
Medically-Related Work		90%
Research		91%

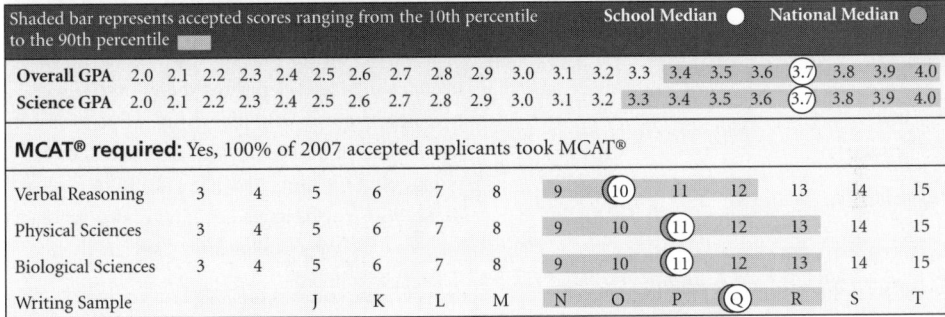

Shaded bar represents accepted scores ranging from the 10th percentile to the 90th percentile. School Median ● National Median ●

Overall GPA	2.0	2.1	2.2	2.3	2.4	2.5	2.6	2.7	2.8	2.9	3.0	3.1	3.2	3.3	3.4	3.5	3.6	(3.7)	3.8	3.9	4.0
Science GPA	2.0	2.1	2.2	2.3	2.4	2.5	2.6	2.7	2.8	2.9	3.0	3.1	3.2	3.3	3.4	3.5	3.6	(3.7)	3.8	3.9	4.0

MCAT® required: Yes, 100% of 2007 accepted applicants took MCAT®

Verbal Reasoning	3	4	5	6	7	8	9	(10)	11	12	13	14	15
Physical Sciences	3	4	5	6	7	8	9	10	(11)	12	13	14	15
Biological Sciences	3	4	5	6	7	8	9	10	(11)	12	13	14	15
Writing Sample			J	K	L	M	N	O	P	(Q)	R	S	T

Acceptance & Matriculation Data for 2007–2008 First Year Class

	Resident	Non-Resident	International	Total
Applied	862	3463	178	4503
Interviewed	321	141	12	474
Deferred	5	0	0	5
Matriculants				
Early Assurance Program	0	0	0	0
Early Decision Program	1	0	0	1
Baccalaureate/MD	n/a	n/a	n/a	n/a
MD/PhD	3	1	1	5
Matriculated	129	30	1	**160**

Applications accepted from International Applicants: Only Canadian

Specialty Choice

2003, 2004, 2005 Graduates, Specialty Choice (As reported by program directors to GME Track™)	
Anesthesiology	4%
Emergency Medicine	8%
Family Practice	8%
Internal Medicine	24%
Obstetrics/Gynecology	2%
Orthopaedic Surgery	3%
Pediatrics	12%
Psychiatry	3%
Radiology	3%
Surgery	8%

Matriculant Demographics: 2007–2008 First Year Class

Men: 67 **Women:** 93

Matriculants' Self-Reported Race/Ethnicity

Mexican American	0	Korean	4
Cuban	0	Vietnamese	3
Puerto Rican	0	Other Asian	8
Other Hispanic	2	Total Asian	47
Total Hispanic	2	Native American	0
Chinese	13	Black	19
Asian Indian	14	Native Hawaiian	1
Pakistani	3	White	100
Filipino	5	Unduplicated Number	
Japanese	0	of Matriculants	160

Science and Math Majors: 73%
Matriculants with:
   Baccalaureate degree: 99%
   Graduate degree(s): 11%

Financial Information

Source: 2006–2007 LCME I-B survey
and 2007–2008 AAMC TSF questionnaire

	Residents	Non-Residents
Total Cost of Attendance	$25,181	$43,416
Tuition and Fees	$21,998	$40,233
Other (includes living expenses)	$1,128	$1,128
Health Insurance (can be waived)	$2,055	$2,055

Average 2007 Graduate Indebtedness: $37,333
% of Enrolled Students Receiving Aid: 84%

Criminal Background Check

This medical school does not require a criminal background check prior to matriculation.

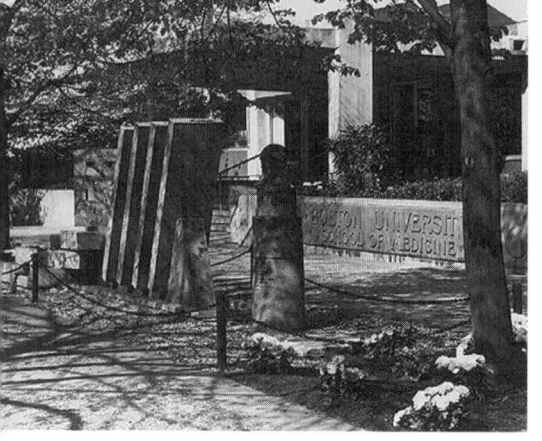

Boston University
School of Medicine
Boston, Massachusetts

Admissions Office, Building L, Rm. 124
Boston University School of Medicine
715 Albany Street
Boston, Massachusetts 02118
T 617 638 4630 **F** 617 638 4718

Admissions medadms@bu.edu
Main www.bumc.bu.edu/busm/
Financial www.bumc.bu.edu/osfs
Email medadms@bu.edu

Private Institution

Dr. Karen Antman, Dean

Dr. Robert A. Witzburg, Associate Dean and Director of Admissions

Dr. Jonathan Woodson, Associate Dean for Student and Minority Affairs

Kathy Stavropoulos, Executive Director for Student Financial Services

Dr. Phyllis L. Carr, Associate Dean for Student Affairs

Ellen Difiore, Registrar

General Information
The New England Female Medical College, founded in 1848, was the first medical college for women in the world. In 1873 the college became the Boston University School of Medicine, the first coeducational medical school in the U.S. The medical campus includes the Schools of Medicine, Dental Medicine, and Public Health, as well as the hospital, Boston Medical Center, the Division of Graduate Medical Sciences, and extensive research facilities.

Mission Statement
To educate and train students, physicians, and scientists who will bring superior qualities to the practice of medicine, biomedical research, and public health, and who will be prepared for changes in the social, legal, and economic climate that will affect the practice of medicine.

Curricular Highlights
Community Service Requirement: Optional. Many students and faculty participate.
Research/Thesis Requirement: Optional. Thesis may be required for dual degree programs.

BUSM offers a flexible program of critical inquiry and rigorous study in the biological, social, and behavioral sciences. The first-year focus is on normal structure and function, unified by Integrated Problems, a problem-based, clinically focused seminar. Introduction to Clinical Medicine has students interviewing and evaluating patients beginning in the first week of school. The basic sciences are linked with applications in clinical

practice, emphasizing multidisciplinary, team-based learning. The second-year focus is on pathophysiology, with an integrated, multidisciplinary format led by basic science and clinical faculty. The core clinical training of the third year includes clerkships in all the major disciplines, with ambulatory and inpatient experience in generalist and subspecialty venues. There is also opportunity for clinical electives. The fourth year includes advanced clerkships and is largely elective. Research opportunities are available in basic science and clinical disciplines, and students may pursue electives in international health. Any academic year may be spread over two calendar years and students may pursue any of several dual degree programs.

USMLE
Step 1: Required. Students must record a passing score for promotion.
Step 2: Clinical Skills (CS): Required. Students must only record a score.
Step 2: Clinical Knowledge (CK): Required. Students must only record a score.

Selection Factors
Applicants are selected not only on the basis of academic record, recommendations, research experience, and involvement in community activities and service, but also by qualities of personality, character, and resilience. A personal interview is an integral part of the admissions process. All interviews are granted at the discretion of the Committee on Admissions.

Financial Aid
BUSM is committed to ensuring that all accepted students can secure the necessary financial resources; need-based aid is available to students in all years. The Office of Student Financial Services administers its portfolio of scholarships and loans, assists students in securing aid from outside sources, conducts debt management seminars, offers entrance and exit counseling, and provides student financial management information. Financial need is not considered in the admissions process. There are no special institutional financial funds disbursed for international students. Unless an international student has an

I-551 or I-151 resident alien card, federally insured loans are not available. Students may secure private educational loans with a co-applicant who is a creditworthy U.S. citizen or resident alien.

Information about Diversity Programs
BUSM is committed to diversity in the faculty and student body. Programs for the recruitment and support of students from groups underrepresented in medicine are managed by the Office of Admissions and the Office of Minority Affairs. All applications to BUSM are processed through the Office of Admissions.

Campus Information

Setting
BU Medical Center is a beautiful urban campus, shared by clinical, educational, and research institutions. The four-square-block campus, located in the heart of Boston, is accessible by public transportation and is within walking distance of residential areas, shops, and cultural institutions.

Enrollment
For 2007, total enrollment was: 652

Special Features
Students complete most of their clinical training at Boston Medical Center Hospital (BMC), a very diverse institution with the busiest emergency department in New England and large programs in both ambulatory and inpatient care. BMC hosts residency training programs in all disciplines. BUSM graduates pursue careers in primary care and in the subspecialties, in full-time clinical practice and in academic centers, in rural and urban settings, in all parts of the U.S., and in international health.

Housing
Limited on-campus housing is available; most students choose to live off-campus. Rents vary, ranging from $650 and up, depending on student choice regarding location and number of roommates.

Satellite Campuses/Facilities
Limited on-campus housing is available, but most students choose to live off-campus. Rents are variable, ranging from $650 and up, depending on student choice regarding location and number of roommates.

Application Process and Requirements 2009–2010

Primary Application Service: AMCAS
Earliest filing date: June 1, 2008
Latest filing date: November 3, 2008

Secondary Application Required?: Yes
Sent to: All applicants
URL: Provided after receipt of initial application.
Contact: Office of Admissions
(617) 638-4630, medadms@bu.edu
Fee: Yes, $100
Fee waiver available: Yes
Earliest filing date: June 2, 2008
Latest filing date: January 2, 2009

Latest MCAT® considered: Any scores available through AMCAS prior to January 2, 2009
Oldest MCAT® considered: 2005

Early Decision Program
School does have EDP
Applicants notified: October 1, 2008
EDP available for: Both Residents and Non-Residents

Regular Acceptance Notice
Earliest date: Early January 2009
Latest date: Until class is full

Applicant's Response to Acceptance Offer – Maximum Time: Two weeks

Requests for Deferred Entrance Considered: No

Deposit to Hold Place in Class: Yes
Deposit (Resident): $500
Deposit (Non-Resident): $500
Deposit due: May 15, 2009
Applied to tuition: Yes
Deposit refundable: Yes
Refundable prior to: May 15, 2009

Estimated number of new entrants: 170
EDP: 3, special program: n/a

Start Month/Year: August 11, 2009

Interview Format: On-campus interview required. Regional interviews are not available.

Other Programs

PREPARATORY PROGRAMS
Postbaccalaureate Program: Yes
Summer Program: No
Early Medical School Selection Program:
www.bumc.bu.edu/Dept/Content.aspx?DepartmentID
=45&PageID=1295, Jonathan Woodson, M.D.,
(617) 638-4163, Jonathan.Woodson@bmc.org
Masters of Arts in Medical Sciences: Yes,
http://cobalt.bumc.bu.edu/current/Catalog/medsci/
intro.htm
COMBINED DEGREE PROGRAMS
Baccalaureate/MD: Yes,
www.bu.edu/admissions/discover/accelerate.html
MD/MPH: Yes, www.bumc.bu.edu/sph
MD/MBA: Yes, http://management.bu.edu/gpo/hc
MD/PhD: Yes, www.bumc.bu.edu/gms

Premedical Coursework

Course	Req.	Rec.	Lab.	Sems.	Course	Req.	Rec.	Lab.	Sems.
Inorganic Chemistry	•		•	2	Genetics		•		1
Behavioral Sciences		•		2	Humanities	•			2
Biochemistry		•		1	Organic Chemistry	•		•	2
Biology	•		•	2	Physics	•			2
Biology/Zoology					Psychology				
Calculus					Social Sciences		•		2
College English	•			2	Molecular Biology		•		1
College Mathematics		•		2	Biostatistics & Epidemiology		•		1
Computer Science									

Selection Factors: 2007 Accepted Applicants

Proportion of Accepted Applicants with Relevant Experience (Data Self-Reported to AMCAS®)		
Community Service/Volunteer		65%
Medically-Related Work		86%
Research		83%

Shaded bar represents accepted scores ranging from the 10th percentile to the 90th percentile. **School Median** ● **National Median** ●

Overall GPA	2.0	2.1	2.2	2.3	2.4	2.5	2.6	2.7	2.8	2.9	3.0	3.1	3.2	3.3	3.4	3.5	3.6	(3.7)	3.8	3.9	4.0
Science GPA	2.0	2.1	2.2	2.3	2.4	2.5	2.6	2.7	2.8	2.9	3.0	3.1	3.2	3.3	3.4	3.5	3.6	(3.7)	3.8	3.9	4.0

MCAT® required: Yes, 100% of 2007 accepted applicants took MCAT®

Verbal Reasoning	3	4	5	6	7	8	9	(10)	11	12	13	14	15
Physical Sciences	3	4	5	6	7	8	9	10	(11)	12	13	14	15
Biological Sciences	3	4	5	6	7	8	9	10	(11)	12	13	14	15
Writing Sample			J	K	L	M	N	O	P	(Q)	R	S	T

Acceptance & Matriculation Data for 2007–2008 First Year Class

	Resident	Non-Resident	International	Total
Applied	730	9796	611	11137
Interviewed	148	890	52	1038
Deferred	0	3	0	3
Matriculants				
Early Assurance Program	3	14	0	17
Early Decision Program	0	0	0	0
Baccalaureate/MD	0	17	0	17
MD/PhD	2	9	0	11
Matriculated	39	119	10	**168**

Applications accepted from International Applicants: Yes

Specialty Choice

2003, 2004, 2005 Graduates, Specialty Choice (As reported by program directors to GME Track™)	
Anesthesiology	3%
Emergency Medicine	6%
Family Practice	5%
Internal Medicine	19%
Obstetrics/Gynecology	6%
Orthopaedic Surgery	3%
Pediatrics	11%
Psychiatry	3%
Radiology	7%
Surgery	8%

Matriculant Demographics: 2007–2008 First Year Class

Men: 79   **Women:** 89

Matriculants' Self-Reported Race/Ethnicity

Mexican American	8	Korean	2
Cuban	1	Vietnamese	3
Puerto Rican	0	Other Asian	3
Other Hispanic	11	**Total Asian**	45
Total Hispanic	20	Native American	1
Chinese	14	Black	18
Asian Indian	21	Native Hawaiian	1
Pakistani	1	White	90
Filipino	0	**Unduplicated Number**	
Japanese	2	**of Matriculants**	168

Science and Math Majors: 73%
Matriculants with:
Baccalaureate degree: 100%
Graduate degree(s): 27%

Financial Information

Source: 2006–2007 LCME I-B survey and 2007–2008 AAMC TSF questionnaire

	Residents	Non-Residents
Total Cost of Attendance	$65,542	$65,542
Tuition and Fees	$43,234	$43,234
Other (includes living expenses)	$19,894	$19,894
Health Insurance (can be waived)	$2,414	$2,414

Average 2007 Graduate Indebtedness: $161,147
% of Enrolled Students Receiving Aid: 83%

Criminal Background Check

This medical school requires a criminal background check prior to matriculation.

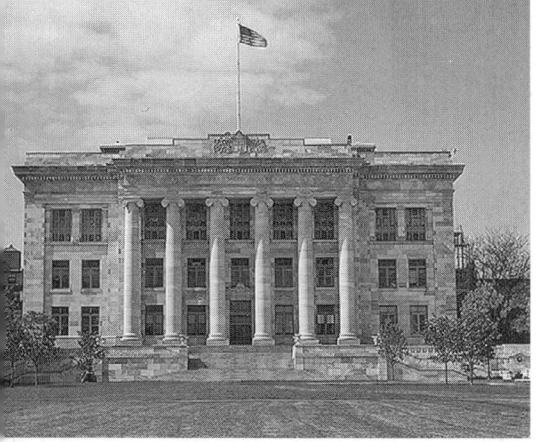

Harvard Medical School

Boston, Massachusetts

Office of the Committee on Admissions
Harvard Medical School
25 Shattuck Street
306 Gordon Hall
Boston, Massachusetts 02115-6092

T 617 432 1550   **F** 617 432 3307
Admissions http://hms.harvard.edu/admissions/
Main http://hms.harvard.edu
Financial www.hms.harvard.edu/finaid/
Email admissions_office@hms.harvard.edu

Private Institution

Dr. Jeffrey S. Flier, Dean

Dr. Robert J. Mayer, Faculty Associate Dean for Admissions

Dr. Darrell N. Smith, Faculty Assistant Dean for Admissions

Dr. Alvin F. Poussaint, Associate Dean for Student Affairs

Robert D. Coughlin, Director of Financial Aid

Joanne M. McEvoy, Director of Admissions

General Information

Harvard Medical School was established in 1782. Clinical teaching is carried out in several hospitals, including Massachusetts General, Brigham and Women's, Children's, Beth Israel Deaconess, Massachusetts Eye and Ear, Mount Auburn, and Cambridge Hospitals. The Massachusetts Mental Health Center and the McLean Hospital are psychiatric facilities. Harvard Vanguard Medical Associates and other community-based health centers provide additional opportunities for patient care, teaching, and research. Other affiliated institutions include the West Roxbury and Brockton VA Medical Centers, the Forsythe Institute, and the Spaulding Rehabilitation Hospital.

Mission Statement

The mission of Harvard Medical School is to create and nurture a diverse community of the best people committed to leadership in alleviating human suffering caused by disease.

Curricular Highlights

Community Service Requirement: Optional.
Research/Thesis Requirement: Encouraged for NP; required for HST.

The New Pathway Program (NP) is a problem-based curriculum that emphasizes small-group tutorials and self-directed learning, complemented by laboratories and lectures. Students are expected to analyze problems, locate relevant material in library and computer-based resources,

and develop habits of lifelong learning and independent study. The NP Program enrolls 135 students each year. A second M.D. pathway is the Harvard-M.I.T. Division of Health Sciences and Technology Program (HST). The HST curriculum is designed for students with a strong interest and background in quantitative science. Courses in the first two years are taught both at HMS and M.I.T. by faculty drawn from both institutions. HST students are expected to become conversant with the underlying quantitative and molecular aspects of medicine and biomedical science, achieved through a deep understanding of the physical and biological sciences, complemented with hands-on experience in the clinic. A thesis is required for graduation. HST enrolls 30 students per year. Basic science and clinical content are interwoven throughout the four years in both programs.

USMLE

Step 1: Required. Students must record a passing score for graduation, but not promotion.
Step 2: Clinical Skills (CS): Required. Students must record a passing total score to graduate.
Step 2: Clinical Knowledge (CK): Required. Students must record a passing total score to graduate.

Selection Factors

Academic excellence is expected. Committee members consider the entire application, including the essay, extracurricular activities, life experiences, research, community work, and the comments contained in letters of recommendation. Harvard Medical School looks for evidence of integrity, maturity, humanitarian concerns, leadership potential, and an aptitude for working with people. The 2007 entering class came from 63 different undergraduate institutions, including representatives from 30 U.S. States and eight foreign countries. Harvard Medical School does not accept applications for advanced standing or transfer.

Financial Aid

All financial aid is awarded on the basis of need. A vigorous effort is made to assist accepted applicants in meeting their medical education costs through loans, medically related employment,

and scholarships. Foreign students are eligible to be considered for need-based institutional scholarships and loans.

Information about Diversity Programs

Harvard Medical School is committed to the enrollment of a diverse body of talented students who will reflect the character of the people whose health needs the medical profession must serve. HMS's commitment to a diverse student population is reflected not only in the variety of institutions from which students are accepted, but also in the ethnic and economic backgrounds of the student body. For over 30 years, HMS has had one of highest minority student enrollment and graduation rates of any United States medical school. The HMS Office of Recruitment and Multicultural Affairs provides support services to individuals from groups under-represented in medicine.

Campus Information

Setting

The Harvard Medical School campus is an integral part of the Longwood Medical and Academic Area (LMA), a community of health and educational institutions located adjacent to Fenway Park in the city of Boston, Massachusetts. Adjoining the medical school are the Harvard School of Public Health, the Harvard School of Dental Medicine, and the Francis A. Countway Library.

Enrollment

For 2007, total enrollment was: 758

Housing

On-campus housing for single students is available in Vanderbilt Hall, a residence complex next to the Harvard Medical School. Students may choose to live in one of the residential communities neighboring the Longwood Medical Area.

Application Process and Requirements 2009–2010

Primary Application Service: AMCAS
Earliest filing date: June 1, 2008
Latest filing date: October 15, 2008

Secondary Application Required?: Yes
Sent to: All applicants
URL: Sent via email after verification of AMCAS application.
Contact: Admissions Office, (617) 432-1550
admissions_office@hms.harvard.edu
Fee: Yes, $85
Fee waiver available: Yes
Earliest filing date: July 1, 2008
Latest filing date: November 1, 2008

Latest MCAT® considered: September 2008
Oldest MCAT® considered: 2005

Early Decision Program
School does not have EDP
Applicants notified: n/a
EDP available for: n/a

Regular Acceptance Notice
Earliest date: February 28, 2009
Latest date: Varies

Applicant's Response to Acceptance Offer – Maximum Time: Three weeks

Requests for Deferred Entrance Considered: Yes

Deposit to Hold Place in Class: No
Deposit (Resident): n/a
Deposit (Non-Resident): n/a
Deposit due: n/a
Applied to tuition: n/a
Deposit refundable: n/a
Refundable by: n/a

Estimated number of new entrants: 165
EDP: n/a, special program: n/a

Start Month/Year: August 2009

Interview Format: On-campus only; scheduled selectively. Regional interviews are not available.

Other Programs

PREPARATORY PROGRAMS
Postbaccalaureate Program: No
Summer Program: No

COMBINED DEGREE PROGRAMS
Baccalaureate/MD: No
MD/MPH: Yes
www.hms.harvard.edu/dualdegrees/index.html
Admissions Office, (617) 432-1550
admissions_office@hms.harvard.edu
MD/MBA: Yes
www.hbs.edu/mba/academics/mdmba.html
(617) 432-1550, admissions_office@hms.harvard.edu
MD/JD: No
MD/PhD: Yes, www.hms.harvard.edu/md_phd/
(617) 432-0991, mdphd@hms.harvard.edu
Additional Program: Yes,
www.hms.harvard.edu/dualdegrees/index.html
(617) 432-1550, admissions_office@hms.harvard.edu

Premedical Coursework

Course	Req.	Rec.	Lab.	Sems.	Course	Req.	Rec.	Lab.	Sems.
Inorganic Chemistry	•		•	2	Computer Science				
Behavioral Sciences					Genetics				
Biochemistry		•		1	Humanities				
Biology	•		•	2	Organic Chemistry	•		•	2
Biology/Zoology					Physics	•			2
Calculus	•			2	Psychology				
College English					Social Sciences				
College Mathematics					Writing		•		2

Selection Factors: 2007 Accepted Applicants

Proportion of Accepted Applicants with Relevant Experience (Data Self-Reported to AMCAS*)		
Community Service/Volunteer		76%
Medically-Related Work		90%
Research		89%

Shaded bar represents accepted scores ranging from the 10th percentile to the 90th percentile. School Median ● National Median ◉

Overall GPA	2.0	2.1	2.2	2.3	2.4	2.5	2.6	2.7	2.8	2.9	3.0	3.1	3.2	3.3	3.4	3.5	3.6	3.7	3.8	(3.9)	4.0
Science GPA	2.0	2.1	2.2	2.3	2.4	2.5	2.6	2.7	2.8	2.9	3.0	3.1	3.2	3.3	3.4	3.5	3.6	3.7	3.8	(3.9)	4.0

MCAT® required: Yes, 100% of 2007 accepted applicants took MCAT®

Verbal Reasoning	3	4	5	6	7	8	9	(10)	(11)	12	13	14	15
Physical Sciences	3	4	5	6	7	8	9	10	(11)	12	(13)	14	15
Biological Sciences	3	4	5	6	7	8	9	10	(11)	12	(13)	14	15
Writing Sample				J	K	L	M	N	O	P	(Q)	R	S	T

Acceptance & Matriculation Data for 2007–2008 First Year Class

	Resident	Non-Resident	International	Total
Applied	417	5792	433	6642
Interviewed	96	885	68	1049
Deferred	1	15	2	18
Matriculants				
Early Assurance Program	n/a	n/a	n/a	n/a
Early Decision Program	0	0	0	0
Baccalaureate/MD	n/a	n/a	n/a	n/a
MD/PhD	1	10	1	12
Matriculated	19	132	14	**165**

Applications accepted from International Applicants: Yes

Specialty Choice

2003, 2004, 2005 Graduates, Specialty Choice (As reported by program directors to GME Track™)	
Anesthesiology	2%
Emergency Medicine	6%
Family Practice	2%
Internal Medicine	20%
Obstetrics/Gynecology	3%
Orthopaedic Surgery	3%
Pediatrics	9%
Psychiatry	5%
Radiology	7%
Surgery	6%

Matriculant Demographics: 2007–2008 First Year Class

Men: 88   **Women:** 77

Matriculants' Self-Reported Race/Ethnicity

Mexican American	4	Korean	2
Cuban	3	Vietnamese	3
Puerto Rican	0	Other Asian	5
Other Hispanic	8	Total Asian	56
Total Hispanic	14	Native American	2
Chinese	22	Black	18
Asian Indian	20	Native Hawaiian	0
Pakistani	2	White	77
Filipino	2	Unduplicated Number	
Japanese	2	of Matriculants	165

Science and Math Majors: 74%
Matriculants with:
Baccalaureate degree: 100%
Graduate degree(s): 11%

Financial Information

Source: 2006–2007 LCME I-B survey and 2007–2008 AAMC TSF questionnaire

	Residents	Non-Residents
Total Cost of Attendance	$60,880	$60,880
Tuition and Fees	$40,499	$40,499
Other (includes living expenses)	$19,019	$19,019
Health Insurance (can be waived)	$1,362	$1,362

Average 2007 Graduate Indebtedness: $98,953
% of Enrolled Students Receiving Aid: 81%

Criminal Background Check

This medical school does not require a criminal background check prior to matriculation.

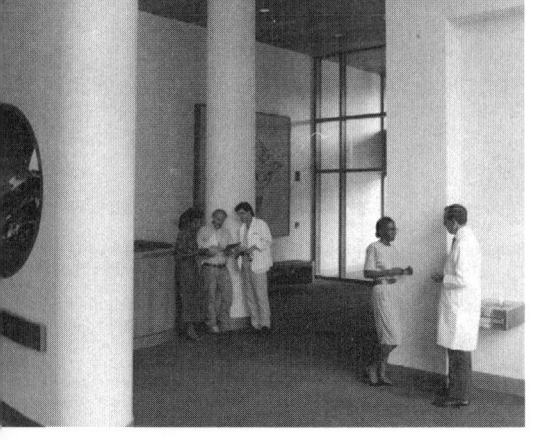

Tufts University School of Medicine
Boston, Massachusetts

Office of Admissions
Tufts University School of Medicine
136 Harrison Avenue
Boston, Massachusetts 02111
T 617 636 6571 **F** unpublished

Admissions www.tufts.edu/med/admissions
Main www.tufts.edu/med
Financial www.tufts.edu/med/about/offices/
finaid/index.html
Email med-admissions@tufts.edu

Private Institution

Dr. Michael Rosenblatt, Dean

Dr. David Neumeyer, Dean for Admissions

Colleen Romain, Director of Minority Affairs

Tara Olsen, Director of Financial Aid

Thomas M. Slavin, Director of Admissions

John Matias, Associate Dean of Admissions

General Information

Tufts University was founded in 1852 in Medford, Massachusetts; the School of Medicine was established in Boston in 1893. Close association of the School of Medicine with 30-plus hospitals currently affords ample facilities for clinical experience.

Mission Statement

To produce a competent, compassionate physician who is skilled and well-educated in a core of general knowledge; one who is capable of building on this core to achieve educational and career goals and to maintain the task of lifelong learning.

Curricular Highlights

Community Service Requirement: Required.
Research/Thesis Requirement: Optional.

Students experience a progressive development of clinical knowledge, skills, and attitudes required as a professional in medicine today. The curriculum emphasizes the basic skills needed by a generalist physician and includes newly expanded topics such as information management, computer literacy, and negotiation/management/team building skills, in addition to integrated topics such as nutrition, gerontology, health care economics, and ethics. Community and ambulatory-based learning experiences are incorporated throughout to reflect the changing environment of health care. In the third year, students develop their clinical skills and learn to take responsibility for patient care under close preceptor supervision at a number of affiliated sites representing

a wide variety of clinical settings. The goal of the fourth year of the curriculum is to expand the basic clinical knowledge and skills acquired in the first three years, enabling the student to manage clinical problems with the degree of independence required of the first-year post-graduate level of medical training.

USMLE

Step 1: Required. Students must record a passing score for promotion.
Step 2: Clinical Skills (CS): Required. Students must only record a score.
Step 2: Clinical Knowledge (CK): Required. Students must only record a score.

Selection Factors

The selection of candidates for admission to the first year is based not only on performance in the required premedical courses, but also on the applicant's entire academic record and extracurricular experiences. Letters of recommendation and additional information supplied by the applicant are reviewed for indications of promise and fitness for a medical career. Personal interviews are a prerequisite for admission and are granted only by invitation of the Admissions Committee. Preference is given to U.S. citizens and permanent residents who will receive a bachelor's degree from an U.S. college or university prior to matriculation. Tufts accepts transfers from other U.S. LCME-accredited medical schools into the second- and third-year classes in years when vacancies have been created by attrition. The number of seats available has traditionally been extremely limited. In some years, no transfer openings are available.

Financial Aid

Up to 75 percent of students participate in the federal government's student loan programs at some time during their four years of study. Additionally, limited scholarship and loan assistance is available directly from Tufts for students who qualify on the basis of need. Approximately 33 percent of the students receive financial aid directly from Tufts at some time during their four years of study.

Information about Diversity Programs

Tufts has a strong commitment to affirmative action and seeks to provide an atmosphere of nondiscrimination for members of groups underrepresented in medicine as well as an accessible campus and support services for persons with disabilities.

Campus Information

Setting

The School of Medicine is located within a health sciences campus that includes the School of Dental Medicine, the Sackler School of Graduate Biomedical Sciences, the Friedman School of Nutrition Science and Policy, the Sackler Center for Health Communications, the Jaharis Center for Biomedical and Nutrition Sciences, the Jean Mayer Nutrition Research Center, and the New England Medical Center.

Enrollment

For 2007, total enrollment was: 705

Special Features

TUSM has created a unique cadre of combined-degree programs by which students can attain an M.D./Ph.D., an M.D./M.P.H, or an M.D./M.B.A. in Health Management.

Housing

A limited amount of on-campus housing is available in Posner Hall, the Health Sciences Campus dormitory. Most TUSM students live off-campus. In the late spring of each year, the Student Affairs Office hires a seasonal off-campus housing coordinator to assist students at the Boston Health Sciences Campus in finding off-campus housing. The coordinator typically distributes general information about the Greater Boston housing market and maintains listings of available housing opportunities.

Satellite Campuses/Facilities

Most of the school's clinical affiliates are located in the metropolitan Boston area. Nevertheless, students should expect to participate in rotations that are located outside of Boston, including some at the Baystate Medical Center (the western campus of TUSM) in Springfield, Massachusetts, and Eastern Maine Medial Center in Bangor, Maine.

Application Process and Requirements 2009–2010

Primary Application Service: AMCAS
Earliest filing date: June 1, 2008
Latest filing date: November 1, 2008

Secondary Application Required?: Yes
Sent to: All applicants
URL: www.tufts.edu/med/admissions/md/howtoapply/secondary.html
Fee: Yes, $105
Fee waiver available: Yes
Earliest filing date: June 1, 2008
Latest filing date: January 15, 2009

Latest MCAT® considered: September 2008
Oldest MCAT® considered: 2006

Early Decision Program
School does have EDP
Applicants notified: October 1, 2008
EDP available for: Both Residents and Non-Residents

Regular Acceptance Notice
Earliest date: October 15, 2008
Latest date: Until class is full

Applicant's Response to Acceptance Offer – Maximum Time: Two weeks

Requests for Deferred Entrance Considered: Yes

Deposit to Hold Place in Class: Yes
Deposit (Resident): $100
Deposit (Non-Resident): $100
Deposit due: With response to acceptance offer
Applied to tuition: Yes
Deposit refundable: Yes
Refundable by: May 15, 2009

Estimated number of new entrants: 173
EDP: 2, special program: 20

Start Month/Year: August 2009

Interview Format: On-campus interviews conducted September–March. Regional interviews are not available.

Other Programs

PREPARATORY PROGRAMS
Postbaccalaureate Program: No
Summer Program: Yes, Colleen Romain
(617) 636-6534, colleen.romain@tufts.edu

COMBINED DEGREE PROGRAMS
Baccalaureate/MD: n/a
MD/MPH: Yes, www.tufts.edu/med/education/phpd/mphdual/mdmph_dvmmph/index.html
MD/MBA: Yes, www.tufts.edu/med/education/combinedmd/mdmba/index.html
MD/JD: No
MD/PhD: Yes, www.tufts.edu/sackler/programs/combined.html

Premedical Coursework

Course	Req.	Rec.	Lab.	Sems.	Course	Req.	Rec.	Lab.	Sems.
Inorganic Chemistry	•		•	2	Computer Science				
Behavioral Sciences					Genetics				
Biochemistry					Humanities				
Biology	•		•	2	Organic Chemistry	•		•	2
Biology/Zoology					Physics	•		•	2
Calculus					Psychology				
College English					Social Sciences				
College Mathematics					Other				

Selection Factors: 2007 Accepted Applicants

Proportion of Accepted Applicants with Relevant Experience (Data Self-Reported to AMCAS)		
Community Service/Volunteer	66%
Medically-Related Work	82%
Research	86%

Shaded bar represents accepted scores ranging from the 10th percentile to the 90th percentile. School Median ● National Median ○

Overall GPA	2.0	2.1	2.2	2.3	2.4	2.5	2.6	2.7	2.8	2.9	3.0	3.1	3.2	3.3	3.4	3.5	3.6	(3.7)	3.8	3.9	4.0
Science GPA	2.0	2.1	2.2	2.3	2.4	2.5	2.6	2.7	2.8	2.9	3.0	3.1	3.2	3.3	3.4	3.5	3.6	(3.7)	3.8	3.9	4.0

MCAT® required: Yes, 100% of 2007 accepted applicants took MCAT®

Verbal Reasoning	3	4	5	6	7	8	9	(10)	(11)	12	13	14	15
Physical Sciences	3	4	5	6	7	8	9	10	(11)	12	13	14	15
Biological Sciences	3	4	5	6	7	8	9	10	(11)	12	13	14	15
Writing Sample					J	K	L	M	N	O	P	(Q)	R	S	T

Acceptance & Matriculation Data for 2007–2008 First Year Class

	Resident	Non-Resident	International	Total
Applied	713	7802	368	8883
Interviewed	164	676	4	844
Deferred	1	6	0	7
Matriculants				
Early Assurance Program	8	13	2	23
Early Decision Program	0	0	0	0
Baccalaureate/MD	n/a	n/a	n/a	n/a
MD/PhD	1	3	0	4
Matriculated	51	119	3	**173**

Applications accepted from International Applicants: Yes

Matriculant Demographics: 2007–2008 First Year Class

Men: 90 **Women:** 83

Matriculants' Self-Reported Race/Ethnicity

Mexican American	1	Korean	6
Cuban	2	Vietnamese	3
Puerto Rican	3	Other Asian	4
Other Hispanic	6	Total Asian	44
Total Hispanic	11	Native American	2
Chinese	13	Black	5
Asian Indian	13	Native Hawaiian	0
Pakistani	1	White	116
Filipino	1	Unduplicated Number	
Japanese	3	of Matriculants	173

Science and Math Majors: 66%
Matriculants with:
   Baccalaureate degree: 100%
   Graduate degree(s): 8%

Specialty Choice

2003, 2004, 2005 Graduates, Specialty Choice (As reported by program directors to GME Track™)

Anesthesiology	7%
Emergency Medicine	7%
Family Practice	7%
Internal Medicine	23%
Obstetrics/Gynecology	3%
Orthopaedic Surgery	4%
Pediatrics	10%
Psychiatry	3%
Radiology	6%
Surgery	9%

Financial Information

Source: 2006–2007 LCME I-B survey and 2007–2008 AAMC TSF questionnaire

	Residents	Non-Residents
Total Cost of Attendance	$67,496	$67,496
Tuition and Fees	$47,116	$47,116
Other (includes living expenses)	$17,440	$17,440
Health Insurance (can be waived)	$2,940	$2,940

Average 2007 Graduate Indebtedness: $179,817
% of Enrolled Students Receiving Aid: 80%

Criminal Background Check

This medical school does not require a criminal background check prior to matriculation.

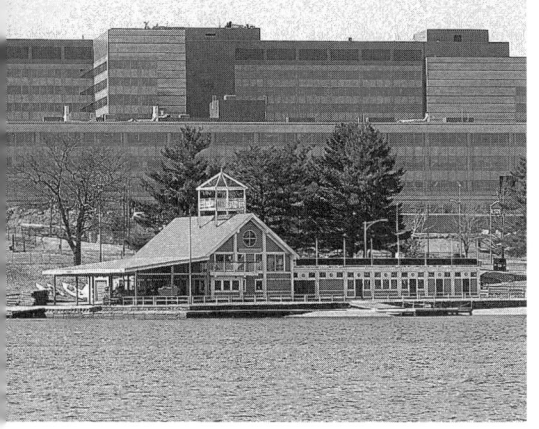

University of Massachusetts Medical School

Worcester, Massachusetts

University of Massachusetts Medical School
Office of Admissions
55 Lake Avenue, North, Room S1-112
Worcester, Massachusetts 01655
T 508 856 2323   F 508 856-3629

Admissions www.umassmed.edu/som/admissions
Main www.umassmed.edu/education
Financial www.umass.edu/financialaid
Email admissions@umassmed.edu

Public Institution

Dr. Terrence Flotte, Dean

*Dr. John Paraskos,
Associate Dean for Admissions*

*Dr. Danna B. Peterson, Assistant Dean of
Student Affairs and Minority Support*

Betsy Groves, Director of Financial Aid

General Information

Established in 1962, the University of Massachusetts Medical School accepted its first class in 1970. UMMS is committed to training physicians in a wide range of medical disciplines and emphasizes training for practice in general medicine and the primary care specialties in the public sector and in underserved areas of Massachusetts. This mission has since been expanded to include graduate education in the biomedical sciences and nursing, graduate medical education, and continuing medical education for health professionals. The school's clinical partner is UMass Memorial Medical Center, consisting of two acute care hospitals with a total of 761 beds. Clinical education is also conducted at a number of affiliated community hospitals and health centers in the region. UMMS Worcester is adjacent to the Massachusetts Biotechnology Research Park, which houses a number of UMass research programs including the Program in Molecular Medicine, the Cancer Center, and the Worcester Foundation for Biomedical Research.

Mission Statement

The mission of the University of Massachusetts Medical School is to serve the people of the Commonwealth through excellence in health sciences education, clinical care, research, and public service.

Curricular Highlights

Community Service Requirement: Optional.
Research/Thesis Requirement: Optional.

The UMMS curriculum encourages interdisciplinary learning and integration of the basic and clinical sciences, with special attention to clinical correlation of subject matter in the preclinical years. Emphasis in the first year is on normal structure and function with a balance of small-group learning and large-group function. Emphasis in the second year is on the etiology of disease, pathophysiology, pharmacology, and clinical diagnosis. The third and fourth years are a continuum of required clerkships and both clinical and research electives. UMMS also encourages students to participate in research programs in basic and clinical science departments.

USMLE

Step 1: Required. Students must record a passing score for graduation, but not promotion.
Step 2: Clinical Skills (CS): Required. Students must only record a score.
Step 2: Clinical Knowledge (CK): Required. Students must only record a score.

Selection Factors

Current policy limits admission to the M.D. program to students who are Massachusetts residents. Residents and non-residents of Massachusetts are eligible for admission to the joint MD/PhD program through the Graduate School of Biomedical Sciences and the Medical School. All applicants must be U.S. citizens or have permanent resident status. The admissions committee bases its evaluation of applicants on academic ability and achievement, MCAT® scores, and such factors as extracurricular achievement, maturity, motivation, and character as these are reflected in letters of recommendation from pre-professional advisory committees and other persons. Interviews are arranged by invitation only. Applicants are selected on the basis of their individual merits without regard to race, sex, creed, national origin, age, or disability. UMMS has a set of technical standards for admission and promotion, which are available upon request.

Financial Aid

Please refer to the UMMS Financial Aid Web page.

Information about Diversity Programs

For additional information, please contact the Associate Vice Chancellor for School Services at 508-856-2444.

Campus Information

Setting

UMMS is in Worcester, MA and thus conveniently located in central Massachusetts. UMass Memorial Health Care is the clinical partner of UMMS and the largest health care system serving central and western Massachusetts. The medical school and clinical affiliate share adjoining buildings. There are several institutions of higher learning in the area offering culturally diverse activities. The campus is accessible by local bus and taxicab services.

Enrollment

For 2007, total enrollment was: 423

Special Features

The UMMS clinical affiliate, UMass Memorial Health Care, houses a regional trauma center and provides specialized education in primary, secondary, tertiary, and quaternary health care. A recently expanded research facility in close proximity to the biotech park has made the campus a focus for biotechnology research in Massachusetts. Students are given the opportunity for international rotations. *U.S. News & World Report* has consistently ranked the medical school as a top school for primary care education.

Housing

On-campus housing is not available. There are many affordable apartments within fifteen minutes of the medical school. Rents average $800-$1,000 per month.

Satellite Campuses/Facilities

Student rotations are divided among multiple campuses of UMass Memorial Health Care: University, Memorial, and Hahnemann Campuses and Clinton, Marlborough, Wing Memorial, and HealthAlliance Hospitals. The school is also affiliated with other suburban medical centers, such as the Berkshire Medical Center, Milford-Whitinsville Regional Hospital, St. Elizabeth's Hospital in Brighton, St. Vincent Hospital at Worcester Medical Center, and the Day Kimball Hospital in Connecticut.

Application Process and Requirements 2009–2010

Primary Application Service: AMCAS
Earliest filing date: June 1, 2008
Latest filing date: November 1, 2008

Secondary Application Required?: Yes
Sent to: All verified applicants
Contact: Admissions Office, 508-856-2323, admissions@umassmed.edu
Fee: Yes, $75
Fee waiver available: Yes
Earliest filing date: After verified application received
Latest filing date: Must be completed by December 15, 2008

Latest MCAT® considered: September 2008
Oldest MCAT® considered: 2005

Early Decision Program
School does have EDP
Applicants notified: October 1, 2008
EDP available for: Residents only

Regular Acceptance Notice
Earliest date: October 15, 2008
Latest date: Until Class is Full

Applicant's Response to Acceptance
Offer – Maximum Time: Two weeks

Requests for Deferred
Entrance Considered: Yes

Deposit to Hold Place in Class: Yes
Deposit (Resident): $100
Deposit (Non-Resident): $100
Deposit due: With response to acceptance offer
Applied to tuition: Yes
Deposit refundable: Yes
Refundable by: May 15, 2009

Estimated number of new entrants: 103
EDP: 10, special program: n/a

Start Month/Year: August 2009

Interview Format: Students meet one-on-one with two interviewers. Off campus interviews are available.

Other Programs

PREPARATORY PROGRAMS
Postbaccalaureate Program: No
Summer Program: Yes, www.umassmed.edu/summer
Summer Enrichment Program
www.umassmed.edu/outreach/sep.aspx
COMBINED DEGREE PROGRAMS
Baccalaureate/MD: No
MD/MPH: No
MD/MBA: No
MD/JD: No
MD/PhD: Yes, www.umassmed.edu/MDPhD/index.aspx

Premedical Coursework

Course	Req.	Rec.	Lab.	Sems.	Course	Req.	Rec.	Lab.	Sems.
Inorganic Chemistry	•		•	2	Computer Science		•		2
Behavioral Sciences					Genetics				
Biochemistry		•			Organic Chemistry	•		•	2
Biology	•		•	2	Physics	•		•	2
Biology/Zoology	•		•	2	Psychology		•		
Calculus		•			Social Sciences				
College English	•			2	Statistics				2
College Mathematics					Other				

Selection Factors: 2007 Accepted Applicants

Proportion of Accepted Applicants with Relevant Experience (Data Self-Reported to AMCAS®)		
Community Service/Volunteer	69%
Medically-Related Work	83%
Research	82%

Shaded bar represents accepted scores ranging from the 10th percentile to the 90th percentile. **School Median** ● **National Median** ●

Overall GPA	2.0	2.1	2.2	2.3	2.4	2.5	2.6	2.7	2.8	2.9	3.0	3.1	3.2	3.3	3.4	3.5	3.6	(3.7)	3.8	3.9	4.0
Science GPA	2.0	2.1	2.2	2.3	2.4	2.5	2.6	2.7	2.8	2.9	3.0	3.1	3.2	3.3	3.4	3.5	3.6	(3.7)	3.8	3.9	4.0

MCAT® required: Yes, 100% of 2007 accepted applicants took MCAT®

Verbal Reasoning	3	4	5	6	7	8	9	(10)	(11)	12	13	14	15
Physical Sciences	3	4	5	6	7	8	9	10	(11)	12	13	14	15
Biological Sciences	3	4	5	6	7	8	9	10	(11)	12	13	14	15
Writing Sample				J	K	L	M	N	O	P	(Q)	R	S	T

Acceptance & Matriculation Data for 2007–2008 First Year Class

	Resident	Non-Resident	International	Total
Applied	750	76	4	830
Interviewed	451	19	0	470
Deferred	4	0	0	4
Matriculants				
Early Assurance Program	n/a	n/a	n/a	n/a
Early Decision Program	5	0	0	5
Baccalaureate/MD	n/a	n/a	n/a	n/a
MD/PhD	6	3	0	9
Matriculated	101	2	0	**103**

Applications accepted from International Applicants: No

Matriculant Demographics: 2007–2008 First Year Class

Men: 46 **Women:** 57

Matriculants' Self-Reported Race/Ethnicity

Mexican American	0	Korean	1
Cuban	0	Vietnamese	1
Puerto Rican	1	Other Asian	0
Other Hispanic	2	Total Asian	13
Total Hispanic	3	Native American	0
Chinese	7	Black	10
Asian Indian	3	Native Hawaiian	0
Pakistani	0	White	81
Filipino	0	Unduplicated Number	
Japanese	1	of Matriculants	103

Science and Math Majors: 64%
Matriculants with:
Baccalaureate degree: 100%
Graduate degree(s): 9%

Specialty Choice

2003, 2004, 2005 Graduates, Specialty Choice (As reported by program directors to GME Track™)	
Anesthesiology	4%
Emergency Medicine	8%
Family Practice	11%
Internal Medicine	23%
Obstetrics/Gynecology	4%
Orthopaedic Surgery	4%
Pediatrics	16%
Psychiatry	4%
Radiology	5%
Surgery	6%

Financial Information

Source: 2006–2007 LCME I-B survey and 2007–2008 AAMC TSF questionnaire

	Residents	Non-Residents
Total Cost of Attendance	$14,087	$0
Tuition and Fees	$13,414	$0
Other (includes living expenses)	$200	$0
Health Insurance (can be waived)	$473	$0

Average 2007 Graduate Indebtedness: $122,227
% of Enrolled Students Receiving Aid: 96%

Criminal Background Check

This medical school does not require a criminal background check prior to matriculation.

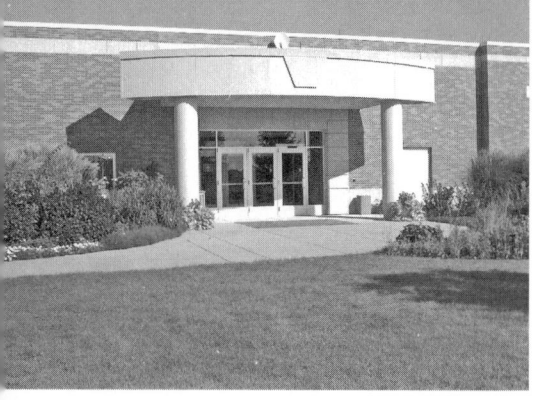

Michigan State University
College of Human Medicine

East Lansing, Michigan

College of Human Medicine, Office of Admissions
A-239 Life Sciences
Michigan State University
East Lansing, Michigan 48824-1317
T 517 353 9620 **F** 517 432 0021

Admissions http://MDadmissions.msu.edu
Main http://humanmedicine.msu.edu
Financial http://finaid.msu.edu/med
Email MDadmissions@msu.edu

Public Institution

Dr. Marsha Rappley, Dean

Dr. Wanda Lipscomb, Associate Dean for Student Affairs, Diversity and Outreach

Dr. Christine Shafer, Assistant Dean for Admissions

Jay Bryde, Admissions Officer

Letitia Fowler, Admissions Senior Counselor

Diane Batten, Coordinator of Medical Student Financial Aid

General Information

The College of Human Medicine (CHM) was founded in response to Michigan's need for primary care physicians. Located on an active Big Ten campus, CHM provides a small college atmosphere. Students begin at the East Lansing campus where they are taught in the classroom, laboratory, and clinical settings before moving on to one of the six community campuses.

Mission Statement

The College of Human Medicine at Michigan State University is committed to educating exemplary physicians and scholars, discovering and disseminating new knowledge, and providing service at home and abroad. We enhance our communities by providing outstanding primary and specialty care, promoting the dignity and inclusion of all people, and responding to the needs of the medically underserved.

Curricular Highlights

Community Service Requirement: Optional. Most are active clinical service and otherwise.
Research/Thesis Requirement: Optional. Various research opportunities exist.

The curriculum provides an integration of the basic biological, behavioral, and social sciences; a developmental approach to learning; early teaching of clinical skills; and clinical training utilizing a community-integrated approach. Grading is on a modified pass/no pass system. Honors-level performance is recognized. Block I is a 2/12 semester experience in which fundamental basic science is presented in a structured, discipline-based format. Basic clinical skills teaching

begins, along with a mentor group, longitudinal patient exposure, and opportunity for independent as well as supplementary learning experiences. A clinical correlations course integrates basic science and medicine. Block II comprises two-semesters of a problem-based format with emphasis on small-group learning and use of a clinical context for basic science concepts. Clinical skills training continues along with special topics seminars. Block III includes 60 weeks of required and 20 weeks of elective clerkships. Required clerkships include a family medicine clerkship. Students have the option to complete elective clerkships in other locations, including third world countries. A Rural Physician Program and a program focused on underserved populations are available.

USMLE

Step 1: Required. Students must record a passing score for promotion.
Step 2: Clinical Skills (CS): Required. Students must record a passing total score to graduate.
Step 2: Clinical Knowledge (CK): Required. Students must record a passing total score to graduate.

Selection Factors

CHM seeks to admit a class that is academically competent, reflective of the rural and urban character of Michigan, and representative of a wide spectrum of personalities, backgrounds, and talents. Disadvantaged students are invited to apply. Ability to pay is not a factor. Selection is based on many factors, including year-to-year and cumulative GPA; MCAT® performance; fit with the school's mission; relevant clinical and community service; assessments of motivation, ability to communicate and problem-solving, maturity, and suitability for the MSU program; state of residence; and potential to contribute to the overall quality of the entering class. CHM considers U.S. and Canadian residents, and applicants with U.S. permanent resident status.

Financial Aid

Information about specific scholarships and financial aid can be obtained from the Office of Financial Aid at *finaid.msu.edu/med.*

Information about Diversity Programs

The Advanced Baccalaureate Learning

Experience (ABLE) is a two semester, enriched academic experience offered to an invited group of disadvantaged students who have applied for admission to CHM. Students who complete the ABLE Program requirements are offered regular admission to CHM's entering class.

Campus Information

Setting

The pre-clinical campus is located in East Lansing, three miles east of Michigan's capitol in Lansing. Students enjoy the 5,200-acre park-like campus, cultural events and entertainment, championship golf courses, and Big Ten athletics. The 9,428 graduate and professional students on campus include law, osteopathic medicine, and veterinary students. Clinical training occurs in one of six fully supported community campuses.

Enrollment

For 2007, total enrollment was: 494

Special Features

Students enjoy a cooperative, service-oriented education where interests and needs are supported by the ABLE program, an extended curriculum option, the Rural Physician Program, and the Leadership in Medicine for the Underserved/Vulnerable Program. The Center for Ethics and Humanities in the Life Sciences makes a strong contribution.

Housing

Options include nearby townhouses and condominiums and subsidized apartment complexes. The University operates three large on-campus apartment complexes and the Owen Graduate Center providing accommodations for graduate and professional students.

Satellite Campuses/Facilities

Clinical campuses (Flint, Grand Rapids, Kalamazoo, Lansing, Saginaw, and the Upper Peninsula) comprise full-time, part-time, and volunteer faculty in the clinical disciplines. Students are connected to an array of health care resources in the community that allow for hands-on learning, exposure to diverse patient problems, and actual medical practice settings. An option to complete both Block II and Block III curriculum is available in Grand Rapids.

Application Process and Requirements 2009–2010

Primary Application Service: AMCAS
Earliest filing date: June 1, 2008
Latest filing date: November 15, 2008

Secondary Application Required?: Yes
Sent to: All applicants with fee paid.
URL: URL provided upon receipt of $60 Secondary Application fee.
Fee: Yes, $60
Fee waiver available: Yes
Earliest filing date: August 2008
Latest filing date: Febuary 2009

Latest MCAT® considered: September 2008
Oldest MCAT® considered: 2005

Early Decision Program
School does have EDP
Applicants notified: October 1, 2008
EDP available for: Both Residents and Non-Residents

Regular Acceptance Notice
Earliest date: October 15, 2008
Latest date: Varies

Applicant's Response to Acceptance Offer – Maximum Time: Two weks

Requests for Deferred Entrance Considered: Yes

Deposit to Hold Place in Class: Yes
Deposit (Resident): $100
Deposit (Non-Resident): $100
Deposit due: With response to acceptance offer
Applied to tuition: Yes
Deposit refundable: Yes
Refundable by: May 15, 2009

Estimated number of new entrants: 156
EDP: 5, special program: 20

Start Month/Year: August 2009

Interview Format: Individual 30 minute student and faculty interviews. Regional interviews are being considered.

Other Programs

PREPARATORY PROGRAMS
Postbaccalaureate Program: Yes.
http://mdadmissions.msu.edu/main/able.htm
Summer Program: No

COMBINED DEGREE PROGRAMS
Baccalaureate/MD: Yes
http://MDadmissions.msu.edu/main/msapplication.htm
MD/MPH: No
MD/MBA: No
MD/JD: No
MD/PhD: Yes,
http://mdadmissions.msu.edu/main/mdphd.htm

Premedical Coursework

Course	Req.	Rec.	Lab.	Sems.	Course	Req.	Rec.	Lab.	Sems.
Inorganic Chemistry	•		•	2	Computer Science		•		
Behavioral Sciences		•			Genetics		•		
Biochemistry		•			Humanities	•			2
Biology	•		•	2	Organic Chemistry	•		•	2
Biology/Zoology					Physics	•		•	2
Calculus					Psychology		•		
College English	•			2	Social Sciences	•	•		
College Mathematics	•			1	1 Upper-Level Biology	•			1

Selection Factors: 2007 Accepted Applicants

Proportion of Accepted Applicants with Relevant Experience (Data Self-Reported to AMCAS)		
Community Service/Volunteer	76%
Medically-Related Work	94%
Research	78%

Shaded bar represents accepted scores ranging from the 10th percentile to the 90th percentile. **School Median** ● **National Median** ●

Overall GPA	2.0	2.1	2.2	2.3	2.4	2.5	2.6	2.7	2.8	2.9	3.0	3.1	3.2	3.3	3.4	3.5	(3.6)	3.7	3.8	3.9	4.0
Science GPA	2.0	2.1	2.2	2.3	2.4	2.5	2.6	2.7	2.8	2.9	3.0	3.1	3.2	3.3	3.4	(3.5)	3.6	3.7	3.8	3.9	4.0

MCAT® required: Yes, 96% of 2007 accepted applicants took MCAT®

Verbal Reasoning	3	4	5	6	7	8	9	(10)	11	12	13	14	15
Physical Sciences	3	4	5	6	7	8	9	(10)	(11)	12	13	14	15
Biological Sciences	3	4	5	6	7	8	9	(10)	(11)	12	13	14	15
Writing Sample			J	K	L	M	N	O	(P)	(Q)	R	S	T

Acceptance & Matriculation Data for 2007–2008 First Year Class

	Resident	Non-Resident	International	Total
Applied	1274	3422	305	5001
Interviewed	272	158	10	440
Deferred	8	5	0	13
Matriculants				
Early Assurance Program	0	0	0	0
Early Decision Program	5	0	0	5
Baccalaureate/MD	10	0	0	10
MD/PhD	n/a	n/a	n/a	n/a
Matriculated	99	54	3	156

Applications accepted from International Applicants: Canadian only

Specialty Choice

2003, 2004, 2005 Graduates, Specialty Choice (As reported by program directors to GME Track™)	
Anesthesiology	6%
Emergency Medicine	8%
Family Practice	18%
Internal Medicine	13%
Obstetrics/Gynecology	10%
Orthopaedic Surgery	2%
Pediatrics	10%
Psychiatry	6%
Radiology	5%
Surgery	7%

Matriculant Demographics: 2007–2008 First Year Class

Men: 73 **Women:** 83

Matriculants' Self-Reported Race/Ethnicity

Mexican American	6	Korean	3
Cuban	0	Vietnamese	2
Puerto Rican	0	Other Asian	2
Other Hispanic	2	Total Asian	30
Total Hispanic	7	Native American	3
Chinese	11	Black	8
Asian Indian	7	Native Hawaiian	0
Pakistani	1	White	108
Filipino	4	Unduplicated Number	
Japanese	1	of Matriculants	156

Science and Math Majors: 65%
Matriculants with:
Baccalaureate degree: 99%
Graduate degree(s): 22%

Financial Information

Source: 2006–2007 LCME I-B survey and 2007–2008 AAMC TSF questionnaire

	Residents	Non-Residents
Total Cost of Attendance	$54,084	$86,966
Tuition and Fees	$28,010	$60,890
Other (includes living expenses)	$24,681	$24,683
Health Insurance (can be waived)	$1,393	$1,393

Average 2007 Graduate Indebtedness: $130,301
% of Enrolled Students Receiving Aid: 95%

Criminal Background Check

This medical school does not require a criminal background check prior to matriculation.

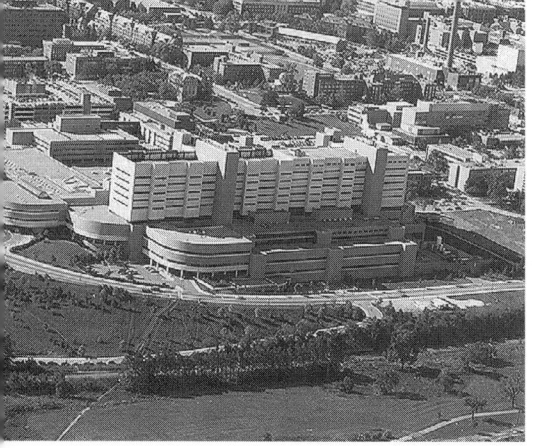

University of Michigan Medical School

Ann Arbor, Michigan

Admissions Office
4303 Medical Science I Building
University of Michigan Medical School
Ann Arbor, Michigan 48109-0624
T 734 764 6317   **F** 734 763 0453

Admissions www.med.umich.edu/medschool/admissions
Main www.med.umich.edu/medschool
Financial www.med.umich.edu/medschool/financialaid
Email umichmedadmiss@umich.edu

Public Institution

Dr. James Woolliscroft, Dean

Dr. Steven Gay, Assistant Dean of Admissions

Dr. David Gordon, Assistant Dean for Diversity and Career Development

Robert F. Ruiz, Director of Admissions

Carmen Colby, Director of Financial Aid

General Information

The University of Michigan Medical School was founded in 1850. This school was the first to establish a university-owned hospital. Today, the medical center occupies more than 30 buildings, the world's largest one-site complex devoted to health care, education, and research. The Health System consistently ranks as one of the top ten in the nation.

Mission Statement

The University of Michigan Medical School seeks to graduate a diverse cohort of physicians who are dedicated to life-long learning. Our goals include educating individuals committed to achieving the highest standards of competency required to provide exemplary patient care. We seek to graduate culturally competent physicians who will assume leadership roles in the areas of clinical medicine, research, and teaching. Physicians who graduate from the University of Michigan will demonstrate a strong foundation in biomedical sciences; empathetic interpersonal skills; an ability to identify and reduce health risk factors; an ability to obtain and interpret relevant patient information and to make effective clinical decisions; a commitment to achieving personal and professional excellence; and the critical attributes of compassion, honesty, and integrity.

Curricular Highlights

Community Service Requirement: Optional.
Research/Thesis Requirement: Optional.

In the first year, the introductory Patients and Populations course acquaints medical students with genetics, principles of disease, epidemiology, and evidence-based medicine. After that, most of the material is structured within Normal Organ Systems sequences and a Microbiology and Infectious Disease course. Clinical skills are taught in focused one- and two-week modules throughout the first and second years, beginning with the medical interview and history-taking skills and moving to physical examination practice. In the two-year Family Centered Experience, pairs of first-year students are assigned to a family in the community. These families will serve as resources to help medical students understand how health changes, chronic conditions, and serious illnesses affect patients and those close to them. The second year curriculum features Abnormal Organ Systems sequences. It includes additional patient cases and continuing reinforcement of information gathering and critical appraisal skills. Clinical skills modules will continue with expectations for mastery of more advanced physical examination, history-taking, and communication skills. Clinical training in the third year includes required rotations, and opportunities for career exploratory electives. Fourth-year requirements include a subinternship and an ICU experience, as well as a course in Advanced Medical Therapeutics. In the subinternship, students are assigned their own patient caseload and they perform with almost the same level of responsibility as a resident. The fourth year includes eight weeks of vacation and interviewing time, as well as 12 weeks of electives, with opportunities for off-campus and international rotations. All courses in the first year are graded pass/fail. In the subsequent years, faculty assign students grades of honors, high pass, pass, or fail.

USMLE

Step 1: Required. Students must record a passing score for promotion.
Step 2: Clinical Skills (CS): Required. Students must record a passing total score to graduate.
Step 2: Clinical Knowledge (CK): Required. Students must record a passing total score to graduate.

Selection Factors

The Admissions Committee is dedicated to matriculating those individuals with the skills, intelligence, and personal attributes to become leaders in medicine. Although admitted students all have demonstrated the ability to succeed academically, other attributes such as compassion, empathy, altruism, leadership, honesty, and communication and interpersonal skills are viewed as being critical to future excellence. The committee considers that all information pertaining to the ability, personality, and character of the applicant is relevant. Although a solid background in science is required, students with expertise in a wide variety of fields, including the humanities, arts, and engineering, are encouraged to apply.

Financial Aid

Application for financial aid may be initiated following acceptance to the medical school.

Information about Diversity Programs

The University of Michigan is committed to training a diverse cohort of physicians who are capable of caring for an increasingly diverse patient population. Medical students of color are very active in organizations such as LANAMA (Latino/a American/Native American Medical Association) and BMA (Black Medical Association). These students are also actively involved in setting the agenda for diversity and cultural competency programs, and participate in the Health System's Multi-cultural Community Health Alliance.

Campus Information

Setting

The University of Michigan Medical School is nestled in a large medical center surrounded by tree-lined streets, city parks and bike paths.

Enrollment

For 2007, total enrollment was: 678

Housing

While some students choose campus housing, most students opt to live in apartments near the medical center.

Application Process and Requirements 2009–2010

Primary Application Service: AMCAS
Earliest filing date: June 1, 2008
Latest filing date: November 15, 2008

Secondary Application Required?: Yes
Sent to: All applicants
URL: n/a
Fee: Yes, $85
Fee waiver available: Yes
Earliest filing date: July 1, 2008
Latest filing date: December 31, 2008

Latest MCAT® considered: September 2008
Oldest MCAT® considered: 2006

Early Decision Program
School does not have EDP
Applicants notified: n/a
EDP available for: n/a

Regular Acceptance Notice
Earliest date: October 15, 2008
Latest date: Until class is full

Applicant's Response to Acceptance Offer – Maximum Time: May 15, 2009

Requests for Deferred Entrance Considered: Yes

Deposit to Hold Place in Class: No
Deposit (Resident): n/a
Deposit (Non-Resident): n/a
Deposit due: n/a
Applied to tuition: n/a
Deposit refundable: n/a
Refundable by: n/a

Estimated number of new entrants: 170
EDP: n/a, special program: n/a

Start Month/Year: August 2009

Interview Format:
Regional interviews are not available.

Other Programs

PREPARATORY PROGRAMS
Postbaccalaureate Program: No
Summer Program: Yes

COMBINED DEGREE PROGRAMS
Baccalaureate/MD: No
MD/MPH: Yes,
www.sph.umich.edu/academics/degrees.html
MD/MBA: Yes, http://med.umich.edu/medstudents/curRes/
dualDegree/mdMBA/index.html
MD/JD: Yes
MD/PhD: Yes, www.med.umich.edu/medschool/mstp/

Premedical Coursework

Course	Req.	Rec.	Lab.	Hrs.
Inorganic Chemistry	•		•	4
Behavioral Sciences				
Biochemistry	•			3
Biology	•		•	6
Biology/Zoology				
Calculus				
College English	•			6
College Mathematics				

Course	Req.	Rec.	Lab.	Hrs.
Computer Science				
Genetics				
Humanities	•			18
Organic Chemistry	•		•	4
Physics	•		•	6
Psychology				
Social Sciences				
Other				

Selection Factors: 2007 Accepted Applicants

Proportion of Accepted Applicants with Relevant Experience (Data Self-Reported to AMCAS)		
Community Service/Volunteer		71%
Medically-Related Work		86%
Research		92%

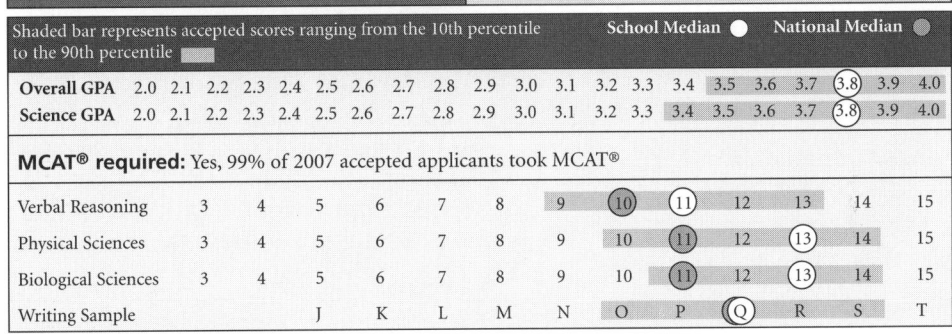

Shaded bar represents accepted scores ranging from the 10th percentile to the 90th percentile. School Median ● National Median ◐

Overall GPA	2.0	2.1	2.2	2.3	2.4	2.5	2.6	2.7	2.8	2.9	3.0	3.1	3.2	3.3	3.4	3.5	3.6	3.7	(3.8)	3.9	4.0
Science GPA	2.0	2.1	2.2	2.3	2.4	2.5	2.6	2.7	2.8	2.9	3.0	3.1	3.2	3.3	3.4	3.5	3.6	3.7	(3.8)	3.9	4.0

MCAT® required: Yes, 99% of 2007 accepted applicants took MCAT®

Verbal Reasoning	3	4	5	6	7	8	9	(10)	(11)	12	13	14	15
Physical Sciences	3	4	5	6	7	8	9	10	(11)	12	(13)	14	15
Biological Sciences	3	4	5	6	7	8	9	10	(11)	12	(13)	14	15
Writing Sample			J	K	L	M	N	O	P	(Q)	R	S	T

Acceptance & Matriculation Data for 2007–2008 First Year Class

	Resident	Non-Resident	International	Total
Applied	1067	4517	85	5669
Interviewed	181	620	0	801
Deferred	7	5	0	12
Matriculants				
Early Assurance Program	0	0	0	0
Early Decision Program	0	0	0	0
Baccalaureate/MD	n/a	n/a	n/a	n/a
MD/PhD	3	7	0	10
Matriculated	76	93	1	**170**

Applications accepted from International Applicants: No

Specialty Choice

2003, 2004, 2005 Graduates, Specialty Choice (As reported by program directors to GME Track™)	
Anesthesiology	7%
Emergency Medicine	8%
Family Practice	5%
Internal Medicine	16%
Obstetrics/Gynecology	4%
Orthopaedic Surgery	4%
Pediatrics	8%
Psychiatry	3%
Radiology	6%
Surgery	8%

Matriculant Demographics: 2007–2008 First Year Class

Men: 77 **Women:** 93

Matriculants' Self-Reported Race/Ethnicity

Mexican American	2	Korean	4
Cuban	1	Vietnamese	2
Puerto Rican	1	Other Asian	1
Other Hispanic	3	Total Asian	43
Total Hispanic	7	Native American	2
Chinese	17	Black	12
Asian Indian	18	Native Hawaiian	0
Pakistani	0	White	117
Filipino	1	**Unduplicated Number**	
Japanese	2	**of Matriculants**	170

Science and Math Majors: 71%
Matriculants with:
Baccalaureate degree: 100%
Graduate degree(s): 9%

Financial Information

Source: 2006–2007 LCME I-B survey
and 2007–2008 AAMC TSF questionnaire

	Residents	Non-Residents
Total Cost of Attendance	$46,445	$61,534
Tuition and Fees	$24,755	$39,119
Other (includes living expenses)	$19,690	$20,415
Health Insurance (can be waived)	$2,000	$2,000

Average 2007 Graduate Indebtedness: $102,383
% of Enrolled Students Receiving Aid: 94%

Criminal Background Check

This medical school requires a criminal background check prior to matriculation.

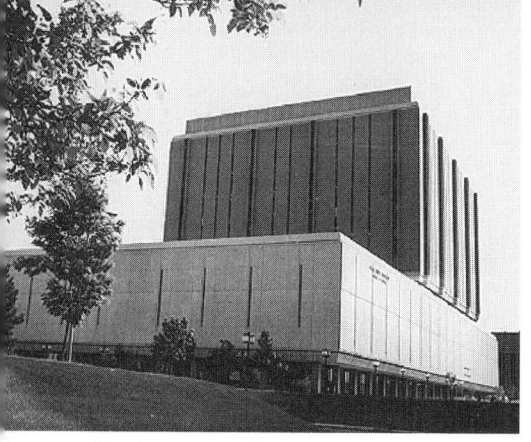

Wayne State University School of Medicine

Detroit, Michigan

Office of Admissions
540 East Canfield, Suite 1310
Detroit, Michigan 48201
T 313 577 1466   F 313 577 9420

Admissions www.med.wayne.edu/admissions
Main www.med.wayne.edu
Financial www.med.wayne.edu/student_affairs/
financial_aid
Email admissions@med.wayne.edu

Public Institution

Dr. Robert M. Mentzer Jr., Dean

Dr. Silas Norman Jr., Assistant Dean for Admissions

Julia Simmons, Director, Diversity and Integrated Student Services Office

Deirdre Moore, Assistant Director, Financial Aid

Dr. Robert R. Frank, Executive Vice Dean

General Information

The School of Medicine, which originated in 1868, is the oldest component of Wayne State University.

Mission Statement

The mission of the Wayne State University School of Medicine is to provide the Michigan community with medical and biotechnical resources, in the form of scientific knowledge and trained professionals, so as to improve the overall health of the community.

Curricular Highlights

Community Service Requirement: Optional. A co-curricular program is available.
Research/Thesis Requirement: Optional.

The curriculum employs a combination of traditional and newer approaches to the teaching of medical students. Year 1 begins with an introductory Clinical Medicine course which runs through all four years including: human sexuality, medical interviewing, physical diagnosis, public health and prevention, and evidence-based medicine. Year 1 is organized around the disciplines of structure (anatomy, histology, and embryology) and function (biochemistry, physiology, genetics, and nutrition), and ends with an integrated neuroscience course. Second year is a completely integrated year focusing on patho-physiology, including immunology/micro-biology and pharmacology. Year 3 is a series of clinical clerkships including medicine, surgery, pediatrics, family medicine, psychiatry, neurology, and obstetrics/gynecology. During Year 3 all students have a six-month Continuity clerkship. Year 4 is predominately an elective year with only

three required one month rotations: emergency medicine, a sub-internship, and an ambulatory block month. The School of Medicine uses traditional lectures, small-group and panel discussions, computer-assisted instruction, and multimedia in its teaching program. Standardized patients are used for student practice and assessment.

USMLE

Step 1: Required. Students must record a passing score for promotion.
Step 2: Clinical Skills (CS): Required. Students must only record a score.
Step 2: Clinical Knowledge (CK): Required. Students must record a passing total score to graduate.

Selection Factors

Consideration is given to the entire record, GPA, MCAT® scores, recommendations, and interview results, as these reflect the applicant's personality, maturity, character, and suitability for medicine. Additionally, the committee regards health care experience as desirable. Following an initial screening process, individuals with competitive applications are selected to complete a secondary application. As a state-supported school, the institution must give preference to Michigan residents; however, out-of-state applicants are encouraged to apply. An applicant's residency is determined by university regulations. Applicants whose educational backgrounds include academic work outside the United States must have completed two years of coursework at a U.S. or Canadian college, including the prerequisite courses. Interviews are required, but scheduled only with those applicants who are given serious consideration. Students are urged to apply by November 1.

Financial Aid

Financial aid awards administered by the School of Medicine are made by the financial aid officer based on federal guidelines and those established by the Committee on Financial Aid and Scholarships, which includes student representation. The College Work-Study Program and other medically oriented jobs are generally available to eligible students for the summer break. Financial aid seminars are held for incoming students and their families. Additional information is

available by calling the Office of Financial Aid at (313) 577-1039 or visiting its Web site.

Information about Diversity Programs

The school supports a one-year postbaccalaureate program for disadvantaged medical school applicants from Michigan who have been denied admission, but who appear to have the potential for academic success. The program consists of premedical science courses, academic skills training, personal adjustment counseling, and academic tutoring. Successful students are guaranteed admission to the School of Medicine. For information, write Julia Simmons, Director, Office of Diversity and Integrated Student Services.

Campus Information

Setting

WSUSOM is located in the 236 acre Detroit Medical Center in Detroit, and consists of Scott Hall, the basic science building, Shiffman Medical Library, Lande Medical Research Building, Elliman Clinical Research Building, and the C.S. Mott Building.

Enrollment

For 2007, total enrollment was: 1167

Special Features

Harper University Hospital, Hutzel Women's Hospital, the Children's Hospital of Michigan, Detroit Receiving Hospital, University Health Center, the Rehabilitation Institute of Michigan, and the John Dingell V.A. Medical Center make up the Detroit Medical Center (DMC). In addition, the SEMCME (SE Michigan Center for Medical Education) brings together Wayne State University, the DMC, and community-based teaching hospitals in the Southeastern Michigan metropolitan area.

Housing

On-campus resident housing is available on the main campus located near the medical center. The Office of Student Organizations maintains a list of affordable apartments located near the medical school.

Application Process and Requirements 2009–2010

Primary Application Service: AMCAS
Earliest filing date: June 1, 2008
Latest filing date: December 15, 2008

Secondary Application Required?: Yes
Sent to: Screened applicants
Contact: Dawn Yargeau
(313) 577-1466, admissions@med.wayne.edu
Fee: Yes, $50
Fee waiver available: Yes
Earliest filing date: August 1, 2008
Latest filing date: March 1, 2009

Latest MCAT® considered: September 2008
Oldest MCAT® considered: 2005

Early Decision Program
School does have EDP
Applicants notified: October 1, 2008
EDP available for: Both Residents
and Non-Residents

Regular Acceptance Notice
Earliest date: October 22, 2008
Latest date: Varies

**Applicant's Response to Acceptance
Offer – Maximum Time:** Three weeks

**Requests for Deferred
Entrance Considered:** Yes

Deposit to Hold Place in Class: Yes
Deposit (Resident): $50
Deposit (Non-Resident): $50
Deposit due: With response to acceptance offer
Applied to tuition: Yes
Deposit refundable: No
Refundable by: n/a

Estimated number of new entrants: 290
EDP: 5, special program: 17

Start Month/Year: August 2009

Interview Format: One-on-one with an
Admission Committee member. Regional
interviews are not available.

Other Programs

PREPARATORY PROGRAMS
Postbaccalaureate Program: Yes,
Julia Simmons, (313) 577-1598
jsimmons@med.wayne.edu
Summer Program: Yes, Julia Simmons,
(313) 577-1598, jsimmons@med.wayne.edu
COMBINED DEGREE PROGRAMS
Baccalaureate/MD: Yes, http://honors.wayne.edu/
medstart.php, Nancy Galster, (313) 577-3030,
ad4469@wayne.edu
MD/MPH: No
MD/MBA: No
MD/JD: No
MD/PhD: Yes, www.med.wayne.edu/gradprog/
md_phd/, Ambika Mathur, Ph.D., (313) 577-1455
amathur@med.wayne.edu

Premedical Coursework

Course	Req.	Rec.	Lab.	Sems.
Inorganic Chemistry	•		•	2
Behavioral Sciences				
Biochemistry		•		1
Biology				
Biology/Zoology	•		•	2
Calculus				
College English	•			2
College Mathematics				

Course	Req.	Rec.	Lab.	Sems.
Computer Science				
Genetics				
Humanities				
Organic Chemistry	•		•	2
Physics	•		•	2
Psychology				
Social Sciences				
Other				

Selection Factors: 2007 Accepted Applicants

Proportion of Accepted Applicants with Relevant Experience (Data Self-Reported to AMCAS)		
Community Service/Volunteer		69%
Medically-Related Work		88%
Research		78%

Shaded bar represents accepted scores ranging from the 10th percentile to the 90th percentile. School Median ● National Median ●

Overall GPA	2.0	2.1	2.2	2.3	2.4	2.5	2.6	2.7	2.8	2.9	3.0	3.1	3.2	3.3	3.4	3.5	3.6	(3.7)	3.8	3.9	4.0
Science GPA	2.0	2.1	2.2	2.3	2.4	2.5	2.6	2.7	2.8	2.9	3.0	3.1	3.2	3.3	3.4	3.5	3.6	(3.7)	3.8	3.9	4.0

MCAT® required: Yes, 100% of 2007 accepted applicants took MCAT®

Verbal Reasoning	3	4	5	6	7	8	9	(10)	11	12	13	14	15
Physical Sciences	3	4	5	6	7	8	9	10	(11)	12	13	14	15
Biological Sciences	3	4	5	6	7	8	9	10	(11)	12	13	14	15
Writing Sample			J	K	L	M	N	O	(P)	(Q)	R	S	T

Acceptance & Matriculation Data for 2007–2008 First Year Class

	Resident	Non-Resident	International	Total
Applied	1376	2189	403	3968
Interviewed	653	219	70	942
Deferred	14	2	0	16
Matriculants				
Early Assurance Program	0	0	0	0
Early Decision Program	1	0	0	1
Baccalaureate/MD	0	0	0	0
MD/PhD	4	0	0	4
Matriculated	272	26	4	**302**

Applications accepted from International Applicants: Canadian Only

Specialty Choice

2003, 2004, 2005 Graduates, Specialty Choice (As reported by program directors to GME Track™)	
Anesthesiology	5%
Emergency Medicine	14%
Family Practice	6%
Internal Medicine	19%
Obstetrics/Gynecology	6%
Orthopaedic Surgery	4%
Pediatrics	9%
Psychiatry	2%
Radiology	7%
Surgery	7%

Matriculant Demographics: 2007–2008 First Year Class

Men: 181   **Women:** 121

Matriculants' Self-Reported Race/Ethnicity

Mexican American	4	Korean	7
Cuban	1	Vietnamese	3
Puerto Rican	1	Other Asian	8
Other Hispanic	2	Total Asian	69
Total Hispanic	8	Native American	2
Chinese	8	Black	24
Asian Indian	37	Native Hawaiian	1
Pakistani	5	White	206
Filipino	2	Unduplicated Number	
Japanese	1	of Matriculants	302

Science and Math Majors: 73%
Matriculants with:
   Baccalaureate degree: 99%
   Graduate degree(s): 15%

Financial Information

Source: 2006–2007 LCME I-B survey
and 2007–2008 AAMC TSF questionnaire

	Residents	Non-Residents
Total Cost of Attendance	$52,588	$81,282
Tuition and Fees	$28,668	$56,656
Other (includes living expenses)	$21,676	$22,382
Health Insurance (can be waived)	$2,244	$2,244

Average 2007 Graduate Indebtedness: $134,258
% of Enrolled Students Receiving Aid: 90%

Criminal Background Check

This medical school does not require a criminal
background check prior to matriculation.

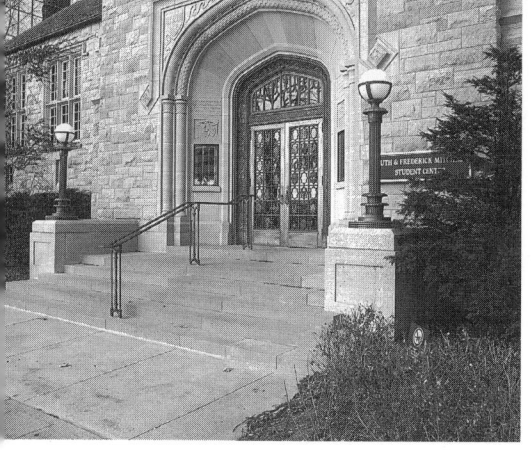

Mayo Clinic College of Medicine
Mayo Medical School
Rochester, Minnesota

Mayo Medical School
200 First Street, SW
Rochester, Minnesota 55905
T 507 284 3671   **F** 507 284 2634

Admissions www.mayo.edu/mms/md-admissions.htm
Main www.mayo.edu/mms
Financial www.mayo.edu/mms/md-tuition.htm
Email medschoolAdmissions@mayo.edu

Private Institution

Dr. Keith D. Lindor, Dean

Dr. Patricia A. Barrier, Associate Dean for Student Affairs

Barbara L. Porter, Assistant Dean for Student Affairs

David L. Dahlen, Director of Financial Aid and Registrar

General Information

Mayo Medical School is an integral part of Mayo Clinic, the world's largest group practice of medicine. Resources of MMS include a diverse patient population of more than 500,000 registrants annually, four affiliated hospitals with facilities for clinical and basic research, primary care facilities including several rural health centers, and affiliations with physicians who practice in surrounding communities and states.

Mission Statement

Mayo Medical School will use the patient-centered focus and strengths of Mayo Clinic to educate physicians to serve society by assuming leadership roles in medical practice, education, and research.

Curricular Highlights

Community Service Requirement: Optional.
Research/Thesis Requirement: Required.

The innovative patient-based curriculum is characterized by extensive early patient interaction and creative integration of sciences in all segments of the curriculum. In the first two years, courses occur in integrated blocks and contain a clinical component with experiences related to topics covered in the classroom. Themes of basic science, clinical experiences, leadership, physician and society, principles of pharmacology, and basic and advanced doctoring are represented throughout the curriculum. First and second year selectives engage students in career exploration, shadowing, and volunteer work. Year three is devoted to developing skills in all of the basic clinical clerkships, moving beyond acquiring information to the level of

synthesis and diagnosis. One quarter of the third year is an opportunity to explore the realm of scientific investigation, as every student completes a research endeavor under the mentorship of an experienced Mayo investigator. Over 80 percent of students publish and/or present their research while in medical school. Year four requirements include a sub-internship and rotations in family medicine, pediatrics, surgery, and emergency medicine. A social medicine rotation is offered to understand the role of community in the mission of medicine. Integrated into the fourth-year curriculum is a three-week return to the classroom to explore preventive medicine, biomedical ethics, palliative medicine, and clinical pharmacology. The remainder of the fourth year is fully elective to allow students to customize their learning.

USMLE

Step 1: Required. Students must record a passing score for promotion.
Step 2: Clinical Skills (CS): Required. Students Must record a passing total score to graduate.
Step 2: Clinical Knowledge (CK): Required. Students Must record a passing total score to graduate.

Selection Factors

Mayo Medical School is dedicated to enrolling students with superior academic credentials who possess leadership characteristics and have a profound desire to commit their lives to service. An evaluation of the entire AMCAS application, including the academic record, MCAT® scores, research, healthcare exploration, and service experiences, is considered in the initial review. For selected candidates an essay specific to Mayo Medical School outcomes and three letters of recommendation will be requested. If the applicant qualifies, an onsite interview is granted. The personal essay is an important part of the final selection process. Appointment notification occurs approximately every four weeks throughout the admissions cycle. Appointments continue to be offered to fill the

class up to the time of matriculation. All matriculates must have completed prerequisite courses and must possess a baccalaureate degree granted from an accredited United States or Canadian college or university; the final two years of coursework must be completed at this school. Mayo does not discriminate on the basis of race, sex, creed, national origin, age, or disability in its educational programs or activities. Mayo Medical School does not accept transfer students.

Financial Aid

A generous scholarship program provides every student significant financial support. Financial aid in the form of loans and need-based grants are also available.

Information about Diversity Programs

Mayo Medical School actively seeks to recruit and matriculate a diverse class of students.

Campus Information

Setting

Mayo Medical School is located in downtown Rochester, Minnesota, a vibrant, friendly city that provides a highly livable environment for more than 26,000 Mayo Clinic staff and students.

Enrollment

For 2007, total enrollment was: 166

Special Features

Mayo Clinic's three practices and regional health system comprise the largest integrated private group practice in the world. Thus, the clinical resources experienced as a Mayo medical student are unparalleled.

Housing

On-campus housing is not available. A list of affordable housing options in areas adjacent to the campus can be provided to new students.

Satellite Campuses/Facilities

In addition to the Mayo Clinic in Rochester, Minnesota, rotations can be completed at Mayo Clinic's group practice sites in Scottsdale, Arizona and Jacksonville, Florida.

Application Process and Requirements 2009–2010

Primary Application Service: AMCAS
Earliest filing date: June 1, 2008
Latest filing date: November 1, 2008

Secondary Application Required?: No
Sent to: n/a
URL: n/a
Fee: Yes, $85
Fee waiver available: Yes
Earliest filing date: n/a
Latest filing date: n/a

Latest MCAT® considered: September 2008
Oldest MCAT® considered: 2006

Early Decision Program
School does not have EDP
Applicants notified: n/a
EDP available for: n/a

Regular Acceptance Notice
Earliest date: October 15, 2008
Latest date: Until class is full

Applicant's Response to Acceptance Offer – Maximum Time: Two weeks

Requests for Deferred Entrance Considered: Yes

Deposit to Hold Place in Class: Yes
Deposit (Resident): $100
Deposit (Non-Resident): $100
Deposit due: With response to acceptance offer
Applied to tuition: No
Deposit refundable: Yes,
Refundable upon matriculation

Estimated number of new entrants: 50
EDP: n/a, special program: n/a

Start Month/Year: July 2009

Interview Format: Two one-on-one interviews with Admissions Committee members. Regional interviews are not available.

Other Programs

PREPARATORY PROGRAMS
Postbaccalaureate Program: No
Summer Program: No

COMBINED DEGREE PROGRAMS
Baccalaureate/MD: No
MD/MPH: Yes, www.mayo.edu/mms/academic-enrichment.html
MD/MBA: No
MD/JD: Yes, www.mayo.edu/mms/academic-enrichment.html
MD/PhD: Yes, www.mayo.edu/mms/md-phd.html

Premedical Coursework

Course	Req.	Rec.	Lab.	Sems.
Inorganic Chemistry	•	•		2
Behavioral Sciences				
Biochemistry	•			1
Biology	•	•		2
Biology/Zoology				
Calculus				
College English				
College Mathematics				

Course	Req.	Rec.	Lab.	Sems.
Computer Science				
Genetics				
Humanities				
Organic Chemistry	•		•	2
Physics	•		•	2
Psychology				
Social Sciences				
Other				

Selection Factors: 2007 Accepted Applicants

Proportion of Accepted Applicants with Relevant Experience (Data Self-Reported to AMCAS®)		
Community Service/Volunteer		78%
Medically-Related Work		92%
Research		92%

Shaded bar represents accepted scores ranging from the 10th percentile to the 90th percentile. **School Median ●** **National Median ●**

Overall GPA	2.0	2.1	2.2	2.3	2.4	2.5	2.6	2.7	2.8	2.9	3.0	3.1	3.2	3.3	3.4	3.5	3.6	3.7	3.8	(3.9) 4.0
Science GPA	2.0	2.1	2.2	2.3	2.4	2.5	2.6	2.7	2.8	2.9	3.0	3.1	3.2	3.3	3.4	3.5	3.6	3.7	(3.8)	3.9 4.0

MCAT® required: Yes, 97% of 2007 accepted applicants took MCAT®

Verbal Reasoning	3	4	5	6	7	8	9	(10)	11	12	13	14	15
Physical Sciences	3	4	5	6	7	8	9	10	(11)	12	13	14	15
Biological Sciences	3	4	5	6	7	8	9	10	(11)	12	13	14	15
Writing Sample			J	K	L	M	N	O	P	(Q)	R	S	T

Acceptance & Matriculation Data for 2007–2008 First Year Class

	Resident	Non-Resident	International	Total
Applied	392	2926	111	3429
Interviewed	45	250	0	295
Deferred	0	0	0	0
Matriculant				
Early Assurance Program	n/a	n/a	n/a	n/a
Early Decision Program	n/a	n/a	n/a	n/a
Baccalaureate/MD	n/a	n/a	n/a	n/a
MD/PhD	1	5	0	6
Matriculated	15	27	0	**42**

Applications accepted from International Applicants: Yes

Specialty Choice

2003, 2004, 2005 Graduates, Specialty Choice (As reported by program directors to GME Track™)	
Anesthesiology	9%
Emergency Medicine	7%
Family Practice	6%
Internal Medicine	16%
Obstetrics/Gynecology	5%
Orthopaedic Surgery	2%
Pediatrics	12%
Psychiatry	2%
Radiology	11%
Surgery	4%

Matriculant Demographics: 2007–2008 First Year Class

Men: 23   **Women:** 19

Matriculants' Self-Reported Race/Ethnicity

Mexican American	1	Korean	0
Cuban	0	Vietnamese	0
Puerto Rican	2	Other Asian	1
Other Hispanic	0	Total Asian	4
Total Hispanic	3	Native American	1
Chinese	1	Black	4
Asian Indian	1	Native Hawaiian	1
Pakistani	0	White	32
Filipino	0	Unduplicated Number	
Japanese	1	of Matriculants	42

Science and Math Majors: 71%
Matriculants with:
　　Baccalaureate degree: 100%
　　Graduate degree(s): 21%

Financial Information

Source: 2006–2007 LCME I-B survey and 2007–2008 AAMC TSF questionnaire

	Residents	Non-Residents
Total Cost of Attendance	$57,055	$57,055
Tuition and Fees	$29,700	$29,700
Other (includes living expenses)	$27,355	$27,355
Health Insurance (can be waived)	$0	$0

Average 2007 Graduate Indebtedness: $68,060
% of Enrolled Students Receiving Aid: 100%

Criminal Background Check

This medical school requires a criminal background check prior to matriculation.

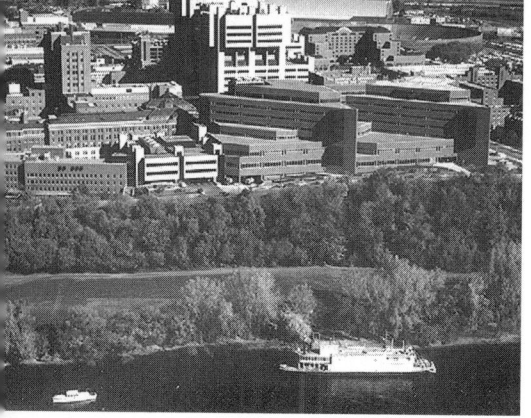

University of Minnesota Medical School
Minneapolis, Minnesota

University of Minnesota
Medical School – Twin Cities
MMC 293, 420 Delaware St SE
Minneapolis, Minnesota 55455
T 612 625 7977   F 612 625 8228
Admissions www.meded.umn.edu/admissions (TC),
www.med.umn.edu/duluth/admissions (DU)

Main www.med.umn.edu/
Financial www.meded.umn.edu/financial (TC),
www.med.umn.edu/duluth/admissions/tuition/home.
html (DU)
Email meded@umn.edu (Twin Cities),
medadmis@d.umn.edu (Duluth)

Public Institution

Dr. Deborah Powell, Dean

Dr. Gary L. Davis, Senior Associate Dean, Duluth Campus

Dr. Lillian A. Repesh, Associate Dean for Admissions and Student Affairs, Duluth

Paul T. White, J.D., Assistant Dean of Admissions, Twin Cities

Dr. Joycelyn Dorscher, Director of Center of American Indian and Minority Health

Mary Tate, Director of Minority Affairs and Diversity, Twin Cities

General Information
Founded in 1888, the University of Minnesota Medical School is located on the Twin Cities campus of the University. A two year basic science regional campus is located in Duluth. The medical school is a unit of the U of M Academic Health Center.

Mission Statement
The mission of the medical school is to be a leader in enhancing the health of people through the education of skilled, compassionate and socially responsible physicians and through research which advances the understanding of health and disease. With two campuses serving diverse populations in rural and urban Minnesota the medical school is dedicated to exemplary primary and specialty care, innovative research and education.

Curricular Highlights
Community Service Requirement: Optional.
Research/Thesis Requirement: Optional.

Minnesota is the first public medical school to offer a flexible MD program with a competency-defined education under the new MED 2010 initiative; students have the option of finishing medical school in as few as 3 1/2 and as many as 6 years. The two-year basic science curriculum on both campuses is designed to prepare students for future medical practice through integrated instruction in basic, clinical, and behavioral sciences. Ample time is devoted to basic science-clinical correlations. Students have early exposure to

patients, learning medical history-taking and physical examination skills; and are paired with preceptors in Years 1 & 2. The third and fourth year medical school program includes 56 weeks of required clerkships, 20 weeks of electives and 25 weeks of unstructured time. Flexibility in scheduling in the 3rd and 4th years provides the opportunity to pursue a wide range of clinical/academic interests.

USMLE
Step 1: Required. Students must record a passing score for promotion.
Step 2: Clinical Skills (CS): Required. Students must record a passing total score to graduate.
Step 2: Clinical Knowledge (CK): Required. Students must record a passing total score to graduate.

Selection Factors
Legal residents of Minnesota are given preference for admission, but qualified out-of-state applicants are also encouraged to apply. Commitment to improving the human condition, unassailable professional conduct, outstanding interpersonal skills, dedication to lifelong learning and cultural sensitivity are evaluated. The medical school seeks to matriculate a diverse student body [*www.meded.umn.edu/admissions/index.cfm*]. Applicant qualifications are evaluated through recommendation letters, post-secondary experiences, undergraduate education, responses to the supplemental application, and on-site interviews. In addition, the medical school's Duluth campus seeks persons with traits that indicate a high potential for becoming a family physician in rural Minnesota or American Indian communities. Duluth applicants must be U.S. citizens or have permanent resident status. Transfer students are rarely accepted into Year 3 on the Twin Cities campus. Students accepted to the Twin Cities and Duluth campuses enter a class of 165 and 56 students, respectively. The University of Minnesota Medical School does not discriminate on the basis of race, gender, creed, sexual orientation, disability, or national origin.

Financial Aid
Financial aid applicants must file the FAFSA. Loans and scholarship aid are available. Tuition rates for new matriculates are fixed through a cost-of-degree tuition policy. For information,

contact B.J. Gibson [TC](612/625-4998, *www.meded.umn.edu/financial*) or Dina Flaherty [DU](218/726-6548, *www.med.umn.edu/duluth/admissions/tuition/home.html*).

Information about Diversity Programs
The U of MN Medical School is committed to the recruitment and education of students from groups underrepresented in medicine. For more information, contact the Office of Minority Affairs (Twin Cities, 612/625-1494), or the Center for American Indian and Minority Health. CAIMH is headquartered in Duluth (218/726-7235) and also has a Twin Cities office (612/624-0465).

Campus Information

Setting
The Twin Cities campus is located on the second largest university campus in the United States. Most major hospitals in the Minneapolis-St. Paul area are affiliated with the Medical School. The Duluth program is located on the U of MN Duluth campus in northeastern Minnesota and has affiliations with Duluth hospitals.

Enrollment
For 2007, total enrollment was: 945

Special Features
The Medical School provides a wide range of clinical and research opportunities [*www.meded.umn.edu/clerkships/index.cfm; www.med.umn.edu/RPAP/; www.med.umn.edu/imer/; www.ahc.umn.edu/; www.meded.umn.edu/resopps/index.cfm*].

Housing
Medical student fraternities [TC] and private housing are available in the campus neighborhoods; both campuses maintain a list of resources for affordable off-campus housing.

Satellite Campuses/Facilities
The two-year program at the Medical School Duluth was established to increase the number of family practice physicians with a commitment to serve in rural Minnesota or American Indian communities. Students transition to the Twin Cities for years 3 and 4 with the opportunity to complete some rotations in Duluth as well as participate in RPAP. For more information: Susan Christensen (218/726-8511; medadmis@d.umn.edu).

Application Process and Requirements 2009–2010

Primary Application Service: AMCAS
Earliest filing date: June 1, 2008
Latest filing date: November 15, 2008

Secondary Application Required?: Yes
Sent to: All
URL: n/a
Fee: Yes, $75
Fee waiver available: Yes
Earliest filing date: n/a
Latest filing date: January 31, 2009 [TC]

Latest MCAT® considered: September 2008
Oldest MCAT® considered: 2005

Early Decision Program
School does have EDP
Applicants notified: October 1, 2008
EDP available for: Both Residents
and Non-Residents

Regular Acceptance Notice
Earliest date: October 15, 2008
Latest date: Until class is full

Applicant's Response to Acceptance
Offer – Maximum Time: Two weeks

Requests for Deferred
Entrance Considered: Yes

Deposit to Hold Place in Class: Yes
Deposit (Resident): $100
Deposit (Non-Resident): $100
Deposit due: With response to acceptance offer
Applied to tuition: Yes
Deposit refundable: Yes
Refundable by: May 15, 2009

Estimated number of new entrants: 221
EDP: 20, special program: 3

Start Month/Year: August 2009

Interview Format: Individual interviews are
conducted. Regional interviews are not available.

Other Programs

PREPARATORY PROGRAMS
Postbaccalaureate Program: No
Summer Program: Yes, www.caimh.org
Pre-matriculation Program: Yes, www.caimh.org

COMBINED DEGREE PROGRAMS
Baccalaureate/MD: Yes,
www.med.umn.edu/duluth/admissions/home.html
Susan Christensen; 218/726-8511
medadmis@d.umn.edu
MD/MPH: Yes, www.sph.umn.edu/education/
degrees/home.html
William Lohman Director, 612/626-0605;
800/774-8636 lohma002@umn.edu
MD/MBA: Yes, www.meded.umn.edu/
admissions/MD-MBA.cfm, Deb Basarich, 612/625-4595
MD/JD: Yes,www.meded.umn.edu/admissions/
JD-MD.cfm, Carol Rachac, 612/625.3356
MD/PhD: Yes, http://mdphd.med.umn.edu/
Additional: Yes, http://ccgb.umn.edu/
~sspeedie/hinf/htdocs/mhi/MD-MHI.html

Premedical Coursework

Course	Req.	Rec.	Lab.	Sems.	Course	Req.	Rec.	Lab.	Sems.
Inorganic Chemistry	•		•	1	Genetics		•		
Behavioral Sciences					Humanities	•			
Biochemistry		•		1	Organic Chemistry		•	•	2
Biology	•		•	1	Physics		•	•	2
Biology/Zoology					Psychology		•		1
Calculus					Social Sciences	•			
College English					Statistics		•		1
College Mathematics					Ethics		•		
Computer Science					Foreign Language		•		

Selection Factors: 2007 Accepted Applicants

Proportion of Accepted Applicants with Relevant Experience (Data Self-Reported to AMCAS®)		
Community Service/Volunteer		70%
Medically-Related Work		87%
Research		78%

Shaded bar represents accepted scores ranging from the 10th percentile to the 90th percentile ▦   School Median ●   National Median ●

Overall GPA	2.0	2.1	2.2	2.3	2.4	2.5	2.6	2.7	2.8	2.9	3.0	3.1	3.2	3.3	3.4	3.5	3.6	③.7	3.8	3.9	4.0
Science GPA	2.0	2.1	2.2	2.3	2.4	2.5	2.6	2.7	2.8	2.9	3.0	3.1	3.2	3.3	3.4	3.5	3.6	③.7	3.8	3.9	4.0

MCAT® required: Yes, 100% of 2007 accepted applicants took MCAT®

Verbal Reasoning	3	4	5	6	7	8	9	⑩	11	12	13	14	15
Physical Sciences	3	4	5	6	7	8	9	⑩	⑪	12	13	14	15
Biological Sciences	3	4	5	6	7	8	9	10	⑪	12	13	14	15
Writing Sample			J	K	L	M	N	O	⑪	⑫	R	S	T

Acceptance & Matriculation Data for 2007–2008 First Year Class

	Resident	Non-Resident	International	Total
Applied	1227	2882	227	4336
Interviewed	403	177	12	592
Deferred	10	0	0	10
Matriculants				
Early Assurance Program	0	0	0	0
Early Decision Program	19	1	0	20
Baccalaureate/MD	2	0	0	2
MD/PhD	3	5	0	8
Matriculated	201	38	2	**241**

Applications accepted from International Applicants: Yes

Matriculant Demographics: 2007–2008 First Year Class

Men: 122   **Women:** 119

Matriculants' Self-Reported Race/Ethnicity

Mexican American	4	**Korean**	1
Cuban	0	**Vietnamese**	3
Puerto Rican	1	**Other Asian**	6
Other Hispanic	4	**Total Asian**	25
Total Hispanic	9	**Native American**	11
Chinese	13	**Black**	5
Asian Indian	4	**Native Hawaiian**	0
Pakistani	0	**White**	198
Filipino	1	**Unduplicated Number**	
Japanese	1	**of Matriculants**	241

Science and Math Majors: 76%
Matriculants with:
        Baccalaureate degree: 100%
        Graduate degree(s): 10%

Specialty Choice

2003, 2004, 2005 Graduates, Specialty Choice (As reported by program directors to GME Track™)	
Anesthesiology	4%
Emergency Medicine	6%
Family Practice	20%
Internal Medicine	19%
Obstetrics/Gynecology	5%
Orthopaedic Surgery	3%
Pediatrics	8%
Psychiatry	3%
Radiology	4%
Surgery	7%

Financial Information

Source: 2006–2007 LCME I-B survey
and 2007–2008 AAMC TSF questionnaire

	Residents	Non-Residents
Total Cost of Attendance	$54,407	$61,721
Tuition and Fees	$31,343	$38,657
Other (includes living expenses)	$21,048	$21,048
Health Insurance (can be waived)	$2,016	$2,016

Average 2007 Graduate Indebtedness: $144,092
% of Enrolled Students Receiving Aid: 94%

Criminal Background Check

This medical school requires a criminal background check prior to matriculation.

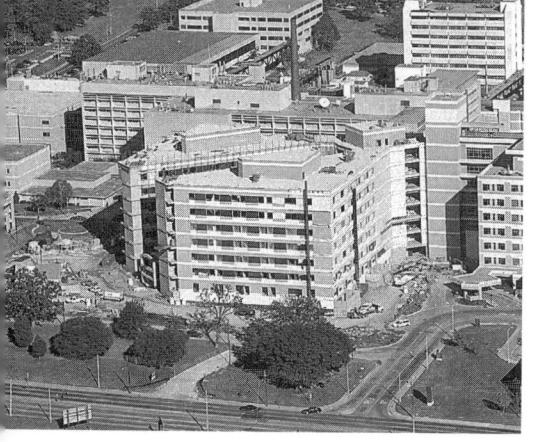

University of Mississippi
School of Medicine

Jackson, Mississippi

Associate Dean for Admissions
University of Mississippi School of Medicine
2500 North State Street
Jackson, Mississippi 39216-4505
T 601 984 5010   **F** 601 984 5008

Admissions http://som.umc.edu/admissions.html
Main http://som.umc.edu
Financial http://som.umc.edu/accepted
Appl.html#FinanAssist
Email AdmitMD@som.umsmed.edu

Public Institution

Dr. Daniel W. Jones, Dean

Dr. Steven T. Case, Associate Dean for Admissions

Dr. Jasmine P. Taylor, Associate Dean for Multicultural Affairs

Stacey Mathews, Director of Student Financial Aid

Dr. Peggy M. Davis, Director of Admissions

Barbara M. Westerfield, Registrar

General Information

The School of Medicine, created by a special act of the Board of Trustees in June 1903, operated as a two-year school in Oxford until 1955, when it expanded to four years and moved to the new University of Mississippi Medical Center in Jackson. The Medical Center now houses the Schools of Medicine, Nursing, Health Related Professions, Dentistry, Graduate Studies in Health Sciences, and the 722-bed University Hospitals and Health System.

Mission Statement

The primary mission of the University of Mississippi School of Medicine is to offer an accredited program of medical education that will provide well-trained physicians and certain supporting health care professionals, in numbers consistent with the health care needs of the state, who are responsive to the health problems of the people and committed to medical education as a continuum, which must prevail throughout professional life.

Curricular Highlights

Community Service Requirement: Optional. Medical students staff the Jackson Free Clinic
Research/Thesis Requirement: Optional.

During the two preclinical years, students learn the sciences basic to the study of medicine and participate in laboratory exercises, small-group discussion, computer-assisted learning, and independent study. The preclinical curriculum was revised to increase integration and improve the sequencing of course content and provide

earlier clinical experience for students. The third year involves full-time clinical study as students rotate through the major clinical disciplines and participate in the team care of patients in the University Hospitals and Clinics, Veterans Affairs Medical Center, and various community settings. The fourth year consists of eight required calendar month blocks that may be taken at any time during the eleven months available from July through May. Fourth-year clinical clerkships provide greater depth of study in core areas of medicine, as well as in a student's anticipated medical specialty. Opportunities exist for advanced study and research in basic science departments and for electives at other institutions in this country or abroad.

USMLE

Step 1: Required. Students must record a passing score for promotion.
Step 2: Clinical Skills (CS): Required. Students must record a passing total score to graduate.
Step 2: Clinical Knowledge (CK): Required. Students must record a passing total score to graduate.

Selection Factors

The Admissions Committee selects applicants on a competitive basis without regard to age, sex, sexual orientation, race, creed, national origin, marital status, handicap, or veteran status. Strong preference is given to legal residents of Mississippi; in recent years, nonresidents have not been admitted. Interviews are arranged at the discretion of the Admissions Committee; major considerations are undergraduate BCPM GPA and MCAT® scores. Interviews are used to assess non-cognitive variables and communication skills. Experiences listed on an AMCAS application document nonacademic and professional attributes, and premedical faculty evaluations reveal an applicant's approach to academic study and professionalism. For details, see *http://som.umc.edu/admissions.html#EvalApps*. Mississippi residents enrolled in other medical schools accredited by the Liaison Committee on Medical Education may be considered for advanced standing transfer.

Financial Aid

Accepted students may apply for financial aid. The school participates in federal scholarship and loan programs (such as Perkins and

Stafford) and state-funded Family Medical Education Loan/Scholarship and State Medical Education Loan/Scholarship programs. Eligible students may qualify for limited scholarship funds provided by private donors. For details, see *http://som.umc.edu/acceptedappl.html# FinanAssist*.

Information about Diversity Programs

The Admissions Committee encourages students from groups underrepresented in medicine to apply for admission. Information about pipeline programs and support provided by the Division of Multicultural Affairs can be obtained at: *http://mca.umc.edu/*.

Campus Information

Setting

The Medical Center is located on a 164 acre campus in Jackson. The state capital and Mississippi's largest city, Jackson offers a wide array of professional arts attractions. Recreational facilities include a 30,000-acre reservoir, just 15 minutes from the campus.

Enrollment

For 2007, total enrollment was: 420

Special Features

The opening of a new adult medical and surgical hospital in 2006 marked the completion of a project to replace the original teaching hospital with four new state-of-the-art hospitals. The Medical Center opened a 57,000 square foot student union – with a state-of-the-art fitness center and gymnasium – in 1999. Medical students sponsor the Jackson Free Clinic that provides medical care to homeless and uninsured patients on Saturdays.

Housing

Rent averages from $450-$750 a month for area apartments.

Satellite Campuses/Facilities

The Jackson Medical Mall, one mile from the campus, houses the hospital's clinics as well as the Medical Center's new Cancer Institute. Originally the city's first shopping mall, the Jackson Medical Mall is recognized as a national model of urban revitalization.

Application Process and Requirements 2009–2010

Primary Application Service: AMCAS
Earliest filing date: June 1, 2008
Latest filing date: October 15, 2008

Secondary Application Required?: Yes
Sent to: URL and password provided after receipt of AMCAS application.
URL: http://som.umc.edu/docs/Secondary Application.pdf
Fee: Yes, $50
Fee waiver available: Yes
Earliest filing date: June 1, 2008
Latest filing date: December 1, 2008

Latest MCAT® considered: September 2008
Oldest MCAT® considered: April 2005

Early Decision Program
School does have EDP
Applicants notified: Not later than October 1, 2008
EDP available for: Residents only

Regular Acceptance Notice
Earliest date: October 16, 2008
Latest date: Until class is full

Applicant's Response to Acceptance Offer – Maximum Time: Two weeks

Requests for Deferred Entrance Considered: Yes

Deposit to Hold Place in Class: Yes
Deposit (Resident): $50
Deposit (Non-Resident): $100
Deposit due: Deposit must accompany response to acceptance offer
Applied to tuition: Yes
Deposit refundable: Yes
Refundable by: May 15, 2009

Estimated number of new entrants: 110
EDP: 10, special program: n/a

Start Month/Year: August 4, 2009

Interview Format: Three semi-structured, one-on-one interviews. Regional interviews are not available.

Other Programs

PREPARATORY PROGRAMS
Postbaccalaureate Program: Yes,
http://som.umc.edu/admissions.html#PPT
Summer Program: Yes,
http://mca.umc.edu/ programs.html
Pre-matriculation Program: Yes,
http://mca.umc.edu/programs.html
MedCorp Program: Yes,
http://mca.umc.edu/ programs.html
COMBINED DEGREE
PROGRAMSBaccalaureate/MD: No
MD/MPH: No
MD/MBA: No
MD/JD: No
MD/PhD: Yes,
http://som.umc.edu/admissions.html#MDPhD

Premedical Coursework

Course	Req.	Rec.	Lab.	Hrs.
Inorganic Chemistry	•		•	8
Behavioral Sciences		•		
Biochemistry		•		
Biology				
Biology/Zoology	•		•	8
Calculus		•		3
College English	•			6
College Mathematics	•			6
Computer Science				

Course	Req.	Rec.	Lab.	Hrs.
Genetics		•		3
Humanities		•		
Organic Chemistry	•		•	8
Physics	•		•	8
Psychology		•		
Social Sciences				
Vertebrate Anatomy		•		3
Histology		•		3
Physiology		•		3

Selection Factors: 2007 Accepted Applicants

Proportion of Accepted Applicants with Relevant Experience (Data Self-Reported to AMCAS®)		Community Service/Volunteer	82%
		Medically-Related Work	75%
		Research	58%

Shaded bar represents accepted scores ranging from the 10th percentile to the 90th percentile. School Median ● National Median ●

Overall GPA	2.0	2.1	2.2	2.3	2.4	2.5	2.6	2.7	2.8	2.9	3.0	3.1	3.2	3.3	3.4	3.5	3.6	3.7	(3.8)	3.9	4.0
Science GPA	2.0	2.1	2.2	2.3	2.4	2.5	2.6	2.7	2.8	2.9	3.0	3.1	3.2	3.3	3.4	3.5	3.6	(3.7)	3.8	3.9	4.0

MCAT® required: Yes, 100% of 2007 accepted applicants took MCAT®

Verbal Reasoning	3	4	5	6	7	8	(9)	(10)	11	12	13	14	15
Physical Sciences	3	4	5	6	7	8	(9)	10	(11)	12	13	14	15
Biological Sciences	3	4	5	6	7	8	9	(10)	(11)	12	13	14	15
Writing Sample				J	K	L	M	N	(O)	P	(Q)	R	S	T

Acceptance & Matriculation Data for 2007–2008 First Year Class

	Resident	Non-Resident	International	Total
Applied	270	0	1	271
Interviewed	195	0	0	195
Deferred	0	0	0	0
Matriculants				
Early Assurance Program	0	0	0	0
Early Decision Program	13	0	0	13
Baccalaureate/MD	n/a	n/a	n/a	n/a
MD/PhD	0	0	0	0
Matriculated	110	0	0	**110**

Applications accepted from International Applicants: No

Matriculant Demographics: 2007–2008 First Year Class

Men: 64   **Women:** 46

Matriculants' Self-Reported Race/Ethnicity

Mexican American	0	Korean	1
Cuban	0	Vietnamese	0
Puerto Rican	0	Other Asian	1
Other Hispanic	0	Total Asian	11
Total Hispanic	0	Native American	0
Chinese	4	Black	11
Asian Indian	4	Native Hawaiian	0
Pakistani	0	White	90
Filipino	1	Unduplicated Number	
Japanese	2	of Matriculants	110

Science and Math Majors: 79%
Matriculants with:
    Baccalaureate degree: 99%
    Graduate degree(s): 12%

Specialty Choice

2003, 2004, 2005 Graduates, Specialty Choice (As reported by program directors to GME Track™)

Anesthesiology	6%
Emergency Medicine	6%
Family Practice	13%
Internal Medicine	21%
Obstetrics/Gynecology	5%
Orthopaedic Surgery	4%
Pediatrics	12%
Psychiatry	4%
Radiology	5%
Surgery	4%

Financial Information

Source: 2006–2007 LCME I-B survey and 2007–2008 AAMC TSF questionnaire

	Residents	Non-Residents
Total Cost of Attendance	$35,164	$45,997
Tuition and Fees	$9,649	$20,482
Other (includes living expenses)	$23,456	$23,456
Health Insurance (can be waived)	$2,059	$2,059

Average 2007 Graduate Indebtedness: $97,047
% of Enrolled Students Receiving Aid: 93%

Criminal Background Check

This medical school requires a criminal background check prior to matriculation.

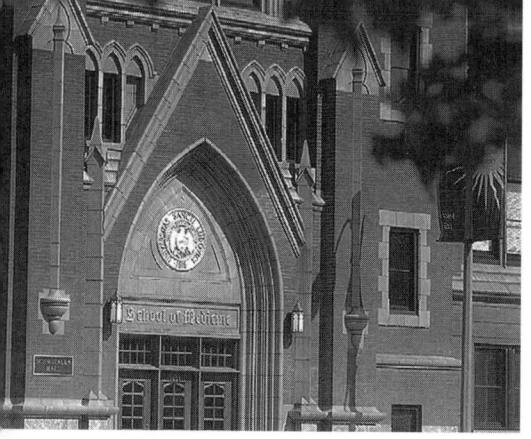

Saint Louis University School of Medicine
St. Louis, Missouri

Saint Louis University School of Medicine
Office of Admissions
1402 S. Grand Blvd. M226
St. Louis, Missouri 63104
T 314 977 9870   F 314 977 9825

Admissions http://medschool.slu.edu/admissions
Main www.slu.edu
Financial http://medschool.slu.edu/sfp
Email slumd@slu.edu

Private Institution

Dr. Philip Alderson, Dean

Dr. L. James Willmore, Associate Dean, Admissions

Dr. George Rausch, Associate Dean Multicultural Affairs

Sandra Pritt, Student Financial Services

General Information

Established in 1836, Saint Louis University School of Medicine has the distinction of awarding the first M.D. degree west of the Mississippi River. The school is recognized as a pioneer in geriatric medicine, organ transplantation, chronic disease prevention, cardiovascular disease, neurosciences, and vaccine research, among others. The School of Medicine trains physicians and biomedical scientists, conducts medical research, and provides health services on a local, national, and international level.

Mission Statement

Beyond the important objective of training physicians who are scholars of human biology, the School of Medicine strives to graduate physicians who manifest in their personal and professional lives an appreciation of humanistic medicine. We regard humanistic medicine as a constellation of ethical and professional attitudes, which affect the physician's interactions with patients, colleagues, and society. Among these attitudes are concern for the sanctity of human life; commitment to dignity and respect in the provision of medical care to all patients; devotion to social justice, especially regarding inequities in the availability of health care; humility and awareness of medicine's limitations in the care of the sick; appreciation of the role of non-medical factors in a patient's state of well-being or illness; and mature, well-balanced professional behavior that derives from comfortable relationships with members of the human family and one's Creator.

Curricular Highlights

Community Service Requirement: Optional.
Distinction in Community Service
Research/Thesis Requirement: Optional.
Distinction in Research

The M.D. curriculum provides coordination and integration of the basic and clinical sciences across all four years. Additionally, it follows established principles of adult learning, and so is a hybrid of lectures, small-group activities, early clinical activities, self-directed learning, and problem-solving exercises. The first two years of the curriculum are devoted to the study of the fundamental sciences basic to medicine. In year two, a series of integrated modules that are organ-based are coupled with the acquisition of fundamental clinical skills required to begin the clinical clerkships that are taught in the Applied Clinical Skills and Patient, Physician, and Society course series. The last two years concentrate on the further development and refinement of essential clinical skills, while also providing ongoing integration of the basic sciences into clinical practice. The grading system consists of the following levels: honors, pass, and fail.

USMLE

Step 1: Required. Students must record a passing score for promotion.
Step 2: Clinical Skills (CS): Required. Students must record a passing total score to graduate.
Step 2: Clinical Knowledge (CK): Required. Students must record a passing total score to graduate.

Selection Factors

Saint Louis University School of Medicine encourages applications from persons who have demonstrated a high level of academic achievement and who manifest in their personal lives those human qualities that are required for a career of service to society.

Financial Aid

The Student Financial Services Office assists students with an aid package to meet educational expenses. Qualified students may be able to receive scholarship and/or loan funds from federal, state, and University programs. Funds based on financial need require the annual filing of the Free Application for Federal Student Aid FAFSA). Parental financial information is required on the FAFSA to be considered for University need-based scholarships and loan programs.

Information about Diversity Programs

The School of Medicine is committed to promoting diversity in the classroom and in the clinics so that all students understand and learn from each other about the practice of medicine in a diverse environment. The Office of Multicultural Affairs (OMA) assists students from diverse backgrounds to be successful as they pursue a career as a physician.

Campus Information

Setting

The medical school is located in the heart of the city's performing arts district and the center of the country and is a five-minute drive from the Gateway Arch on the Mississippi Riverfront.

Enrollment

For 2007, total enrollment was: 676

Special Features

An Anesthesiology Laboratory and a Clinical Skills Center provide the latest methodology for instruction and evaluation using standardized patients and other devices to learn clinical skills, in addition to the regular training sites. The new research building provides state-of-the-art facilities for health sciences research that touches lives and provides service to the community.

Housing

St. Louis and the surrounding area offer plenty of affordable housing.

Satellite Campuses/Facilities

Major teaching affiliations include The University Hospital, Cardinal Glennon Medical Center for Children, Wohl Memorial Institute, St. Elizabeth's Hospital, St. John's Mercy Medical Center, St. Mary's Hospital, Bethesda Cancer Research Center, and St. Louis Veterans Affairs Hospitals.

Application Process and Requirements 2009–2010

Primary Application Service: AMCAS
Earliest filing date: June 1, 2008
Latest filing date: December 14, 2008

Secondary Application Required?: Yes
Sent to: All applicants
URL: www.oasprod3.com/schools/slusom
Fee: Yes, $100
Fee waiver available: Yes
Earliest filing date: June 1, 2008
Latest filing date: February 15, 2009

Latest MCAT® considered: September 2008
Oldest MCAT® considered: April 2005

Early Decision Program
School does have EDP
Applicants notified: October 1, 2008
EDP available for: Both Residents
and Non-Residents

Regular Acceptance Notice
Earliest date: October 15, 2008
Latest date: Until class is full

**Applicant's Response to Acceptance
Offer – Maximum Time:** Two weeks

**Requests for Deferred
Entrance Considered:** Yes

Deposit to Hold Place in Class: Yes
Deposit (Resident): $100
Deposit (Non-Resident): $100
Deposit due: With response to acceptance offer
Applied to tuition: Yes
Deposit refundable: Yes
Refundable by: May 15, 2009

Estimated number of new entrants: 175
EDP: 3, special program: 30

Start Month/Year: August 2009

Interview Format: A single one-on-one interview. Some regional interviews may be offered.

Other Programs

PREPARATORY PROGRAMS
Postbaccalaureate Program: No
Summer Program: No

COMBINED DEGREE PROGRAMS
Baccalaureate/MD: Yes,
www.slu.edu/colleges/AS/phs/medScholars.html
MD/MPH: Yes,
http://publichealth.slu.edu/programs/
mph/mdmph.html, Bernard Backer,
(314) 977-8144, backerb@slu.edu
MD/MBA: Yes, www.slu.edu/x16691.xml
MD/JD: No
MD/PhD: Yes, http://medschool.slu.edu/
admissions/index.phtml?page=mdphd,
Andrew Lechner, Ph.D., (314) 977-9877,
lechnera@slu.edu

Premedical Coursework

Course	Req.	Rec.	Lab.	Hrs.
Inorganic Chemistry	•		•	8
Behavioral Sciences				
Biochemistry		•		
Biology				
Biology/Zoology	•		•	8
Calculus				
College English	•			6
College Mathematics				

Course	Req.	Rec.	Lab.	Hrs.
Computer Science				
Genetics				
Humanities	•			12
Organic Chemistry	•		•	8
Physics	•		•	8
Psychology				
Social Sciences				
Other				

Selection Factors: 2007 Accepted Applicants

Proportion of Accepted Applicants with Relevant Experience (Data Self-Reported to AMCAS®)		
Community Service/Volunteer		72%
Medically-Related Work		85%
Research		77%

Shaded bar represents accepted scores ranging from the 10th percentile to the 90th percentile — School Median ● National Median ●

Overall GPA	2.0	2.1	2.2	2.3	2.4	2.5	2.6	2.7	2.8	2.9	3.0	3.1	3.2	3.3	3.4	3.5	3.6	3.7	(3.8)	3.9	4.0
Science GPA	2.0	2.1	2.2	2.3	2.4	2.5	2.6	2.7	2.8	2.9	3.0	3.1	3.2	3.3	3.4	3.5	3.6	3.7	(3.8)	3.9	4.0

MCAT® required: Yes, 100% of 2007 accepted applicants took MCAT®

Verbal Reasoning	3	4	5	6	7	8	9	(10)	11	12	13	14	15
Physical Sciences	3	4	5	6	7	8	9	(10)	(11)	12	13	14	15
Biological Sciences	3	4	5	6	7	8	9	10	(11)	12	13	14	15
Writing Sample				J	K	L	M	N	O	(P)	(Q)	R	S	T

Acceptance & Matriculation Data for 2007–2008 First Year Class

	Resident	Non-Resident	International	Total
Applied	383	5722	254	6359
Interviewed	110	788	39	937
Deferred	0	6	1	7
Matriculants				
Early Assurance Program	0	0	0	0
Early Decision Program	1	0	0	1
Baccalaureate/MD	12	15	0	27
MD/PhD	0	1	0	1
Matriculated	35	144	0	**179**

Applications accepted from International Applicants: Yes

Matriculant Demographics: 2007–2008 First Year Class

Men: 106   **Women:** 73

Matriculants' Self-Reported Race/Ethnicity

Mexican American	1	Korean	5
Cuban	0	Vietnamese	6
Puerto Rican	0	Other Asian	5
Other Hispanic	0	Total Asian	46
Total Hispanic	1	Native American	1
Chinese	9	Black	5
Asian Indian	18	Native Hawaiian	0
Pakistani	3	White	128
Filipino	1	**Unduplicated Number**	
Japanese	2	**of Matriculants**	179

Science and Math Majors: 76%
Matriculants with:
   Baccalaureate degree: 99%
   Graduate degree(s): 8%

Specialty Choice

2003, 2004, 2005 Graduates, Specialty Choice (As reported by program directors to GME Track™)	
Anesthesiology	7%
Emergency Medicine	6%
Family Practice	7%
Internal Medicine	20%
Obstetrics/Gynecology	6%
Orthopaedic Surgery	4%
Pediatrics	14%
Psychiatry	4%
Radiology	5%
Surgery	5%

Financial Information

Source: 2006–2007 LCME I-B survey and 2007–2008 AAMC TSF questionnaire

	Residents	Non-Residents
Total Cost of Attendance	$64,806	$64,806
Tuition and Fees	$42,783	$42,783
Other (includes living expenses)	$19,919	$19,919
Health Insurance (can be waived)	$2,104	$2,104

Average 2007 Graduate Indebtedness: $173,984
% of Enrolled Students Receiving Aid: 84%

Criminal Background Check

This medical school requires a criminal background check prior to matriculation.

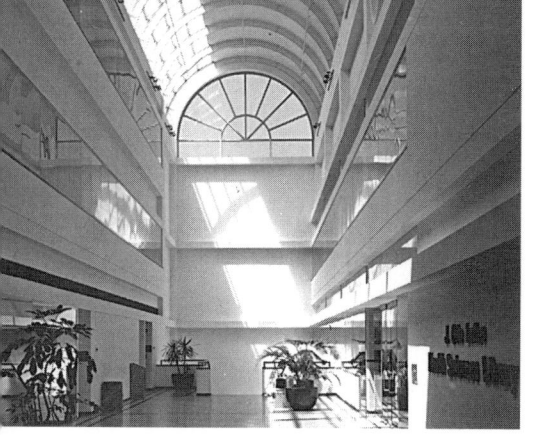

University of Missouri — Columbia School of Medicine

Columbia, Missouri

Marivern Easton, Admissions, Recruitment & Records
Office of Med. Education, MA215 Med. Sci. Bldg
Univ. of Missouri — Columbia School of Medicine
One Hospital Drive, Columbia, Missouri 65212
T 573 882 9219   **F** 573 884 2988

Admissions http://som.missouri.edu/admit.shtml/
Main http://som.missouri.edu/
Financial http://som.missouri.edu/financial/
Email MizzouMed@missouri.edu

Public Institution

Dr. William Crist, Dean

*Dr. Linda Headrick, Senior Associate
Dean for Education*

Cheri Marks, Coordinator of Financial Aid

*Dr. Rachel Brown, Associate Dean
for Student Programs*

*Dr. Michael Hosokawa,
Associate Dean for Curriculum*

General Information

The University of Missouri-Columbia School
of Medicine was established in 1872. The MU
Health Sciences Center includes the University
Hospital, and multiple specialized and community clinics, both inpatient and outpatient. The
MU School of Medicine has additional affiliations with other hospitals and clinics across
the state.

Mission Statement

The mission of MU School of Medicine is to educate physicians to provide effective patient-centered care for the people of Missouri and beyond.
Patient-centered care reflects a respect for individual patient's values, preferences, and expressed
needs. This care is grounded in the best available
evidence and conserves limited resources, and it
depends on shared decision-making and active
patient participation. Our graduates' care will be
marked by compassion, empathy, and patient
advocacy. Our graduates also will be: honest, with
high ethical standards; knowledgeable in biomedical sciences, evidence-based practice, and societal
and cultural issues; critical-thinkers and problem-
solvers; able to communicate with patients and
other health-care team members; committed to
improving quality and safety; and committed to
lifelong learning and mastering information.

Curricular Highlights

Community Service Requirement: Optional.
Research/Thesis Requirement: Optional.

MU emphasizes a strong foundation in the basic
sciences, problem-solving, clinical skills, early
experiences with patients and role-model physicians, self-directed learning/lifelong learning, and
attitudes essential for competent and compassionate patient care. The first two years offer eight 10-
week blocks with three components: Basic Science/
Problem-Based Learning, Introduction to Patient
Care, and Ambulatory Care Experience. Students
work in groups of eight with a faculty tutor in the
first two components and individual physicians for
ACE. The third year features seven required clerkships. The fourth year has three required clinical
electives, one advanced basic science rotation, and
four general electives. A multilevel grading system
is used, with satisfactory/ unsatisfactory used in
year one and satisfactory/ unsatisfactory/letters of
commendation/honors used in the fourth year.

USMLE

Step 1: Required. Students must record a
passing score for promotion.
Step 2: Clinical Skills (CS): Required. Students
must record a passing total score to graduate.
Step 2: Clinical Knowledge (CK): Required. Students must record a passing total score to graduate.

Selection Factors

The Admissions Committee conducts required
on-campus personal interviews. Strong preference is given to Missouri residents. Exceptional
residents of other states may also be admitted.
Non-Missouri residents are evaluated on an individual basis, and may be asked to provide evidence of Missouri ties, diversity, and/or exceptional academics. Selection for interview is based
upon academic performance; personal qualities
such as motivation, social concern, and integrity;
and tested motivation for medicine. Early
Decision Program applicants must be Missouri
residents with 3.75 cum GPA and MCAT® sum
of 30 with no individual section score below 9.
Transfer students (primarily Missouri residents)
are occasionally admitted into the third year
from U.S. and/or foreign allopathic medical
schools. The School of Medicine does not
discriminate on the basis of race, sex, creed,
national origin, age, handicap, religion, or status
as a Vietnam-era veteran in admission or access
to or treatment or employment in its programs
and activities.

Financial Aid

Students are admitted to the School of Medicine
without regard to financial circumstances. MU
participates in federal scholarship and loan programs. The institutional scholarship program is
primarily need-based. Institutional long-term
loans are available and MU also operates an
emergency short-term loan program.

Information about Diversity Programs

The University of Missouri is committed to the
recruitment and education of disadvantaged and
nontraditional applicants and applicants from
groups underrepresented in medicine. The
School of Medicine sponsors summer programs
targeting rural and disadvantaged high school
students, although students from across Missouri
may participate.

Campus Information

Setting

The University of Missouri-Columbia School of
Medicine is located in the heart of the University
of Missouri's main campus, allowing students
to use its programs and facilities. MU has affiliations with all five hospitals in the city and a
number of satellite and specialty clinics in the
mid-Missouri area.

Enrollment

For 2007, total enrollment was: 370

Housing

Most medical students live in privately-owned
apartments, condominiums, and townhouses;
some purchase their own homes.

Satellite Campuses/Facilities

Students may choose to complete all elective
clinical rotations in and around Columbia,
or off-site in Missouri or across the country.
Students may participate in the Rural Track
Program, which offers three rural sites for both
clerkship and elective experiences.

Application Process and Requirements 2009–2010

Primary Application Service: AMCAS
Earliest filing date: June 1, 2008
Latest filing date: November 1, 2008

Secondary Application Required?: Yes
Sent to: All Missouri residents and screened out-of-state applicants
Marivern Easton, (573) 882-9219
eastonm@health.missouri.edu
URL: n/a
Fee: Yes, $75
Fee waiver available: Yes
Earliest filing date: July 1, 2008
Latest filing date: January 15, 2009

Latest MCAT® considered: September 2008
Oldest MCAT® considered: 2005

Early Decision Program
School does have EDP
Applicants notified: October 1, 2008
EDP available for: Residents only

Regular Acceptance Notice
Earliest date: October 15, 2008
Latest date: Until class is full

Applicant's Response to Acceptance Offer – Maximum Time: 30 days

Requests for Deferred Entrance Considered: Yes

Deposit to Hold Place in Class: Yes
Deposit (Resident): $100
Deposit (Non-Resident): $100
Deposit due: Within 30 days of acceptance offer until July, after which less time is given.
Applied to tuition: Yes
Deposit refundable: Yes
Refundable by: May 15, 2009

Estimated number of new entrants: 96
EDP: 4, special program: n/a

Start Month/Year: August 2009

Interview Format: Two open file, one-on-one interviews by Admissions Committee members are required. Regional interviews are not available.

Other Programs

PREPARATORY PROGRAMS
Postbaccalaureate Program: No
Summer Program: No

COMBINED DEGREE PROGRAMS
Baccalaureate/MD: No
MD/MPH: No
MD/MBA: No
MD/JD: No
MD/PhD: Yes,
Douglas Anthony, M.D., Ph.D., (573) 884-4074

Premedical Coursework

Course	Req.	Rec.	Lab.	Hrs.
Inorganic Chemistry	•		•	8
Behavioral Sciences				
Biochemistry		•		
Biology	•		•	8
Biology/Zoology				
Calculus				
College English				
College Mathematics	•			3

Course	Req.	Rec.	Lab.	Hrs.
Computer Science				
Genetics				
Humanities		•		
Organic Chemistry	•		•	8
Physics	•		•	8
Psychology				
Social Sciences		•		
English Composition	•			6

Selection Factors: 2007 Accepted Applicants

Proportion of Accepted Applicants with Relevant Experience (Data Self-Reported to AMCAS®)		
Community Service/Volunteer		65%
Medically-Related Work		71%
Research		69%

Shaded bar represents accepted scores ranging from the 10th percentile to the 90th percentile. School Median ● National Median ●

Overall GPA	2.0	2.1	2.2	2.3	2.4	2.5	2.6	2.7	2.8	2.9	3.0	3.1	3.2	3.3	3.4	3.5	3.6	3.7	(3.8)	3.9	4.0
Science GPA	2.0	2.1	2.2	2.3	2.4	2.5	2.6	2.7	2.8	2.9	3.0	3.1	3.2	3.3	3.4	3.5	3.6	3.7	(3.8)	3.9	4.0

MCAT® required: Yes, 85% of 2007 accepted applicants took MCAT®

Verbal Reasoning	3	4	5	6	7	8	9	(10)	11	12	13	14	15
Physical Sciences	3	4	5	6	7	8	9	(10)	(11)	12	13	14	15
Biological Sciences	3	4	5	6	7	8	9	10	(11)	12	13	14	15
Writing Sample				J	K	L	M	N	O	(P)	(Q)	R	S	T

Acceptance & Matriculation Data for 2007–2008 First Year Class

	Resident	Non-Resident	International	Total
Applied	456	793	15	1264
Interviewed	216	67	0	283
Deferred	4	1	0	5
Matriculants				
Early Assurance Program	n/a	n/a	n/a	n/a
Early Decision Program	10	0	0	10
Baccalaureate/MD	n/a	n/a	n/a	n/a
MD/PhD	n/a	n/a	n/a	n/a
Matriculated	91	5	0	**96**

Applications accepted from International Applicants: No

Specialty Choice

2003, 2004, 2005 Graduates, Specialty Choice (As reported by program directors to GME Track™)	
Anesthesiology	6%
Emergency Medicine	6%
Family Practice	16%
Internal Medicine	15%
Obstetrics/Gynecology	6%
Orthopaedic Surgery	3%
Pediatrics	13%
Psychiatry	4%
Radiology	6%
Surgery	4%

Matriculant Demographics: 2007–2008 First Year Class

Men: 52 **Women:** 44

Matriculants' Self-Reported Race/Ethnicity

Mexican American	3	**Korean**	0
Cuban	0	**Vietnamese**	0
Puerto Rican	0	**Other Asian**	1
Other Hispanic	0	**Total Asian**	3
Total Hispanic	3	**Native American**	0
Chinese	0	**Black**	0
Asian Indian	1	**Native Hawaiian**	0
Pakistani	0	**White**	92
Filipino	1	**Unduplicated Number**	
Japanese	0	**of Matriculants**	96

Science and Math Majors: 81%
Matriculants with:
Baccalaureate degree: 100%
Graduate degree(s): 10%

Financial Information

Source: 2006–2007 LCME I-B survey and 2007–2008 AAMC TSF questionnaire

	Residents	Non-Residents
Total Cost of Attendance	$41,354	$63,940
Tuition and Fees	$23,846	$46,432
Other (includes living expenses)	$15,729	$15,729
Health Insurance (can be waived)	$1,779	$1,779

Average 2007 Graduate Indebtedness: $130,015
% of Enrolled Students Receiving Aid: 96%

Criminal Background Check

This medical school requires a criminal background check prior to matriculation.

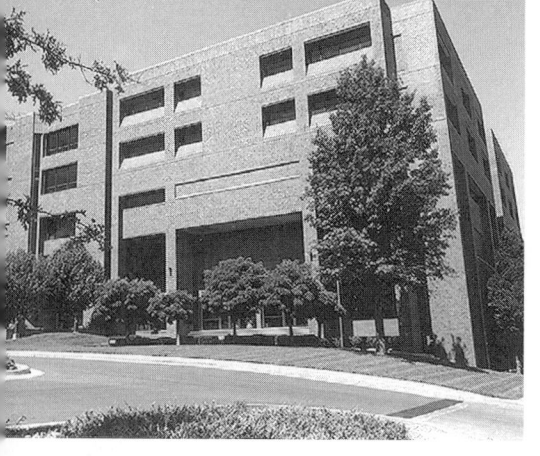

University of Missouri — Kansas City School of Medicine

Kansas City, Missouri

Council on Selection
University of Missouri — Kansas City
School of Medicine
2411 Holmes
Kansas City, Missouri 64108-2792
T 816 235 1870   F 816 235 6579

Admissions www.umkc.edu/admissions
Main www.med.umkc.edu
Financial www.sfa.umkc.edu
Email umkcmedweb@umkc.edu

Public Institution

Dr. Betty Drees, Dean

Dr. Christine Sullivan, Interim Chair, Council on Selection

Dr. Reaner Shannon, Associate Dean, Cultural Enhancement and Diversity

Jan Brandow, Director of Student Financial Aid

General Information

The Board of Curators of the University of Missouri authorized the establishment of a medical school at the University of Missouri-Kansas City in 1969. Located on a 135-acre Hospital Hill campus, the medical school is near both the schools and colleges of the university and affiliated community hospitals.

Mission Statement

The mission of the University of Missouri-Kansas City School of Medicine is to prepare graduates so that they are able to enter and complete graduate programs in medical education, qualify for medical licensure, provide competent medical care, and have the educational background necessary for lifelong learning in order to address the health care needs of our state and nation.

Curricular Highlights

Community Service Requirement: Optional.
Research/Thesis Requirement: Optional.

The School of Medicine, in combination with the College of Arts and Sciences and the School of Biological Sciences, offers a year-round program leading to baccalaureate and M.D. degrees in six calendar years. The student is required to complete both degrees and has the freedom to major in any department of the School of Biological Sciences or the College of Arts and Sciences. The program is designed primarily for high school seniors who are entering college. To receive the baccalaureate degree, the student must complete 120 semester hours of credit. The fundamental objective of the program is to provide students with a broad liberal arts education and to prepare physicians who are committed to providing comprehensive health care. Under the guidance of a clinician-scholar, called a docent, small groups of first- and second-year students are introduced to medicine in several community hospitals where they can observe patients and their problems. During the first two years of the program, the student is occupied predominantly with arts and sciences coursework, with about one-fourth of the time being devoted to introduction to medicine courses. After these two years the student advances, with the approval of the Council on Evaluation, to Year 3 of the six-year program. During the last four years of the curriculum, the student, with guidance from a docent and education team coordinator, plans a program for meeting the curricular requirements. Two months of Years 4 through 6 are spent with the docent on an inpatient internal medicine rotation. The remaining months of each year are spent in a number of other required and elective course offerings in the basic and clinical sciences and the humanities and social sciences. Students spend two academic terms in arts and sciences coursework during the last four years of the program. Basic, clinical, and behavioral science information is presented and emphasized throughout the six-year program. Thus, each student is expected to acquire a firm and broad base of information in each of these major content areas. The academic program provides the medical student with a realistic working knowledge of community health problems and resources. The school provides an environment for learning medicine, which is enhanced by the strong student support system. An alternative path is available for extended study.

USMLE

Step 1: Required. Students must record a passing score for promotion.
Step 2: Clinical Skills (CS): Required. Students must record a passing total score to graduate.
Step 2: Clinical Knowledge (CK): Required. Students must record a passing total score to graduate.

Selection Factors

The criteria for selection are: (1) the applicant's academic potential as judged by quality of high school courses, rank in high school class, and scores on the ACT. In the 2007-2008 entering class, the average ACT score fell at the 92nd percentile, and the average rank-in-class was at the 93rd percentile; (2) personal qualities, including maturity, leadership, stamina, reliability, motivation for medicine, range of interests, interpersonal skills, compassion, and job experience. The Council on Selection carefully reviews all applicants to this program. Applicants who appear to be well qualified are invited for interviews at the medical school campus. If invited, the applicant is notified by phone or email and is required to be present at the scheduled date and time of the interview. Students are considered on the basis of their individual qualifications without regard to race, creed, sex, or national origin. Effective in 2007, the program may accept transfer students.

Financial Aid

A variety of financial assistance is available to all medical students. Additional information and applications for financial aid may be obtained from: Student Financial Aid Office, University of Missouri-Kansas City, 5115 Oak, Kansas City, Missouri 64110. Priority application should be made prior to March 1.

Information about Diversity Programs

Information for students from groups underrepresented in medicine is available from Dr. Reaner Shannon, Associate Dean for Cultural Enhancement and Diversity, or Mary Anne Morgenegg, Coordinator, Council on Selection at the School of Medicine.

Campus Information

Enrollment

For 2007, total enrollment was: 624

Application Process and Requirements 2009–2010

Primary Application Service: School Specific
Earliest filing date: August 1, 2008
Latest filing date: November 15, 2008

Secondary Application Required?: Yes
Sent to: All applicants
URL: n/a
Fee: No
Fee waiver available: n/a
Earliest filing date: n/a
Latest filing date: n/a

Latest MCAT® considered: n/a
Oldest MCAT® considered: n/a

Early Decision Program
School does not have EDP
Applicants notified: n/a
EDP available for: n/a

Regular Acceptance Notice
Earliest date: April 1, 2009
Latest date: Varies

Applicant's Response to Acceptance Offer – Maximum Time: 30 days

Requests for Deferred Entrance Considered: No

Deposit to Hold Place in Class: Yes
Deposit (Resident): $100
Deposit (Non-Resident): $100
Deposit due: With response to acceptance offer
Applied to tuition: Yes
Deposit refundable: Yes
Refundable by: May 14, 2009

Estimated number of new entrants: 100
EDP: n/a, special program: 100

Start Month/Year: August 2009

Interview Format: Two thirty-minute interviews. Regional interviews are not available.

Other Programs

PREPARATORY PROGRAMS
Postbaccalaureate Program: No
Summer Program: No

COMBINED DEGREE PROGRAMS
Baccalaureate/MD: Yes, www.med.umkc.edu
MD/MPH: No
MD/MBA: No
MD/JD: No
MD/PhD: No

Premedical Coursework

Course	Req.	Rec.	Lab.	Hrs.	Course	Req.	Rec.	Lab.	Hrs.
Inorganic Chemistry					Computer Science				
Behavioral Sciences					Genetics				
Biochemistry					Humanities				
Biology					Organic Chemistry				
Biology/Zoology					Physics				
Calculus					Psychology				
College English					Social Sciences				
College Mathematics					Other				

Selection Factors: 2007 Accepted Applicants

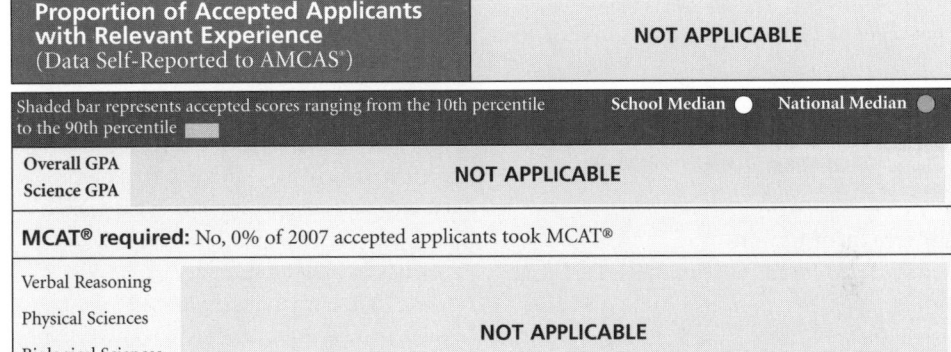

Proportion of Accepted Applicants with Relevant Experience (Data Self-Reported to AMCAS®)	**NOT APPLICABLE**

Shaded bar represents accepted scores ranging from the 10th percentile to the 90th percentile. School Median ● National Median ●

Overall GPA / Science GPA	**NOT APPLICABLE**

MCAT® required: No, 0% of 2007 accepted applicants took MCAT®

Verbal Reasoning / Physical Sciences / Biological Sciences / Writing Sample	**NOT APPLICABLE**

Acceptance & Matriculation Data for 2007–2008 First Year Class

	Resident	Non-Resident	International	Total
Applied	54	40	0	94
Interviewed	165	76	0	241
Deferred	0	0	0	0
Matriculants				
Early Assurance Program	n/a	n/a	n/a	n/a
Early Decision Program	0	0	0	0
Baccalaureate/MD	93	31	0	124
MD/PhD	n/a	n/a	n/a	n/a
Matriculated	54	40	0	**94**

Applications accepted from International Applicants: No

Matriculant Demographics: 2007–2008 First Year Class

Men: 38 **Women:** 56

Matriculants' Self-Reported Race/Ethnicity

Mexican American	0	Korean	0
Cuban	0	Vietnamese	0
Puerto Rican	0	Other Asian	0
Other Hispanic	0	Total Asian	0
Total Hispanic	0	Native American	0
Chinese	0	Black	0
Asian Indian	0	Native Hawaiian	0
Pakistani	0	White	0
Filipino	0	Unduplicated Number	
Japanese	0	of Matriculants	94

Science and Math Majors: n/a
Matriculants with:
  Baccalaureate degree: n/a
  Graduate degree(s): n/a

Specialty Choice

2003, 2004, 2005 Graduates, Specialty Choice (As reported by program directors to GME Track™)	
Anesthesiology	7%
Emergency Medicine	5%
Family Practice	10%
Internal Medicine	22%
Obstetrics/Gynecology	6%
Orthopaedic Surgery	3%
Pediatrics	11%
Psychiatry	3%
Radiology	2%
Surgery	6%

Financial Information

Source: 2006–2007 LCME I-B survey and 2007–2008 AAMC TSF questionnaire

	Residents	Non-Residents
Total Cost of Attendance	$54,397	$81,330
Tuition and Fees	$28,228	$55,161
Other (includes living expenses)	$25,202	$25,202
Health Insurance (not applicable)	$967	$967

Average 2007 Graduate Indebtedness: $145,568
% of Enrolled Students Receiving Aid: 83%

Criminal Background Check

This medical school requires a criminal background check prior to matriculation.

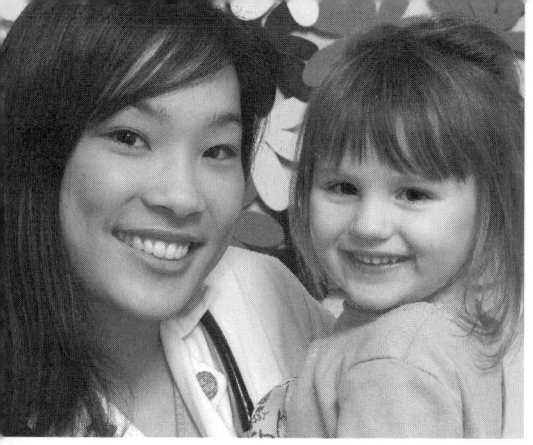

Washington University School of Medicine

St. Louis, Missouri

Office of Admissions
Washington University in St. Louis School of Medicine
660 South Euclid Avenue, #8107
St. Louis, Missouri 63110
T 314 362 6858 **F** 314 362 4658

Admissions medschool.wustl.edu/admissions
Main medschool.wustl.edu
Financial www.wusmfinaid.wustl.edu
Email wumscoa@wustl.edu

Private Institution

Dr. Larry J. Shapiro, Dean and Executive Vice Chancellor for Medical Affairs

Dr. W. Edwin Dodson, Associate Vice Chancellor and Associate Dean for Admissions

Dr. Will Ross, Associate Dean, Diversity Programs

Robert McCormack, Assistant Dean and Director of Financial Aid

General Information

Dedicated solely to education, the Farrell Learning and Teaching Center opened in 2005 to provide a state-of-the-art facility for medical education and to advance learning the compassionate delivery of scientific medicine. It is located at the heart of the 230-acre Washington Univer-sity Medical Center in which the School of Medicine occupies more than 4 million square feet of space. This new facility complements the outstanding clinical educational resources at Barnes-Jewish Hospital, the largest hospital in the region, and at St. Louis Children's Hospital, one of the top pediatric centers in the country, both of which are members of BJC Health System, the largest academically linked health care system in the nation.

Mission Statement

The mission of Washington University is the promotion of learning by students and by faculty. Teaching, the transmission of knowledge, is central to our mission, as is research, the creation of new knowledge. Our goals are: to foster excellence in our teaching, research, scholarship, and service; to prepare students with attitudes, skills, and habits of lifelong learning and with leadership skills, enabling them to be useful members of a global society; and to be an exemplary institution in our home community, St. Louis, as well as in the nation and the world.

Curricular Highlights

Community Service Requirement: Optional.
Research/Thesis Requirement: Optional.

The curriculum provides a state-of-the-art foundation in the science and the art of medicine.

Instruction is by lecture and small-group interactive sessions, and includes problem-based exercises and self-directed learning using computers and other resources led by faculty facilitators. Medical humanities and ethics are integrated into the four years of medical training, with emphasis given to the sociological and cultural concerns of patients and to the adaptation of medical care to their needs. Patient contact begins in the first semester of the first year and the fourth year is all electives. There are abundant opportunities in basic and clinical research. A five-year M.A. and M.D. degree program is available for students desiring one or two years of research training, while a Medical Scientist Training Program leads to both M.D. and Ph.D. degrees. A pass/fail grading system is used in the first year.

USMLE

Step 1: Optional.
Step 2: Clinical Skills (CS): Optional.
Step 2: Clinical Knowledge (CK): Optional.

Selection Factors

A good doctor must be compassionate and understanding, as well as a good scientist. To this end, the School of Medicine selects students who, in addition to possessing keen minds, demonstrate sensitivity and a commitment to serve others. Hence, students are selected on the basis of character, attitude, interest, intellectual ability, motivation, maturity, and achievement as indicated by superior academic and extracurricular accomplishments. Policies and programs are nondiscriminatory, and full consideration is given to all applicants without regard to sex, age, race, handicap, sexual preference, creed, or national or ethnic origin. Students from groups underrepresented in medicine are encouraged to apply. Selected applicants are invited to interview, which is required for acceptance.

Financial Aid

The financial resources of an applicant do not enter into the selection process. Tuition is established upon entry and does not increase during the four years of medical school. Need-based financial aid comprised of both scholarships

and loans is awarded to students who document financial need. Merit-based full-tuition scholarships are awarded to selected students in each entering class and are renewable.

Information about Diversity Programs

Washington University is strongly committed to the recruitment, selection, education, and graduation of an increased number of students from groups underrepresented in medicine. Students are supported by an active chapter of the Student National Medical Association and a network of faculty from diverse groups.

Campus Information

Setting

The Washington University Medical Center extends over 12 city blocks and is adjacent to the 1,371 acre Forest Park.

Enrollment

For 2007, total enrollment was: 591

Special Features

An education from Washington University School of Medicine prepares graduates for leadership and readies them for rigorous post-graduate clinical training, leading edge research, and rewarding medical careers. Learning takes place at the edge of what is known alongside exceptional colleagues and in state-of-the-art facilities. There are abundant clinical and research opportunities, including one of the largest genome sequencing facilities in the world. Newly completed in August 2005, the Farrell Learning and Teaching Center features state-of-the-art learning technology and facilities.

Housing

St. Louis is nationally recognized for its abundant, convenient, safe, and affordable housing. The bus and light rail system are free to students. The on-campus Spencer T. Olin Residence Hall is connected to the medical school buildings.

Application Process and Requirements 2009–2010

Primary Application Service: AMCAS
Earliest filing date: June 1, 2008
Latest filing date: December 1, 2008

Secondary Application Required?: Yes
Sent to: All applicants
URL: http://wumsapply.wustl.edu
Fee: Yes, $50
Fee waiver available: Yes
Earliest filing date: July 1, 2008
Latest filing date: December 31, 2008

Latest MCAT® considered: September 2008
Oldest MCAT® considered: 2005

Early Decision Program
School does not have EDP
Applicants notified: n/a
EDP available for: n/a

Regular Acceptance Notice
Earliest date: November 1, 2008
Latest date: Until class is full

Applicant's Response to Acceptance
Offer – Maximum Time: Two weeks

Requests for Deferred
Entrance Considered: Yes

Deposit to Hold Place in Class: Yes
Deposit (Resident): $100
Deposit (Non-Resident): $100
Deposit due: With response to acceptance offer
Applied to tuition: Yes
Deposit refundable: Yes
Refundable by: May 15, 2009

Estimated number of new entrants: 120
EDP: n/a, special program: 20

Start Month/Year: August 2009

Interview Format: Open, unstructured, one-on-one. Regional interviews are not available.

Other Programs

PREPARATORY PROGRAMS
Postbaccalaureate Program: Yes
http://ucollege.artsci.wustl.edu/postbacc.php
Steve Ehrlich, Associate Dean, (314) 935-6759,
ehrlich@wustl.edu
Summer Program: No

COMBINED DEGREE PROGRAMS
Baccalaureate/MD: Yes,
http://uscholars.wustl.edu
MD/MPH: No
MD/MBA: No
MD/JD: No
MD/PhD: Yes, http://mstp.wustl.edu

Premedical Coursework

Course	Req.	Rec.	Lab.	Sems.	Course	Req.	Rec.	Lab.	Sems.
Inorganic Chemistry	•			2	Computer Science				
Behavioral Sciences					Genetics				
Biochemistry					Humanities				
Biology	•			2	Organic Chemistry	•			2
Biology/Zoology					Physics	•			2
Calculus	•			2	Psychology				
College English					Social Sciences				
College Mathematics					Other				

Selection Factors: 2007 Accepted Applicants

Proportion of Accepted Applicants with Relevant Experience (Data Self-Reported to AMCAS®)		
Community Service/Volunteer		70%
Medically-Related Work		84%
Research		93%

Shaded bar represents accepted scores ranging from the 10th percentile to the 90th percentile. School Median ● National Median ◐

Overall GPA	2.0	2.1	2.2	2.3	2.4	2.5	2.6	2.7	2.8	2.9	3.0	3.1	3.2	3.3	3.4	3.5	3.6	3.7	3.8	(3.9)	4.0
Science GPA	2.0	2.1	2.2	2.3	2.4	2.5	2.6	2.7	2.8	2.9	3.0	3.1	3.2	3.3	3.4	3.5	3.6	3.7	3.8	(3.9)	4.0

MCAT® required: Yes, 100% of 2007 accepted applicants took MCAT®

Verbal Reasoning	3	4	5	6	7	8	9	⑩	11	⑫	13	14	15
Physical Sciences	3	4	5	6	7	8	9	10	⑪	12	⑬	14	15
Biological Sciences	3	4	5	6	7	8	9	10	⑪	12	⑬	14	15
Writing Sample			J	K	L	M	N	O	P	ⓠ	R	S	T

Acceptance & Matriculation Data for 2007–2008 First Year Class

	Resident	Non-Resident	International	Total
Applied	190	3657	265	4112
Interviewed	58	964	65	1087
Deferred	1	6	1	8
Matriculants				
Early Assurance Program	n/a	n/a	n/a	n/a
Early Decision Program	0	0	0	0
Baccalaureate/MD	0	0	0	0
MD/PhD	2	19	3	24
Matriculated	9	109	4	**122**

Applications accepted from International Applicants: Yes

Specialty Choice

2003, 2004, 2005 Graduates, Specialty Choice (As reported by program directors to GME Track™)	
Anesthesiology	6%
Emergency Medicine	6%
Family Practice	1%
Internal Medicine	16%
Obstetrics/Gynecology	3%
Orthopaedic Surgery	7%
Pediatrics	20%
Psychiatry	3%
Radiology Diagnostic	6%
Surgery General	7%

Matriculant Demographics: 2007–2008 First Year Class

Men: 62 **Women:** 60

Matriculants' Self-Reported Race/Ethnicity

Mexican American	2	Korean	6
Cuban	0	Vietnamese	0
Puerto Rican	1	Other Asian	1
Other Hispanic	1	Total Asian	39
Total Hispanic	4	Native American	1
Chinese	18	Black	7
Asian Indian	12	Native Hawaiian	1
Pakistani	1	White	74
Filipino	0	Unduplicated Number	
Japanese	1	of Matriculants	122

Science and Math Majors: 80%
Matriculants with:
　　Baccalaureate degree: 100%
　　Graduate degree(s): 2%

Financial Information

Source: 2006–2007 LCME I-B survey
and 2007–2008 AAMC TSF questionnaire

	Residents	Non-Residents
Total Cost of Attendance	$58,564	$58,564
Tuition and Fees	$43,380	$43,380
Other (includes living expenses)	$15,184	$15,184
Health Insurance (can not be waived)	$0	$0

Average 2007 Graduate Indebtedness: $100,975
% of Enrolled Students Receiving Aid: 88%

Criminal Background Check

This medical school requires a criminal background check prior to matriculation.

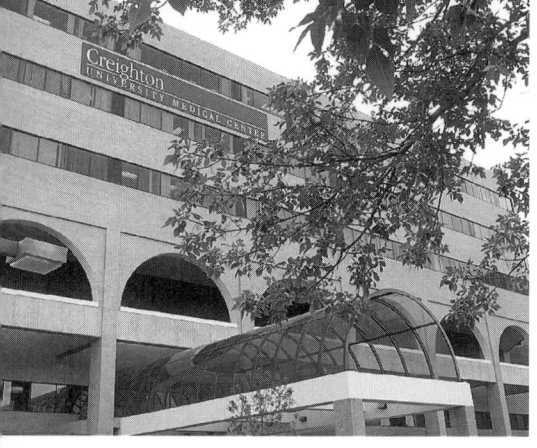

Creighton University School of Medicine

Omaha, Nebraska

Creighton University School of Medicine
Office of Medical Admissions
2500 California Plaza
Omaha, Nebraska 68178
T 402 280 2799   **F** 402 280 1241

Admissions http://medicine.creighton.edu/
medschool/admissions
Main http://medicine.creighton.edu
Financial www.creighton.edu/finaid
Email medschadm@creighton.edu

Private Institution

Dr. Cam E. Enarson, Dean,
Vice President for Health Sciences

Dr. Henry C. Nipper,
Assistant Dean for Admissions

Dr. Sade Kosoko-Lasaki, Associate Vice President
for Multicultural and Community Affairs

Karen Malloy, Financial Aid Coordinator

Garland Jarmon, Jr., Director of Admissions

General Information

Creighton University School of Medicine opened in October 1892, 14 years after the opening of the parent university, a Jesuit, catholic institution. The newly remodeled Criss Complex includes a new Medical Education Center offering state-of-the-art small-group rooms, lecture halls, anatomy suites, and a 60-seat computer classroom. Clinical instruction is at Creighton University Medical Center, a Level 1 trauma center, and other area hospitals and clinics. Ranked 5th nationally in PC Magazine's "Top Wired Colleges", we podcast all lectures in the M1 & M2 years, administer all exams on computer and lead in many other educational innovations.

Mission Statement

In the Catholic, Jesuit tradition of Creighton University, the mission of the School of Medicine is to improve the human condition through excellence in educating students, physicians and the public, advancing knowledge, and providing comprehensive patient care. We will be a School of Medicine respected by our peers for excellence in teaching, research, and clinical care. We will be distinguished for preparing graduates who achieve excellence in their chosen fields and who demonstrate extraordinary compassion and commitment to the service of others.

Curricular Highlights

Community Service Requirement: Optional. See the Web site for ILAC and Magis Clinic
Research/Thesis Requirement: Optional.

The curriculum integrates basic and clinical science in all four years. Year one combines strong

basic science content with the fundamentals of physical diagnosis and interviewing techniques. Year two is organized around a series of organ system-based courses and clinical skills training, including longitudinal clinics. Year three is comprised of core clerkships in a variety of inpatient and ambulatory settings. In year four students continue clinical training in critical care, surgery, and primary care and explore their own interests through electives. Clinical experiences, and ethical and societal issues, are prominent parts of the curriculum in all years. Instructional methodology uses case-based small-group sessions and computer-assisted instruction. Close faculty/student relationships provide for mentoring and advising of students. Students are graded against curriculum standards on an honors/satisfactory/unsatisfactory system, so they do not compete against each other.

USMLE

Step 1: Required. Students must record a passing score for promotion.
Step 2: Clinical Skills (CS) Required. Students must only record a score.
Step 2: Clinical Knowledge (CK): Required. Students must only record a score.

Selection Factors

The qualities of intellectual ability and curiosity, emotional maturity, honesty, proper motivation, proven scholastic ability, significant service to humanity, and documented medical experience are of highest importance. A formal interview on campus is required prior to acceptance. No restrictions are placed on applicants due to race, religion, sex, national or ethnic origin, age, disability, veteran status, or state of residence. Creighton values diversity in its medical classes. Advantage is given to applicants who complete their pre-professional education at Creighton. Both the AMCAS and Creighton's secondary applications are required of all applicants.

Financial Aid

In addition to student loans and other government programs, a limited number of scholarships are available for applicants who are academically well-qualified and have strong records of service to others.

Information about Diversity Programs

Qualified candidates from groups who are underrepresented in medicine are encouraged to apply. Creighton's Office of Health Sciences Multicultural and Community Affairs has several active programs to increase diversity and provide appropriate support services. The office administers several diversity programs, including pipeline and premedical postbaccalaureate programs.

Campus Information

Setting

Creighton's 100-acre campus and medical center are near Omaha's revitalized downtown and new arena. All of Creighton's schools and colleges are located on one campus.

Enrollment

For 2007, total enrollment was: 500

Special Features

"...service is a primary goal of education...our graduates and their mentors should be advocates of justice and crafters of a social order." – John Schlegel, S.J., President. Student life at the School of Medicine is personified by "balance" between academics and service to others. Activities include the Institute for Latin American Concern in the Dominican Republic, Project CURA, Habitat for Humanity, and the student-operated Magis Clinic. Although not required, all students do community service. The school also supports a student Wellness Council that organizes such events as picnics, movie nights, and stress management sessions; a Wellness Center; and the Wellness Chronicle. A variety of sports, music, and recreational activities is available on campus or nearby.

Housing

Safe, affordable housing is available on campus or nearby. Creighton offers two student parking garages which ease parking for commuters.

Satellite Campuses/Facilities

Satellite Campuses/Facilities: Opportunities for off-campus experiences exist in Phoenix, San Francisco, Indian Health Service hospitals, and the Dominican Republic.

Application Process and Requirements 2009–2010

Primary Application Service: AMCAS
Earliest filing date: July 1, 2008
Latest filing date: November 1, 2008

Secondary Application Required?: Yes
Sent to: All applicants
URL: www2.creighton.edu/medschool/medicine/oma/index.php
Fee: Yes, $95
Fee waiver available: Yes
Earliest filing date: July 1, 2008
Latest filing date: January 15, 2009

Latest MCAT® considered: September 2008
Oldest MCAT® considered: April 2006

Early Decision Program
School does have EDP
Applicants notified: October 1, 2008
EDP available for: Both Residents and Non-Residents

Regular Acceptance Notice
Earliest date: October 16, 2008
Latest date: Until class is full

Applicant's Response to Acceptance Offer – Maximum Time: Two weeks

Requests for Deferred Entrance Considered: Yes

Deposit to Hold Place in Class: Yes
Deposit (Resident): $100
Deposit (Non-Resident): $100
Deposit due: With response to acceptance offer
Applied to tuition: Yes
Deposit refundable: Yes
Refundable by: May 15, 2009

Estimated number of new entrants: 126
EDP: 1, special program: n/a

Start Month/Year: August 2009

Interview Format: Two open-file, one-on-one, non-stress interviews with faculty and medical students. Regional interviews are not available.

Other Programs

PREPARATORY PROGRAMS
Postbaccalaureate Program: Yes, http://www2.creighton.edu/health/hsmaca/premedicalpost-bacprogram/index.php
Summer Program: No
Premedical Pre-matriculation Program: Becky Messenger, BSW, (402) 280-2910, bmessenger@creighton.edu
Summer Research Program: http://medicine.creighton.edu/research/student_research_opportunities.htm
COMBINED DEGREE PROGRAMS
Baccalaureate/MD: No
MD/MPH: No
MD/MBA: No
MD/JD: No
MD/PhD: Yes, www2.creighton.edu/fileadmin/user/Registrar/docs/archive/MD_06-08.pdf

Premedical Coursework

Course	Req.	Rec.	Lab.	Hrs.	Course	Req.	Rec.	Lab.	Hrs.
Inorganic Chemistry	•		•	8	Computer Science				
Behavioral Sciences					Genetics		•		
Biochemistry		•			Humanities				
Biology	•		•	8	Organic Chemistry	•		•	8
Biology/Zoology					Physics	•		•	8
Calculus					Psychology				
College English				6	Social Sciences				
College Mathematics					Other				

Selection Factors: 2007 Accepted Applicants

Proportion of Accepted Applicants with Relevant Experience (Data Self-Reported to AMCAS)		
Community Service/Volunteer		77%
Medically-Related Work		86%
Research		78%

Shaded bar represents accepted scores ranging from the 10th percentile to the 90th percentile. School Median ● National Median ●

Overall GPA	2.0	2.1	2.2	2.3	2.4	2.5	2.6	2.7	2.8	2.9	3.0	3.1	3.2	3.3	3.4	3.5	3.6	3.7	(3.8)	3.9	4.0
Science GPA	2.0	2.1	2.2	2.3	2.4	2.5	2.6	2.7	2.8	2.9	3.0	3.1	3.2	3.3	3.4	3.5	3.6	3.7	(3.8)	3.9	4.0

MCAT® required: Yes, 100% of 2007 accepted applicants took MCAT®

Verbal Reasoning	3	4	5	6	7	8	9	(10)	11	12	13	14	15
Physical Sciences	3	4	5	6	7	8	9	(10)	(11)	12	13	14	15
Biological Sciences	3	4	5	6	7	8	9	(10)	(11)	12	13	14	15
Writing Sample				J	K	L	M	N	O	(P)	(Q)	R	S	T

Acceptance & Matriculation Data for 2007–2008 First Year Class

	Resident	Non-Resident	International	Total
Applied	221	5049	163	5433
Interviewed	66	525	2	593
Deferred	0	2	0	2
Matriculants				
Early Assurance Program	0	4	0	4
Early Decision Program	0	2	0	2
Baccalaureate/MD	n/a	n/a	n/a	n/a
MD/PhD	0	0	0	0
Matriculated	14	111	1	**126**

Applications accepted from International Applicants: Yes

Specialty Choice

2003, 2004, 2005 Graduates, Specialty Choice (As reported by program directors to GME Track™)	
Anesthesiology	13%
Emergency Medicine	3%
Family Practice	8%
Internal Medicine	18%
Obstetrics/Gynecology	10%
Orthopaedic Surgery	6%
Pediatrics	10%
Psychiatry	5%
Radiology	8%
Surgery	6%

Matriculant Demographics: 2007–2008 First Year Class

Men: 69 **Women:** 57

Matriculants' Self-Reported Race/Ethnicity

Mexican American	1	Korean	5
Cuban	1	Vietnamese	6
Puerto Rican	0	Other Asian	4
Other Hispanic	2	Total Asian	19
Total Hispanic	4	Native American	2
Chinese	1	Black	4
Asian Indian	2	Native Hawaiian	1
Pakistani	0	White	100
Filipino	1	Unduplicated Number	
Japanese	0	of Matriculants	126

Science and Math Majors: 75%
Matriculants with:
Baccalaureate degree: 100%
Graduate degree(s): 10%

Financial Information
Source: 2006–2007 LCME I-B survey and 2007–2008 AAMC TSF questionnaire

	Residents	Non-Residents
Total Cost of Attendance	$62,858	$62,858
Tuition and Fees	$41,778	$41,778
Other (includes living expenses)	$19,348	$19,348
Health Insurance (can be waived)	$1,732	$1,732

Average 2007 Graduate Indebtedness: $177,972
% of Enrolled Students Receiving Aid: 94%

Criminal Background Check

This medical school requires a criminal background check prior to matriculation.

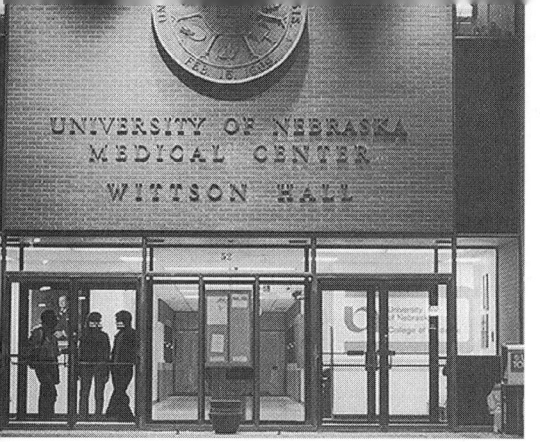

University of Nebraska College of Medicine
Omaha, Nebraska

Office of Admissions and Students
University of Nebraska Medical Center
College of Medicine
986585 Nebraska Medical Center
Omaha, Nebraska 68198-6585
T 402 559 2259   **F** 402 559 6840

Admissions www.unmc.edu/uncom
Main www.unmc.edu/uncom
Financial www.unmc.edu/student/
studentservices/financialaid
Email grrogers@unmc.edu

Public Institution

Dr. John L. Gollan, Dean

*Dr. Jeffrey W. Hill, Associate Dean,
Office of Admissions and Students*

*Dr. Kristie D. Hayes, Assistant Dean for
Student and Multicultural Affairs*

*Judith Walker, Assistant Director
of Financial Aid*

Gigi Rogers, Administrative Coordinator

General Information

Medical education has been continuous in Omaha since students first entered the Omaha Medical College in the fall of 1880. The medical college includes the Colleges of Medicine, Nursing, Pharmacy, and Dentistry; the School of Allied Health Professions; University Psychiatric Services; Eppley Cancer Center; and Munroe-Meyer Institute. These facilities are supplemented by direct teaching affiliations with the Veterans Affairs Medical Center and eight community hospitals. Students have access to facilities with a total of approximately 2,800 teaching beds.

Mission Statement

The mission of the University of Nebraska Medical Center is to improve the health of Nebraska through premier educational programs, innovative research, the highest quality patient care, and outreach to underserved populations.

Curricular Highlights

Community Service Requirement: Required.
Research/Thesis Requirement: Optional.

Students of the College of Medicine are recognized throughout the country as highly skilled practitioners. The education students receive provides a sound basis for support of career choices in medical practice, teaching, research, or administration. The college is particularly oriented toward training physicians to meet all the health care needs of the citizens of Nebraska. The curriculum ensures that students develop the understanding, clinical skills, and knowledge needed for residency training and practice.

USMLE

Step 1: Required. Students must record a passing score for promotion.
Step 2: Clinical Skills (CS): Required. Students must only record a score.
Step 2: Clinical Knowledge (CK): Required. Students must only record a score.

Selection Factors

Selection is based on a total assessment of each candidate's motivation, interests, character, demonstrated intellectual ability, previous academic record and its trends, personal interview, scores on the MCAT, and general fitness and promise for a career in medicine. Admission is based on individual qualifications without regard to age, sex, sexual preference, race, national origin, handicap, or religious or political beliefs. Strong preference is given to residents of Nebraska, but a number of students from other states may be accepted. The University of Nebraska encourages students from rural areas or disadvantaged backgrounds to apply. The potential for service to underserved communities is taken into consideration during the preadmission evaluation.

Financial Aid

Some scholarships are available each year. Several fellowships and assistantships are available to students who desire to take one or two years of graduate study or research in the basic sciences.

Information about Diversity Programs

The University of Nebraska College of Medicine is committed to increasing the number of physicians from groups currently underrepresented in the medical profession. Information is available through the Office of Student Equity and Multicultural Affairs at (402) 559-4437.

Campus Information

Setting

The University of Nebraska College of Medicine is located in the heart of Omaha. UNMC is a 60 acre campus and growing. Recreational and cultural activities include the Omaha Symphony Orchestra, the Old Market, the Joslyn Art Museum, the Omaha Community Playhouse, and the nationally recognized Opera Omaha. The Henry Doorly Zoo contains the world's largest indoor tropical rain forest and an IMAX theater. Spectator sports in Omaha include a full range of high school and collegiate sports and minor league teams. Omaha is the home of the College Baseball World Series.

Enrollment

For 2007, total enrollment was: 476

Special Features

The University of Nebraska College of Medicine strives to be a regional and national leader in the education of primary care health professionals, in the application of information technology to health care, and in research and clinical services related to cancer, transplantation, neurosciences, cardiovascular disease, genetics, rural health, and other major areas of healthcare need. The Lied Transplant Center and transplant programs have become national leaders in patient care and research, and they draw patients from all over the world. The LifeNet helicopter transport service transfers acutely ill patients from distances up to 200 miles from Omaha to the teaching services of the Nebraska Medical Center.

Housing

Campus housing is available and many affordable apartments are within walking distance.

Satellite Campuses/Facilities

The clinical facilities at the University of Nebraska Medical Center include the Nebraska Medical Center, University Medical Associates, and the Meyer Rehabilitation Institute. The Nebraska Medical Center is the primary teaching hospital for the College of Medicine. The College has affiliations with community hospitals throughout the state. The Omaha Veterans Affairs Medical Center is fully integrated into the educational programs of the College of Medicine.

Application Process and Requirements 2009–2010

Primary Application Service: AMCAS
Earliest filing date: June 1, 2008
Latest filing date: November 1, 2008

Secondary Application Required?: Yes
Sent to: Invited applicants only
URL: http://net.unmc.edu/apply
Contact: Jackie O'Hara, (402) 559-2259
johara@unmc.edu
Fee: Yes, $45
Fee waiver available: Yes
Earliest filing date: n/a
Latest filing date: January 15, 2009

Latest MCAT® considered: September 2008
Oldest MCAT® considered: 2006

Early Decision Program
School does have EDP
Applicants notified: October 1, 2008
EDP available for: Both Residents and
Non-Residents

Regular Acceptance Notice
Earliest date: December 2008
Latest date: Until class is full

Applicant's Response to Acceptance
Offer – Maximum Time: Two weeks

Requests for Deferred
Entrance Considered: No

Deposit to Hold Place in Class: Yes
Deposit (Resident): $100
Deposit (Non-Resident): $100
Deposit due: With response to acceptance offer
Applied to tuition: Yes
Deposit refundable: Yes
Refundable by: May 15, 2009

Estimated number of new entrants: 130
EDP: 35, special program: n/a

Start Month/Year: August 2009

Interview Format: By invitation only;
one-one-one interviews. Regional interviews
are not available.

Other Programs

PREPARATORY PROGRAMS
Postbaccalaureate Program: No
Summer Program: Yes, www.unmc.edu/dept/
cce/smdep, Giovanni Jones, (800) 701-9665,
smdep@unmc.edu
Summer Undergraduate Research: Yes,
www.unmc.edu/dept/summerresearch,
Jeanne Ferbrache, (402)559-3937,
jferbrache@unmc.edu
Baccalaureate/MD: No
MD/MPH: Yes, Jessica B. Tschirren, MPA,
(402) 561-7586, jtschirren@unmc.edu
MD/MBA: No
MD/JD: No
MD/PhD Summer Undergraduate
Research: Yes, www.unmc.edu/UNCOM/summer
Sonja Cox, (402) 559-8242, sacox@unmc.edu

Premedical Coursework

Course	Req.	Rec.	Lab.	Hrs.	Course	Req.	Rec.	Lab.	Hrs.
Inorganic Chemistry	•		•	8	Computer Science				
Behavioral Sciences					Genetics		•		3
Biochemistry	•			3	Humanities		•		12
Biology	•		•	8	Organic Chemistry	•		•	8
Biology/Zoology					Physics	•		•	8
Calculus	•			3	Psychology				
College English	•			3	Social Sciences				
College Mathematics	•			3	Other				

Selection Factors: 2007 Accepted Applicants

Proportion of Accepted Applicants with Relevant Experience (Data Self-Reported to AMCAS®)		
Community Service/Volunteer		66%
Medically-Related Work		75%
Research		74%

Shaded bar represents accepted scores ranging from the 10th percentile to the 90th percentile   School Median ○   National Median ◉

Overall GPA	2.0	2.1	2.2	2.3	2.4	2.5	2.6	2.7	2.8	2.9	3.0	3.1	3.2	3.3	3.4	3.5	3.6	3.7	(3.8)	3.9	4.0
Science GPA	2.0	2.1	2.2	2.3	2.4	2.5	2.6	2.7	2.8	2.9	3.0	3.1	3.2	3.3	3.4	3.5	3.6	3.7	(3.8)	3.9	4.0

MCAT® required: Yes, 99% of 2007 accepted applicants took MCAT®

Verbal Reasoning	3	4	5	6	7	8	9	(10)	11	12	13	14	15
Physical Sciences	3	4	5	6	7	8	9	(10)	(11)	12	13	14	15
Biological Sciences	3	4	5	6	7	8	9	(10)	(11)	12	13	14	15
Writing Sample				J	K	L	M	N	(O)	P	(Q)	R	S	T

Acceptance & Matriculation Data for 2007–2008 First Year Class

	Resident	Non-Resident	International	Total
Applied	318	1031	21	1370
Interviewed	255	153	0	408
Deferred	5	2	0	7
Matriculants				
Early Assurance Program	n/a	n/a	n/a	n/a
Early Decision Program	22	0	0	22
Baccalaureate/MD	n/a	n/a	n/a	n/a
MD/PhD	1	4	0	5
Matriculated	97	20	2	**119**

Applications accepted from International Applicants: No

Matriculant Demographics: 2007–2008 First Year Class

Men: 73   **Women:** 46

Matriculants' Self-Reported Race/Ethnicity

Mexican American	3	Korean	0
Cuban	0	Vietnamese	0
Puerto Rican	0	Other Asian	0
Other Hispanic	1	**Total Asian**	5
Total Hispanic	4	Native American	1
Chinese	2	Black	2
Asian Indian	3	Native Hawaiian	1
Pakistani	0	White	109
Filipino	0	**Unduplicated Number**	
Japanese	0	**of Matriculants**	119

Science and Math Majors: 77%
Matriculants with:
    Baccalaureate degree: 97%
    Graduate degree(s): 8%

Specialty Choice

2003, 2004, 2005 Graduates, Specialty Choice (As reported by program directors to GME Track™)	
Anesthesiology	10%
Emergency Medicine	7%
Family Practice	14%
Internal Medicine	15%
Obstetrics/Gynecology	3%
Orthopaedic Surgery	3%
Pediatrics	11%
Psychiatry	7%
Radiology	3%
Surgery	6%

Financial Information

Source: 2006–2007 LCME I-B survey
and 2007–2008 AAMC TSF questionnaire

	Residents	Non-Residents
Total Cost of Attendance	$38,056	$67,628
Tuition and Fees	$22,572	$52,144
Other (includes living expenses)	$14,520	$14,520
Health Insurance (can be waived)	$964	$964

Average 2007 Graduate Indebtedness: $122,050
% of Enrolled Students Receiving Aid: 98%

Criminal Background Check

This medical school requires a criminal background check prior to matriculation.

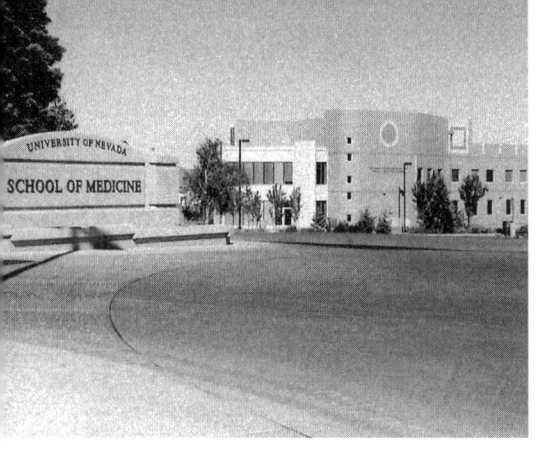

University of Nevada School of Medicine

Reno, Nevada

Office of Admissions and Student Affairs
University of Nevada School of Medicine
Mail Stop 0357
Reno, Nevada 89557-0357
T 775 784 6063   F 775 784 6194

Admissions www.medicine.nevada.edu/dept/asa/
default.asp
Main www.medicine.nevada.edu/
Financial www.medicine.nevada.edu/dept/asa/
students/financial_assistance_home.htm
Email asa@med.unr.edu

Public Institution

*Dr. John A. McDonald, Dean and
Vice President for Health Sciences*

*Dr. Cheryl Hug-English, Associate Dean
for Admissions and Student Affairs*

*Dr. Peggy Dupey, Assistant Dean for Student
Affairs*

*Ann Diggins, Director of Recruitment and
Student Services*

General Information

The University of Nevada School of Medicine is
a state-supported, community-based, university-
integrated school which relies heavily on community physicians as teachers and community
health facilities as sites for the majority of its
clinical education. The school is dedicated to
selecting individuals with diverse backgrounds
who will learn to be compassionate and competent physicians. Students study comprehensive
health care delivery considering the needs of
the individual, the family, and the community.

Mission Statement

To provide educational opportunities for
Nevadans, to improve the quality of healthcare
for citizens of Nevada, to create new biomedical
knowledge through education, research, patient
care and community service, and to provide
continuing medical education.

Curricular Highlights

Community Service Requirement: Optional.
Research/Thesis Requirement: Optional.

The first two years of the program are concen-
trated in classrooms and laboratories on the
Reno campus. The curriculum emphasizes the
biomedical and behavioral sciences basic to
medicine. Basic science disciplines are integrated with each other and with clinical problems to promote the learning of problem-solving skills. A clinical correlation course, which
explores the basics of bio-medical ethics, is
taught. Early clinical training is provided for
students to learn patient interviewing and doctor-patient relationship skills and the basics
of physical examination and diagnosis.

Throughout the first and second years, students
spend time with a physician to observe medical
practice in the office setting and clinic settings.
There are also opportunities to participate in
basic and clinical science research throughout
the curriculum. The third and fourth years
emphasize a balance of ambulatory and inpatient medical education designed to better prepare students for residency. Third and fourth
year students study clinical medicine in Reno,
Las Vegas, and rural Nevada.

USMLE

Step 1: Required. Students must record a passing
score for promotion.
Step 2: Clinical Skills (CS): Required. Students
must record a passing total score to graduate.
Step 2: Clinical Knowledge (CK): Required. Students must record a passing total score to graduate.

Selection Factors

Candidates are evaluated on the basis of academic performance; results of the MCAT®; the
nature and depth of scholarly, extracurricular,
and health care-related activities during college
years (excellence and balance of the natural sciences, social sciences, and humanities); academic
letters of evaluation; and the personal interview.
A small number of nonresident applicants from
Alaska, Idaho, Montana, or Wyoming or residents of northern California counties bordering
Nevada (medical catchment area) are considered.
Applicants from other western states should contact the office of admissions for updated eligibility information. Applicants are required to be
U.S. citizens or have a permanent resident visa.
Only those students who are currently enrolled
and in good academic standing at LCME-accredited medical schools and have a strong residential
tie to Nevada are considered for transfer to the
second and third years. The number of positions
available for transfer is strictly limited by attrition and compatibility to the school's curriculum. Only U.S. citizens are considered. Transfer
applications from students attending foreign
medical schools are not considered. Completion
of a criminal background check is required of all
accepted applicants. The fee for this background
check is $51.25.

Financial Aid

Every attempt is made to assist students and their
families in meeting both their financial obligations
to the School of Medicine and the student's essential personal needs. Financial status is not a determinant in selecting qualified applicants. A limited
number of loans and scholarships are available on
the basis of need and merit. Determination of
financial aid awards is made after acceptance.

Information about Diversity Programs

The School of Medicine is committed to the
recruitment, selection, and retention of individuals who are members of groups traditionally underrepresented in American medicine.
Residents of the state of Nevada and individuals who meet the nonresident criteria and who
are from such backgrounds are encouraged to
apply. The University of Nevada, Reno, does
not discriminate on the basis of race, color,
religion, sex, age, creed, national origin, veteran
status, physical or mental disability, and in
accordance with university policy, sexual orientation, in any program or activity it operates.

Campus Information

Enrollment

For 2007, total enrollment was: 224

Special Features

The Reno campus features state-of-the art
research facilities, a new medical education
building with the latest wireless technology,
and a Human Patient Simulator (S.T.A.N.).
Students have opportunities to work in several
clinical facilities. The Las Vegas campus features a Level I trauma center.

Housing

Housing is available within short distances
of campuses.

Satellite Campuses/Facilities

The University of Nevada School of Medicine is
a state-wide institution with varied clinical sites
including a Level I trauma center and numerous research and rural clinical opportunities.

Application Process and Requirements 2009–2010

Primary Application Service: AMCAS
Earliest filing date: June 1, 2008
Latest filing date: November 1, 2008

Secondary Application Required?: Yes
Sent to: Screened applicants
Contact: Kristine Nelson, (775) 784-6063, knelson@medicine.nevada.edu
Fee: Yes, $45
Fee waiver available: Yes
Earliest filing date: August 1, 2008
Latest filing date: December 1, 2008

Latest MCAT® considered: September 2008
Oldest MCAT® considered: 2005

Early Decision Program
School does have EDP
Applicants notified: October 1, 2008
EDP available for: Both Residents and Non-Residents

Regular Acceptance Notice
Earliest date: January 15, 2009
Latest date: Varies

Applicant's Response to Acceptance Offer – Maximum Time: Two weeks

Requests for Deferred Entrance Considered: Yes

Deposit to Hold Place in Class: No
Deposit (Resident): n/a
Deposit (Non-Resident): n/a
Deposit due: n/a
Applied to tuition: n/a
Deposit refundable: n/a
Refundable by: n/a

Estimated number of new entrants: 62
EDP: 5, special program: n/a

Start Month/Year: August 2009

Interview Format: Interviews are blind and semi-structured. Applicants are interviewed in Reno and Las Vegas.

Other Programs

PREPARATORY PROGRAMS
Postbaccalaureate Program: No
Summer Program: No

COMBINED DEGREE PROGRAMS
Baccalaureate/MD: Yes
MD/MPH: No
MD/MBA: No
MD/JD: No
MD/PhD: Yes,
David Lupan, Ph.D., (775) 784-4908
asa@med.unr.edu

Premedical Coursework

Course	Req.	Rec.	Lab.	Hrs.	Course	Req.	Rec.	Lab.	Hrs.
Inorganic Chemistry	•		•	8	Computer Science		•		
Behavioral Sciences	•			6	Genetics		•		
Biochemistry		•			Humanities		•		
Biology	•		•	12	Organic Chemistry	•		•	8
Biology/Zoology					Physics	•		•	8
Calculus		•			Psychology				
College English		•			Social Sciences		•		
College Mathematics		•			Other 1, 2, & 3		•		

Selection Factors: 2007 Accepted Applicants

Proportion of Accepted Applicants with Relevant Experience (Data Self-Reported to AMCAS®)	Community Service/Volunteer	72%
	Medically-Related Work	93%
	Research	84%

Shaded bar represents accepted scores ranging from the 10th percentile to the 90th percentile. School Median ● National Median ●

Overall GPA	2.0	2.1	2.2	2.3	2.4	2.5	2.6	2.7	2.8	2.9	3.0	3.1	3.2	3.3	3.4	3.5	3.6	(3.7)	3.8	3.9	4.0
Science GPA	2.0	2.1	2.2	2.3	2.4	2.5	2.6	2.7	2.8	2.9	3.0	3.1	3.2	3.3	3.4	3.5	(3.6)	3.7	3.8	3.9	4.0

MCAT® required: Yes, 100% of 2007 accepted applicants took MCAT®

Verbal Reasoning	3	4	5	6	7	8	9	(10)	11	12	13	14	15
Physical Sciences	3	4	5	6	7	8	9	(10)	(11)	12	13	14	15
Biological Sciences	3	4	5	6	7	8	9	(10)	(11)	12	13	14	15
Writing Sample			J	K	L	M	N	O	(P)	(Q)	R	S	T

Acceptance & Matriculation Data for 2007–2008 First Year Class

	Resident	Non-Resident	International	Total
Applied	164	930	15	1109
Interviewed	153	84	0	237
Deferred	0	0	0	0
Matriculants				
Early Assurance Program	n/a	n/a	n/a	n/a
Early Decision Program	4	1	0	5
Baccalaureate/MD	n/a	n/a	n/a	n/a
MD/PhD	n/a	n/a	n/a	n/a
Matriculated	51	11	0	**62**

Applications accepted from International Applicants: No

Specialty Choice

2003, 2004, 2005 Graduates, Specialty Choice (As reported by program directors to GME Track™)	
Anesthesiology	6%
Emergency Medicine	13%
Family Practice	16%
Internal Medicine	17%
Obstetrics/Gynecology	6%
Orthopaedic Surgery	3%
Pediatrics	11%
Psychiatry	7%
Radiology	3%
Surgery	3%

Matriculant Demographics: 2007–2008 First Year Class

Men: 34   **Women:** 28

Matriculants' Self-Reported Race/Ethnicity

Mexican American	2	Korean	0
Cuban	0	Vietnamese	1
Puerto Rican	0	Other Asian	3
Other Hispanic	2	Total Asian	13
Total Hispanic	4	Native American	2
Chinese	3	Black	0
Asian Indian	3	Native Hawaiian	0
Pakistani	1	White	50
Filipino	2	Unduplicated Number	
Japanese	1	of Matriculants	62

Science and Math Majors: 79%
Matriculants with:
 Baccalaureate degree: 98%
 Graduate degree(s): 11%

Financial Information
Source: 2006–2007 LCME I-B survey and 2007–2008 AAMC TSF questionnaire

	Residents	Non-Residents
Total Cost of Attendance	$36,973	$56,829
Tuition and Fees	$13,075	$32,931
Other (includes living expenses)	$21,896	$21,896
Health Insurance (can be waived)	$2,002	$2,002

Average 2007 Graduate Indebtedness: $116,119
% of Enrolled Students Receiving Aid: 91%

Criminal Background Check

This medical school requires a criminal background check prior to matriculation.

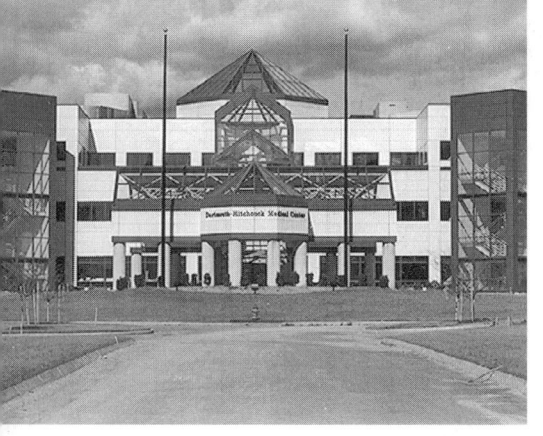

Dartmouth Medical School
Hanover, New Hampshire

Dartmouth Medical School
Office of Admissions
3 Rope Ferry Road
Hanover, New Hampshire 03755-1404
T 603 650 1505 **F** 603 650 1560

Admissions http://dms.dartmouth.edu/admissions/
Main http://dms.dartmouth.edu/
Financial http://dms.dartmouth.edu
admissions/financial_aid/
Email dms.admissions@dartmouth.edu

Private Institution

Dr. William Green, Dean

Andrew G. Welch, Director of Admissions

Dr. Lori Alvord, Associate Dean of Student and Multicultural Affairs

Sally Kelley, Acting Director of Financial Aid

General Information

Dartmouth Medical School, the fourth oldest U.S. medical school, is a partner of Dartmouth-Hitchcock Medical Center (DHMC). DHMC serves a patient population of 1.6 million and includes Mary Hitchcock Memorial Hospital, Dartmouth-Hitchcock Clinic, and the Veterans Affairs Hospital. Other facilities contributing to the integration of advanced research and quality care within DHMC include the Norris Cotton Cancer Center, Children's Hospital at Dartmouth, and the Borwell Research Building; DHMC is a major force for medical treatment and discovery and is the site of numerous clinical trials. Additional teaching sites span nationally and internationally from the New England states to California to Tanzania. A faculty of approximately 2,000 affords ample opportunity for individual instruction.

Mission Statement

Dartmouth Medical School educates outstanding leaders prepared to transform medicine and science. The school aspires to be the best in the world at expanding knowledge and using it wisely to improve health, all done in the context of the tradition of collegiality of Dartmouth and the values its community honors. We are committed to the challenges of discovery and innovation and to their application to health care that meets the needs and wants of patients and society.

Curricular Highlights

Community Service Requirement: Optional.
Research/Thesis Requirement: Optional.

The DMS curriculum integrates basic and clinical sciences throughout medical school. Its hallmarks are longitudinal experiences in the basic and clinical sciences, early introduction to patient care, small-group instruction, close relationships with faculty, and opportunities for independent learning. DMS uses various pedagogies, including problem-based learning, lectures, and small elective courses. Year One includes On Doctoring, a course that pairs students with faculty practitioners in the clinical environment. The Scientific Basis of Medicine, an interdisciplinary pathophysiology course combined with an introduction to the mechanisms of disease and the principles of clinical medicine, is a feature of Year Two. Six eight-week clerkships and opportunities to practice in diverse settings shape the third year. The fourth year includes two required clerkships, a sub-internship, and four short courses, but students largely spend this year refining their interests through electives.

USMLE

Step 1: Required. Students must only record a score.
Step 2: Clinical Skills (CS): Required. Students must only record a score.
Step 2: Clinical Knowledge (CK): Required. Students must only record a score.

Selection Factors

The admissions committee carefully reviews the entire application with attention to personal, scholastic, and scientific qualifications. DMS does not employ numeric cutoffs or inflexible criteria. Selected applicants interview in Hanover from September to March. DMS supports equal opportunity for all persons. No student shall be denied admission or financial aid or be otherwise discriminated against because of age, disability, race, creed, religion, sex, sexual orientation, or national origin.

Financial Aid

DMS practices need-blind admissions. Application fee waivers are granted to individuals who have received an AMCAS fee waiver. All accepted U.S. citizens and permanent residents with documented need are offered financial aid packages. DMS awards scholarships and loans on the basis of need as indicated by the FAFSA, the Need Access form, the DMS financial aid application, and supporting documentation. Financial support for foreign students is limited.

Information about Diversity Programs

DMS seeks to enroll a talented and diverse class of students from various racial, ethnic, cultural, religious, and socio-economic backgrounds. Lori Alvord, M.D., is Associate Dean of Student and Multicultural Affairs.

Campus Information

Setting

DMS is located in Hanover, NH, on the campus of a well-resourced institution in a classic New England town. DMS and the surrounding communities provide abundant cultural and recreational opportunities. A sample of venues includes the Hopkins Center, with frequent concerts, films, lectures, and artistic performances, and the Hood Museum, which boasts impressive permanent and temporary exhibits.

Enrollment

For 2007, total enrollment was: 316

Special Features

DMS offers both small classes and one of the nation's top 16 major teaching hospitals. With a patient population of nearly 1.6 million people, Dartmouth medical students gain exposure to a broad spectrum of patients and treatments and are well-prepared for residency training.

Housing

Housing is available on and off-campus.

Satellite Campuses/Facilities

DMS provides a variety of clinical training opportunities; students gain exposure to various patient populations, healthcare delivery systems, and management models. Locations such as Tuba City, AZ; Orange County, CA; San Francisco, CA; Bethel, AK; the Florida Keys, Dar es Salaam, Tanzania; and every New England state (except Massachusetts) are only some of the possibilities. Students may also study on-campus at the internationally known Dartmouth Institute for Health Policy and Clinical Practice (formerly CECS).

Application Process and Requirements 2009–2010

Primary Application Service: AMCAS
Earliest filing date: June 1, 2008
Latest filing date: November 1, 2008

Secondary Application Required?: Yes
Sent to: All applicants
URL: http://dms.dartmouth.edu/admissions/instrs_to_applicants.shtml
Fee: Yes, $85
Fee waiver available: Yes
Earliest filing date: June 1, 2008
Latest filing date: January 2, 2009

Latest MCAT® considered: September 2008
Oldest MCAT® considered: 2006

Early Decision Program
School does not have EDP
Applicants notified: n/a
EDP available for: n/a

Regular Acceptance Notice
Earliest date: November 1, 2008
Latest date: Until class is full

Applicant's Response to Acceptance Offer – Maximum Time: Two weeks

Requests for Deferred Entrance Considered: Yes

Deposit to Hold Place in Class: No
Deposit (Resident): n/a
Deposit (Non-Resident): n/a
Deposit due: n/a
Applied to tuition: n/a
Deposit refundable: n/a
Refundable by: n/a

Estimated number of new entrants: 73
EDP: 0, special program: n/a

Start Month/Year: August 2009

Interview Format: Two half-hour interviews. Regional interviews are not available.

Other Programs

PREPARATORY PROGRAMS
Postbaccalaureate Program: No
Summer Program: Yes,
Kalindi Trietley, (603) 650-6535
Kalindi.E.Trietley@Dartmouth.edu

COMBINED DEGREE PROGRAMS
Baccalaureate/MD: No
MD/MPH: Yes,
http://dms.dartmouth.edu/cfm/education/joint.php
MD/MBA: Yes, www.tuck.dartmouth.edu/
MD/JD: No
MD/PhD: Yes, http://dms.dartmouth.edu/admissions/curriculum/mdphd/

Premedical Coursework

Course	Req.	Rec.	Lab.	Hrs.	Course	Req.	Rec.	Lab.	Hrs.
Inorganic Chemistry	•			8	Computer Science				
Behavioral Sciences					Genetics				
Biochemistry		•		3	Humanities				
Biology	•			8	Organic Chemistry	•			8
Biology/Zoology					Physics	•			8
Calculus	•			3	Psychology				
College English					Social Sciences				
College Mathematics					Other				

Selection Factors: 2007 Accepted Applicants

Proportion of Accepted Applicants with Relevant Experience (Data Self-Reported to AMCAS®)		
Community Service/Volunteer	70%	
Medically-Related Work	91%	
Research	90%	

Shaded bar represents accepted scores ranging from the 10th percentile to the 90th percentile ▬ School Median ● National Median ●

Overall GPA	2.0	2.1	2.2	2.3	2.4	2.5	2.6	2.7	2.8	2.9	3.0	3.1	3.2	3.3	3.4	3.5	3.6	3.7	(3.8)	3.9	4.0
Science GPA	2.0	2.1	2.2	2.3	2.4	2.5	2.6	2.7	2.8	2.9	3.0	3.1	3.2	3.3	3.4	3.5	3.6	3.7	(3.8)	3.9	4.0

MCAT® required: No, 98% of 2007 accepted applicants took MCAT®

Verbal Reasoning	3	4	5	6	7	8	9	(10)	(11)	12	13	14	15
Physical Sciences	3	4	5	6	7	8	9	10	(11)	(12)	13	14	15
Biological Sciences	3	4	5	6	7	8	9	10	(11)	(12)	13	14	15
Writing Sample			J	K	L	M	N	O	P	(Q)	R	S	T

Acceptance & Matriculation Data for 2007–2008 First Year Class

	Resident	Non-Resident	International	Total
Applied	71	4796	443	5310
Interviewed	31	649	N/A	680
Deferred	0	0	0	0
Matriculants				
Early Assurance Program	0	0	0	0
Early Decision Program	0	0	0	0
Baccalaureate/MD	n/a	n/a	n/a	n/a
MD/PhD	0	2	3	5
Matriculated	5	56	12	**73**

Applications accepted from International Applicants: Yes

Specialty Choice

2003, 2004, 2005 Graduates, Specialty Choice (As reported by program directors to GME Track™)	
Anesthesiology	7%
Emergency Medicine	5%
Family Practice	8%
Internal Medicine	16%
Obstetrics/Gynecology	3%
Orthopaedic Surgery	5%
Pediatrics	11%
Psychiatry	5%
Radiology	6%
Surgery	11%

Matriculant Demographics: 2007–2008 First Year Class

Men: 32   **Women:** 41

Matriculants' Self-Reported Race/Ethnicity

Mexican American	3	Korean	0
Cuban	1	Vietnamese	1
Puerto Rican	0	Other Asian	1
Other Hispanic	1	Total Asian	17
Total Hispanic	5	Native American	0
Chinese	7	Black	0
Asian Indian	6	Native Hawaiian	0
Pakistani	0	White	39
Filipino	0	Unduplicated Number	
Japanese	2	of Matriculants	73

Science and Math Majors: 75%
Matriculants with:
Baccalaureate degree: 100%
Graduate degree(s): 4%

Financial Information

Source: 2006–2007 LCME I-B survey and 2007–2008 AAMC TSF questionnaire

	Residents	Non-Residents
Total Cost of Attendance	$56,075	$56,075
Tuition and Fees	$38,675	$38,675
Other (includes living expenses)	$15,400	$15,400
Health Insurance (can be waived)	$2,000	$2,000

Average 2007 Graduate Indebtedness: $119,389
% of Enrolled Students Receiving Aid: 84%

Criminal Background Check

This medical school does not require a criminal background check prior to matriculation.

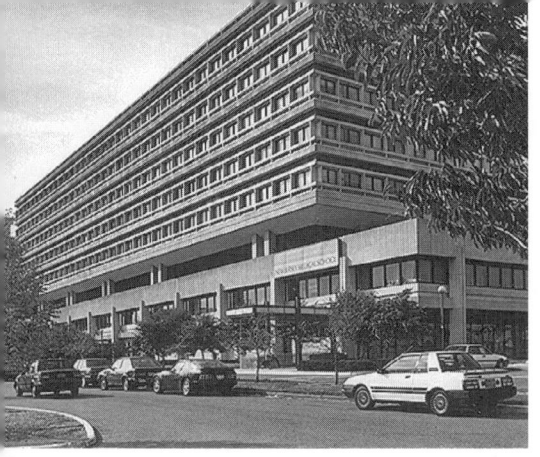

University of Medicine and Dentistry of New Jersey — New Jersey Medical School
Newark, New Jersey

Director of Admissions
UMDNJ — New Jersey Medical School
185 South Orange Avenue C-653
Newark, New Jersey 07103
T 973 972 4631 **F** 973 972 7986

Admissions http://njms.umdnj.edu/education/admissions
Main http://njms.umdnj.edu
Financial www.umdnj.edu/studentfinancialaid
Email njmsadmiss@umdnj.edu

Public Institution

Dr. Robert L. Johnson, Interim Dean

Dr. Maria Soto-Greene, Vice Dean

Dr. George F. Heinrich, Associate Dean for Admissions and Special Programs

Elaine Varas, University Director of Student Financial Aid

Mercedes M. Rivero, Director of Admissions

General Information

New Jersey Medical School (NJMS), formerly Seton Hall College of Medicine and Dentistry, is the state's oldest academic medical institution. More than 700 faculty and 1,300 volunteer faculty in our 19 academic departments play a critical role in transforming our students into qualified clinicians who will meet and exceed the healthcare needs of New Jersey and the nation. Major clinical instruction is carried out at the University Hospital, Hackensack University Medical Center, Veterans Affairs Medical Center, St. Barnabus Medical Center, Newark Beth Israel Medical Center, Morristown Memorial Hospital, Overlook Hospital, Mountainside Hospital and Kessler Institute for Rehabilitation.

Mission Statement

To educate students, physicians, and scientists to meet society's current and future healthcare needs through patient-centered education; pioneering research; innovative clinical, rehabilitative and preventive care; and collaborative community outreach.

Curricular Highlights
Community Service Requirement: Optional.
Research/Thesis Requirement: Optional.

Years 1 and 2 are devoted to providing an understanding of the basic sciences integrated with early clinical exposure and a comprehensive introduction to the field of medicine through a course called the "Physician's Core." The basic sciences are taught utilizing a variety of teaching modalities, including lectures, laboratories and small-group sessions. Students receive components of their clinical training in the Clinical Skills Training Center, which features 12 simulated patient examination rooms equipped to monitor mock patient encounters with standardized patients. Years 3 and 4 are devoted to providing in-depth exposure to clinical medicine. In Year 3, students rotate through the major disciplines in medicine (internal medicine, surgery, family medicine, pediatrics, psychiatry and obstetrics-gynecology)and in Year 4, students will assume a higher degree of autonomy and responsibility as they rotate through acting internships and an emergency medicine rotation, and select from a wide range of electives, both at NJMS and throughout the country.

USMLE
Step 1: Required. Students must record a passing score for promotion.
Step 2: Clinical Skills (CS): Required. Students must record a passing total score to graduate.
Step 2: Clinical Knowledge (CK): Required. Students must record a passing total score to graduate.

Selection Factors

Applicants are selected on the basis of academic excellence, leadership qualities, demonstrated compassion for others and broad extracurricular experiences. Related factors such as passion, perseverance, special aptitudes and stamina are also considered. Intense competition tends to favor those with stronger credentials. Out-of-state residents are encouraged to apply.

Financial Aid

The student financial aid programs are a centrally managed operation at UMDNJ and not considered in the admissions process. Financial Aid Professionals meet and advise accepted students regarding the financial aspects of their medical education.

Information about Diversity Programs

NJMS is committed to the recruitment of a diverse student body as well as enhancing the cultural competency of all its medical students in order to improve access to care for underserved populations. Several programs have been established to support these goals. Information may be obtained by contacting the Office of Special Programs at (973) 972-3762.

Campus Information

Setting

NJMS is located in University Heights near the Newark Bears Riverfront Stadium, NJPAC, Ironbound district, Weequahic Golf Course and Branch Brook Park. Manhattan is just a 15-minute train ride away. Many buildings on the 65-acre campus are connected, making it convenient to travel from classrooms and labs to the library and University Hospital. Many students live on and around campus in the university apartments, as well as townhomes located directly across from the school.

Enrollment

For 2007, total enrollment was: 708

Special Features

In 2004, NJMS received $104 million in extramural grants supporting basic, clinical and translational research. NJMS is also home to the Global Tuberculosis Institute, The Institute for Ophthalmology and Visual Science, and the Center for Emerging and Reemerging Pathogens. NJMS is a charter member of the New Jersey Stem Cell Research and Education Foundation. Designated Areas of Excellence include: Brain Injury and Stroke, Cancer/Oncology, Cardiovascular Biology, Cellular Signal Transduction, Immunology, Infectious Diseases, Neurosciences, Psychiatry/Behavioral Sciences. NJMS faculty contributions include: the development of the worldwide standard in knee replacement, the New Jersey Knee; a patented method for the early detection of Lyme disease; the identification of pediatric AIDS and the development of drug-therapy to reduce the likelihood of pre-natal transmission; and proof of the connection between smoking and cancer resulting in the warning message printed on cigarette packages.

Housing

Our on-campus student housing facility houses 465 students in 234 residential apartments. The 14-story building includes a private exterior courtyard, a fitness center and several retail establishments, as well as a parking garage.

Application Process and Requirements 2009–2010

Primary Application Service: AMCAS
Earliest filing date: June 1, 2008
Latest filing date: December 1, 2008

Secondary Application Required?: Yes
Sent to: All applicants
Contact: njmsadmiss@umdnj.edu
Fee: Yes, $75
Fee waiver available: Yes
Earliest filing date: July 1, 2008
Latest filing date: January 1, 2009

Latest MCAT® considered: Any MCAT® taken in 2008 or before
Oldest MCAT® considered: Any

Early Decision Program
School does have EDP
Applicants notified: October 1, 2008
EDP available for: Both Residents and Non-Residents

Regular Acceptance Notice
Earliest date: October 15, 2008
Latest date: Until class is full

Applicant's Response to Acceptance
Offer – Maximum Time: Two weeks

Requests for Deferred
Entrance Considered: Yes

Deposit to Hold Place in Class: Yes
Deposit (Resident): $100
Deposit (Non-Resident): $100
Deposit due: Within two weeks of acceptance
Applied to tuition: Yes
Deposit refundable: Yes
Refundable by: May 15, 2009

Estimated number of new entrants: 170
EDP: 20, special program: 25

Start Month/Year: August 2009

Interview Format: One-to-one, non-stress interview with faculty.

Other Programs

PREPARATORY PROGRAMS
Postbaccalaureate Program: No
Summer Program: Yes
Dolores Anthony, (973) 972-3762
anthondd@umdnj.edu

COMBINED DEGREE PROGRAMS
Baccalaureate/MD: Yes,
http://njms.umdnj.edu/education/admissions/
seven_year_ba_md.cfm
MD/MPH: Yes, http://sph.umdnj.edu
MD/MBA: Yes,
http://njms.umdnj.edu/education/
admissions/md_mba.cfm
MD/JD: No
MD/PhD: Yes, http://njms.umdnj.edu/
education/admissions/md_phd.cfm

Premedical Coursework

Course	Req.	Rec.	Lab.	Hrs.
Inorganic Chemistry	•		•	8
Behavioral Sciences				
Biochemistry				
Biology		•		
Biology/Zoology	•		•	8
Calculus				
College English	•			6
College Mathematics		•		3

Course	Req.	Rec.	Lab.	Hrs.
Computer Science				
Genetics				
Humanities				
Organic Chemistry	•		•	8
Physics	•		•	8
Psychology				
Social Sciences				
Other				

Selection Factors: 2007 Accepted Applicants

Proportion of Accepted Applicants with Relevant Experience (Data Self-Reported to AMCAS®)		
Community Service/Volunteer		57%
Medically-Related Work		81%
Research		82%

Shaded bar represents accepted scores ranging from the 10th percentile to the 90th percentile. **School Median** ● **National Median** ●

Overall GPA	2.0	2.1	2.2	2.3	2.4	2.5	2.6	2.7	2.8	2.9	3.0	3.1	3.2	3.3	3.4	3.5	3.6	(3.7)	3.8	3.9	4.0
Science GPA	2.0	2.1	2.2	2.3	2.4	2.5	2.6	2.7	2.8	2.9	3.0	3.1	3.2	3.3	3.4	3.5	(3.6)	3.7	3.8	3.9	4.0

MCAT® required: Yes, 99% of 2007 accepted applicants took MCAT®

Verbal Reasoning	3	4	5	6	7	8	9	(10)	11	12	13	14	15
Physical Sciences	3	4	5	6	7	8	9	10	(11)	12	13	14	15
Biological Sciences	3	4	5	6	7	8	9	10	(11)	12	13	14	15
Writing Sample			J	K	L	M	N	O	(P)	(Q)	R	S	T

Acceptance & Matriculation Data for 2007–2008 First Year Class

	Resident	Non-Resident	International	Total
Applied	1210	3470	15	4695
Interviewed	706	134	0	840
Deferred	2	0	0	2
Matriculants				
Early Assurance Program	3	0	0	3
Early Decision Program	25	0	0	25
Baccalaureate/MD	19	0	0	19
MD/PhD	3	0	0	3
Matriculated	163	15	0	**178**

Applications accepted from International Applicants: No

Specialty Choice

2003, 2004, 2005 Graduates, Specialty Choice (As reported by program directors to GME Track™)	
Anesthesiology	7%
Emergency Medicine	8%
Family Practice	4%
Internal Medicine	16%
Obstetrics/Gynecology	4%
Orthopaedic Surgery	6%
Pediatrics	14%
Psychiatry	4%
Radiology	7%
Surgery	6%

Matriculant Demographics: 2007–2008 First Year Class

Men: 95 **Women:** 83

Matriculants' Self-Reported Race/Ethnicity

Mexican American	0	Korean	11
Cuban	8	Vietnamese	2
Puerto Rican	5	Other Asian	4
Other Hispanic	10	Total Asian	78
Total Hispanic	22	Native American	0
Chinese	16	Black	16
Asian Indian	35	Native Hawaiian	1
Pakistani	7	White	78
Filipino	6	Unduplicated Number	
Japanese	1	of Matriculants	178

Science and Math Majors: 72%
Matriculants with:
　　Baccalaureate degree: 98%
　　Graduate degree(s): 12%

Financial Information

Source: 2006–2007 LCME I-B survey and 2007–2008 AAMC TSF questionnaire

	Residents	Non-Residents
Total Cost of Attendance	$47,897	$60,964
Tuition and Fees	$24,121	$37,188
Other (includes living expenses)	$21,955	$21,955
Health Insurance (can be waived)	$1,821	$1,821

Average 2007 Graduate Indebtedness: $127,203
% of Enrolled Students Receiving Aid: 84%

Criminal Background Check

This medical school requires a criminal background check prior to matriculation.

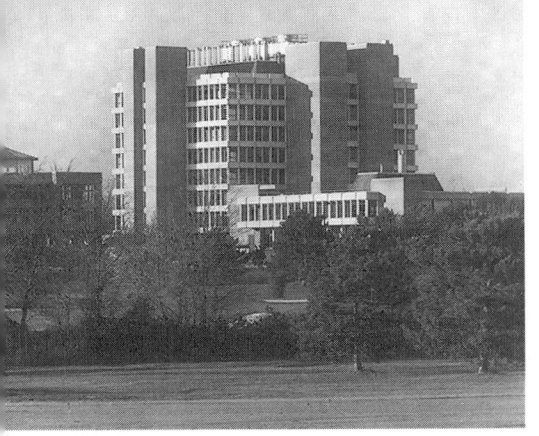

University of Medicine and Dentistry of New Jersey — Robert Wood Johnson Medical School

Piscataway, New Jersey

Associate Dean for Admissions
University of Medicine and Dentistry of New Jersey
Robert Wood Johnson Medical School
675 Hoes Lane
Piscataway, New Jersey 08854-5635
T 732 235 4576 F 732 235 5078

Admissions http://rwjms.umdnj.edu/admissions
Main http://rwjms.umdnj.edu
Financial www.umdnj.edu/studentfinancialaid
Email rwjapadm@umdnj.edu

Public Institution

Dr. Peter S. Amenta, Interim Dean

Dr. Carol A. Terregino, Associate Dean for Admissions

Dr. Cheryl Dickson, Assistant Dean for Multicultural Affairs

Marshall Anthony, Associate Director of Financial Aid

Meryle Kramer, Admissions Officer

Betty Oglesby, Minority Recruiter/Counselor

General Information

Robert Wood Johnson Medical School, formerly Rutgers Medical School, has campuses in Piscataway, New Brunswick and Camden. A full complement of clinical training facilities including Robert Wood Johnson University Hospital, Bristol Myers Squibb Children's Hospital, Cooper University Hospital and numerous ambulatory sites provide outstanding educational experiences. The medical school encompasses 22 basic science and clinical departments and more than 2,500 full-time and volunteer faculty members.

Mission Statement

The medical school is dedicated to the pursuit of excellence in education, research, health care delivery and the promotion of community health. Excellence is achieved through the work of a scholarly and creative faculty and a high-achieving and diverse student body.

Curricular Highlights

Community Service Requirement: Optional. Distinction in Service to the Community
Research/Thesis Requirement: Optional. Distinction in Research

The preclerkship pass/fail curriculum provides for early introduction to patient care via the Patient Centered Medicine course, integration of clinical skills into the basic sciences, and opportunity for self-directed learning. There is ample elective time in the third year. In the fourth year students rotate in emergency medicine and critical care, a sub-internship, outpatient subspecialties and 20 weeks of electives. A longitudinal primary care experience and an independent project round out the clinical curriculum. The Clinical Skills Center runs a formative and summative clinical skills assessment. Each clerkship has an OSCE, and grading is on a 5-point scale. There are a number of dual degree options. The MD/PhD is a tri-institutional program with Princeton University and Rutgers University.

USMLE

Step 1: Required. Students must record a passing score for promotion.
Step 2: Clinical Skills (CS): Required. Students must record a passing total score to graduate.
Step 2: Clinical Knowledge (CK): Required. Students must record a passing total score to graduate.

Selection Factors

Preference is given to New Jersey residents. Out-of-state applicants are encouraged to apply. Admission is determined on the basis of academics, MCAT®, preprofessional evaluations, character, motivation, and interview. We believe that a diverse student body contributes to the educational program of all students. Selection and recruitment is based on a holistic review of each applicant's experiences, personal qualities and potential to enhance the learning environment. Applications from members of groups underrepresented in medicine are encouraged. Interviews are by invitation. Matriculants must submit to a criminal background check.

Financial Aid

Financial aid is awarded on the basis of evaluated need. All awards consist of a package of loans and grants when funds are available. New funds have been allocated for scholarships. Counseling services are available.

Information about Diversity Programs

Robert Wood Johnson Medical School is committed to the education of physicians from groups underrepresented in medicine. Applications from in-state and out-of-state candidates are welcome. Numerous support services are available for disadvantaged students, including a pre-matriculation summer program.

Campus Information

Setting

The facilities of the Piscataway campus include the Kessler Teaching Labs/Clinical Skills Center and the Research Tower, University Behavioral Health Care Center, the Center for Advanced Biotechnology and Medicine and the Environmental and Occupational health Sciences Institute, UMDNJ School of Public Health and the Robert Wood Johnson Medical School Research Building, the current site for the Stem Cell Institute. The New Brunswick campus includes the Cancer Hospital, BMS Children's Hospital, Children's Specialized Hospital, the Child Health Institute, the Cancer Institute of New Jersey. A groundbreaking ceremony for the Stem Cell Institute and Cardio-vascular Institute took place in the Fall of 2007. The Camden Regional Campus is close to the historic river front, and across the river from Philadelphia. The medical school and Cooper University Hospital facilities are adjacent to each other and a new Education/Research Building is planned.

Enrollment

For 2007, total enrollment was: 659

Special Features

The medical school hosts 85 centers and institutes including the Cancer Institute of New Jersey, the Cardiovascular Institute, the Child Health Institute of New Jersey, the Center for Advanced Biotechnology and Medicine, and the Environmental and Occupational Health Sciences Institute. Students provide continuity care to the community in Urban Health Initiatives, the Promise Clinic and the Homeless and Indigent Population Health Outreach Project. They tailor their medical school experiences as Student Scholars, researchers, leaders of organizations and non-credit electives and as international travelers. Scholarly and social lives are rich.

Housing

On-campus housing is currently not available. Students are assisted in finding affordable housing.

Satellite Campuses/Facilities

Camden is a regional campus. One third of the class completes clinical training at this a single-hospital site. Students in the New Brunswick program rotate among three hospital sites.

Application Process and Requirements 2009–2010

Primary Application Service: AMCAS
Earliest filing date: June 1, 2008
Latest filing date: December 1, 2008

Secondary Application Required?: n/a
Sent to: n/a
URL: n/a
Fee: Yes, $75
Fee waiver available: Yes
Earliest filing date: n/a
Latest filing date: n/a

Latest MCAT® considered: September 2008
Oldest MCAT® considered: 2006

Early Decision Program
School does have EDP
Applicants notified: October 1, 2008
EDP available for: Both Residents and Non-Residents

Regular Acceptance Notice
Earliest date: October 15, 2008
Latest date: Until class is full

Applicant's Response to Acceptance Offer – Maximum Time: Two weeks

Requests for Deferred Entrance Considered: Yes

Deposit to Hold Place in Class: Yes
Deposit (Resident): $50
Deposit (Non-Resident): $50
Deposit due: With response to acceptance offer
Applied to tuition: Yes
Deposit refundable: Yes
Refundable by: May 15, 2009

Estimated number of new entrants: 156
EDP: 5, special program: 10

Start Month/Year: August 2009

Interview Format: One (faculty) or two (faculty and student) interviews. Applicants can interview on any of the campuses.

Other Programs

PREPARATORY PROGRAMS
Postbaccalaureate Program: No
Summer Program: Yes, Cheryl Dickson, M.D.
(732) 235-2144, dicksoca@umdnj.edu

COMBINED DEGREE PROGRAMS
Baccalaureate/MD: Yes,
http://lifesci.rutgers.edu/~hpo/
MD/MPH: Yes, http://sph.umdnj.edu
Tina Greco, (732) 235-4017, grecotm@umdnj.edu
MD/MBA: Yes, David Seiden Ph.D.
(732) 235-4577, seiden@umdnj.edu
MD/JD: Yes, Carol A. Terregino, M.D.
(732) 235-4577, terregca@umdnj.edu
MD/PhD: Yes, http://rwjms.umdnj.edu/research/scientist_training/
Terri Kinzy Ph.D., (732) 235-5450
kinzytg@umdnj.edu

Premedical Coursework

Course	Req.	Rec.	Lab.	Sems.
Inorganic Chemistry	•		•	2
Behavioral Sciences		•		
Biochemistry		•		
Biology				
Biology/Zoology	•		•	2
Calculus				
College English	•			2
College Mathematics	•			1
Computer Science				

Course	Req.	Rec.	Lab.	Sems.
Genetics				
Humanities		•		
Organic Chemistry	•		•	2
Physics	•		•	2
Psychology		•		
Social Sciences		•		
Molecular Biology		•		
Statistics		•		
Cell Biology		•		

Selection Factors: 2007 Accepted Applicants

Proportion of Accepted Applicants with Relevant Experience (Data Self-Reported to AMCAS®)		
Community Service/Volunteer		60%
Medically-Related Work		86%
Research		85%

Shaded bar represents accepted scores ranging from the 10th percentile to the 90th percentile   **School Median ●   National Median ●**

Overall GPA	2.0	2.1	2.2	2.3	2.4	2.5	2.6	2.7	2.8	2.9	3.0	3.1	3.2	3.3	3.4	3.5	3.6	③.7	3.8	3.9	4.0
Science GPA	2.0	2.1	2.2	2.3	2.4	2.5	2.6	2.7	2.8	2.9	3.0	3.1	3.2	3.3	3.4	3.5	3.6	③.7	3.8	3.9	4.0

MCAT® required: Yes, 96% of 2007 accepted applicants took MCAT®

Verbal Reasoning	3	4	5	6	7	8	9	⑩	11	12	13	14	15
Physical Sciences	3	4	5	6	7	8	9	10	⑪	12	13	14	15
Biological Sciences	3	4	5	6	7	8	9	10	⑪	12	13	14	15
Writing Sample			J	K	L	M	N	O	⑫	⑫	R	S	T

Acceptance & Matriculation Data for 2007–2008 First Year Class

	Resident	Non-Resident	International	Total
Applied	1208	2300	43	3551
Interviewed	418	97	0	515
Deferred	3	0	0	3
Matriculants				
Early Assurance Program	0	0	0	0
Early Decision Program	5	0	0	5
Baccalaureate/MD	10	0	0	10
MD/PhD	3	3	0	6
Matriculated	142	24	0	**166**

Applications accepted from International Applicants: No

Matriculant Demographics: 2007–2008 First Year Class

Men: 68   **Women:** 98

Matriculants' Self-Reported Race/Ethnicity

Mexican American	0	Korean	9
Cuban	1	Vietnamese	0
Puerto Rican	3	Other Asian	7
Other Hispanic	9	Total Asian	65
Total Hispanic	11	Native American	0
Chinese	15	Black	14
Asian Indian	29	Native Hawaiian	0
Pakistani	1	White	80
Filipino	4	Unduplicated Number	
Japanese	2	of Matriculants	166

Science and Math Majors: 63%
Matriculants with:
Baccalaureate degree: 99%
Graduate degree(s): 8%

Specialty Choice

2003, 2004, 2005 Graduates, Specialty Choice (As reported by program directors to GME Track™)	
Anesthesiology	6%
Emergency Medicine	5%
Family Practice	6%
Internal Medicine	20%
Obstetrics/Gynecology	4%
Orthopaedic Surgery	4%
Pediatrics	10%
Psychiatry	7%
Radiology	9%
Surgery	8%

Financial Information

Source: 2006–2007 LCME I-B survey and 2007–2008 AAMC TSF questionnaire

	Residents	Non-Residents
Total Cost of Attendance	$50,579	$63,646
Tuition and Fees	$24,296	$37,363
Other (includes living expenses)	$24,462	$24,462
Health Insurance (can be waived)	$1,821	$1,821

Average 2007 Graduate Indebtedness: $121,096
% of Enrolled Students Receiving Aid: 86%

Criminal Background Check

This medical school requires a criminal background check prior to matriculation.

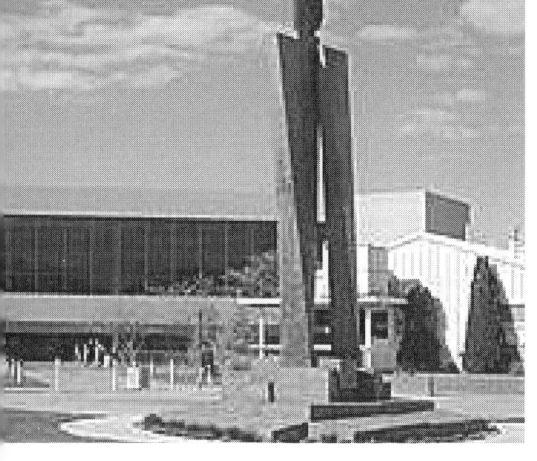

University of New Mexico School of Medicine
Albuquerque, New Mexico

University of New Mexico Health Sciences Center
School of Medicine, Office of Admissions,
MSC09 5085, Health Sciences Library and
Informatics Center, Room 125
Albuquerque, New Mexico 87131-0001
T 505 272 4766   **F** 505 925 6031

Admissions http://hsc.unm.edu/som/admissions
Main http://hsc.unm.edu/som
Financial http://hsc.unm.edu/som/admissions/aid.shtml
Email somadmissions@salud.unm.edu

Public Institution

Dr. Paul B. Roth, Dean

*Dr. David G. Bear, Assistant Dean
for Admissions*

*Dr. Valerie Romero-Leggott, Associate Dean
for Office of Diversity*

Janell Valdez, Supervisor, Financial Aid

Marlene Ballejos, Admissions Director

General Information
The establishment of a school of the basic medical sciences was authorized by the regents and the faculty of the University of New Mexico in 1961. The first class of 24 students was enrolled in September 1964. The School of Medicine is a professional and graduate school where students may earn the MD degree, a combined MD/PhD degree, a PhD degree, or BS or MS degrees in several allied health science fields. Medical education at the resident and postgraduate levels is offered through the university's teaching hospitals.

Mission Statement
The mission of the University of New Mexico is to educate students, scientists, physicians and other health professionals through the transmission of biomedical knowledge acquired from research and patient care. We aspire to improve the health of all New Mexicans by being a model of excellence in educating students, scientists, physicians and other health professionals, in creating new knowledge and in providing patient care.

Curricular Highlights
Community Service Requirement: Required. A community research project is required.
Research/Thesis Requirement: Required. A research project and report is required.

The University of New Mexico School of Medicine adopted a new hybrid curriculum in 1993 incorporating aspects of its prior educational innovations. The goals of the new curriculum are to graduate physicians who are enthusiastic and responsible for their continued

learning; have the ability to define problems, formulate questions, and carry out scholarly inquiry; are skilled in self and peer assessment; and have a broad perspective on the importance of human biology, behavior, environment, culture, and social setting in the health of individuals and of populations. Educational innovations include the integration of the basic and clinical sciences throughout undergraduate medical education, early clinical skills-training and community-based learning, and the incorporation of a population and behavioral perspective into the clinical years. Student assessment will be competency-based and will value mastery of knowledge, critical appraisal, interpersonal and clinical skills, and peer and self-assessment.

USMLE
Step 1: Required. Students must record a passing score for promotion.
Step 2: Clinical Skills (CS): Required. Students must record a passing total score to graduate.
Step 2: Clinical Knowledge (CK): Required. Students must only record a score.

Selection Factors
Selected applicants will be sent a supplemental application upon receipt of their AMCAS application. In general, only those applicants with ties to the state of New Mexico or residents of the WICHE states (Montana or Wyoming) will receive consideration for admission. Those who pass initial screening will be sent a supplemental application and interviewed. Selection is based upon scholastic achievement, performance on the MCAT®, personal interviews with members of the Admissions Committee, and recommendations.

Financial Aid
The school makes accessible federal, state and institutional aid in the form of scholarships, grants, and loans. Both need-based and merit-based funding are available to students. The amount of an award varies according to the student's need and the level of funding available. The Office of Financial Aid assists all students in locating necessary funds to support their medical education.

Information about Diversity Programs
The mission of the Office of Diversity is to promote racial, ethnic, socio-economic, and geographic diversity in the UNM Health Sciences Center and to develop a variety of opportunities addressing key issues in diversity. Strategies to achieve this mission include creating college awareness and identifying, recruiting, and supporting students, residents, and faculty from these diverse backgrounds.

Campus Information
Setting
Albuquerque is home to a blend of culture and cuisine, styles and stories, peoples, pursuits, and panoramas.

Enrollment
For 2007, total enrollment was: 315

Special Features
The School of Medicine facilities include a Basic Medical Sciences Building, a Biomedical Research Facility, the Health Sciences Library and Informatics Center, the Mental Health Center, the UNM Children's Hospital, the Children's Psychiatric Center, the Family Practice Center, the Mind Imaging Center, Clinical and Translational Science Center, and the Cancer Research and Treatment Center. Other components include: Addiction and Substance Abuse Programs, Brain Imaging Center, Center for Disease Medicine, Center for Environmental Health Sciences, Center for Telehealth, Center on Aging, Children's Hospital Heart Center, Clinical Trials Center, General Clinical Research Center, Geriatric Education Center, HSC Institute for Ethics, New Mexico AIDS Education and Training Center, New Mexico Immunization Coalition, New Mexico Poison Control Center, Sleep Disorders Center, School of Medicine Center for Community partnerships and Speech/Language/Swallow Center.

Housing
On-campus housing is not available.

Satellite Campuses/Facilities
Student clinical rotations are divided among University Hospital and several other locations in the Albuquerque area.

Application Process and Requirements 2009–2010

Primary Application Service: AMCAS
Earliest filing date: June 1, 2008
Latest filing date: November 15, 2008

Secondary Application Required?: Yes
Sent to: Screened applicants
URL: http://hsc.unm.edu/som/admissions
Fee: Yes, $50
Fee waiver available: Yes
Earliest filing date: August 1, 2008
Latest filing date: February 1, 2009

Latest MCAT® considered: September 2008
Oldest MCAT® considered: 2004

Early Decision Program
School does have EDP
Applicants notified: October 1, 2008
EDP available for: Both Residents and Non-Residents

Regular Acceptance Notice
Earliest date: March 15, 2009
Latest date: Until class is full

Applicant's Response to Acceptance Offer – Maximum Time: Two weeks

Requests for Deferred Entrance Considered: Yes

Deposit to Hold Place in Class: Yes
Deposit (Resident): $200
Deposit (Non-Resident): $200
Deposit due: May 15, 2009
Applied to tuition: Yes
Deposit refundable: Yes
Refundable by: May 15, 2009

Estimated number of new entrants: 75
EDP: n/a, special program: 7

Start Month/Year: August 2009

Interview Format: Two one-on-one interviews by committee members.

Other Programs

PREPARATORY PROGRAMS
Postbaccalaureate Program: Yes,
http://hsc.unm.edu/som/asc/
Steven Mitchell, (505) 925-4441,
smitchell@salud.unm.edu
Summer Program: No

COMBINED DEGREE PROGRAMS
Baccalaureate/MD: Yes,
http://hsc.unm.edu/som/combinedbamd
Kathy Kersting, (505) 925-4500
combinedbamd@salud.unm.edu
MD/MPH: No
MD/MBA: No
MD/JD: No
MD/PhD: Yes, http://hsc.unm.edu/som/
programs/mdphd, Fernando Valenzuela,
(505) 272-1887, bsgp@salud.unm.edu

Premedical Coursework

Course	Req.	Rec.	Lab.	Hrs.
Inorganic Chemistry	•	•		8
Behavioral Sciences				
Biochemistry	•			3
Biology				
Biology/Zoology	•	•		8
Calculus				
College English				
College Mathematics				
Computer Science				

Course	Req.	Rec.	Lab.	Hrs.
Genetics				
Humanities				
Organic Chemistry	•		•	8
Physics	•			6
Psychology				
Anatomy & Physiology		•	•	
Microbiology		•		
Immunology		•		

Selection Factors: 2007 Accepted Applicants

Proportion of Accepted Applicants with Relevant Experience (Data Self-Reported to AMCAS®)		
Community Service/Volunteer		69%
Medically-Related Work		86%
Research		79%

Shaded bar represents accepted scores ranging from the 10th percentile to the 90th percentile. School Median ● National Median ●

Overall GPA	2.0	2.1	2.2	2.3	2.4	2.5	2.6	2.7	2.8	2.9	3.0	3.1	3.2	3.3	3.4	3.5	3.6	(3.7)	3.8	3.9	4.0
Science GPA	2.0	2.1	2.2	2.3	2.4	2.5	2.6	2.7	2.8	2.9	3.0	3.1	3.2	3.3	3.4	3.5	(3.6)	3.7	3.8	3.9	4.0

MCAT® required: Yes, 100% of 2007 accepted applicants took MCAT®

Verbal Reasoning	3	4	5	6	7	8	(9)	(10)	11	12	13	14	15
Physical Sciences	3	4	5	6	7	8	(9)	10	(11)	12	13	14	15
Biological Sciences	3	4	5	6	7	8	9	(10)	(11)	12	13	14	15
Writing Sample			J	K	L	M	N	O	(P)	(Q)	R	S	T

Acceptance & Matriculation Data for 2007–2008 First Year Class

	Resident	Non-Resident	International	Total
Applied	210	818	13	1041
Interviewed	190	21	0	211
Deferred	4	0	0	4
Matriculants				
Early Assurance Program	n/a	n/a	n/a	n/a
Early Decision Program	9	0	0	9
Baccalaureate/MD	n/a	n/a	n/a	n/a
MD/PhD	0	0	0	0
Matriculated	72	3	0	**75**

Applications accepted from International Applicants: No

Matriculant Demographics: 2007–2008 First Year Class

Men: 35   **Women:** 40

Matriculants' Self-Reported Race/Ethnicity

Mexican American	12	**Korean**	1
Cuban	0	**Vietnamese**	0
Puerto Rican	0	**Other Asian**	2
Other Hispanic	8	**Total Asian**	9
Total Hispanic	20	**Native American**	4
Chinese	3	**Black**	1
Asian Indian	3	**Native Hawaiian**	1
Pakistani	0	**White**	55
Filipino	0	**Unduplicated Number**	
Japanese	1	**of Matriculants**	75

Science and Math Majors: 80%
Matriculants with:
      Baccalaureate degree: 100%
      Graduate degree(s): 11%

Specialty Choice

2003, 2004, 2005 Graduates, Specialty Choice (As reported by program directors to GME Track™)	
Anesthesiology	6%
Emergency Medicine	7%
Family Practice	13%
Internal Medicine	18%
Obstetrics/Gynecology	8%
Orthopaedic Surgery	4%
Pediatrics	12%
Psychiatry	4%
Radiology	4%
Surgery	7%

Financial Information

Source: 2006–2007 LCME I-B survey and 2007–2008 AAMC TSF questionnaire

	Residents	Non-Residents
Total Cost of Attendance	$36,416	$62,522
Tuition and Fees	$16,795	$42,901
Other (includes living expenses)	$19,512	$19,512
Health Insurance (cannot be waived)	$109	$109

Average 2007 Graduate Indebtedness: $94,639
% of Enrolled Students Receiving Aid: 90%

Criminal Background Check

This medical school does not require a criminal background check prior to matriculation.

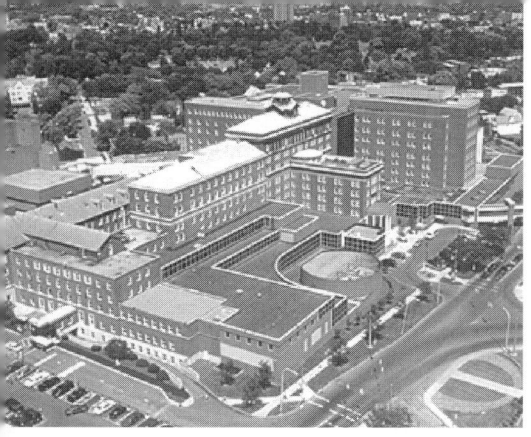

Albany Medical College
Albany, New York

Office of Admissions, Mail Code 3
Albany Medical College
47 New Scotland Avenue
Albany, New York 12208
T 518 262 5521 **F** 518 262 5887

Admissions www.amc.edu/academic/Undergraduate_Admissions/
Main www.amc.edu/Academic/
Financial www.amc.edu/academic/Undergraduate/FinancialAid.html
Email admissions@mail.amc.edu

Private Institution

Dr. Vincent Verdile, Dean

Joanne H. Nanos, Director, Admissions and Student Records

Ann Loughman, Director of Financial Aid

Dr. Henry Pohl, Vice Dean for Academic Administration

General Information

Founded in 1839, Albany Medical College is one of the oldest medical schools in the country and one of the largest teaching hospitals in New York State. The college is coeducational, nondenominational, and privately supported. The college and the 650-bed Albany Medical Center Hospital comprise Albany Medical Center. Patient care, from primary to tertiary, is provided for over 2.5 million residents of eastern New York and western New England.

Mission Statement

The mission of the Albany Medical College is to: (1) educate medical students, all physicians, biomedical scientists, and other health professionals to meet future primary and specialty health care needs, (2) foster biomedical research that leads to scientific advances and improvement of public health, and (3) provide a broad range of patient services.

Curricular Highlights

Community Service Requirement: Optional. MD with Distinction Biomedical Ethics
Research/Thesis Requirement: Optional. MD with Distinction in Research

Basic and clinical sciences are integrated into themes stressing normal function in Year 1 and pathological processes in Year 2. There are also five longitudinal themes integrated throughout the curriculum: clinical skills, ethical and health systems issues, evidence-based medicine, nutrition, and informatics. In every theme, learning focuses on clinical presentations. Beginning in Year 1, students learn to interview and examine both real and standardized patients. Clinical skills competence is highlighted throughout the four years. Basic science knowledge is reinforced during years 3 and 4. Primary care is emphasized

throughout the four years. Year 3 clerkships focus on care in ambulatory settings. Year 4 required rotations concentrate on care in hospital-based settings, preparing students for residency and practice. The remainder of fourth year includes electives chosen by the students and a required course in learning how to teach.

USMLE

Step 1: Required. Students must record a passing score for graduation, but not promotion.
Step 2: Clinical Skills (CS): Required. Students must record a passing total score to graduate.
Step 2: Clinical Knowledge (CK): Required. Students must record a passing total score to graduate.

Selection Factors

In selecting students, emphasis is placed upon integrity, character, academic achievement, motivation, emotional stability, and social and intellectual suitability. The college is committed to the belief that educational opportunities should be available to all eligible persons without regard to race, creed, age, gender, religion, marital status, handicap, national origin, or sexual orientation. Admission is not restricted to state residents. The committee evaluates applications based on a number of factors in addition to MCAT® scores and GPAs. Invitations for interview are made at the discretion of the committee. Preapplication inquiries or questions concerning the status of applications are always welcome.

Financial Aid

The mission of the Financial Aid Office is to be the primary source of information and education about financing a degree. Outreach events and media are provided to guide the development of students' immediate and long-range spending plans that secure their financial future. The office awards and certifies need-based aid for 88% of enrolled students and provides lifetime service to graduated students.

Information about Diversity Programs

The Office of Minority Affairs is actively involved in the recruitment and retention of qualified applicants from groups underrepresented in medicine. With a firm commitment to educating and

graduating a diverse group of students, guidance is offered to students from the application stage forward. The Assistant Dean for Student and Minority Affairs is available for counseling and assistance at any time. This office also coordinates academic, social, and cultural support services.

Campus Information

Setting

Albany is the capital of New York and a part of the tri-city area which includes Schenectady and Troy. Rich in history, Albany has diverse cultural and recreational opportunities. Fifteen area colleges and universities add to the region's eclectic appeal.

Enrollment

For 2007, total enrollment was: 565

Special Features

Albany Medical Center Hospital provides sophisticated health care to more than 2 million people in 24 counties. A recently completed renovation invested approximately $15 million and added 45,000 square feet of new construction. The new addition permitted several outpatient services and all physician offices to move to one location and opened space within the hospital to add 25 additional inpatient beds.

Housing

On-campus housing is not available. The college maintains a list of affordable apartments within a 5-mile radius. Rents average $500-$850 per month.

Satellite Campuses/Facilities

The medical college is affiliated with other hospitals in New York State. Clinical departments utilize a network of community physicians to serve the ambulatory care educational needs of students. The college, which is combined with Albany Medical Center Hospital on its campus, is also affiliated with the Veterans Administration Hospital, community hospitals, and private and community clinics in surrounding counties.

Application Process and Requirements 2009–2010

Primary Application Service: AMCAS
Earliest filing date: June 1, 2008
Latest filing date: November 15, 2008

Secondary Application Required?: Yes
Sent to: All applicants
Contact: Admissions Staff
(518) 262-5521, admissions@mail.amc.edu
Fee: Yes, $105
Fee waiver available: Yes
Earliest filing date: June 2008
Latest filing date: January 14, 2009

Latest MCAT® considered: September 2008
Oldest MCAT® considered: 2005

Early Decision Program
School does not have EDP
Applicants notified: n/a
EDP available for: n/a

Regular Acceptance Notice
Earliest date: December 15, 2008
Latest date: Until class is full

Applicant's Response to Acceptance Offer – Maximum Time: Two weeks

Requests for Deferred Entrance Considered: Yes

Deposit to Hold Place in Class: Yes
Deposit (Resident): $100
Deposit (Non-Resident): $100
Deposit due: With response to acceptance offer
Applied to tuition: Yes
Deposit refundable: Yes
Refundable by: May 15, 2009

Estimated number of new entrants: 138
EDP: n/a, special program: n/a

Start Month/Year: August 2009

Interview Format: Individual interviews by Admissions Committee. Regional interviews are not available.

Other Programs

PREPARATORY PROGRAMS
Postbaccalaureate Program: No
Summer Program: No

COMBINED DEGREE PROGRAMS
Baccalaureate/MD: Yes,
Johanna Comanzo, (518) 262-5529
combineddegreeprograms@mail.amc.edu
MD/MPH: No
MD/MBA: No
MD/JD: No
MD/PhD: No
Additional Program: Yes, MD with Distinction in Health Systems Analysis, MD with Distinction in Service

Premedical Coursework

Course	Req.	Rec.	Lab.	Hrs.	Course	Req.	Rec.	Lab.	Hrs.
Inorganic Chemistry	•		•	6	Computer Science				
Behavioral Sciences					Genetics				
Biochemistry					Humanities				
Biology	•		•	6	Organic Chemistry	•		•	6
Biology/Zoology	•		•	6	Physics	•		•	6
Calculus					Psychology				
College English					Social Sciences				
College Mathematics					Other				

Selection Factors: 2007 Accepted Applicants

Proportion of Accepted Applicants with Relevant Experience (Data Self-Reported to AMCAS®)		
Community Service/Volunteer	62%
Medically-Related Work	83%
Research	72%

Shaded bar represents accepted scores ranging from the 10th percentile to the 90th percentile. **School Median** ● **National Median** ●

	2.0	2.1	2.2	2.3	2.4	2.5	2.6	2.7	2.8	2.9	3.0	3.1	3.2	3.3	3.4	3.5	3.6	3.7	3.8	3.9	4.0
Overall GPA	2.0	2.1	2.2	2.3	2.4	2.5	2.6	2.7	2.8	2.9	3.0	3.1	3.2	3.3	3.4	3.5	(3.6)	3.7	3.8	3.9	4.0
Science GPA	2.0	2.1	2.2	2.3	2.4	2.5	2.6	2.7	2.8	2.9	3.0	3.1	3.2	3.3	3.4	(3.5)	3.6	3.7	3.8	3.9	4.0

MCAT® required: Yes, 86% of 2007 accepted applicants took MCAT®

Verbal Reasoning	3	4	5	6	7	8	9	(10)	11	12	13	14	15
Physical Sciences	3	4	5	6	7	8	9	(10)	(11)	12	13	14	15
Biological Sciences	3	4	5	6	7	8	9	10	(11)	12	13	14	15
Writing Sample			J	K	L	M	N	O	(P)	(Q)	R	S	T

Acceptance & Matriculation Data for 2007–2008 First Year Class

	Resident	Non-Resident	International	Total
Applied	1581	6710	606	8897
Interviewed	166	379	27	572
Deferred	1	0	0	1
Matriculants				
Early Assurance Program	1	0	0	1
Early Decision Program	0	0	0	0
Baccalaureate/MD	28	19	0	47
MD/PhD	n/a	n/a	n/a	n/a
Matriculated	55	86	3	**144**

Applications accepted from International Applicants: Yes

Specialty Choice

2003, 2004, 2005 Graduates, Specialty Choice (As reported by program directors to GME Track™)	
Anesthesiology	4%
Emergency Medicine	10%
Family Practice	9%
Internal Medicine	13%
Obstetrics/Gynecology	4%
Orthopaedic Surgery	4%
Pediatrics	14%
Psychiatry	6%
Radiology	4%
Surgery	8%

Matriculant Demographics: 2007–2008 First Year Class

Men: 71   **Women:** 73

Matriculants' Self-Reported Race/Ethnicity

Mexican American	2	Korean	4
Cuban	0	Vietnamese	1
Puerto Rican	1	Other Asian	4
Other Hispanic	2	Total Asian	42
Total Hispanic	4	Native American	2
Chinese	8	Black	5
Asian Indian	22	Native Hawaiian	0
Pakistani	2	White	82
Filipino	1	Unduplicated Number	
Japanese	1	of Matriculants	144

Science and Math Majors: 79%
Matriculants with:
Baccalaureate degree: 97%
Graduate degree(s): 22%

Financial Information

Source: 2006–2007 LCME I-B survey and 2007–2008 AAMC TSF questionnaire

	Residents	Non-Residents
Total Cost of Attendance	$61,145	$61,845
Tuition and Fees	$43,008	$43,008
Other (includes living expenses)	$15,350	$16,050
Health Insurance (can be waived)	$2,787	$2,787

Average 2007 Graduate Indebtedness: $168,804
% of Enrolled Students Receiving Aid: 88%

Criminal Background Check

This medical school requires a criminal background check prior to matriculation.

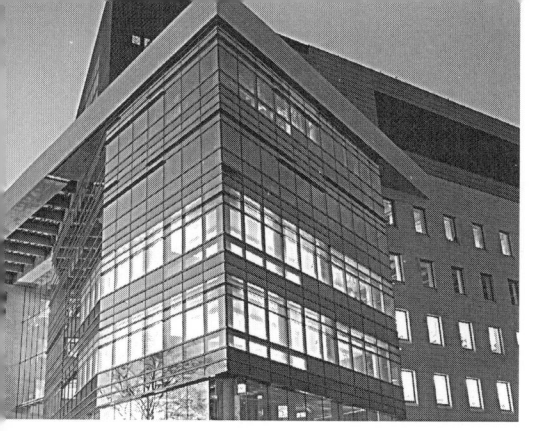

Albert Einstein College of Medicine of Yeshiva University
Bronx, New York

Office of Admissions, Albert Einstein College of
Medicine of Yeshiva U Jack and Pearl Resnick Campus
1300 Morris Park Avenue
Bronx, New York 10461
T 718 430 2106   **F** 718 430 8840

Admissions www.aecom.yu.edu/home/admissions
Main www.aecom.yu.edu
Financial www.aecom.yu.edu/home/admissions/
financial_aid.htm
Email admissions@aecom.yu.edu

Private Institution

Dr. Allen M. Spiegel, Dean

*Noreen Kerrigan, Assistant Dean for
Student Admissions*

*Dr. Milton A. Gumbs, Associate Dean
for Cultural Diversity*

Carl Nykaza, Financial Aid Officer

*Dr. Albert Kuperman, Associate Dean for
Educational Affairs*

*Dr. Paul Marantz, Associate Dean for Clinical
Research Education*

General Information
Clinical education takes place in acute care hospitals, long-term care and skilled nursing facilities, hospices, and neighborhood health centers that serve a diverse population of patients in and around the NY metropolitan area. There are many facilities devoted to biomedical research and teaching, and a new building for genetic and translational research.

Mission Statement
To conduct educational programs of the highest quality in the biomedical and clinical sciences. To conduct fundamental biomedical and clinical research related to health and disease and health policy. To maintain excellent patient care in association with the education and training of medical students and postgraduate physicians. To conduct collaborative educational, research, and training programs with affiliated institutions. To provide, sustain, and improve health care in our community. To encourage widespread participation in the evolution of public policy in biomedical science, education, and health care.

Curricular Highlights
Community Service Requirement: Optional.
Research/Thesis Requirement: Required.

Years 1 and 2 are interdisciplinary courses with self-directed case-based learning in small groups, and the "Introduction to Clinical Medicine" in which students see patients three weeks after matriculation. Year 3 consists of clerkship rotations. Year 4 provides experience in ambulatory care, Neurology and a hospital-based subinternship.

4th year electives include overseas exchange programs, global health fellowships, and research. Many students do a tuition-free/fellowship supported fifth year, to conduct year-long projects, or to study for the MPH Degree. Performance is Pass/Fail in Years 1 and 2, supplemented by Honors and detailed narrative reports in Years 3 and 4.

USMLE
Step 1: Required. Students must record a passing score for promotion.
Step 2: Clinical Skills (CS): Required. Students must record a passing total score to graduate.
Step 2: Clinical Knowledge (CK): Required. Students must record a passing total score to graduate.

Selection Factors
In addition to the usual selection factors, attention is paid to community service, potential for professional achievement, motivation, and evidence of other personal qualities deemed essential for the study and practice of medicine. Einstein seeks traditional and non-traditional applicants who add diversity to the class and bring various perspectives to the study and practice of medicine. (Non-discrimination statement at: *www.aecom.yu.edu/admissions/page.aspx?id=568*).

Financial Aid
Every attempt is made to assist students in meeting their financial obligations to the college and their essential personal needs. About 50% of students receive institutional loans and/or scholarships; about 80% qualify for outside loans and/or grants.

Information about Diversity Programs
The College of Medicine welcomes applications from students who are from groups underrepresented in medicine and/or who are economically disadvantaged. The College's Office of Diversity Enhancement provides opportunities for students to participate in special programs for high school and college students. Individual counseling is provided to students in need of long-term assistance to assure retention. The Office offers a summer research program to college students. Information on a summer research program can be obtained at 718-430-3091.

Campus Information

Setting
Located in a residential area of the northeast Bronx, surrounded by private homes and apartment buildings and near the Westchester County border, the area combines small-town living with easy access to Manhattan. Close by are the Bronx Zoo, Botanical Gardens, Yankee Stadium, City Island (a fishing and sailing community), Orchard Beach, and the sprawling Pelham Bay Park, where there is hiking, swimming, horseback riding, golfing, and bicycling.

Enrollment
For 2007, total enrollment was: 759

Special Features
There are fellowships for projects in basic and clinical research, global health, community and population health, and ethics and humanism. There is an Alternative Pathway to the M.D.-Ph.D. after Year 2, overseas exchange programs, a Clinical Research MD/MS Program, a stipend for the MPH Degree (anywhere in the world), a Medical Spanish Program, and a program for Personal Wellness.

Housing
Housing at Einstein is outstanding. Apartments are large. Rents are low. Security is excellent. There are studios, one-and two-bedroom apartments with a/c, fully equipped eat-in-kitchens, and ample closet space. Parking, laundry facilities, children's playground, and a large athletic facility are on the premises. Housing is available to all Einstein students and to their spouses or committed partners.

Satellite Campuses/Facilities
Facilities include:Beth Israel Medical Center, Bronx-Lebanon Hospital, Jacobi Medical Center, North Shore/Long Island Jewish Medical Center, Montefiore and the Jack D. Weiler Hospitals, Bronx Children's Psychiatric Center, Bronx Psychiatric Center, Four Winds Hospital, Beth Abraham Hospital, Hebrew Home for the Aged, Morningside House, the Parker Jewish Geriatric Institute, the Children's Evaluation and Rehabilitation Center, the Division of Substance Abuse, and the Sound View Throgs Neck Community Mental Health Center.

Application Process and Requirements 2009–2010

Primary Application Service: AMCAS
Earliest filing date: June 1, 2008
Latest filing date: November 1, 2008

Secondary Application Required?: Yes
Sent to: All applicants
URL: www.aecom.yu.edu/admissions/page.aspx?
ID= 626
Fee: Yes, $110
Fee waiver available: Yes
Earliest filing date: July 1, 2008
Latest filing date: March 15, 2009

Latest MCAT® considered: September 2008
Oldest MCAT® considered: 2005

Early Decision Program
School does have EDP
Applicants notified: October 1, 2008
EDP available for: Both Residents
and Non-Residents

Regular Acceptance Notice
Earliest date: January 15, 2009
Latest date: Until class is full

**Applicant's Response to Acceptance
Offer – Maximum Time:** Two weeks
until May 1, 2009; one week thereafter

**Requests for Deferred
Entrance Considered:** Yes

Deposit to Hold Place in Class: Yes
Deposit (Resident): $100
Deposit (Non-Resident): $100
Deposit due: With response to acceptance offer
Applied to tuition: Yes
Deposit refundable: Yes
Refundable by: June 1, 2009

Estimated number of new entrants: 183
EDP: 2, special program: 5

Start Month/Year: August 2009

Interview Format: One interview with a faculty
member only. Regional interviews are not available.

Other Programs

PREPARATORY PROGRAMS
Postbaccalaureate Program: No
Summer Program: Yes
**Summer Undergraduate Research
Program (SURP)**
**Minority Student Summer Research
Opportunity Program**
**Hispanic Center of Excellence Summer
Undergraduate Mentorship Program**
Mentoring in Medicine Program
COMBINED DEGREE PROGRAMS
Baccalaureate/MD: No
MD/MPH: Yes, Dr. Paul Marantz,
(718) 430-4187, marantz@aecom.yu.edu
MD/MBA: No
MD/JD: No
MD/PhD: Yes, mstp.aecom.yu.edu/
Clinical Research Program: Yes, www.aecom.
yu.edu/ooe/special_programs/clinical_research_
md_ms_program.htm

Premedical Coursework

Course	Req.	Rec.	Lab.	Hrs.	Course	Req.	Rec.	Lab.	Hrs.
Inorganic Chemistry	•		•	8	Computer Science		•		
Behavioral Sciences					Genetics				
Biochemistry		•	•	4	Humanities		•		
Biology	•		•	8	Organic Chemistry	•		•	8
Biology/Zoology					Physics	•		•	8
Calculus					Psychology				
College English	•			6	Social Sciences		•		
College Mathematics	•			6	Other				

Selection Factors: 2007 Accepted Applicants

Proportion of Accepted Applicants with Relevant Experience (Data Self-Reported to AMCAS*)		
Community Service/Volunteer		62%
Medically-Related Work		88%
Research		91%

Shaded bar represents accepted scores ranging from the 10th percentile to the 90th percentile   School Median ●   National Median ●

Overall GPA	2.0	2.1	2.2	2.3	2.4	2.5	2.6	2.7	2.8	2.9	3.0	3.1	3.2	3.3	3.4	3.5	3.6	3.7	(3.8)	3.9	4.0
Science GPA	2.0	2.1	2.2	2.3	2.4	2.5	2.6	2.7	2.8	2.9	3.0	3.1	3.2	3.3	3.4	3.5	3.6	3.7	(3.8)	3.9	4.0

MCAT® required: Yes, 100% of 2007 accepted applicants took MCAT®

Verbal Reasoning	3	4	5	6	7	8	9	(10)	(11)	12	13	14	15
Physical Sciences	3	4	5	6	7	8	9	10	(11)	12	13	14	15
Biological Sciences	3	4	5	6	7	8	9	10	(11)	12	13	14	15
Writing Sample			J	K	L	M	N	O	P	(Q)	R	S	T

Acceptance & Matriculation Data for 2007–2008 First Year Class

	Resident	Non-Resident	International	Total
Applied	1552	5351	513	7416
Interviewed	423	911	112	1446
Deferred	1	2	0	3
Matriculants				
Early Assurance Program	0	0	0	0
Early Decision Program	1	0	0	1
Baccalaureate/MD	n/a	n/a	n/a	n/a
MD/PhD	48	148	39	235
Matriculated	78	99	7	**184**

Applications accepted from International Applicants: Yes

Specialty Choice

2003, 2004, 2005 Graduates, Specialty Choice (As reported by program directors to GME Track™)	
Anesthesiology	4%
Emergency Medicine	7%
Family Practice	2%
Internal Medicine	28%
Obstetrics/Gynecology	3%
Orthopaedic Surgery	3%
Pediatrics	14%
Psychiatry	5%
Radiology	7%
Surgery	5%

Matriculant Demographics: 2007–2008 First Year Class

Men: 96   **Women:** 88

Matriculants' Self-Reported Race/Ethnicity

Mexican American	2	Korean	6
Cuban	1	Vietnamese	3
Puerto Rican	1	Other Asian	3
Other Hispanic	1	Total Asian	42
Total Hispanic	5	Native American	0
Chinese	20	Black	12
Asian Indian	8	Native Hawaiian	1
Pakistani	1	White	118
Filipino	2	Unduplicated Number	
Japanese	2	of Matriculants	184

Science and Math Majors: 72%
Matriculants with:
Baccalaureate degree: 100%
Graduate degree(s): 3%

Financial Information

Source: 2006–2007 LCME I-B survey
and 2007–2008 AAMC TSF questionnaire

	Residents	Non-Residents
Total Cost of Attendance	$58,420	$58,420
Tuition and Fees	$43,370	$43,370
Other (includes living expenses)	$15,050	$15,050
Health Insurance (not applicable)	$0	$0

Average 2007 Graduate Indebtedness: $150,090
% of Enrolled Students Receiving Aid: 73%

Criminal Background Check

This medical school does not require a criminal
background check prior to matriculation.

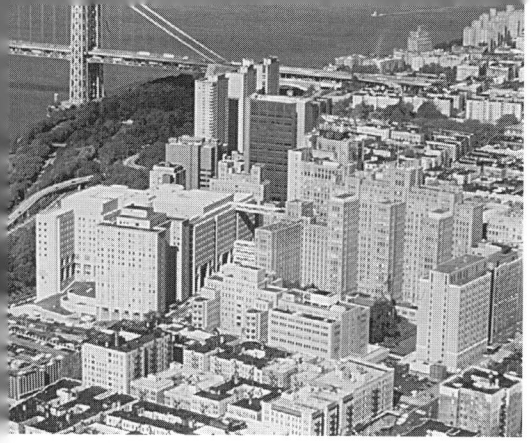

Columbia University
College of Physicians and Surgeons

New York, New York

Columbia University
College of Physicians and Surgeons
Admissions Office, Room 1-416
630 West 168th Street
New York, New York 10032
T 212 305 3595   **F** 212 305 3601

Admissions www.cumc.columbia.edu/dept/
ps/admissions
Main http://cumc.columbia.edu/dept/ps
Financial http://cumc.columbia.edu/student/finaid
Email psadmissions@columbia.edu

Private Institution

Dr. Lee Goldman, Dean, Executive Vice President for Health and Biomedical Sciences

Dr. Andrew G. Frantz, Associate Dean for Admissions

Dr. Hilda Y. Hutcherson, Associate Dean, Office of Diversity

Ellen Spilker, Director, Office of Student Financial Planning

General Information

The College of Physicians and Surgeons originated in 1767 as the Medical Faculty of King's College and was the first school to award an earned doctor of medicine degree in the American colonies. The college is part of the Columbia University Medical Center. Clinical teaching is provided at CUMC; Roosevelt-St. Luke's Hospital Center and Harlem Hospital Center in Manhattan; Bassett Hospital in Cooperstown, NY; and Stamford Hospital in Connecticut.

Mission Statement

The mission of Columbia is to produce physicians who excel in both the science and art of medicine, and who will become leaders in their fields. It seeks to do this by providing an atmosphere that is collegial rather than competitive, and by offering students opportunities to express their interests in a wide variety of humanistic as well as scientific activities.

Curricular Highlights

Community Service Requirement: Optional.
Research/Thesis Requirement: Optional.
Numerous opportunities available.

The curriculum has a solid foundation in basic sciences as well as in the art and practice of clinical medicine. The updated curriculum develops an interdisciplinary and integrative approach to the basic science subjects taught in the first two years. Small groups are emphasized. Patient contact begins in the 1st year in a variety of settings. Clinical correlation with basic sciences is emphasized, and, in the second year, all topics in pathophysiology are studied by means of

case-based histories led by preceptors in small-discussion groups. The program is designed to teach that the patient is not simply a disease entity and is being improperly cared for if treated as such. Ethical problems as well as topics in health care are discussed in this course. Clerkships begin in year two. Students follow an individually selected program of studies in year four. A variety of electives are offered, including research electives and opportunities for study abroad.

USMLE

Step 1: Required. Students must record a passing score for promotion.
Step 2: Clinical Skills (CS): Required. Students must record a passing total score to graduate.
Step 2: Clinical Knowledge (CK): Required. Students must record a passing total score to graduate.

Selection Factors

We seek applicants who have shown the greatest evidence of excellence and leadership potential in the science and art of medicine. Beyond academic ability, medicine also demands integrity, the ability to relate easily to others, and concern for their welfare. The school evaluates by several means: letters of recommendation, participation in extracurricular and summer activities, breadth of interests and undergraduate education, and the personal interview. Each year, some applicants are accepted who display extraordinary promise with regard to either the science or the art of medicine, even though they do not meet, in optimal measure, all of the criteria described above. CUMC seeks diversity of background among its applicants, geographical and otherwise; no preference is given to state of residence. Admission is possible for all qualified applicants regardless of sex, race, age, religion, sexual orientation, national origin, or handicap.

Financial Aid

Admission is not based on an applicant's ability to pay for medical school. The College makes every effort to help accepted students finance their medical education. Federal and private student loan programs are available to cover educational expenses that cannot be met by family resources. More than $8 million in need-based

grants and low-cost loans are awarded annually. To be considered for need-based funds, financial data for oneself and one's parents must be provided. After subtracting "calculated family resources" from the student budget, remaining need is met first with a package of low-cost loans, then with school grants and scholarships. Students who do not qualify for need-based funds from the school can access Federal Stafford, Graduate PLUS, and private loans.

Information about Diversity Programs

The College has a strong commitment to increase the numbers of medical students from groups underrepresented in medicine. There is a highly diverse student body and faculty. For additional information, call (212) 305-4157.

Campus Information

Setting

Located on the Upper West Side of New York City, the CUMC is on a large multi-acre campus. Two subway lines stop at the Medical Center and afford rapid access to the entire city. The main campus is a short bus or subway ride away.

Enrollment

For 2007, total enrollment was: 155

Special Features

The Russ Berrie Pavilion and Center for diabetes research and treatment was recently renovated. The New York State Psychiatric Institute building and Morgan Stanley Children's Hospital were recently opened. MS Children's Hospital is ranked among the top five pediatric hospitals in the nation. Faculty members Dr. Eric Kandel and Dr. Richard Axel were recently awarded Nobel Prizes in Neural Science.

Housing

On-campus housing is available for single students, married couples, and domestic partnerships. First-year accommodations are guaranteed in Bard Hall.

Satellite Campuses/Facilities

Students may train at some–or all–of P&S's affiliated hospitals in rural and urban settings.

Application Process and Requirements 2009–2010

Primary Application Service: AMCAS
Earliest filing date: June 1, 2008
Latest filing date: October 15, 2008

Secondary Application Required?: Yes
Sent to: All applicants
URL: https://app.applyyourself.com/?id=COL-MED
Fee: Yes, $85
Fee waiver available: Yes
Earliest filing date: June 1, 2008
Latest filing date: November 15, 2008

Latest MCAT® considered: September 2008
Oldest MCAT® considered: 2005

Early Decision Program
School does not have EDP
Applicants notified: n/a
EDP available for: n/a

Regular Acceptance Notice
Earliest date: March 2, 2009
Latest date: Varies

Applicant's Response to Acceptance Offer – Maximum Time: Three weeks

Requests for Deferred Entrance Considered: Yes

Deposit to Hold Place in Class: No
Deposit (Resident): n/a
Deposit (Non-Resident): n/a
Deposit due: n/a
Applied to tuition: n/a
Deposit refundable: n/a
Refundable by: n/a

Estimated number of new entrants: 153
EDP: n/a, special program: n/a

Start Month/Year: August 2009

Interview Format: Monday-Friday, September through February. Regional interviews are very rarely available.

Other Programs

PREPARATORY PROGRAMS
Postbaccalaureate Program: Yes,
www.columbia.edu/cu/gs/postbacc,
(212) 854-2881, pmaofficers@columbia.edu
Summer Program: Yes,
www.oda-ps.cumc.columbia.edu

COMBINED DEGREE PROGRAMS
Baccalaureate/MD: No
MD/MPH: Yes, www.mailman.hs.columbia.edu,
(212) 305-3927
MD/MBA: Yes, www.gsb.columbia.edu/mba ,
Susan Sullivan, (212) 854-4557,
sms12@columbia.edu
MD/JD: No
MD/PhD: Yes, http://mdphd.columbia.edu,
Stacy Warren, (212) 342-5653,
MD-PhD@columbia.edu

Premedical Coursework

Course	Req.	Rec.	Lab.	Sems.
Inorganic Chemistry	•	•		2
Behavioral Sciences				
Biochemistry				
Biology	•	•		2
Biology/Zoology				
Calculus				
College English	•			2
College Mathematics				

Course	Req.	Rec.	Lab.	Sems.
Computer Science				
Genetics				
Humanities				
Organic Chemistry	•		•	2
Physics	•			2
Psychology				
Social Sciences				
Other				

Selection Factors: 2007 Accepted Applicants

Proportion of Accepted Applicants with Relevant Experience (Data Self-Reported to AMCAS®)		
Community Service/Volunteer	71%	
Medically-Related Work	83%	
Research	89%	

Shaded bar represents accepted scores ranging from the 10th percentile to the 90th percentile. **School Median** ● **National Median** ●

	2.0	2.1	2.2	2.3	2.4	2.5	2.6	2.7	2.8	2.9	3.0	3.1	3.2	3.3	3.4	3.5	3.6	3.7	3.8	3.9	4.0
Overall GPA	2.0	2.1	2.2	2.3	2.4	2.5	2.6	2.7	2.8	2.9	3.0	3.1	3.2	3.3	3.4	**3.5**	**3.6**	**3.7**	**(3.8)**	3.9	4.0
Science GPA	2.0	2.1	2.2	2.3	2.4	2.5	2.6	2.7	2.8	2.9	3.0	3.1	3.2	3.3	**3.4**	**3.5**	**3.6**	**3.7**	**(3.8)**	3.9	4.0

MCAT® required: Yes, 100% of 2007 accepted applicants took MCAT®

	3	4	5	6	7	8	9	10	11	12	13	14	15
Verbal Reasoning	3	4	5	6	7	8	9	(10)	(11)	12	13	14	15
Physical Sciences	3	4	5	6	7	8	9	10	(11)	(12)	13	14	15
Biological Sciences	3	4	5	6	7	8	9	10	(11)	(12)	13	14	15
Writing Sample			J	K	L	M	N	O	P	(Q)	R	S	T

Acceptance & Matriculation Data for 2007–2008 First Year Class

	Resident	Non-Resident	International	Total
Applied	1098	5315	426	6839
Interviewed	229	953	12	1194
Deferred	0	1	0	1
Matriculants				
Early Assurance Program	0	0	0	0
Early Decision Program	0	0	0	0
Baccalaureate/MD	n/a	n/a	n/a	n/a
MD/PhD	4	13	0	17
Matriculated	46	100	9	**155**

Applications accepted from International Applicants: Yes

Matriculant Demographics: 2007–2008 First Year Class

Men: 78 **Women:** 77

Matriculants' Self-Reported Race/Ethnicity

Mexican American	4	Korean	1
Cuban	2	Vietnamese	0
Puerto Rican	2	Other Asian	2
Other Hispanic	8	Total Asian	23
Total Hispanic	16	Native American	0
Chinese	14	Black	14
Asian Indian	5	Native Hawaiian	0
Pakistani	0	White	107
Filipino	0	Unduplicated Number	
Japanese	1	of Matriculants	155

Science and Math Majors: 57%
Matriculants with:
Baccalaureate degree: 99%
Graduate degree(s): 8%

Specialty Choice

2003, 2004, 2005 Graduates, Specialty Choice (As reported by program directors to GME Track™)	
Anesthesiology	4%
Emergency Medicine	5%
Family Practice	0%
Internal Medicine	19%
Obstetrics/Gynecology	5%
Orthopaedic Surgery	7%
Pediatrics	11%
Psychiatry	6%
Radiology	5%
Surgery	5%

Financial Information

Source: 2006–2007 LCME I-B survey and 2007–2008 AAMC TSF questionnaire

	Residents	Non-Residents
Total Cost of Attendance	$61,178	$61,178
Tuition and Fees	$42,848	$42,848
Other (includes living expenses)	$15,965	$15,965
Health Insurance (can be waived)	$2,365	$2,365

Average 2007 Graduate Indebtedness: $112,649
% of Enrolled Students Receiving Aid: 82%

Criminal Background Check

This medical school does not require a criminal background check prior to matriculation.

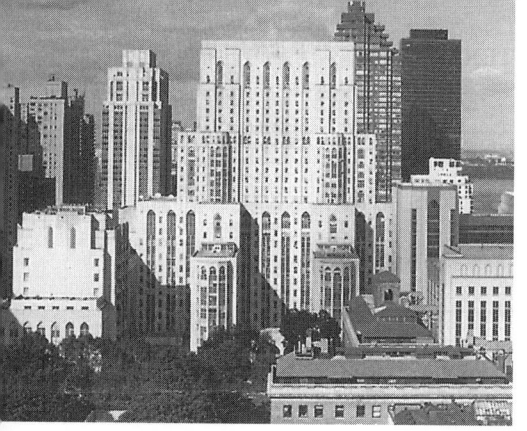

Joan & Sanford I. Weill Medical College of Cornell University

New York, New York

Office of Admissions
Weill Cornell Medical College
445 East 69th Street
New York, New York 10021
T 212 746 1067   F 212 746 8052

Admissions www.med.cornell.edu/
education/admissions
Main www.med.cornell.edu
Financial www.med.cornell.edu/education/
admissions/app_fin_aid.html
Email wcmc-admissions@med.cornell.edu

Private Institution

Dr. Antonio M. Gotto Jr., Dean

Dr. Charles L. Bardes, Associate Dean and Chair, Committee on Admissions

Dr. Carlyle H. Miller, Associate Dean for Student Affairs

Gladys Laden, Director of Financial Aid

Liliana Montano, Assistant Dean of Admissions

General Information

Founded in 1898 as Cornell University Medical College, the school's name was changed to the Joan and Sanford I. Weill Medical College of Cornell University in 1998. The medical school campus embraces the New York-Presbyterian Hospital, Memorial Sloan-Kettering Cancer Center, Rockefeller University, and the Hospital for Special Surgery. In addition, students train in clinical care throughout an affiliated network, including public, private, research, tertiary care, and community hospitals, as well as primary care sites.

Mission Statement

WMC is committed to excellence in research, teaching, patient care, and the advancement of the art and science of medicine. To this end, our mission is to provide the finest education possible for medical students, to provide superior continuing medical education for the lifelong education of physicians throughout their careers, to conduct research at the cutting edge of knowledge, to improve the health care of the nation and world both now and for further generations, and to provide the highest level of clinical care for the communities we serve.

Curricular Highlights

Community Service Requirement: Optional.
Special degree program: M.D. with Honors in Service
Research/Thesis Requirement: Optional.
Special degree program: M.D. with Honors in Research

The first two years center on problem-based learning (PBL), in which students learn by

actively solving problems with the faculty in small group seminars. Lectures, anatomic dissection, experimental laboratories and journal clubs augment the learning experience. Basic science courses are integrated and multidisciplinary. Students begin to work with patients immediately during the three-year sequence of Medicine, Patients, and Society, which focuses on clinical skills, the doctor-patient relationship, health care systems, and ultimately ethics and end-of-life care. The core clinical clerkships include medicine, neurology, obstetrics and gynecology, pediatrics, primary care, psychiatry, public health, and surgery. Year 4 provides the major time block for electives in clinical medicine, research, and international health experiences, as well as a return to advanced biomedical science.

USMLE

Step 1: Optional.
Step 2: Clinical Skills (CS): Optional.
Step 2: Clinical Knowledge (CK): Optional.

Selection Factors

WMC considers each applicant on an individual basis and welcomes those with backgrounds in the basic sciences, social sciences, and liberal arts. We encourage applicants to sample a broad range of academic disciplines and to explore one or more areas in depth. Participation in other activities should demonstrate commitment and initiative. We encourage applicants to explore medicine via research, clinical work, and volunteer service. We seek students who demonstrate emotional maturity, personal depth, commitment to others' well-being, and ethical and moral integrity. We seek to build a diverse class and emphasize diversity in all its dimensions, including race, ethnicity, educational background, personal experiences, and fields of interest. For the class entering in 2007, the mean science GPA was 3.70, and the mean MCAT® scores were as follows: Verbal Reasoning 11, Physical Sciences 11.6, Biological Sciences 11.8. Two-thirds were science majors, and one-third was liberal arts or dual majors.

Financial Aid

Admissions decisions are made without regard to applicants' financial status. All financial aid is

based on need. Some 85% of the class receives financial aid, and about 50% receives grants from the College. Housing is guaranteed for all students and priced well below market rate. Financial support for community service, summer research, and international electives is available for all students. The application fee will be waived if it represents a financial hardship to the applicant. Students who are not citizens or permanent residents of the United States are not eligible for Weill Cornell financial aid.

Information about Diversity Programs

Cornell University has been deeply committed to diversity from its very founding, and the Medical College upholds this principle. WMC's educational mission is dedicated to the inclusion of students from diverse ethnic, racial, social, economic, and educational backgrounds. Special summer research programs are available for college undergraduates who have a major interest in the medical problems of the underserved. Further information is available at *www.med. cornell.education/student/min_aff.html*.

Campus Information

Setting

Weill Cornell is located in the heart of New York City in the Upper East Side of Manhattan, a lovely residential neighborhood. Many of the city's cultural resources are a short walk away, including the Metropolitan Museum of Art, The Museum of Modern Art, Carnegie Hall, Central Park, among others.

Enrollment

For 2007, total enrollment was: 410

Special Features

Most students participate in international electives.

Housing

Modern, reduced-cost on-campus housing is guaranteed for all students.

Satellite Campuses/Facilities

Students rotate throughout New York City at public, private, community, research, and tertiary care hospitals, as well as primary care sites.

Application Process and Requirements 2009–2010

Primary Application Service: AMCAS
Earliest filing date: June 2008
Latest filing date: October 15, 2008

Secondary Application Required?: Yes
Sent to: All applicants
URL: Sent to verified applicants only.
Contact: Office of Admissions
(212) 746-1067, wcmc-admissions@med.cornell.edu
Fee: Yes, $75
Fee waiver available: Yes
Earliest filing date: Depends on release of AMCAS application.
Latest filing date: November 17, 2008

Latest MCAT® considered: September 2008
Oldest MCAT® considered: 2006

Early Decision Program
School does have EDP
Applicants notified: October 1, 2008
EDP available for: Both Residents and Non-Residents

Regular Acceptance Notice
Earliest date: December 2008
Latest date: Until class is full

Applicant's Response to Acceptance Offer – Maximum Time: Two weeks

Requests for Deferred Entrance Considered: Yes

Deposit to Hold Place in Class: Yes
Deposit (Resident): $100
Deposit (Non-Resident): $100
Deposit due: May 15, 2009
Applied to tuition: Yes
Deposit refundable: Yes
Refundable by: May 15, 2009

Estimated number of new entrants: 101
EDP: 1, special program: 3

Start Month/Year: August 2009

Interview Format: Two individual interviews with admissions committee members. No regional interviews.

Other Programs

PREPARATORY PROGRAMS
Postbaccalaureate Program: No
Summer Program: Yes,
www.med.cornell.edu/education/student/min_sum_pro.html, Elizabeth Wilson-Anstey, (212) 746-1058, eaanstey@med.cornell.edu

COMBINED DEGREE PROGRAMS
Baccalaureate/MD: No
MD/MPH: No
MD/MBA: Yes, www.med.cornell.edu/education
MD/JD: No
MD/PhD: Yes, www.med.cornell.edu/mdphd, (212) 746-6023, mdphd@med.cornell.edu

Premedical Coursework

Course	Req.	Rec.	Lab.	Hrs.
Inorganic Chemistry	•		•	8
Behavioral Sciences				
Biochemistry				
Biology				
Biology/Zoology	•		•	8
Calculus				
College English	•			6
College Mathematics				

Course	Req.	Rec.	Lab.	Hrs.
Computer Science				
Genetics				
Humanities				
Organic Chemistry	•		•	8
Physics	•		•	8
Psychology				
Social Sciences				
Other				

Selection Factors: 2007 Accepted Applicants

Proportion of Accepted Applicants with Relevant Experience (Data Self-Reported to AMCAS®)

Community Service/Volunteer	75%
Medically-Related Work	89%
Research	90%

Shaded bar represents accepted scores ranging from the 10th percentile to the 90th percentile. School Median ● National Median ●

Overall GPA: median 3.8 (national 3.9)
Science GPA: median 3.9

MCAT® required: Yes, 100% of 2007 accepted applicants took MCAT®

Verbal Reasoning: School median 10, National median 11
Physical Sciences: School median 11, National median 12
Biological Sciences: School median 11, National median 12
Writing Sample: School median Q

Acceptance & Matriculation Data for 2007–2008 First Year Class

	Resident	Non-Resident	International	Total
Applied	1162	4369	322	5853
Interviewed	170	565	18	753
Deferred	0	5	0	5
Matriculants				
Early Assurance Program	n/a	n/a	n/a	n/a
Early Decision Program	0	1	0	1
Baccalaureate/MD	n/a	n/a	n/a	n/a
MD/PhD	4	10	0	14
Matriculated	35	64	2	**101**

Applications accepted from International Applicants: Yes

Matriculant Demographics: 2007–2008 First Year Class

Men: 48 **Women:** 53

Matriculants' Self-Reported Race/Ethnicity

Mexican American	2	Korean	5
Cuban	0	Vietnamese	0
Puerto Rican	1	Other Asian	1
Other Hispanic	6	Total Asian	18
Total Hispanic	9	Native American	1
Chinese	9	Black	18
Asian Indian	1	Native Hawaiian	0
Pakistani	0	White	61
Filipino	1	Unduplicated Number	
Japanese	2	of Matriculants	101

Science and Math Majors: 66%
Matriculants with:
Baccalaureate degree: 100%
Graduate degree(s): 8%

Specialty Choice

2003, 2004, 2005 Graduates, Specialty Choice (As reported by program directors to GME Track™)

Anesthesiology	5%
Emergency Medicine	6%
Family Practice	1%
Internal Medicine	21%
Obstetrics/Gynecology	2%
Orthopaedic Surgery	4%
Pediatrics	11%
Psychiatry	8%
Radiology	5%
Surgery	9%

Financial Information

Source: 2006–2007 LCME I-B survey and 2007–2008 AAMC TSF questionnaire

	Residents	Non-Residents
Total Cost of Attendance	$ 62,995	$ 62,995
Tuition and Fees	$ 40,890	$ 40,890
Other (includes living expenses)	$ 17,652	$ 17,652
Health Insurance (can be waived)	$ 4,453	$ 4,453

Average 2007 Graduate Indebtedness: $106,905
% of Enrolled Students Receiving Aid: 84%

Criminal Background Check

This medical school does not require a criminal background check prior to matriculation.

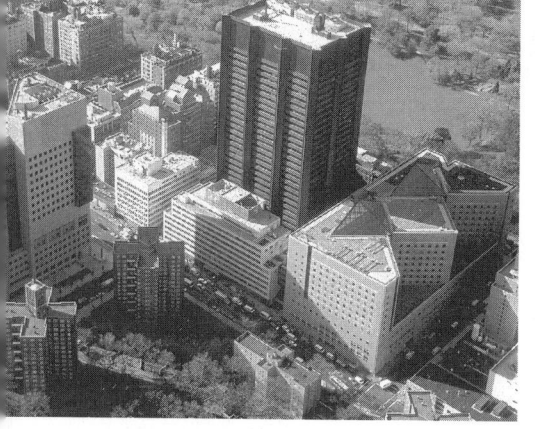

Mount Sinai School of Medicine of New York University

New York, New York

Office of Admissions, Mount Sinai School of Medicine
Annenberg Building, Room 5-04
One Gustave L. Levy Place – Box 1002
New York, New York 10029-6574
T 212 241 6696   F 212 828 4135

Admissions www.mssm.edu/bulletin/admissions/admissions.htm
Main www.mssm.edu
Financial www.mssm.edu/bulletin/admissions/financial_aid.htm
Email admissions@mssm.edu

Private Institution

Dr. Dennis Charney, Dean

*Dr. Scott H. Barnett,
Associate Dean for Admissions*

*Dr. Gary C. Butts, Associate Dean for
Multicultural and Community Affairs*

*Dale Fuller, Director of
Student Financial Services*

General Information

Mount Sinai School of Medicine is privately endowed and affiliated with New York University. The medical center campus includes The Mount Sinai Hospital, research and service laboratories, teaching facilities, and the Graduate School of Biological Sciences. The school recently completed Phase II/IV of the total renovation of its educational space, and will soon start construction that will expand its research space by approximately thirty percent. Additional clinical training sites extend throughout New York City, New Jersey, Westchester County, and Long Island.

Mission Statement

The school is committed to serving science and society through outstanding research, education, patient care, and community service. We strive to develop new approaches to teaching, translate scientific discoveries into improvements in patient care, and identify new ways to enhance the health and educational opportunities of the communities we serve.

Curricular Highlights

Community Service Requirement: Optional.
Research/Thesis Requirement: Optional.

Mount Sinai School of Medicine's curriculum is designed to teach a core knowledge of the biological basis of health and disease, skills in critical thinking, life-long learning skills, professional and humanistic attitudes, a scientific approach to medicine, and an appreciation of the physician's obligations to society and the community. The curriculum emphasizes the interdisciplinary nature of the basic and clinical sciences; it utilizes lectures and small group, case-based seminars and laboratory exercises. Courses are graded pass/fail during the first two years, and honors/high pass/pass/fail in the last two years.

USMLE

Step 1: Required. Students must record a passing score for promotion.
Step 2: Clinical Skills (CS): Required. Students must record a passing total score to graduate.
Step 2: Clinical Knowledge (CK): Required. Students must record a passing total score to graduate.

Selection Factors

Excellence in scholarship, personal maturity, integrity, intellectual creativity, and motivation for medicine are important factors. The interview, recommendations, and MCAT® scores are criteria for evaluation. All applicants are considered, regardless of race, sex, color, creed, age, national origin, handicap, veteran status, marital status, or sexual orientation.

Financial Aid

Applications for financial aid are treated confidentially, and awards are made by a faculty committee on financial aid. Each applicant is considered on an individual basis so that the school can provide maximal support for those who most need it. Financial aid may be offered in the form of a scholarship, a loan, or both, in accordance with the requirements of the individual situation and the availability of funds. Students who are not citizens or permanent residents of the United States are not eligible for financial assistance.

Information about Diversity Programs

Strongly motivated students from groups underrepresented in medicine are actively sought and encouraged to apply. A pre-entrance summer enrichment program is available for students who are accepted to the first-year class. Tutorial assistance is available for all students. The school's Center for Multicultural and Community Affairs provides leadership and coordination for minority affairs activities, multicultural diversity program activities, a variety of enrichment programs, and advisory and career counseling services.

Campus Information

Setting

The campus sits on the border between the Upper East Side of Manhattan and the thriving and vibrant community of East Harlem. Student housing is located across the street from the campus, as is Central Park. The Museum Mile, restaurants, shopping, and public transportation are all convenient to the campus.

Enrollment

For 2007, total enrollment was: 506

Special Features

The hospital and the school work together to remain at the cutting-edge of modern medicine, and to maintain regional and national leadership. Mount Sinai was the first U.S. medical school to establish academic Departments of Geriatrics and Environmental and Occupational Medicine, and is one of the few schools of medicine in the United States to have a Department of Health Policy. MD, MD/PhD, MD/MPH and MD/MBA degrees are offered. There is extensive online support for the curriculum. Student feedback is highly valued. Special features include: a standardized patient facility, human simulator center, the Global Health Center, the Office of Research Opportunities, and the Center for Multicultural and Community Affairs.

Housing

Students are guaranteed housing. Single students are housed in Aron Hall, located across the street from the school, and couples housing is within easy walking distance of the campus.

Satellite Campuses/Facilities

The main teaching site is the Mount Sinai Hospital, located on the main campus. Students also rotate to inpatient and ambulatory sites within a teaching consortium, among the largest in the country, which consists of outstanding public and private institutions in New York City and the suburbs of New Jersey.

Application Process and Requirements 2009–2010

Primary Application Service: AMCAS
Earliest filing date: June 1, 2008
Latest filing date: November 1, 2008

Secondary Application Required?: Yes
Sent to: All applicants
Contact: (212) 241-6996
admissions@mssm.edu
Fee: Yes, $105
Fee waiver available: Yes
Earliest filing date: August 1, 2008
Latest filing date: December 1, 2008

Latest MCAT® considered: September 2008
Oldest MCAT® considered: 2007

Early Decision Program
School does have EDP
Applicants notified: October 1, 2008
EDP available for: Both Residents
and Non-Residents

Regular Acceptance Notice
Earliest date: November 1, 2008
Latest date: Until class is full

Applicant's Response to Acceptance
Offer – Maximum Time: Two weeks

Requests for Deferred
Entrance Considered: Yes

Deposit to Hold Place in Class: No
Deposit (Resident): n/a
Deposit (Non-Resident): n/a
Deposit due: n/a
Applied to tuition: n/a
Deposit refundable: n/a
Refundable by: n/a

Estimated number of new entrants: 128
EDP: 1, special program: 12

Start Month/Year: August 14, 2009

Interview Format: Two thirty-minute interviews.
Regional interviews are not available.

Other Programs

PREPARATORY PROGRAMS
Postbaccalaureate Program: Yes
(212) 241-6546, www.mssm.edu/gradschool/
prepmed/index.shtml
Summer Program: Yes
grads@mssm.edu, (212) 241-6546
COMBINED DEGREE PROGRAMS
Baccalaureate/MD: No
MD/MPH: Yes, (212) 241-7941
www.mssm.edu/cpm/mph/
MD/MBA: Yes, (212) 241-2260
www.mssm.edu/medschool/md_mba/
ray.cornbill@mssm.edu
MD/JD: No
MD/PhD: Yes, mstp@mssm.edu
www.mssm.edu/gradschool/mstp/

Premedical Coursework

Course	Req.	Rec.	Lab.	Sems.	Course	Req.	Rec.	Lab.	Sems.
Inorganic Chemistry	•		•	2	Computer Science				
Behavioral Sciences					Genetics		•		
Biochemistry		•			Humanities				
Biology	•		•	2	Organic Chemistry	•		•	2
Biology/Zoology					Physics	•		•	2
Calculus					Psychology				
College English	•			2	Social Sciences				
College Mathematics	•			2	Other				

Selection Factors: 2007 Accepted Applicants

Proportion of Accepted Applicants with Relevant Experience (Data Self-Reported to AMCAS®)		
Community Service/Volunteer		68%
Medically-Related Work		85%
Research		87%

Shaded bar represents accepted scores ranging from the 10th percentile to the 90th percentile   **School Median** ●   **National Median** ●

Overall GPA	2.0	2.1	2.2	2.3	2.4	2.5	2.6	2.7	2.8	2.9	3.0	3.1	3.2	3.3	3.4	3.5	3.6	3.7	(3.8)	3.9	4.0
Science GPA	2.0	2.1	2.2	2.3	2.4	2.5	2.6	2.7	2.8	2.9	3.0	3.1	3.2	3.3	3.4	3.5	3.6	3.7	(3.8)	3.9	4.0

MCAT® required: Yes, 94% of 2007 accepted applicants took MCAT®

Verbal Reasoning	3	4	5	6	7	8	9	(10)	(11)	12	13	14	15
Physical Sciences	3	4	5	6	7	8	9	10	(11)	(12)	13	14	15
Biological Sciences	3	4	5	6	7	8	9	10	(11)	(12)	13	14	15
Writing Sample			J	K	L	M	N	O	P	(Q)	R	S	T

Acceptance & Matriculation Data for 2007–2008 First Year Class

	Resident	Non-Resident	International	Total
Applied	1498	4785	375	6658
Interviewed	341	446	20	807
Deferred	5	3	0	8
Matriculants				
Early Assurance Program	9	13	0	22
Early Decision Program	0	0	0	0
Baccalaureate/MD	n/a	n/a	n/a	n/a
MD/PhD	6	6	0	12
Matriculated	48	86	7	**141**

Applications accepted from International Applicants: Yes

Specialty Choice

2003, 2004, 2005 Graduates, Specialty Choice (As reported by program directors to GME Track™)	
Anesthesiology	9%
Emergency Medicine	4%
Family Practice	2%
Internal Medicine	24%
Obstetrics/Gynecology	4%
Orthopaedic Surgery	2%
Pediatrics	9%
Psychiatry	9%
Radiology	5%
Surgery	8%

Matriculant Demographics: 2007–2008 First Year Class

Men: 67   **Women:** 74

Matriculants' Self-Reported Race/Ethnicity

Mexican American	3	Korean	2
Cuban	4	Vietnamese	1
Puerto Rican	6	Other Asian	1
Other Hispanic	6	Total Asian	30
Total Hispanic	**19**	Native American	2
Chinese	17	Black	8
Asian Indian	9	Native Hawaiian	0
Pakistani	0	White	87
Filipino	0	**Unduplicated Number**	
Japanese	0	**of Matriculants**	**141**

Science and Math Majors: 57%
Matriculants with:
    Baccalaureate degree: 99%
    Graduate degree(s): 10%

Financial Information
Source: 2006–2007 LCME I-B survey
and 2007–2008 AAMC TSF questionnaire

	Residents	Non-Residents
Total Cost of Attendance	$55,508	$55,508
Tuition and Fees	$35,850	$35,850
Other (includes living expenses)	$16,980	$16,980
Health Insurance (can be waived)	$2,678	$2,678

Average 2007 Graduate Indebtedness: $136,338
% of Enrolled Students Receiving Aid: 74%

Criminal Background Check

This medical school requires a criminal background check prior to matriculation.

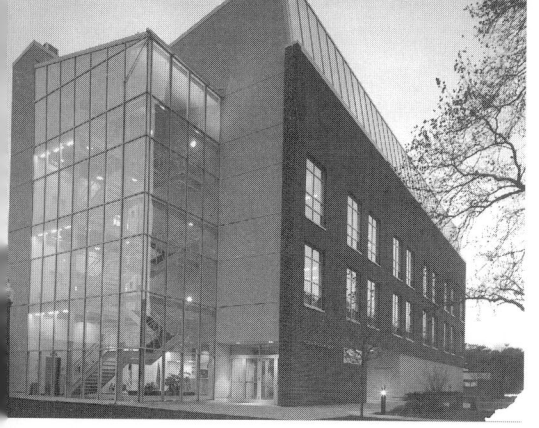

New York Medical College
Valhalla, New York

Office of Admissions
Administration Building
New York Medical College
Valhalla, New York 10595
T 914 594 4507   F 914 594 4976

Admissions www.nymc.edu/admit/
medical/info/index.asp
Main www.nymc.edu
Financial www.nymc.edu/studentlife/sfs.htm
Email mdadmit@nymc.edu

Private Institution

Dr. Ralph A. O'Connell, Provost and Dean

Dr. Fern R. Juster, Associate Dean and Chair, Committee on Admissions

Dr. Gladys M. Ayala, Associate Dean, Student and Minority Affairs

Anthony M. Sozzo, Associate Dean and Director of Student Financial Planning

Dr. Laurie Sullivan, Assistant Dean of Admissions

General Information

Founded in 1860, New York Medical College is located in suburban Westchester County, 25 miles from New York City. The university educates students for careers in medicine, biomedical science, and the health professions through its School of Medicine, Graduate School of Basic Medical Sciences, and School of Public Health.

Mission Statement

New York Medical College, a health sciences university in the Catholic tradition, exists to advance your health. We educate physicians, scientists, and healthcare professionals. We conduct research and provide service. We have one goal: your well-being. Our academic community provides programs that improve the health of the population. We join with many partners, among them people like you whom we educate and encourage to adopt healthier lifestyles, whom we treat during times of illness, and who benefit from our scientific progress. We are a university with a special responsibility to the underserved and with a deep awareness and recognition of the sacredness of all human life. Our programs are vital to the quality of health care throughout the Hudson Valley and the New York metropolitan area.

Curricular Highlights

Community Service Requirement: Optional.
Research/Thesis Requirement: Optional.

NYMC's goal is to provide a general professional education that prepares students for all career options in medicine. There is emphasis on critical thinking, evidence-based decision-making, and cultural humility throughout the curriculum.

Clinical exposure begins in the first year with a longitudinal assignment to a primary care physician where students focus on communication skills, history-taking, and preventive medicine. In addition to traditional lectures and laboratory exercises, basic science courses utilize self-directed study, small-group discussion, computer-assisted instruction, and problem-based learning. Clerkships in seven disciplines at a wide variety of hospitals and community-based clinical settings comprise the third year. In the required fourth-year sub-internships, students are expected to function at the level of a beginning resident in required rotations and electives at medical institutions around the country and the world. Highlights of the curriculum include an optional Summer Research Fellowship Program between the first and second years; exposure to medical informatics; an integrated curriculum in biomedical ethics; rigorous sub-internships in Medicine or Pediatrics; palliative care components in the medicine clerkship; and a required fourth-year rotation in Geriatric Medicine or Chronic Care Pediatrics.

USMLE

Step 1: Required. Students must record a passing score for promotion.
Step 2: Clinical Skills (CS): Required. Students must only record a score.
Step 2: Clinical Knowledge (CK): Students must record a passing total score to graduate.

Selection Factors

The Admissions Committee selects students after considering factors of intellect, character, and personality pointing toward their ability to become informed and caring physicians. A history of academic excellence is essential. Undergraduate major is not a factor in selection. Clear evidence of a strong motivation toward medicine and a sense of dedication to the service of others is encouraged. Qualities of character and personality are evaluated from letters of evaluation, personal statements, and the interview. The school does not deny admission to any applicant on the basis of any legally prohibited discrimination involving, but not limited to, such factors as race, color, creed, religion, national or ethnic origin, age, sex, sexual orientation, or disability.

Financial Aid

Financial aid is awarded on the basis of need; scholarships, based on academic merit and need, are available to entering students. The college provides debt management and loan counseling services.

Information about Diversity Programs

New York Medical College seeks to admit a diverse class, including diversity of gender, race, ethnicity, cultural and economic background, and life experience. A diverse student body provides a valuable educational experience that prepares medical students for the real world of medical practice in a multicultural society.

Campus Information

Setting

NYMC, Westchester Medical Center, and Maria Fareri Children's Hospital/Regional Trauma Center are located on a 22-acre suburban campus. Affiliated hospitals and clinical sites are located in NYC and lower Hudson Valley.

Enrollment

For 2007, total enrollment was: 786

Special Features

New York Medical College is the only academic biomedical research institution between New York City and Albany, with $46 million in sponsored programs of research, training, and service.

Housing

On-campus housing is available on the main campus in Valhalla. Most first and second-year students live on campus. Half of third and fourth-year students live in Manhattan. The Housing Office maintains a list of off-campus housing opportunities.

Satellite Campuses/Facilities

New York Medical College's wide range of affiliated hospitals, including large urban medical centers, small suburban hospitals, and technologically advanced regional tertiary care facilities, provide extensive resources and educational opportunities.

Application Process and Requirements 2009–2010

Primary Application Service: AMCAS
Earliest filing date: June 1, 2008
Latest filing date: December 15, 2008

Secondary Application Required?: Yes
Sent to: All applicants
URL: www.nymc.edu/medadmission/
Instructions.html
Fee: Yes, $100
Fee waiver available: No
Earliest filing date: July 21, 2008
Latest filing date: January 31, 2009

Latest MCAT® considered: September 2008
Oldest MCAT® considered: April 2006

Early Decision Program
School does have EDP
Applicants notified: October 1, 2008
EDP available for: Both Residents
and Non-Residents

Regular Acceptance Notice
Earliest date: December 8, 2008
Latest date: Until class is full

Applicant's Response to Acceptance
Offer – Maximum Time: Two weeks

Requests for Deferred
Entrance Considered: Yes

Deposit to Hold Place in Class: Yes
Deposit (Resident): $100
Deposit (Non-Resident): $100
Deposit due: Within two weeks of acceptance
Applied to tuition: Yes
Deposit refundable: Yes
Refundable by: May 15, 2009

Estimated number of new entrants: 190
EDP: 2, special program: n/a

Start Month/Year: August 2009

Interview Format: One-on-one blind
and minimally structured interviews. Regional
interviews are not available.

Other Programs

PREPARATORY PROGRAMS
Postbaccalaureate Program: Yes,
www.nymc.edu/gsbms/interdisciplinary.asp
Summer Program: No

COMBINED DEGREE PROGRAMS
Baccalaureate/MD: No
MD/MPH: Yes, www.nymc.edu/sph/admissions.asp
MD/MBA: No
MD/JD: No
MD/PhD: Yes,
www.nymc.edu/gsbms/md-phd-program.asp

Premedical Coursework

Course	Req.	Rec.	Lab.	Sems.
Inorganic Chemistry	•		•	2
Behavioral Sciences				
Biochemistry		•		
Biology	•		•	2
Biology/Zoology				
Calculus				
College English	•			2
College Mathematics				

Course	Req.	Rec.	Lab.	Sems.
Computer Science				
Genetics				
Humanities				
Organic Chemistry	•		•	2
Physics	•		•	2
Psychology				
Social Sciences				
Other				

Selection Factors: 2007 Accepted Applicants

Proportion of Accepted Applicants with Relevant Experience (Data Self-Reported to AMCAS®)		Community Service/Volunteer	61%
		Medically-Related Work	92%
		Research	89%

Shaded bar represents accepted scores ranging from the 10th percentile to the 90th percentile ▓   School Median ●   National Median ●

Overall GPA	2.0	2.1	2.2	2.3	2.4	2.5	2.6	2.7	2.8	2.9	3.0	3.1	3.2	3.3	**3.4**	**3.5**	**(3.6)**	**3.7**	3.8	3.9	4.0
Science GPA	2.0	2.1	2.2	2.3	2.4	2.5	2.6	2.7	2.8	2.9	3.0	3.1	3.2	**3.3**	**3.4**	**3.5**	**(3.6)**	**3.7**	3.8	3.9	4.0

MCAT® required: Yes, 100% of 2007 accepted applicants took MCAT®

Verbal Reasoning	3	4	5	6	7	8	9	(10)	11	12	13	14	15
Physical Sciences	3	4	5	6	7	8	9	(10)	(11)	12	13	14	15
Biological Sciences	3	4	5	6	7	8	9	10	(11)	12	13	14	15
Writing Sample				J	K	L	M	N	O	(P)	(Q)	R	S	T

Acceptance & Matriculation Data for 2007–2008 First Year Class

	Resident	Non-Resident	International	Total
Applied	1785	8288	579	10652
Interviewed	378	724	22	1394
Deferred	0	7	0	7
Matriculants				
Early Assurance Program	n/a	n/a	n/a	n/a
Early Decision Program	1	0	0	1
Baccalaureate/MD	n/a	n/a	n/a	n/a
MD/PhD	n/a	n/a	n/a	n/a
Matriculated	48	143	4	**195**

Applications accepted from International Applicants: Yes

Specialty Choice

2003, 2004, 2005 Graduates, Specialty Choice (As reported by program directors to GME Track™)	
Anesthesiology	7%
Emergency Medicine	4%
Family Practice	4%
Internal Medicine	24%
Obstetrics/Gynecology	4%
Orthopaedic Surgery	3%
Pediatrics	13%
Psychiatry	4%
Radiology	11%
Surgery	8%

Matriculant Demographics: 2007–2008 First Year Class

Men: 85   **Women:** 110

Matriculants' Self-Reported Race/Ethnicity

Mexican American	0	**Korean**	13
Cuban	0	**Vietnamese**	7
Puerto Rican	0	**Other Asian**	9
Other Hispanic	2	**Total Asian**	74
Total Hispanic	2	**Native American**	1
Chinese	28	**Black**	2
Asian Indian	15	**Native Hawaiian**	2
Pakistani	0	**White**	114
Filipino	2	**Unduplicated Number**	
Japanese	3	**of Matriculants**	195

Science and Math Majors: 71%
Matriculants with:
    Baccalaureate degree: 99%
    Graduate degree(s): 11%

Financial Information

Source: 2006–2007 LCME I-B survey
and 2007–2008 AAMC TSF questionnaire

	Residents	Non-Residents
Total Cost of Attendance	$62,368	$67,076
Tuition and Fees	$41,036	$40,736
Other (includes living expenses)	$18,372	$23,380
Health Insurance (can be waived)	$2,960	$2,960

Average 2007 Graduate Indebtedness: $178,943
% of Enrolled Students Receiving Aid: 88%

Criminal Background Check

This medical school does not require a criminal background check prior to matriculation.

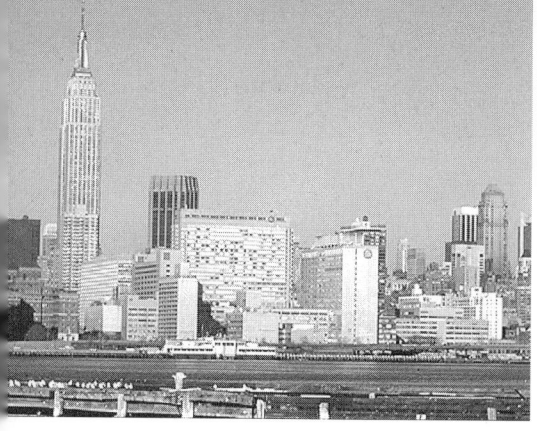

New York University School of Medicine
New York, New York

Office of Admissions
New York University School of Medicine
550 First Avenue
New York, New York 10016
T 212 263 5290   **F** 212 263 0720

Admissions www.med.nyu.edu/admissions
Main www.med.nyu.edu
Financial www.med.nyu.edu/medicaldegree/fees
Email admissions@med.nyu.edu

Private Institution

Dr. Robert I. Grossman, Dean

Dr. Nancy B. Genieser,
Associate Dean of Admissions and Financial Aid

Mekbib Gemeda, Assistant Dean of
Diversity Affairs

Joanne McGrath, Assistant Dean of Admissions

General Information
Founded in 1841, NYU School of Medicine is one of the nation's preeminent academic institutions. For over 150 years, NYU has trained thousands of physician-scientists who have enriched countless lives and helped shape medical history. Through scientific research, medical education, and patient care, NYU continues its deep, abiding commitment to improve the human condition. NYU is among the nation's leaders in consistently producing physician graduates who go on to become full-time members of medical school faculties. Students train at Bellevue, the nation's first hospital. NYU is a "private university in the public service." The School of Medicine combines the best of modern biomedical science with a rich tradition of caring for all populations at the highest level of human achievement.

Mission Statement
NYU has a threefold mission: the education and training of physicians and scientists, the search for new knowledge, and the care of the sick. The three are inseparable. Medicine can be handed on to succeeding generations only by long training in the scientific method of investigation and by the actual care of patients. Progress in medicine, which is medical research, must look constantly to the school for its investigators, and to the patient for its problems, whereas the whole future of medical care rests upon a continuing supply of physicians and upon the promise of new discovery. The purpose, then, can only be achieved by endeavor in all three directions — medical education, research, and patient care — and they must be carried on simultaneously, for they are wholly dependent upon each other, not only for inspiration, but also for their very means of success.

Curricular Highlights
Community Service Requirement: Optional. Most students participate in community service.
Research/Thesis Requirement: Optional. M.D. with honors given upon completion.

The newly launched curriculum innovates basic science teaching and promotes independent, interdisciplinary learning through small-group seminars, problem-solving activities, and computer-assisted instruction. Interdepartmental faculty instruct students in thematic curricular modules during the first two years, providing students with the essential information base, concepts, and skills necessary to understand, apply, and continually build upon the foundation of clinical medicine. Clinical sciences study continues though the four years. Advanced biomedical concepts are brought forward during clerkships through palindromic case studies stressing the translation of molecular biological and molecular genetic knowledge into decision-making and clinical care. Required clerkships and electives throughout the third and fourth years allow students to design specific courses in line with their educational and career goals. Through the honors research program, independent study projects, and the Masters Scholars program, students forge mentored relationships and cultivate their interests including public health, bioethics, human rights, biomedical health sciences, and medical informatics.

USMLE
Step 1: Required. Students must only record a score.
Step 2: Clinical Skills (CS): Required. Students must only record a score.
Step 2: Clinical Knowledge (CK): Required. Students Must only record a score.

Selection Factors
Applicants are considered from several viewpoints: excellence in coursework, premedical committee evaluation, interview, trends in the student's college progress, and the MCAT®. The committee does not rely solely on MCAT® scores and GPAs. Volunteer activities, independent research, and accomplishments in the humanities and liberal arts fields are also strongly considered. Only international applicants who hold a permanent resident visa will be considered for admission.

Financial Aid
The Financial Aid Office reviews all applications for financial assistance. Enrolled students and new accepts are eligible to file applications for assistance. For more information, see *www.med.nyu.edu/ medicaldegree/fees.*

Information about Diversity Programs
The School of Medicine is committed to admitting a diverse class. The Office of Diversity Affairs and Advisory Council has established programs and services to meet the academic, educational, personal, and cultural needs of students from groups underrepresented in medicine. See: *www.med.nyu.edu/diversity_affairs/index.html.*

Campus Information

Setting
NYUSOM lies at the heart of NYU Medical Center, which embraces NYU Hospitals Center (Tisch Hospital and the Rusk Institute for Rehabilitation Medicine,) and NYU's major hospital affiliates (Bellevue, Hospital for Joint Diseases, and the VA Hospital).

Enrollment
For 2007, total enrollment was: 716

Special Features
Bellevue is the primary location of clinical instruction and is also a significant research hub. Students complete much of their third-year clinical clerkships there, and many complete their fourth-year subinternships and clinical electives there, as well. Bellevue's Level I Treatment Center is an internationally recognized model for ER development.

Housing
There are three residence halls for students, ranging from single rooms to two bedroom apartments. All buildings are protected by security systems.

Application Process and Requirements 2009–2010

Primary Application Service: AMCAS
Earliest filing date: June 1, 2008
Latest filing date: October 15, 2008

Secondary Application Required?: Yes
Sent to: All applicants
URL: www.med.nyu.edu/medicaldegree/admissions
Fee: Yes, $100
Fee waiver available: Yes
Earliest filing date: July 1, 2008
Latest filing date: December 1, 2008

Latest MCAT® considered: September 2008
Oldest MCAT® considered: 2005

Early Decision Program
School does not have EDP
Applicants notified: n/a
EDP available for: n/a

Regular Acceptance Notice
Earliest date: March 1, 2009
Latest date: Until class is full

Applicant's Response to Acceptance
Offer – Maximum Time: Two weeks

Requests for Deferred
Entrance Considered: Yes

Deposit to Hold Place in Class: Yes
Deposit (Resident): $100
Deposit (Non-Resident): $100
Deposit due: With response to acceptance offer
Applied to tuition: Yes
Deposit refundable: Yes
Refundable by: May 15, 2009

Estimated number of new entrants: 160
EDP: 0, special program: n/a

Start Month/Year: August 2009

Interview Format: One-on-one interview with a faculty member. Regional interviews are not available.

Other Programs

PREPARATORY PROGRAMS
Postbaccalaureate Program: Yes
www.nyu.edu/cas/prehealth/
Summer Program: Yes, www.med.nyu.edu/sackler/programs/summer.html

COMBINED DEGREE PROGRAMS
Baccalaureate/MD: No
MD/MPH: Yes, www.nyu.edu/mph
MD/MBA: No
MD/JD: No
MD/PhD: Yes, www.med.nyu.edu/sackler/mdphd
MD/MPA: Yes, http://wagner.nyu.edu/dualdegrees/dual3.php

Premedical Coursework

Course	Req.	Rec.	Lab.	Hrs.	Course	Req.	Rec.	Lab.	Hrs.
Inorganic Chemistry	•		•	6	Computer Science				
Behavioral Sciences					Genetics		•		
Biochemistry		•			Humanities				
Biology	•		•	6	Organic Chemistry	•		•	6
Biology/Zoology					Physics	•		•	6
Calculus					Psychology				
College English	•			6	Social Sciences				
College Mathematics					Other				

Selection Factors: 2007 Accepted Applicants

Proportion of Accepted Applicants with Relevant Experience (Data Self-Reported to AMCAS®)	Community Service/Volunteer	64%
	Medically-Related Work	86%
	Research	92%

Shaded bar represents accepted scores ranging from the 10th percentile to the 90th percentile ▨ — School Median ● — National Median ●

Overall GPA	2.0	2.1	2.2	2.3	2.4	2.5	2.6	2.7	2.8	2.9	3.0	3.1	3.2	3.3	3.4	3.5	3.6	3.7	(3.8)	3.9	4.0
Science GPA	2.0	2.1	2.2	2.3	2.4	2.5	2.6	2.7	2.8	2.9	3.0	3.1	3.2	3.3	3.4	3.5	3.6	3.7	(3.8)	3.9	4.0

MCAT® required: Yes, 99% of 2007 accepted applicants took MCAT®

Verbal Reasoning	3	4	5	6	7	8	9	(10)	(11)	12	13	14	15
Physical Sciences	3	4	5	6	7	8	9	10	(11)	(12)	13	14	15
Biological Sciences	3	4	5	6	7	8	9	10	(11)	(12)	13	14	15
Writing Sample				J	K	L	M	N	O	P	(Q)	R	S	T

Acceptance & Matriculation Data for 2007–2008 First Year Class

	Resident	Non-Resident	International	Total
Applied	1430	5945	198	7573
Interviewed	273	676	11	960
Deferred	2	1	0	3
Matriculants				
Early Assurance Program	0	0	0	0
Early Decision Program	0	0	0	0
Baccalaureate/MD	n/a	n/a	n/a	n/a
MD/PhD	1	8	0	9
Matriculated	69	90	1	**160**

Applications accepted from International Applicants: Only Canadian

Specialty Choice

2003, 2004, 2005 Graduates, Specialty Choice (As reported by program directors to GME Track™)	
Anesthesiology	4%
Emergency Medicine	5%
Family Practice	0%
Internal Medicine	29%
Obstetrics/Gynecology	4%
Orthopaedic Surgery	5%
Pediatrics	8%
Psychiatry	4%
Radiology	9%
Surgery	6%

Matriculant Demographics: 2007–2008 First Year Class

Men: 80 | **Women:** 80

Matriculants' Self-Reported Race/Ethnicity

Mexican American	2	Korean	4
Cuban	2	Vietnamese	1
Puerto Rican	4	Other Asian	2
Other Hispanic	11	Total Asian	45
Total Hispanic	17	Native American	0
Chinese	17	Black	8
Asian Indian	17	Native Hawaiian	1
Pakistani	1	White	104
Filipino	4	**Unduplicated Number**	
Japanese	0	**of Matriculants**	160

Science and Math Majors: 70%
Matriculants with:
   Baccalaureate degree: 100%
   Graduate degree(s): 2%

Financial Information

Source: 2006–2007 LCME I-B survey and 2007–2008 AAMC TSF questionnaire

	Residents	Non-Residents
Total Cost of Attendance	$58,729	$58,729
Tuition and Fees	$40,729	$40,729
Other (includes living expenses)	$14,800	$14,800
Health Insurance (can be waived)	$3,200	$3,200

Average 2007 Graduate Indebtedness: $124,351
% of Enrolled Students Receiving Aid: 75%

Criminal Background Check

This medical school does not require a criminal background check prior to matriculation.

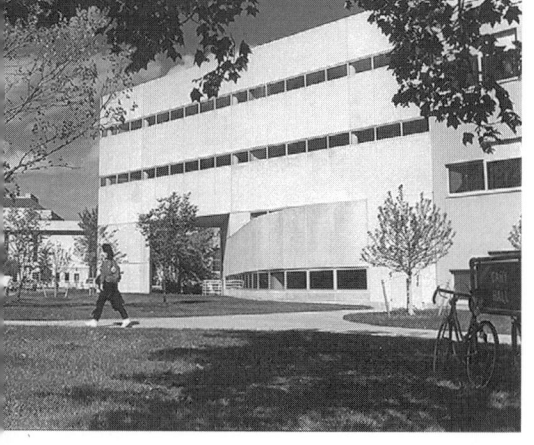

University at Buffalo School of Medicine & Biomedical Sciences

Buffalo, New York

Office of Medical Admissions
University at Buffalo
131 Biomedical Education Building
Buffalo, New York 14214-3013
T 716 829 3466   **F** 716 829 3849

Admissions www.smbs.buffalo.edu/
ome/ome_admission.htm
Main www.smbs.buffalo.edu
Financial src.buffalo.edu/financialaid
Email jjrosso@buffalo.edu

Public Institution

Dr. Michael Cain, Dean

Dr. Nancy Nielsen, Senior Associate Dean of Medical Education

Dr. Charles M. Severin, Associate Dean for Medical Education and Admissions

Dr. David A. Milling, Assistant Dean, Multicultural Affairs

General Information

The School of Medicine was founded in 1846 by Millard Fillmore and a group of physicians. In 1962 the University of Buffalo joined the State University of New York (SUNY) system. The University at Buffalo has the most comprehensive campus in the SUNY system and was honored in 1989 with election to the Association of American Universities. The clinical education program is conducted in cooperation with nine area hospitals.

Mission Statement

To provide well-trained physicians and other health care professionals who will attend to the health needs of citizens.To offer a source of continuing education to the community of health care providers, To provide a center of research and scholarship that will advance and promote health-related services As a public institution, the mission places particular emphasis on diversity, inclusion, and the special needs of New York State such as minority recruitment and retention, and the underserved urban and rural health populations.

Curricular Highlights

Community Service Requirement: Optional.
Research/Thesis Requirement: Optional.

The curriculum emphasizes the relevance of medical education to the practice of medicine and the relevance of basic science to clinical practice. It introduces patient contact and patient-centered learning in the first year of medical school, and it increases ambulatory care experiences in the clinical years. The first two years contain an integrated curriculum that includes the Introduction to Clinical Medicine course continuum, which prepares students in the knowledge, skills, and attitudes required for third-year clinical clerkships and provides the foundation for a medical career. Ethics, the doctor-patient relationship, principles of health promotion, disease prevention, and promotion of self-learning and inquiry are emphasized, in addition to extensive education in the skills basic to medical practice and patient care. The clinical years include required clerkships and electives. There is ample time for additional electives during the senior year.

USMLE

Step 1: Required. Students must record a passing score for promotion.
Step 2: Clinical Skills (CS): Required. Students must record a passing total score to graduate.
Step 2: Clinical Knowledge (CK): Required. Students must record a passing total score to graduate.

Selection Factors

The Admissions Committee seeks to identify and select students who display favorable qualities deemed important for the pursuit of a career in medicine. In making its assessments and determinations, the committee relies on information contained in the application and in documents submitted in support of the applicant. Based on careful screening, applicants are invited to appear for an interview. Reapplications are treated no differently than initial applications. Rejected applicants should seek the advice and counsel of their premedical advisor. Students are accepted without regard to race, sex, creed, national origin, age, sexual preference, or handicap. All applicants will receive the "Technical Standards of the Medical School Curriculum" with the secondary application. Some preference is given to qualified residents of New York State. Competitive out-of-state applicants are encouraged to apply.

Financial Aid

The priority due date for receipt of the Free Application for Federal Student Aid (FAFSA) is March 1, 2009. Forms received after the deadline are subject to funds available. Financial aid requests are considered after admission. Awards are made based on need. In most requests, parental income information is required regardless of dependency status. A limited number of scholarships based on academic merit and financial need are provided each year.

Information about Diversity Programs

The Summer Enrichment and Support Program helps facilitate students' retention in medical school. It is designed for admitted first-year educationally and socioeconomically disadvantaged students. Tutorial and counseling services are available throughout the summer and academic year.

Campus Information

Setting

The medical school is located on a recently renovated 33-acre campus on Main Street, in the northeast corner of the city of Buffalo. The world-renowned Shock Trauma Center is located two miles from the main medical school building. There are several public parks, cultural institutions, and shopping areas located in the vicinity. The "Main Street Campus" is accessible by subway to downtown Buffalo and is within walking distance of the VA Medical Center.

Enrollment

For 2007, total enrollment was: 560

Special Features

Students receive training in world-renowned clinical centers, including the Children's Hospital Trauma Center and Roswell Park Memorial Cancer Institute. There are also numerous opportunities for clinical and basic science research and varied international clinical experiences.

Housing

While on-campus housing is not available, the University maintains a list of affordable apartments and homes within a 10-mile radius of the campus. Rents average $500-$700 per month.

Satellite Campuses/Facilities

Student rotations are divided among nine teaching hospitals and several clinics in the metro Buffalo area. The medical school is also affiliated with ambulatory care centers in outlying suburban areas.

Application Process and Requirements 2009–2010

Primary Application Service: AMCAS
Earliest filing date: June 1, 2008
Latest filing date: November 15, 2008

Secondary Application Required?: Yes
Sent to: All applicants
Contact: James J. Rosso
(716) 829-3466, jjrosso@buffalo.edu
Fee: Yes, $65
Fee waiver available: Yes
Earliest filing date: June 1, 2008
Latest filing date: December 15, 2008

Latest MCAT® considered: 2008
Oldest MCAT® considered: 2005

Early Decision Program
School does have EDP
Applicants notified: October 1, 2008
EDP available for: Both Residents
and Non-Residents

Regular Acceptance Notice
Earliest date: October 15, 2008
Latest date: Until class is full

Applicant's Response to Acceptance
Offer – Maximum Time: Two weeks

Requests for Deferred
Entrance Considered: Yes

Deposit to Hold Place in Class: Yes
Deposit (Resident): $100
Deposit (Non-Resident): $100
Deposit due: With response to acceptance offer
Applied to tuition: Yes
Deposit refundable: Yes
Refundable by: May 15, 2009

Estimated number of new entrants: 135
EDP: 2, special program: 4

Start Month/Year: August 2009

Interview Format: Two, one-on-one
interviews. Regional interviews are not available.

Other Programs

PREPARATORY PROGRAMS
Postbaccalaureate Program: No
Summer Program: No

COMBINED DEGREE PROGRAMS
Baccalaureate/MD: No
MD/MPH: Yes, James J. Rosso
(716) 829-3466, jjrosso@buffalo.edu
MD/MBA: Yes, James J. Rosso
(716) 829-3466, jjrosso@buffalo.edu
MD/JD: No
MD/PhD: Yes, Arlene Albrecht
(716) 829-3398, ama7@buffalo.edu

Premedical Coursework

Course	Req.	Rec.	Lab.	Sems.
Inorganic Chemistry	•	•		2
Behavioral Sciences				
Biochemistry		•		
Biology	•		•	2
Biology/Zoology				
Calculus				
College English	•			2
College Mathematics				

Course	Req.	Rec.	Lab.	Sems.
Computer Science				
Genetics		•		
Humanities		•		
Organic Chemistry	•		•	2
Physics	•			2
Psychology				
Social Sciences		•		
Other				

Selection Factors: 2007 Accepted Applicants

Proportion of Accepted Applicants with Relevant Experience (Data Self-Reported to AMCAS®)		
Community Service/Volunteer		59%
Medically-Related Work		89%
Research		81%

Shaded bar represents accepted scores ranging from the 10th percentile to the 90th percentile. School Median ● National Median ●

Overall GPA	2.0	2.1	2.2	2.3	2.4	2.5	2.6	2.7	2.8	2.9	3.0	3.1	3.2	3.3	3.4	3.5	3.6	(3.7)	3.8	3.9	4.0
Science GPA	2.0	2.1	2.2	2.3	2.4	2.5	2.6	2.7	2.8	2.9	3.0	3.1	3.2	3.3	3.4	3.5	(3.6)	3.7	3.8	3.9	4.0

MCAT® required: Yes, 97% of 2007 accepted applicants took MCAT®

Verbal Reasoning	3	4	5	6	7	8	9	(10)	11	12	13	14	15
Physical Sciences	3	4	5	6	7	8	9	10	(11)	12	13	14	15
Biological Sciences	3	4	5	6	7	8	9	(10)	(11)	12	13	14	15
Writing Sample				J	K	L	M	N	O	P	(Q)	R	S	T

Acceptance & Matriculation Data for 2007–2008 First Year Class

	Resident	Non-Resident	International	Total
Applied	1762	1961	103	3826
Interviewed	404	225	0	629
Deferred	2	2	0	4
Matriculants				
Early Assurance Program	6	3	0	9
Early Decision Program	2	0	0	2
Baccalaureate/MD	n/a	n/a	n/a	n/a
MD/PhD	2	2	0	4
Matriculated	115	24	0	**139**

Applications accepted from International Applicants: No

Matriculant Demographics: 2007–2008 First Year Class

Men: 64 **Women:** 75

Matriculants' Self-Reported Race/Ethnicity

Mexican American	0	Korean	6
Cuban	1	Vietnamese	6
Puerto Rican	0	Other Asian	3
Other Hispanic	1	Total Asian	43
Total Hispanic	2	Native American	0
Chinese	14	Black	4
Asian Indian	9	Native Hawaiian	0
Pakistani	4	White	93
Filipino	2	Unduplicated Number	
Japanese	0	of Matriculants	139

Science and Math Majors: 71%
Matriculants with:
Baccalaureate degree: 100%
Graduate degree(s): 16%

Specialty Choice

2003, 2004, 2005 Graduates, Specialty Choice (As reported by program directors to GME Track™)	
Anesthesiology	6%
Emergency Medicine	8%
Family Practice	6%
Internal Medicine	16%
Obstetrics/Gynecology	6%
Orthopaedic Surgery	3%
Pediatrics	12%
Psychiatry	7%
Radiology	7%
Surgery	5%

Financial Information

Source: 2006–2007 LCME I-B survey
and 2007–2008 AAMC TSF questionnaire

	Residents	Non-Residents
Total Cost of Attendance	$44,290	$58,990
Tuition and Fees	$20,218	$34,918
Other (includes living expenses)	$22,622	$22,622
Health Insurance (can be waived)	$1,450	$1,450

Average 2007 Graduate Indebtedness: $122,378
% of Enrolled Students Receiving Aid: 84%

Criminal Background Check

This medical school requires a criminal background check prior to matriculation.

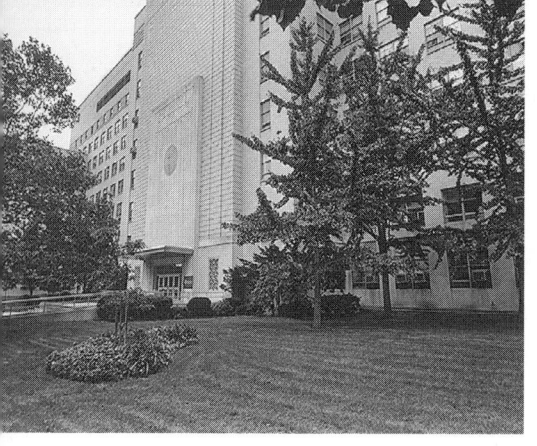

State University of New York
Downstate Medical Center College of Medicine
Brooklyn, New York

Admissions Office, State University of New York
Downstate Medical Center
450 Clarkson Avenue — Box 60
Brooklyn, New York 11203-2098
T 718 270 2446   F 718 270 4775

Admissions www.downstate.edu/college_of_medicine/
pages/admissions.htm
Main www.downstate.edu/college_of_medicine/
default.html
Financial http://sls.downstate.edu/admissions/medicine/
financial_aid.html
Email admissions@downstate.edu

Public Institution

*Dr. Ian L. Taylor, Dean and Senior
Vice President for Biomedical Education
and Research*

*Dr. Constance Hill, Associate Dean for
Minority Affairs*

General Information
Current information about the college, curriculum, and admissions is available on the Web site at *www.downstate.edu*.

Mission Statement
To provide high quality education for the next generation of health professionals. Integral to our concept of professional education are both a commitment to confront the health problems of urban communities and a responsibility to advance the state of knowledge and practice in the health disciplines through basic and applied clinical research.

Curricular Highlights
Community Service Requirement: Optional.
Research/Thesis Requirement: Optional.

In preparing physicians to practice in the future health care system, the medical education process in under constant evaluation. The main goals of the curriculum are to improve the integration of basic and clinical science throughout the four years of medical school; to provide earlier exposure to patient care by introducing clinical experiences in the first and second years of medical school; to provide for small-group, self-directed and case-based learning; and to foster life-long learning skills through the introduction of new applications of information science, outcomes studies, and evidence-based medicine. An organ system approach is followed. The emphasis is on the development of clinical reasoning and problem-solving skills. During the first year, attention is focused on the basic components of human biology and behavior, as well as on the essential aspects of the physician-patient relationship. The second year begins the study of human disease. The third and fourth years provide integrated clerkships and electives. See the Web site for more details. All courses are graded fail, conditional, pass, high pass and honors.

USMLE
Step 1: Required. Students must record a passing score for promotion.
Step 2: Clinical Skills (CS): Required. Students must only record a score.
Step 2: Clinical Knowledge (CK): Required. Students must only record a score.

Selection Factors
The Committee on Admissions considers the total qualifications of each applicant without regard to sex, sexual orientation, race, color, creed, religion, national origin, age, marital status, or disability. Decisions are based on multiple factors, including but not limited to, prior academic performance; completion of required courses for admission; the potential for academic success, including performance on standardized tests such as the MCAT®; communication skills, character, and personal skills; health-related experiences; and motivation for medicine. The 2007 entering class attended 70 different colleges and universities. Matriculants' ages ranged from 18 to 43 years, with a mean age on matriculation of 24 years.

Financial Aid
The college is committed to help students meet their educational expenses. Aid is granted on the basis of need, and, for some scholarships, on academic achievement. The major portion of assistance is derived from federal and state allocations: grants, scholarships, loans, and/or college work-study. Loans are the most common form of assistance. Financial aid application materials are sent to all accepted applicants, and students' financial aid needs are reviewed annually.

Information about Diversity Programs
SUNY Downstate maintains a tradition of commitment to the enrollment of students from groups underrepresented in medicine. The Office of Minority Affairs directs several programs targeted to furnish information and support to students from underrepresented and disadvantaged backgrounds. Entering students from groups underrepresented in medicine are matched with a faculty mentor. The Daniel Hale Williams Society also provides peer support for underrepresented students. Contact the Office of Minority Affairs at: oma@downstate.edu.

Campus Information

Setting
In NYC, 2.4 million people reside in Brooklyn. Downstate is located in central Brooklyn on an urban campus that includes a Basic Science Building, a Health Science Education Building, University Hospital, two residence halls, a student center, and a Biotech Center. The school is across the street from Kings County Hospital and three blocks from a subway station. More information is on the Web site.

Enrollment
For 2007, total enrollment was: 776

Special Features
The curriculum includes clinical exposure starting in the first year. Varied clinical settings throughout the curriculum prepare students superbly for their residency training (see Web site for more information). During the fourth year, 20-25 students participate in an international elective entitled, "Health Care in Developing Countries." A Clinical Neuroscience Pathway is available to provide enhanced exposure to neurosciences throughout the four years. Research opportunities are available throughout the four years and may lead to graduation honors. MD/MPH degrees may be earned concurrently within four years.

Housing
Two on-campus residence halls offer three different housing accommodations (see Web site for more information), while being conveniently located across the street from both academic buildings and recreational activities in the Student Center.

Application Process and Requirements 2009–2010

Primary Application Service: AMCAS
Earliest filing date: June 2, 2008
Latest filing date: December 15, 2008

Secondary Application Required?: Yes
Sent to: All applicants – download from Web site
URL: http://sls.downstate.edu/admissions/medicine/programs/index.html
Fee: Yes, $80
Fee waiver available: Yes
Earliest filing date: June 2, 2008
Latest filing date: February 2, 2009

Latest MCAT® considered: September 2008
Oldest MCAT® considered: 2006

Early Decision Program
School does have EDP
Applicants notified: October 1, 2008
EDP available for: Both Residents and Non-Residents

Regular Acceptance Notice
Earliest date: October 15, 2008
Latest date: Until class is full

Applicant's Response to Acceptance
Offer – Maximum Time: Two weeks

Requests for Deferred
Entrance Considered: Yes

Deposit to Hold Place in Class: Yes
Deposit (Resident): $100
Deposit (Non-Resident): $100
Deposit due: Within two weeks of acceptance
Applied to tuition: Yes
Deposit refundable: Yes
Refundable by: May 15, 2009

Estimated number of new entrants: 185
EDP: 5, special program: n/a

Start Month/Year: August 2009

Interview Format: One-on-one, about one hour in length. Regional interviews are not available.

Other Programs

PREPARATORY PROGRAMS
Postbaccalaureate Program: No
Summer Program: n/a

COMBINED DEGREE PROGRAMS
Baccalaureate/MD: Yes, http://depthome.brooklyn.cuny.edu/bamd/bamdmain.html
Dr. Raymond Weston, (718) 951-4706, RWeston@brooklyn.cuny.edu
MD/MPH: Yes, www.downstate.edu/mphprogram/concurrentdegree.html
(718) 270-1065, mphprogram@downstate.edu
MD/MBA: No
MD/JD: No
MD/PhD: Yes, http://sls.downstate.edu/admissions/medicine/mdpdh_program.html
Dr. Stanley Friedman, (718) 270 1335
sfriedman@downstate.edu

Premedical Coursework

Course	Req.	Rec.	Lab.	Sems.	Course	Req.	Rec.	Lab.	Sems.
Inorganic Chemistry	•		•	8	Computer Science				
Behavioral Sciences					Genetics				
Biochemistry		•		4	Humanities				
Biology	•		•	8	Organic Chemistry	•		•	8
Biology/Zoology					Physics	•		•	8
Calculus					Psychology				
College English	•			6	Social Sciences				
College Mathematics					See website for recom.			•	

Selection Factors: 2007 Accepted Applicants

Proportion of Accepted Applicants with Relevant Experience (Data Self-Reported to AMCAS')		Community Service/Volunteer	62%
		Medically-Related Work	88%
		Research	82%

Shaded bar represents accepted scores ranging from the 10th percentile to the 90th percentile   School Median ● National Median ●

Overall GPA	2.0	2.1	2.2	2.3	2.4	2.5	2.6	2.7	2.8	2.9	3.0	3.1	3.2	3.3	3.4	3.5	3.6	(3.7)	3.8	3.9	4.0
Science GPA	2.0	2.1	2.2	2.3	2.4	2.5	2.6	2.7	2.8	2.9	3.0	3.1	3.2	3.3	3.4	3.5	3.6	(3.7)	3.8	3.9	4.0

MCAT® required: Yes, 100% of 2007 accepted applicants took MCAT®

Verbal Reasoning	3	4	5	6	7	8	9	(10)	11	12	13	14	15
Physical Sciences	3	4	5	6	7	8	9	10	(11)	12	13	14	15
Biological Sciences	3	4	5	6	7	8	9	10	(11)	12	13	14	15
Writing Sample			J	K	L	M	N	O	P	(Q)	R	S	T

Acceptance & Matriculation Data for 2007–2008 First Year Class

	Resident	Non-Resident	International	Total
Applied	2157	2296	112	4565
Interviewed	732	265	0	997
Deferred	2	2	0	4
Matriculants				
Early Assurance Program	n/a	n/a	n/a	n/a
Early Decision Program	1	0	0	1
Baccalaureate/MD	14	0	0	14
MD/PhD	5	1	0	6
Matriculated	145	25	0	**170**
Applications accepted from International Applicants: No				

Specialty Choice

2003, 2004, 2005 Graduates, Specialty Choice (As reported by program directors to GME Track™)	
Anesthesiology	8%
Emergency Medicine	7%
Family Practice	2%
Internal Medicine	27%
Obstetrics/Gynecology	4%
Orthopaedic Surgery	2%
Pediatrics	14%
Psychiatry	4%
Radiology	4%
Surgery	6%

Matriculant Demographics: 2007–2008 First Year Class

Men: 85   **Women:** 85

Matriculants' Self-Reported Race/Ethnicity

Mexican American	2	Korean	8
Cuban	1	Vietnamese	1
Puerto Rican	2	Other Asian	9
Other Hispanic	9	Total Asian	54
Total Hispanic	13	Native American	1
Chinese	15	Black	17
Asian Indian	17	Native Hawaiian	1
Pakistani	1	White	94
Filipino	3	Unduplicated Number	
Japanese	1	of Matriculants	170

Science and Math Majors: 63%
Matriculants with:
　　Baccalaureate degree: 100%
　　Graduate degree(s): 12%

Financial Information

Source: 2006–2007 LCME I-B survey and 2007–2008 AAMC TSF questionnaire

	Residents	Non-Residents
Total Cost of Attendance	$49,815	$64,515
Tuition and Fees	$19,370	$34,070
Other (includes living expenses)	$27,176	$27,176
Health Insurance (can be waived)	$3,269	$3,269

Average 2007 Graduate Indebtedness: $101,502
% of Enrolled Students Receiving Aid: 89%

Criminal Background Check

This medical school does not require a criminal background check prior to matriculation.

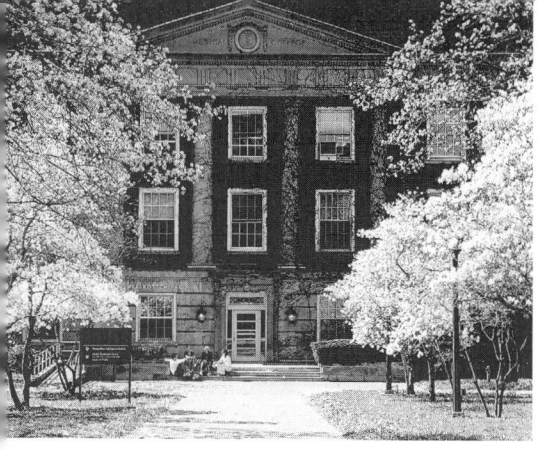

State University of New York
Upstate Medical University College of Medicine
Syracuse, New York

Admissions Office
SUNY Upstate Medical University
766 Irving Ave.
Syracuse, New York 13210
T 315 464 4570   F 315 464 8867

Admissions www.upstate.edu/com/admissions.shtml
Main www.upstate.edu/com
Financial www.upstate.edu/prospective/tuition.php
Email admiss@upstate.edu

Public Institution

Dr. Steven J. Scheinman, Dean

Jennifer Welch, Director of Admissions

Dr. Gregory Threatte, Interim Assistant Dean of Multicultural Resources

Mike Pede, Director of Financial Aid

Dr. Julie White, Dean, Student Affairs

General Information
The College of Medicine was established in 1834 as the Geneva Medical College. The college was transferred to the State University of New York (SUNY) system in 1950. In 1999, its name changed to SUNY Upstate Medical University to best reflect the college's academic mission in medical care, research, and education.

Mission Statement
The main mission of SUNY Upstate is the education of health professionals and to conduct biomedical research. Upstate's clinical faculty and health care professionals commit themselves to education and patient care, demonstrating excellence and compassion. In pursuing its mission, Upstate provides its faculty, staff, students, and volunteers an environment of mutual trust and respect, with opportunities to grow personally, and professionally and to make a positive difference in the lives of others.

Curricular Highlights
Community Service Requirement: Optional.
Research/Thesis Requirement: Optional.

The curriculum integrates the basic and clinical sciences and provides clinical exposure in the first semester. All courses are aligned by organ systems. The curriculum also addresses the humanistic aspects of medicine, including its ethical, legal, and social implications. During the third year, the students apply the principles of basic science to clinical problem-solving. Clerkships in subspecialty services are required. A research track is available, in which students spend the first two summers and elective time on a research project. Another interesting opportunity is the Rural Medical Education Program, which places students in rural communities for nine consecutive months of clinical and didactic education during the 3rd and 4th year. A modified pass/fail grading system is used.

USMLE
Step 1: Required. Students must record a passing score for promotion.
Step 2: Clinical Skills (CS): Required. Students must only record a score.
Step 2: Clinical Knowledge (CK): Required. Students must only record a score.

Selection Factors
The Admissions Committee takes an applicant's total qualifications into consideration for the study and practice of medicine. Major factors in the selection of applicants include: review of college records, MCAT® scores, letters of recommendation from premedical advisory committees, personal interview, communication skills, character, and motivation.

Financial Aid
Accepted applicants who are US citizens or permanent residents are eligible to apply for financial aid. The Financial Aid Office generally sends out financial aid award letters beginning in March.

Information about Diversity Programs
Upstate is committed to making student enrollment reflective of the diverse New York State population. Disadvantaged students and students from groups underrepresented in medicine are actively sought. A summer Human Anatomy program is available for all students. For more information, please contact the Office of Admissions.

Campus Information

Setting
Located in Syracuse, New York's fourth largest city, SUNY Upstate is a compact, easy-to-navigate campus. We have a new human anatomy lab, an excellent library, and a teaching hospital that is connected to our main academic building. Syracuse is an affordable, medium-sized city with big-city sports, arts, and recreation. Just outside the city, you will find numerous parks, lakes, mountains, golf courses, ski slopes, hiking trails and beaches. University Hospital is a level-one trauma center and tertiary care hospital that services 17 different counties.

Enrollment
For 2007, total enrollment was: 623

Special Features
SUNY Upstate's teaching hospital, University Hospital, is the main clinical site in Syracuse. As the only Level I trauma and burn center in the region, University Hospital treats the most seriously ill and injured patients. University Hospital offers hundreds of specialty services and programs, including the Center for Children's Cancer and Blood Disorders, Clark Burn Center, CNY Gamma Knife Center, and the Joslin Diabetes Center. In 2009, we will open a Children's Hospital at University Hospital, the first children's hospital in the region. We also have a clinical campus in the city of Binghamton, which offers clinical training in a community-based setting.

Housing
Clark Tower, SUNY Upstate's residence hall, houses approximately 170 students from all four colleges in fully-furnished standard rooms, studio apartments, and two-bedroom suites. Clark Tower is located next door to the Campus Activities Building, one block from University Hospital and a short walk from the Library and the academic buildings.

Satellite Campuses/Facilities
At the beginning of the third year, one quarter of the class moves from SUNY Upstate's main campus in Syracuse to the Binghamton Campus. The Binghamton Campus is located 70 miles south of Syracuse. There, clinical training occurs in a community-based setting similar to the environment in which most physicians practice.

Application Process and Requirements 2009–2010

Primary Application Service: AMCAS
Earliest filing date: June 1, 2008
Latest filing date: October 15, 2008

Secondary Application Required?: Yes
Sent to: Information on how to access secondary application materials is sent to all verified AMCAS applicants.
URL: n/a
Fee: Yes, $100
Fee waiver available: Yes
Earliest filing date: Upon receipt of verified AMCAS application.
Latest filing date: December 1, 2008

Latest MCAT® considered: September 2008
Oldest MCAT® considered: 2005

Early Decision Program
School does have EDP
Applicants notified: October 1, 2008
EDP available for: Both Residents and Non-Residents

Regular Acceptance Notice
Earliest date: October 15, 2008
Latest date: Until class is full

Applicant's Response to Acceptance Offer – Maximum Time: Two weeks

Requests for Deferred Entrance Considered: Yes

Deposit to Hold Place in Class: Yes
Deposit (Resident): $100
Deposit (Non-Resident): $100
Deposit due: With response to acceptance offer
Applied to tuition: Yes
Deposit refundable: Yes
Refundable by: May 15, 2009

Estimated number of new entrants: 160
EDP: 2, special program: 15

Start Month/Year: August 2009

Interview Format: On campus with two individual interviewers. Regional interviews are not available.

Other Programs

PREPARATORY PROGRAMS
Postbaccalaureate Program: No
Summer Program: Yes, Jennifer Welch
(315) 464-4570, admiss@upstate.edu

COMBINED DEGREE PROGRAMS
Baccalaureate/MD: Yes
www.upstate.edu/com/admissions/options.php
MD/MPH: No
MD/MBA: No
MD/JD: No
MD/PhD: Yes
www.upstate.edu/mdphd/

Premedical Coursework

Course	Req.	Rec.	Lab.	Hrs.	Course	Req.	Rec.	Lab.	Hrs.
Inorganic Chemistry	•		•	6-8	Computer Science				
Behavioral Sciences					Genetics		•		
Biochemistry		•			Humanities		•		
Biology					Organic Chemistry	•		•	6-8
Biology/Zoology	•		•	6-8	Physics	•		•	6-8
Calculus		•			Psychology		•		
College English	•			6	Social Sciences		•		
College Mathematics		•			Other				

Selection Factors: 2007 Accepted Applicants

Proportion of Accepted Applicants with Relevant Experience (Data Self-Reported to AMCAS®)		Community Service/Volunteer	65%
		Medically-Related Work	88%
		Research	78%

Shaded bar represents accepted scores ranging from the 10th percentile to the 90th percentile   School Median ●   National Median ●

Overall GPA	2.0	2.1	2.2	2.3	2.4	2.5	2.6	2.7	2.8	2.9	3.0	3.1	3.2	3.3	3.4	3.5	3.6	3.7	(3.8)	3.9	4.0
Science GPA	2.0	2.1	2.2	2.3	2.4	2.5	2.6	2.7	2.8	2.9	3.0	3.1	3.2	3.3	3.4	3.5	3.6	(3.7)	3.8	3.9	4.0

MCAT® required: Yes, 93% of 2007 accepted applicants took MCAT®

Verbal Reasoning	3	4	5	6	7	8	9	(10)	11	12	13	14	15
Physical Sciences	3	4	5	6	7	8	9	10	(11)	12	13	14	15
Biological Sciences	3	4	5	6	7	8	9	10	(11)	12	13	14	15
Writing Sample			J	K	L	M	N	O	(P)	(Q)	R	S	T

Acceptance & Matriculation Data for 2007–2008 First Year Class

	Resident	Non-Resident	International	Total
Applied	1853	2218	410	4481
Interviewed	292	292	84	668
Deferred	2	2	1	5
Matriculants				
Early Assurance Program	18	3	2	23
Early Decision Program	0	0	0	0
Baccalaureate/MD	8	0	0	8
MD/PhD	1	1	1	3
Matriculated	100	43	17	**160**

Applications accepted from International Applicants: Yes

Matriculant Demographics: 2007–2008 First Year Class

Men: 79   **Women:** 81

Matriculants' Self-Reported Race/Ethnicity

Mexican American	0	Korean	3
Cuban	0	Vietnamese	0
Puerto Rican	0	Other Asian	5
Other Hispanic	0	Total Asian	34
Total Hispanic	0	Native American	1
Chinese	8	Black	17
Asian Indian	16	Native Hawaiian	0
Pakistani	3	White	88
Filipino	0	Unduplicated Number	
Japanese	0	of Matriculants	160

Science and Math Majors: 77%
Matriculants with:
Baccalaureate degree: 100%
Graduate degree(s): 14%

Specialty Choice

2003, 2004, 2005 Graduates, Specialty Choice (As reported by program directors to GME Track™)	
Anesthesiology	6%
Emergency Medicine	7%
Family Practice	6%
Internal Medicine	20%
Obstetrics/Gynecology	5%
Orthopaedic Surgery	4%
Pediatrics	14%
Psychiatry	3%
Radiology	7%
Surgery	7%

Financial Information

Source: 2006–2007 LCME I-B survey and 2007–2008 AAMC TSF questionnaire

	Residents	Non-Residents
Total Cost of Attendance	$37,996	$52,696
Tuition and Fees	$19,956	$34,656
Other (includes living expenses)	$15,730	$15,730
Health Insurance (can be waived)	$2,310	$2,310

Average 2007 Graduate Indebtedness: $122,765
% of Enrolled Students Receiving Aid: 87%

Criminal Background Check

This medical school does not require a criminal background check prior to matriculation.

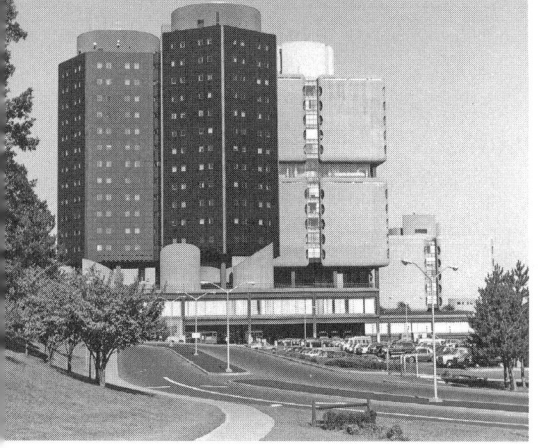

Stony Brook University School of Medicine
Stony Brook, New York

Committee on Admissions
Level 4 Health Sciences Center
Stony Brook University School of Medicine
Stony Brook, New York 11794-8434
T 631 444 2113   F 631 444 6032

Admissions www.stonybrookmedicalcenter.org/
education/som_admissions.cfm
Main www.stonybrookmedicalcenter.org/
Financial
www.hsc.stonybrook.edu/som/student_affairs/index.cfm
Email somadmissions@stonybrook.edu

Public Institution

Dr. Richard N. Fine, Dean

Dr. Jack Fuhrer, Associate Dean for Admissions

Dr. Aldustus E. Jordan, Associate Dean for Student and Minority Affairs

Mary Jean Allen, Director of Financial Aid

Grace S. Agnetti, Assistant Dean for Admissions

General Information
Stony Brook University's School of Medicine accepted its first class in 1971. It is part of the Stony Brook University Medical, which includes the 540-bed University Hospital.

Mission Statement
The School of Medicine strives to improve the quality of health care by demonstrating national leadership in education, research, patient care, and community service. The School of Medicine prepares its students for careers in medical practice or research through its state-of-the-art curriculum and clinical and research opportunities.

Curricular Highlights
Community Service Requirement: Optional.
Research/Thesis Requirement: Optional.

The curriculum of the School of Medicine provides the opportunity for extensive training in the basic medical sciences and teaching in the clinical disciplines of medicine. The curriculum requires the acquisition and utilization of a variety of skills in basic and clinical sciences. The official grading system is honors/pass/fail. The first two years are devoted to basic sciences and the integrated Foundations of Medicine course. The Foundations course teaches medical ethics, patient assessment skills, preventive medicine, human behavior, and nutrition. The second year focuses on an organ system-based pathophysiology and therapeutics course. Third year students complete core clerkships in medicine, pediatrics, family medicine, obstetrics-gynecology, psychiatry, ambulatory medicine and surgery. One month of elective time is available. Fourth year students are offered selectives and electives. Core clerkships are completed at University Hospital or one of three teaching affiliates. Electives can be completed at other sites.

USMLE
Step 1: Required. Students must record a passing score for promotion.
Step 2: Clinical Skills (CS): Required. Students must only record a score.
Step 2: Clinical Knowledge (CK): Required. Students must record a passing total score to graduate.

Selection Factors
Grades, MCAT® scores, letters of evaluation, and extracurricular and work experiences are carefully examined. Motivational and personal characteristics as indicated in the application and a personal interview are also a major part of the admissions assessment. There is no discrimination in the admissions process on the basis of sex, race, religion, national origin, age, marital status, or handicap. The school attempts to enroll a class representative of a variety of backgrounds and academic interests. Stony Brook hopes to attract a significant representation of persons from groups that have historically been underrepresented in medicine. Premedical coursework must be completed at an American college or university. While residents of New York constitute the majority of the applicants and entrants, out-of-state applicants are given due consideration. Required supporting documentation includes official transcripts of all college work and official letters of evaluation. Personal interviews will be arranged at the initiative of the school for candidates who appear to be serious contenders for admission. Stony Brook does not utilize a "cut-off" in grades or MCAT® scores in making admission decisions. The school is committed to giving all applicants the individualized attention that they merit.

Financial Aid
Stony Brook participates in all financial aid programs available at the medical schools of the SUNY system. Financial aid and counseling are available through the Office of Student Affairs, as is assistance in securing housing and in meeting other personal needs. On-campus housing is available. Students are advised to have transportation available because there is no public transportation to outlying clinical facilities.

Information about Diversity Programs
Stony Brook is committed to admitting a diverse class each year. The school makes a concerted effort to enroll qualified students from groups underrepresented in medicine.

Campus Information

Setting
Stony Brook University and the School of Medicine are located 60 miles east of NYC on the north shore of Long Island. The campus is surrounded by a picturesque and historic community. The campus provides a wide spectrum of activities ranging from NCAA Division I sporting events to professional theatre and fine arts. Students can participate in a wide range of intramural athletic activities. The clinical campus includes Stony Brook University Hospital and three affiliates.

Enrollment
For 2007, total enrollment was: 449

Special Features
Stony Brook offers excellent research and clinical opportunities and has attracted a faculty of national and international renown. The University enjoys an outstanding research relationship with Cold Spring Harbor and Brookhaven National Laboratories. State-of-the-art Cancer and Heart Centers serve the needs of Long Islanders and a NIH-funded General Clinical Research Center offers cutting edge clinical research.

Housing
There is limited on-campus housing and most medical students share apartments or houses in the surrounding communities. Housing costs range from $400-$900 per month with a median rent of $600.

Application Process and Requirements 2009–2010

Primary Application Service: AMCAS
Earliest filing date: June 1, 2008
Latest filing date: December 15, 2008

Secondary Application Required?: Yes
Sent to: All applicants
URL: www.stonybrookmedicalcenter.org/education/som_admissions.cfm
Fee: Yes, $75
Fee waiver available: Yes
Earliest filing date: June 15, 2008
Latest filing date: December 26, 2008

Latest MCAT® considered: September 2008
Oldest MCAT® considered: 2004

Early Decision Program
School does have EDP
Applicants notified: October 1, 2008
EDP available for: Both Residents and Non-Residents

Regular Acceptance Notice
Earliest date: October 15, 2008
Latest date: Until class is full

Applicant's Response to Acceptance Offer – Maximum Time: 15 days, unless otherwise specified

Requests for Deferred Entrance Considered: Yes

Deposit to Hold Place in Class: Yes
Deposit (Resident): $100
Deposit (Non-Resident): $100
Deposit due: With response to acceptance offer
Applied to tuition: Yes
Deposit refundable: Yes
Refundable by: May 15, 2009

Estimated number of new entrants: 116
EDP: 2, special program: 8

Start Month/Year: August 2009

Interview Format: Two individual interviews with admission committee members.

Other Programs

PREPARATORY PROGRAMS
Postbaccalaureate Program: Yes
Summer Program: No

COMBINED DEGREE PROGRAMS
Baccalaureate/MD: Yes,
www.stonybrook.edu/honors,
www.wise.sunysb.edu/,
ugadmissions/programs/engsfmed.shtml
MD/MPH: Yes, stonybrookmedicalcenter.org/education/public_health/
MD/MBA: No
MD/JD: No
MD/PhD: Yes, www.pharm.stonybrook.edu/mstp/index.html

Premedical Coursework

Course	Req.	Rec.	Lab.	Sems.
Inorganic Chemistry	•	•		2
Behavioral Sciences				
Biochemistry		•		1
Biology	•	•		2
Biology/Zoology				
Calculus				
College English	•			2
College Mathematics				

Course	Req.	Rec.	Lab.	Sems.
Computer Science				
Genetics				
Humanities				
Organic Chemistry	•	•		2
Physics	•	•		2
Psychology				
Social Sciences				
Other				

Selection Factors: 2007 Accepted Applicants

Proportion of Accepted Applicants with Relevant Experience (Data Self-Reported to AMCAS®)		
Community Service/Volunteer	61%
Medically-Related Work	88%
Research	85%

Shaded bar represents accepted scores ranging from the 10th percentile to the 90th percentile. School Median ● National Median ●

Overall GPA	2.0	2.1	2.2	2.3	2.4	2.5	2.6	2.7	2.8	2.9	3.0	3.1	3.2	3.3	3.4	3.5	3.6	(3.7)	3.8	3.9	4.0
Science GPA	2.0	2.1	2.2	2.3	2.4	2.5	2.6	2.7	2.8	2.9	3.0	3.1	3.2	3.3	3.4	3.5	3.6	(3.7)	3.8	3.9	4.0

MCAT® required: Yes, 100% of 2007 accepted applicants took MCAT®

Verbal Reasoning	3	4	5	6	7	8	9	(10)	11	12	13	14	15
Physical Sciences	3	4	5	6	7	8	9	10	(11)	12	13	14	15
Biological Sciences	3	4	5	6	7	8	9	10	(11)	12	13	14	15
Writing Sample			J	K	L	M	N	O	P	(Q)	R	S	T

Acceptance & Matriculation Data for 2007–2008 First Year Class

	Resident	Non-Resident	International	Total
Applied	2026	1299	206	3531
Interviewed	498	95	4	597
Deferred	4	0	0	4
Matriculants				
Early Assurance Program	n/a	n/a	n/a	n/a
Early Decision Program	0	0	0	0
Baccalaureate/MD	3	0	0	3
MD/PhD	3	2	0	5
Matriculated	100	14	2	**116**

Applications accepted from International Applicants: Yes

Matriculant Demographics: 2007–2008 First Year Class

Men: 59 **Women:** 57

Matriculants' Self-Reported Race/Ethnicity

Mexican American	2	Korean	10
Cuban	1	Vietnamese	1
Puerto Rican	2	Other Asian	4
Other Hispanic	2	Total Asian	46
Total Hispanic	7	Native American	1
Chinese	20	Black	3
Asian Indian	10	Native Hawaiian	0
Pakistani	3	White	60
Filipino	0	Unduplicated Number	
Japanese	1	of Matriculants	116

Science and Math Majors: 69%
Matriculants with:
   Baccalaureate degree: 100%
   Graduate degree(s): 11%

Specialty Choice

2003, 2004, 2005 Graduates, Specialty Choice (As reported by program directors to GME Track™)	
Anesthesiology	6%
Emergency Medicine	8%
Family Practice	2%
Internal Medicine	25%
Obstetrics/Gynecology	6%
Orthopaedic Surgery	3%
Pediatrics	11%
Psychiatry	5%
Radiology	4%
Surgery	9%

Financial Information

Source: 2006–2007 LCME I-B survey and 2007–2008 AAMC TSF questionnaire

	Residents	Non-Residents
Total Cost of Attendance	$42,690	$57,390
Tuition and Fees	$19,889	$34,589
Other (includes living expenses)	$20,025	$20,025
Health Insurance (can be waived)	$2,776	$2,776

Average 2007 Graduate Indebtedness: $130,513
% of Enrolled Students Receiving Aid: 86%

Criminal Background Check

This medical school requires a criminal background check prior to matriculation.

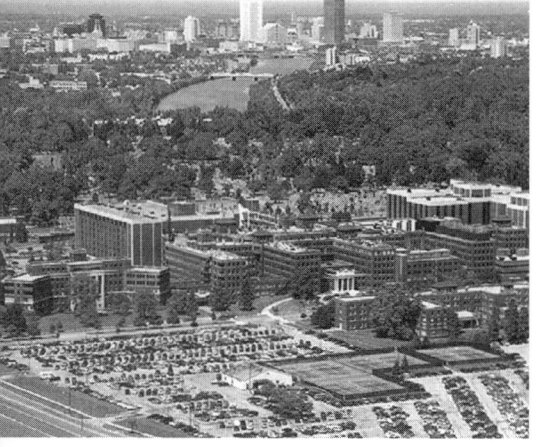

University of Rochester School of Medicine and Dentistry

Rochester, New York

Director of Admissions, University of Rochester
School of Medicine and Dentistry
601 Elmwood Avenue, Box 601A
Rochester, New York 14642
T 585 275 4539   F 585 756 5479

Admissions www.urmc.rochester.edu/smd/admissions
Main www.urmc.rochester.edu/SMD
Financial www.urmc.rochester.edu/smd/admissions/
financial_aid
Email mdadmish@urmc.rochester.edu

Private Institution

Dr. David S. Guzick, Dean

Dr. John T. Hansen, Associate Dean for Admissions

Gladys Pedraza-Burgos, Co-Director, Center for Advocacy, Community Health, Education and Diversity

Nancy Janson, Director, Financial Aid

Patricia Samuelson, Director of Admissions

General Information

The School of Medicine and Dentistry is an academic division of the University of Rochester, a privately endowed institution founded in 1850. The Medical Center includes the School of Medicine and Dentistry, School of Nursing, Eastman Dental Center, Strong Memorial Hospital, and Golisano Children's Hospital at Strong.

Mission Statement

As the home of the biopsychosocial model, Rochester offers a student-centered educational program that prepares physicians for the 21st century. The curriculum fosters knowledge, skills, attitudes, and behaviors of the physician/ scientist/humanist by combining cutting-edge, evidence-based medical science with the relationship-centered art that is medicine's distinctive trademark.

Curricular Highlights

Community Service Requirement: Required. Community Health Improvement Clerkship. **Research/Thesis Requirement:** Optional. Graduate with "Distinction in Research" honors.

Rochester's Double Helix Curriculum captures the integrated strands of basic science and clinical medicine as they are woven throughout the four-year curriculum. The focus of the educational program is not merely the transfer of information, but the transformation of the learner in a culture providing that ingenious combination of support and challenge, which leads to education. Courses are interdisciplinary and clinical exposure begins during the first week of school with an introduction to clinical

medicine and the start of the ambulatory care clerkship during the first spring semester. Inpatient clerkships focus on acute care experiences in adult medicine, women's and children's health, mind/ brain/behavior, and urgent/emergent care. A formal tutoring system and assistance programs are available. A rich menu of opportunities is available to students, including a strong M.D./Ph.D. program (MSTP), a five-year Academic Research Track, Medical Humanities selectives, and community and international medicine experiences.

USMLE

Step 1: Required. Students must only record a score.
Step 2: Clinical Skills (CS): Required. Students must only record a score.
Step 2: Clinical Knowledge (CK): Required. Students must only record a score.

Selection Factors

Evaluation of applicants includes a careful examination of the entire academic record, letters of recommendation, and the candidate's personal statement. Demonstrated excellence in a demanding academic program, including a high level of achievement in the natural sciences, is a requirement for acceptance. Evidence of intrinsic intellectual drive and curiosity is highly valued since the program at Rochester emphasizes independent learning opportunities for individual students. Particular attention is given to achievements that demonstrate breadth and commitment, especially in areas of research, outreach, and clinical experience.

Financial Aid

The medical school offers scholarships and long-term loans to those students who demonstrate financial need. Entering students applying for institutional financial aid are required to provide a FAFSA, a more detailed financial statement including parent information, and the School of Medicine's financial aid application.

Information about Diversity Programs

The Center for Advocacy, Community Health, Education and Diversity represents a serious commitment on the part of the School of

Medicine and Dentistry to meet the urgent need for diverse physicians in all aspects of the medical profession. Rochester believes that a diverse class enriches the educational environment for all of its students. The office also coordinates numerous academic and cultural events for the education of all students.

Campus Information

Setting

The Medical Center is located adjacent to the University of Rochester which enrolls about 4,450 undergraduates and 3,890 graduate students. The Medical Center has new education and research facilities. Three affiliated hospitals, regional Veterans Affairs clinics, and community health centers are in close proximity to the Medical Center. The metropolitan area includes 1.1 million residents and is located in the scenic Finger Lakes region of upstate New York.

Enrollment

For 2007, total enrollment was: 391

Special Features

The University is consistently ranked among the top 30 institutions in federal funding for research and development, and it owns the Strong Memorial Hospital, which is a major referral center for upstate New York.

Housing

Campus housing is available and assigned by lottery; high quality, affordable housing is also located within a short distance of the Medical Center.

Satellite Campuses/Facilities

Students also rotate through three affiliated hospitals and community and private ambulatory clinics within a short distance of the Medical Center. Both inner city and rural clinic/hospital experiences are offered.

Application Process and Requirements 2009–2010

Primary Application Service: AMCAS
Earliest filing date: June 1, 2008
Latest filing date: October 15, 2008

Secondary Application Required?: Yes
Sent to: All applicants
URL: www.urmc.rochester.edu/smd/education/secapp
Fee: Yes, $75
Fee waiver available: Yes, (AMCAS FAP)
Earliest filing date: July 7, 2008
Latest filing date: November 15, 2008

Latest MCAT® considered: September 2008
Oldest MCAT® considered: 2005

Early Decision Program
School does not have EDP
Applicants notified: n/a
EDP available for: n/a

Regular Acceptance Notice
Earliest date: October 15, 2008
Latest date: Until class is full

Applicant's Response to Acceptance
Offer – Maximum Time: Two weeks

Requests for Deferred
Entrance Considered: Yes

Deposit to Hold Place in Class: Yes
Deposit (Resident): $100
Deposit (Non-Resident): $100
Deposit due: With response to acceptance offer
Applied to tuition: Yes
Deposit refundable: Yes
Refundable by: May 15, 2009

Estimated number of new entrants: 100
EDP: 0, special program: 12

Start Month/Year: August 2009

Interview Format: Two interviews.
Regional interviews are not available.

Other Programs

PREPARATORY PROGRAMS
Postbaccalaureate Program: No
Summer Program: No
One week pre-matriculation course:
John Hansen, (585) 275-4606
John_Hansen@urmc.rochester.edu

COMBINED DEGREE PROGRAMS
Baccalaureate/MD: Yes,
http://enrollment.rochester.edu/admissions/learning/programs.shtm
MD/MPH: Yes,
www.urmc.rochester.edu/smd/grad/joint_degree.cfm
MD/MBA: Yes,
www.urmc.rochester.edu/smd/grad/joint_degree.cfm
MD/JD: No
MD/PhD: Yes,
www.urmc.rochester.edu/smd/grad/joint_degree.cfm

Premedical Coursework

Course	Req.	Rec.	Lab.	Sems.	Course	Req.	Rec.	Lab.	Sems.
Inorganic Chemistry	•		•	2	Genetics				
Behavioral Sciences					Humanities	•			3
Biochemistry		•		1	Organic Chemistry	•		•	2
Biology	•		•	2	Physics	•		•	2
Biology/Zoology					Psychology				
Calculus		•		1	Social Sciences	•			2
College English	•			2	Anatomy/Physiology			•	1
College Mathematics					Biostatistics			•	1

Selection Factors: 2007 Accepted Applicants

Proportion of Accepted Applicants with Relevant Experience (Data Self-Reported to AMCAS®)		Community Service/Volunteer	66%
		Medically-Related Work	87%
		Research	85%

Shaded bar represents accepted scores ranging from the 10th percentile to the 90th percentile ▪   School Median ●   National Median ●

Overall GPA	2.0	2.1	2.2	2.3	2.4	2.5	2.6	2.7	2.8	2.9	3.0	3.1	3.2	3.3	3.4	3.5	3.6	⦿3.7	3.8	3.9	4.0
Science GPA	2.0	2.1	2.2	2.3	2.4	2.5	2.6	2.7	2.8	2.9	3.0	3.1	3.2	3.3	3.4	3.5	3.6	⦿3.7	3.8	3.9	4.0

MCAT® required: Yes, 96% of 2007 accepted applicants took MCAT®

Verbal Reasoning	3	4	5	6	7	8	9	⑩	⑪	12	13	14	15
Physical Sciences	3	4	5	6	7	8	9	10	⑪	12	13	14	15
Biological Sciences	3	4	5	6	7	8	9	10	⑪	12	13	14	15
Writing Sample			J	K	L	M	N	O	P	ⓆQ	R	S	T

Acceptance & Matriculation Data for 2007–2008 First Year Class

	Resident	Non-Resident	International	Total
Applied	1123	3221	9	4353
Interviewed	255	469	0	724
Deferred	0	3	0	3
Matriculants				
Early Assurance Program	n/a	n/a	n/a	n/a
Early Decision Program	0	0	0	0
Baccalaureate/MD	2	0	0	2
MD/PhD	2	4	0	6
Matriculated	46	55	0	**101**

Applications accepted from International Applicants: No

Matriculant Demographics: 2007–2008 First Year Class

Men: 53   **Women:** 48

Matriculants' Self-Reported Race/Ethnicity

Mexican American	2	Korean	2
Cuban	0	Vietnamese	1
Puerto Rican	1	Other Asian	2
Other Hispanic	1	**Total Asian**	22
Total Hispanic	4	Native American	2
Chinese	10	Black	11
Asian Indian	4	Native Hawaiian	0
Pakistani	2	White	63
Filipino	1	**Unduplicated Number**	
Japanese	2	**of Matriculants**	101

Science and Math Majors: 71%
Matriculants with:
          Baccalaureate degree: 99%
          Graduate degree(s): 13%

Specialty Choice

2003, 2004, 2005 Graduates, Specialty Choice (As reported by program directors to GME Track™)	
Anesthesiology	6%
Emergency Medicine	4%
Family Practice	5%
Internal Medicine	17%
Obstetrics/Gynecology	5%
Orthopaedic Surgery	2%
Pediatrics	11%
Psychiatry	6%
Radiology	4%
Surgery	8%

Financial Information

Source: 2006–2007 LCME I-B survey and 2007–2008 AAMC TSF questionnaire

	Residents	Non-Residents
Total Cost of Attendance	$55,799	$55,799
Tuition and Fees	$38,657	$38,657
Other (includes living expenses)	$16,000	$16,000
Health Insurance (can be waived)	$1,142	$1,142

Average 2007 Graduate Indebtedness: $131,881
% of Enrolled Students Receiving Aid: 91%

Criminal Background Check

This medical school requires a criminal background check prior to matriculation.

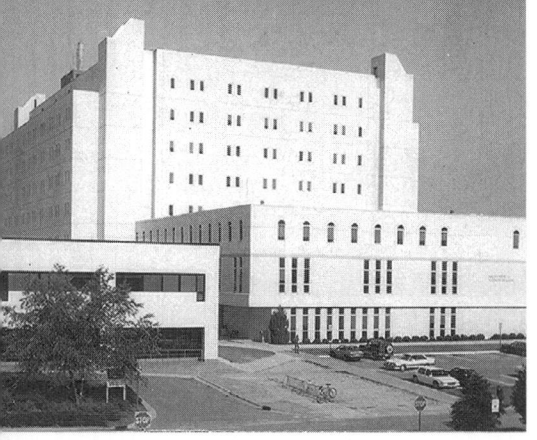

The Brody School of Medicine at East Carolina University

Greenville, North Carolina

Associate Dean, Office of Admissions
The Brody School of Medicine
at East Carolina University
Greenville, North Carolina 27834
T 252 744 2202   **F** 252 744 1926

Admissions www.ecu.edu/bsomadmissions
Main www.ecu.edu/med
Financial www.ecu.edu/bsomstudentaffairs/
FinancialAid/Aid.htm
Email somadmissions@ecu.edu

Public Institution

Dr. Phyllis N. Horns, Interim Dean

*Dr. James G. Peden Jr.,
Associate Dean for Admissions*

*Dr. Virginia D. Hardy, Senior Associate
Dean for Academic Affairs*

*Kelly Lancaster, Director of
Financial Aid and Student Services*

General Information

In 1972, East Carolina University enrolled students in the First-Year Program in Medical Education. The Board of Governors and the State General Assembly authorized the expansion to a degree-granting School of Medicine in 1975, and the first class was enrolled in August 1977. The school's educational facilities are located in the nine-story Brody Medical Sciences Building on the 100-acre Health Sciences Center campus.

Mission Statement

Our mission is threefold: educating primary care physicians, making medical care more readily available to the people of eastern North Carolina, and providing opportunities for disadvantaged students.

Curricular Highlights

Community Service Requirement: Optional.
Research/Thesis Requirement: Optional.

The first year of the four-year curriculum is devoted to the study of the body through courses in anatomy, biochemistry, physiology, microbiology/immunology, and genetics. Courses in clinical skills, the psychosocial basis of medicine, and ethical and social issues in medicine and a primary care preceptorship are also presented. The second-year curriculum is directed toward clinical medicine, with courses including microbiology, pharmacology, pathology, psychiatry (including human sexuality and lifestyle abuse), ethical and social issues, clinical skills, and a primary care preceptorship. The third year is composed of six required clerkships in family medicine, internal medicine, obstetrics and gynecology, pediatrics, psychiatry, and surgery and a two-week clinical elective. The fourth year is composed of 36 weeks of clinical and basic science electives, which must include blocks in primary care, medicine, and surgery. Student performance is evaluated by letter grade, and promotion to the next year's class is recommended to the dean by the Promotions Committee of the respective year.

USMLE

Step 1: Required. Students must record a passing score for promotion.
Step 2: Clinical Skills (CS): Required. Students must record a passing total score to graduate.
Step 2: Clinical Knowledge (CK): Required. Students must record a passing total score to graduate.

Selection Factors

Factors considered in the selection process encompass the social, personal, and intellectual development of each applicant. All available application data are evaluated: MCAT scores; academic performance; comments contained in letters of reference/recommendation; and (for invited applicants) the results of two personal interviews, conducted only at the medical school campus, with two members of the Admissions committee. The Brody School of Medicine at East Carolina University seeks competent students of diverse personalities and backgrounds, and all applicants are evaluated without discrimination based on race, religion, sex, color, national origin, age, or disability. Very strong preference is given to qualified residents of North Carolina. In conjunction with the undergraduate Office of Admissions, the Brody School of Medicine offers an Early Assurance Program for highly qualified high school seniors. Selected scholars enroll in the University and are assured of a spot in the medical school class after receiving their baccalaureate degree (provided certain academic standards are maintained). Qualified North Carolina residents from schools with similar medical curricula may be considered for transfer into the second- or third-year classes, but advanced standing positions are dependent on the very limited number of seats that become available through attrition. Interested students should send letters describing their circumstances to the Office of Admissions for further information.

Financial Aid

Many resources are available for loans and scholarships. A member of the Financial Aid Office meets with every interviewee to provide financial aid information, and assists accepted students who demonstrate need for financial assistance in acquiring funds to meet the costs of their educational and living expenses. Awards are based on need as determined by confidential information supplied by the student. Merit awards, such as the Brody Medical Scholars Program, are also available.

Information about Diversity Programs

Persons from groups underrepresented in medicine who hold residence in North Carolina are encouraged to apply. There is diverse membership on the Admissions Committee, and the Academic Support and Enrichment Center offers a wide range of services to students desiring assistance or guidance.

Campus Information

Setting

The medical school is located in the 100-acre medical district and is adjacent to the primary clinical training site, Pitt County Memorial Hospital. Greenville is a short drive from several beaches, sounds, and other recreational areas.

Enrollment

For 2007, total enrollment was: 293

Special Features

The medical school houses an international robotic surgery training center. A $150 million regional research center for cardiovascular disease, the East Carolina Heart Institute, will be completed in 2008. The NC Legislature has recently approved funding for a dental school.

Housing

There are many apartments, duplexes, and houses near the medical school.

Application Process and Requirements 2009–2010

Primary Application Service: AMCAS
Earliest filing date: June 1, 2008
Latest filing date: November 15, 2008

Secondary Application Required?: Yes
Sent to: All NC applicants
Contact: somadmissions@ecu.edu
Fee: Yes, $60
Fee waiver available: Yes
Earliest filing date: July 1, 2008
Latest filing date: November 15, 2008 or 2 weeks after receipt of AMCAS

Latest MCAT® considered: September 2008
Oldest MCAT® considered: 2005

Early Decision Program
School does have EDP
Applicants notified: October 1, 2008
EDP available for: Residents only

Regular Acceptance Notice
Earliest date: October 15, 2008
Latest date: Varies

Applicant's Response to Acceptance Offer – Maximum Time: Three weeks

Requests for Deferred Entrance Considered: No

Deposit to Hold Place in Class: Yes
Deposit (Resident): $100
Deposit (Non-Resident): $100
Deposit due: With response to acceptance offer
Applied to tuition: Yes
Deposit refundable: Yes
Refundable by: May 15, 2009

Estimated number of new entrants: 76
EDP: 8, special program: n/a

Start Month/Year: August 2009

Interview Format: Two semi-blind interviews by committee members. All interviews are conducted at the medical school.

Other Programs

PREPARATORY PROGRAMS
Postbaccalaureate Program: No
Summer Program: Yes
www.ecu.edu/ascc/SPFD06.htm

COMBINED DEGREE PROGRAMS
Baccalaureate/MD: No
MD/MPH: Yes, www.ecu.edu/mph
MD/MBA: Yes, www.ecu.edu/cs-dhs/med/MD_MBA.cfm
MD/JD: No
MD/PhD: Yes, www.ecu.edu/cs-dhs/med/MD_PhD.cfm

Premedical Coursework

Course	Req.	Rec.	Lab.	Hrs.	Course	Req.	Rec.	Lab.	Hrs.
Inorganic Chemistry	•		•	8	Computer Science				
Behavioral Sciences					Genetics		•		
Biochemistry					Humanities		•		
Biology					Organic Chemistry	•		•	8
Biology/Zoology	•		•	8	Physics	•		•	8
Calculus					Psychology				
College English	•			6	Social Sciences		•		
College Mathematics					Biostatistics		•		

Selection Factors: 2007 Accepted Applicants

Proportion of Accepted Applicants with Relevant Experience (Data Self-Reported to AMCAS®)		
Community Service/Volunteer		79%
Medically-Related Work		92%
Research		74%

Shaded bar represents accepted scores ranging from the 10th percentile to the 90th percentile. School Median ● National Median ●

Overall GPA	2.0	2.1	2.2	2.3	2.4	2.5	2.6	2.7	2.8	2.9	3.0	3.1	3.2	3.3	3.4	(3.5)	3.6	3.7	3.8	3.9	4.0
Science GPA	2.0	2.1	2.2	2.3	2.4	2.5	2.6	2.7	2.8	2.9	3.0	3.1	3.2	3.3	3.4	(3.5)	3.6	3.7	3.8	3.9	4.0

MCAT® required: Yes, 97% of 2007 accepted applicants took MCAT®

Verbal Reasoning	3	4	5	6	7	8	9	(10)	11	12	13	14	15
Physical Sciences	3	4	5	6	7	8	(9)	10	(11)	12	13	14	15
Biological Sciences	3	4	5	6	7	8	9	(10)	(11)	12	13	14	15
Writing Sample			J	K	L	M	N	(O)	P	(Q)	R	S	T

Acceptance & Matriculation Data for 2007–2008 First Year Class

	Resident	Non-Resident	International	Total
Applied	815	0	0	815
Interviewed	450	0	0	450
Deferred	0	0	0	0
Matriculants				
Early Assurance Program	3	0	0	3
Early Decision Program	12	0	0	12
Baccalaureate/MD	n/a	n/a	n/a	n/a
MD/PhD	0	0	0	0
Matriculated	73	0	0	**73**

Applications accepted from International Applicants: No

Matriculant Demographics: 2007–2008 First Year Class

Men: 36 **Women:** 37

Matriculants' Self-Reported Race/Ethnicity

Mexican American	0	Korean	1
Cuban	0	Vietnamese	2
Puerto Rican	0	Other Asian	1
Other Hispanic	4	Total Asian	11
Total Hispanic	4	Native American	2
Chinese	2	Black	9
Asian Indian	3	Native Hawaiian	0
Pakistani	1	White	53
Filipino	0	Unduplicated Number	
Japanese	1	of Matriculants	73

Science and Math Majors: 68%
Matriculants with:
    Baccalaureate degree: 99%
    Graduate degree(s): 22%

Specialty Choice

2003, 2004, 2005 Graduates, Specialty Choice (As reported by program directors to GME Track™)	
Anesthesiology	1%
Emergency Medicine	7%
Family Practice	21%
Internal Medicine	17%
Obstetrics/Gynecology	5%
Orthopaedic Surgery	3%
Pediatrics	13%
Psychiatry	2%
Radiology	1%
Surgery	5%

Financial Information

Source: 2006–2007 LCME I-B survey and 2007–2008 AAMC TSF questionnaire

	Residents	Non-Residents
Total Cost of Attendance	$27,911	$52,901
Tuition and Fees	$9,066	$34,056
Other (includes living expenses)	$17,045	$17,045
Health Insurance (can be waived)	$1,800	$1,800

Average 2007 Graduate Indebtedness: $81,212
% of Enrolled Students Receiving Aid: 86%

Criminal Background Check

This medical school requires a criminal background check prior to matriculation.

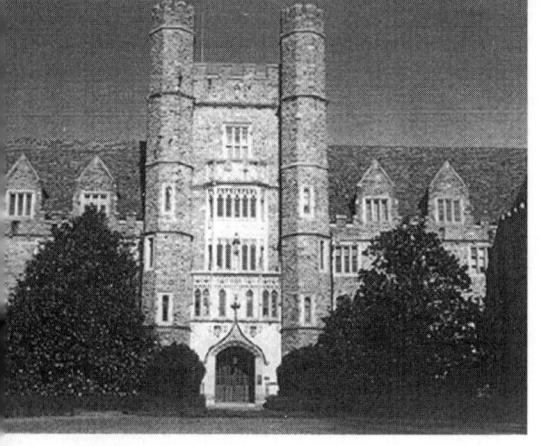

Duke University School of Medicine
Durham, North Carolina

Committee on Admissions
Duke University School of Medicine
DUMC 3710
Durham, North Carolina 27710
T 919 684 2985 F 919 684 8893

Admissions http://dukemed.duke.edu/Admissions
FinancialAid/index.cfm?method=HowToApply
Main http://dukemed.duke.edu
Financial http://dukemed.duke.edu/Admissions
FinancialAid/index.cfm?method=FinancialAid
Email medadm@mc.duke.edu

Private Institution

Dr. Nancy Andrews, Dean

Dr. Brenda E. Armstrong, Associate Dean and Director of Admissions

Dr. Delbert R. Wigfall, Associate Dean, Director, Multicultural Resource Center

Stacey R. McCorison, Associate Dean of Medical Education, Director of Financial Aid and Registrar

Richard S. Wallace, Associate Director of Admissions

General Information

Duke University Health System is a world-class health care network dedicated to outstanding patient care, innovative medical education and biomedical research.

Mission Statement

DukeMed is a community of scholars devoted to understanding the causes, prevention and treatment of human disease. Our missions are to train scholars and leaders across a broad spectrum of careers in medicine and are undertaken by students from diverse communities committed to the highest of academic goals: the generation, conservation, and dissemination of knowledge leading to the prevention and eradication of human disease throughout the world through innovative curricula, outstanding resources in education, clinical care, and basic and clinical research.

Curricular Highlights

Community Service Requirement: Optional.
Research/Thesis Requirement: Required. Required to complete the third year of medical school.

The curriculum stimulates rapid expansion of medical knowledge. First-year students study basic science principles alongside the first of two-years' introduction to clinical medicine. The second year is the clinical clerkship year. The third and fourth years are elective including half basic science/half clinical coursework with opportunities for mentored research. Students also elect from a number of dual-degree programs which begin during the

third year. The fourth year is an advanced clinical clerkship year to prepare for post-graduate study. The MST Program provides MD/Ph.D degrees over a six-to-seven-year period. It is expected that candidates for this combined degree plan will have careers in academic medicine.

USMLE
Step 1: Required. Students must only record a score.
Step 2: Clinical Skills (CS): Required. Students must only record a score.
Step 2: Clinical Knowledge (CK): Required. Students must only record a score.

Selection Factors

Selection is based evidence of outstanding academic and experiential preparation, including but not limited to outstanding curricular/extracurricular achievement, evidence of leadership, participation in volunteer/community service activities, excellent communications skills, supportive letters of recommendations from teachers/advisors, strong MCAT® scores, and the applicant's interview evaluation. Successful students have high GPAs/MCAT® scores, demonstrated leadership on campus and in their respective communities. Duke Med does not discriminate on the basis of sex, race, religion, sexual orientation, creed, age, handicap, or national origin.

Financial Aid

The Office of Financial Aid requires the Need Access, the federal government's FAFSA obtained via Internet. Students applying for only Federal Stafford Loans only complete the FAFSA. Students are encouraged to submit the applications as soon as possible after acceptance. Prior year tax returns should be submitted. Accepted students receive award notices once all forms are received. Students with demonstrated need applying for institutional funds will receive approximately 55% Stafford and/or Duke loans and 45% institutional grants. 85% of currently enrolled medical students receive some type of financial aid. Admissions is need-blind. Seven Dean's Tuition Scholarships are awarded to academically excellent students from groups underrepresented in

medicine. Financially needy/disadvantaged students and students from groups underrepresented in medicine selected for the North Carolina Board of Governor's Medical Scholarship will receive full tuition, fees, and a stipend. Students who enter the Medical Scientist Training Program receive full tuition, fees, and a stipend.

Information about Diversity Programs

The Multicultural Resource Center is a resource-intensive repository providing opportunities for diverse learning experiences for all students and targeted pipeline programs for women, URM/disadvantaged, and students interested in biomedical research beginning as early as elementary school through undergraduate and graduate education. MRC integrates cross-cultural issues in medicine to the medical school curriculum.

Campus Information

Setting

DukeMed is physically contiguous with the main campus of Duke University. Durham is one of three communities part of the Research Triangle Park, one of the nation's most prolific research centers and one rich in cultural, educational, and recreational opportunities.

Enrollment

For 2007, total enrollment was: 408

Special Features

DukeMed is consistently ranked among the top ten academic health centers in the country and has a national and international reputation for innovation and excellence.

Housing

Students choose from a number of affordable on- and off-campus housing units. Housing costs are extremely affordable.

Satellite Campuses/Facilities

Students are based throughout the Duke Health System at Duke University Hospital, the VA Hospital, Durham Regional Hospital, Lennox Baker Children's Hospital, Duke Children's Hospital, and more than 70 outpatient clinics located in Durham, Raleigh, Chapel Hill and surrounding communities.

Application Process and Requirements 2009–2010

Primary Application Service: AMCAS
Earliest filing date: June 1, 2008
Latest filing date: November 15, 2008

Secondary Application Required?: Yes
Sent to: All applicants
URL: http://dukemed.duke.edu
Fee: Yes, $80
Fee waiver available: Yes
Earliest filing date: Once AMCAS has verified application.
Latest filing date: December 1, 2008

Latest MCAT® considered: September 2008
Oldest MCAT® considered: 2005

Early Decision Program
School does not have EDP
Applicants notified: n/a
EDP available for: n/a

Regular Acceptance Notice
Earliest date: March 1, 2009
Latest date: Until class is full

Applicant's Response to Acceptance Offer – Maximum Time: Two weeks

Requests for Deferred Entrance Considered: Yes

Deposit to Hold Place in Class: Yes
Deposit (Resident): $100
Deposit (Non-Resident): $100
Deposit due: May 15, 2009
Applied to tuition: Yes
Deposit refundable: Yes
Refundable by: May 15, 2009

Estimated number of new entrants: 100
EDP: n/a, special program: n/a

Start Month/Year: August 3, 2009

Interview Format: One-on-one interviews on campus. Regional interviews are available.

Other Programs

PREPARATORY PROGRAMS
Postbaccalaureate Program: No
Summer Program: Yes, www.smdep.org
Maureen Cullins, (919) 684-5882 mcullins@duke.edu

COMBINED DEGREE PROGRAMS
Baccalaureate/MD: No
MD/MPH: Yes,
http://dukemed.duke.edu
MD/MBA: Yes,
http://dukemed.duke.edu
MD/JD: Yes,
http://dukemed.duke.edu
MD/PhD: Yes,
http://dukemed.duke.edu

Premedical Coursework

Course	Req.	Rec.	Lab.	Sems.
Inorganic Chemistry	•		•	2
Behavioral Sciences				
Biochemistry		•		1
Biology	•		•	1
Biology/Zoology	•			1
Calculus	•			1
College English	•			2
College Mathematics	•			1
Computer Science				

Course	Req.	Rec.	Lab.	Sems.
Genetics		•		1
Humanities				
Organic Chemistry	•		•	2
Physics	•		•	2
Psychology				
Social Sciences				
Statistics/Biostatistics		•		1
Spanish		•		1
Cell Biology		•		1

Selection Factors: 2007 Accepted Applicants

Proportion of Accepted Applicants with Relevant Experience (Data Self-Reported to AMCAS)		
Community Service/Volunteer		68%
Medically-Related Work		87%
Research		92%

Shaded bar represents accepted scores ranging from the 10th percentile to the 90th percentile. School Median ● National Median ●

Overall GPA	2.0	2.1	2.2	2.3	2.4	2.5	2.6	2.7	2.8	2.9	3.0	3.1	3.2	3.3	3.4	3.5	3.6	3.7	(3.8)	3.9	4.0
Science GPA	2.0	2.1	2.2	2.3	2.4	2.5	2.6	2.7	2.8	2.9	3.0	3.1	3.2	3.3	3.4	3.5	3.6	3.7	(3.8)	3.9	4.0

MCAT® required: Yes, 100% of 2007 accepted applicants took MCAT®

Verbal Reasoning	3	4	5	6	7	8	9	(10)	(11)	12	13	14	15
Physical Sciences	3	4	5	6	7	8	9	10	(11)	12	(13)	14	15
Biological Sciences	3	4	5	6	7	8	9	10	(11)	12	(13)	14	15
Writing Sample			J	K	L	M	N	O	P	(Q)	R	S	T

Acceptance & Matriculation Data for 2007–2008 First Year Class

	Resident	Non-Resident	International	Total
Applied	398	4611	300	5309
Interviewed	69	692	19	780
Deferred	1	2	1	4
Matriculants				
Early Assurance Program	0	0	0	0
Early Decision Program	0	0	0	0
Baccalaureate/MD	n/a	n/a	n/a	n/a
MD/PhD	11	121	0	132
Matriculated	16	80	4	**100**

Applications accepted from International Applicants: Yes

Specialty Choice

2003, 2004, 2005 Graduates, Specialty Choice (As reported by program directors to GME Track™)	
Anesthesiology	2%
Emergency Medicine	5%
Family Practice	3%
Internal Medicine	23%
Obstetrics/Gynecology	3%
Orthopaedic Surgery	6%
Pediatrics	7%
Psychiatry	2%
Radiology	10%
Surgery	6%

Matriculant Demographics: 2007–2008 First Year Class

Men: 51   **Women:** 49

Matriculants' Self-Reported Race/Ethnicity

Mexican American	0	Korean	4
Cuban	2	Vietnamese	1
Puerto Rican	0	Other Asian	1
Other Hispanic	0	Total Asian	24
Total Hispanic	2	Native American	1
Chinese	11	Black	22
Asian Indian	6	Native Hawaiian	0
Pakistani	0	White	51
Filipino	1	Unduplicated Number	
Japanese	0	of Matriculants	100

Science and Math Majors: 77%
Matriculants with:
    Baccalaureate degree: 100%
    Graduate degree(s): 11%

Financial Information

Source: 2006–2007 LCME I-B survey and 2007–2008 AAMC TSF questionnaire

	Residents	Non-Residents
Total Cost of Attendance	$64,028	$64,028
Tuition and Fees	$41,839	$41,839
Other (includes living expenses)	$20,625	$20,625
Health Insurance (can be waived)	$1,564	$1,564

Average 2007 Graduate Indebtedness: $93,976
% of Enrolled Students Receiving Aid: 75%

Criminal Background Check

This medical school requires a criminal background check prior to matriculation.

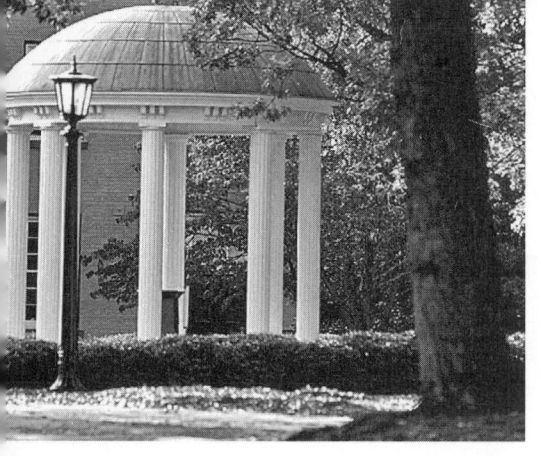

University of North Carolina at Chapel Hill School of Medicine

Chapel Hill, North Carolina

Office of Admissions
CB #9500 1001 Bondurant Hall, First Floor
University of North Carolina at Chapel Hill
School of Medicine
Chapel Hill, North Carolina 27599-9500
T 919 962 8331   F 919 966 9930

Admissions www.med.unc.edu/admit
Main www.med.unc.edu
Financial www.med.unc.edu/md/financial-aid
Email Admis_UNC-SOM@listserv.med.unc.edu

Public Institution

Dr. William L. Roper, Dean,
Vice Chancellor for Medical Affairs

Dr. Axalla J. Hoole,
Associate Dean for Admissions

Sheila M. Graham-McDonald,
Financial Aid Officer

Larry D. Keith, Assistant Dean for Admissions

General Information

The School of Medicine was established in 1879 and expanded to a four-year school in 1952. Other schools of health sciences are adjacent, allowing easy interaction and collaboration. The School of Medicine is continuing a major expansion and renovation of teaching and clinical facilities. Among other projects, three hospitals, Women's, Children's, and Neuroscience recently have been completed, and the North Carolina Cancer Hospital will be completed in 2009. Additional educational and clinical facilities are available throughout the State in Area Health Education Centers (AHEC) established in 1972 to provide clinical experiences and educational opportunities in community settings.

Mission Statement

The School of Medicine of the University of North Carolina at Chapel Hill exists to educate students and professionals of the health and biomedical sciences, to conduct scholarly investigation in biomedical, behavioral, and social sciences, and to render service to the people and institutions of the state, the region, the nation, and, as appropriate, throughout the world.

Curricular Highlights

Community Service Requirement: Optional.
Research/Thesis Requirement: Optional.

The curriculum offers an education that reflects our mission. The first year presents courses in basic biomedical science. Presentation is through a compilation of lectures, problem and case based small-group sessions, and electronic resource materials. Introduction to the profession of medicine begins in the first week of the first year through Introduction to Clinical Medicine (ICM). ICM provides a two-year continuum of weekly small-group seminars and experience with simulated and real patients. A second weekly first year seminar, Medicine and Society, focuses on health care issues. The second year presents the pathophysiology of disease in organ-based courses. Clinical skills development continues through the second year of ICM, and issues in social aspects of health care are presented through selectives offered by the Department of Social Medicine. The third and fourth year present a 2-year continuum of instruction in clinical medicine. Core clinical rotations, which are primarily completed in the third year, include internal medicine, surgery, family medicine, obstetrics and gynecology, pediatrics, and psychiatry. Some rotations are at AHEC sites. The advanced clinical curriculum of the 4th year builds more independence and increased responsibility into the base of the core. Students are assisted in choosing their interest in post graduate training through counseling and a broad choice of electives. Students conduct research with faculty mentorship support by school or grant funding, or through selection to the Distinguished Medical Scholars or Doris Duke programs (a year of funded study and research). Students pursue interests in rural and community medicine, public policy, or public health through Social Medicine selectives, fourth year Advance Practice Selectives, and Community Health Projects. The grading system is honors/pass/fail.

USMLE

Step 1: Required. Students must record a passing score for promotion.
Step 2: Clinical Skills (CS): Required. Students must only record a score.
Step 2: Clinical Knowledge (CK): Required. Students must record a passing total score to graduate.

Selection Factors

The Committee on Admissions evaluates the qualifications of all applicants to select those with the greatest potential for accomplishment in one of the many careers open to medical graduates. Preference is given to North Carolina residents. UNC does not discriminate on the basis of race, national origin, religion, sex, age, or handicap. In making its final selections from the group of qualified applicants, the committee considers evidence of each candidate's motivation, maturity, leadership, integrity, and a variety of other personal qualifications and accomplishments in addition to the scholastic record. All information available about each applicant is considered without assigning priority to any single factor. No special admission tracks or quotas are applied among applicants. Undergraduate major is not an important consideration, but excellence in the chosen field is expected. Re-applications are compared to those previously submitted to determine if there is sufficient evidence to warrant an interview.

Financial Aid

Grants, school-based and Stafford loans are available to students with financial need. Awards are based on information obtained from the Free Application for Federal Student Aid (FAFSA) submitted by the student. A few scholarships are awarded for academic achievement and promise. Economically or environmentally disadvantaged state residents are eligible to apply to the Board of Governors Medical Scholarship-Loan Program. For more information call (919) 962-6118.

Information about Diversity Programs

The Medical Education Development Program acquaints disadvantaged students with the medical school curriculum and faculty. Academic counseling, including tutorial programs, the Learning and Assessment Laboratory, and other resources, are available. Summer review programs are also available.

Campus Information

Enrollment

For 2007, total enrollment was: 736

Application Process and Requirements 2009–2010

Primary Application Service: AMCAS
Earliest filing date: June 1, 2008
Latest filing date: November 15, 2008

Secondary Application Required?: Yes
Sent to: Screened applicants
URL: n/a
Fee: Yes, $68
Fee waiver available: Yes
Earliest filing date: August 1, 2008
Latest filing date: January 1, 2009

Latest MCAT® considered: September 2008
Oldest MCAT® considered: 2004

Early Decision Program
School does have EDP
Applicants notified: October 1, 2008
EDP available for: Both Residents and Non-Residents

Regular Acceptance Notice
Earliest date: October 15, 2008
Latest date: Varies

Applicant's Response to Acceptance Offer – Maximum Time: Three weeks

Requests for Deferred Entrance Considered: Yes

Deposit to Hold Place in Class: Yes
Deposit (Resident): $100
Deposit (Non-Resident): $100
Deposit due: With response to acceptance offer
Applied to tuition: Yes
Deposit refundable: Yes
Refundable by: May 15, 2009

Estimated number of new entrants: 160
EDP: 7, special program: n/a

Start Month/Year: August 2009

Interview Format: One-on-one, open file. Regional interviews are not available.

Other Programs

PREPARATORY PROGRAMS
Postbaccalaureate Program: No
Summer Program: No

COMBINED DEGREE PROGRAMS
Baccalaureate/MD: No
MD/MPH: Yes,
Available after completion of first two years.
MD/MBA: No
MD/JD: No
MD/PhD: Yes, www.med.unc.edu/mdphd
Elizabeth Garman, (919) 843-6507
Elizabeth_Garman@med.unc.edu

Premedical Coursework

Course	Req.	Rec.	Lab.	Hrs.	Course	Req.	Rec.	Lab.	Hrs.
Inorganic Chemistry	•		•	8	Computer Science				
Behavioral Sciences					Genetics		•		
Biochemistry		•			Humanities		•		
Biology	•		•	7	Organic Chemistry	•		•	8
Biology/Zoology					Physics	•		•	8
Calculus					Psychology				
College English	•			6	Social Sciences		•		
College Mathematics					Other		•		

Selection Factors: 2007 Accepted Applicants

Proportion of Accepted Applicants with Relevant Experience (Data Self-Reported to AMCAS®)		
Community Service/Volunteer		74%
Medically-Related Work		85%
Research		80%

Shaded bar represents accepted scores ranging from the 10th percentile to the 90th percentile. **School Median** ● **National Median** ●

Overall GPA	2.0	2.1	2.2	2.3	2.4	2.5	2.6	2.7	2.8	2.9	3.0	3.1	3.2	3.3	3.4	3.5	3.6	3.7	(3.8)	3.9	4.0
Science GPA	2.0	2.1	2.2	2.3	2.4	2.5	2.6	2.7	2.8	2.9	3.0	3.1	3.2	3.3	3.4	3.5	3.6	(3.7)	3.8	3.9	4.0

MCAT® required: Yes, 100% of 2007 accepted applicants took MCAT®

Verbal Reasoning	3	4	5	6	7	8	9	(10)	(11)	12	13	14	15
Physical Sciences	3	4	5	6	7	8	9	10	(11)	12	13	14	15
Biological Sciences	3	4	5	6	7	8	9	10	(11)	12	13	14	15
Writing Sample				J	K	L	M	N	O	P	(Q)	R	S	T

Acceptance & Matriculation Data for 2007–2008 First Year Class

	Resident	Non-Resident	International	Total
Applied	886	2949	130	3965
Interviewed	458	98	25	581
Deferred	9	0	0	9
Matriculants				
Early Assurance Program	n/a	n/a	n/a	n/a
Early Decision Program	5	1	0	6
Baccalaureate/MD	n/a	n/a	n/a	n/a
MD/PhD	3	4	0	7
Matriculated	136	25	0	**161**

Applications accepted from International Applicants: Yes

Specialty Choice

2003, 2004, 2005 Graduates, Specialty Choice (As reported by program directors to GME Track™)	
Anesthesiology	7%
Emergency Medicine	8%
Family Practice	12%
Internal Medicine	18%
Obstetrics/Gynecology	5%
Orthopaedic Surgery	3%
Pediatrics	12%
Psychiatry	5%
Radiology	3%
Surgery	4%

Matriculant Demographics: 2007–2008 First Year Class

Men: 79   **Women:** 82

Matriculants' Self-Reported Race/Ethnicity

Mexican American	1	**Korean**	0
Cuban	0	**Vietnamese**	0
Puerto Rican	1	**Other Asian**	1
Other Hispanic	1	**Total Asian**	26
Total Hispanic	3	**Native American**	1
Chinese	8	**Black**	20
Asian Indian	16	**Native Hawaiian**	0
Pakistani	1	**White**	118
Filipino	0	**Unduplicated Number**	
Japanese	0	**of Matriculants**	161

Science and Math Majors: 77%
Matriculants with:
    Baccalaureate degree: 100%
    Graduate degree(s): 10%

Financial Information

Source: 2006–2007 LCME I-B survey and 2007–2008 AAMC TSF questionnaire

	Residents	Non-Residents
Total Cost of Attendance	$39,016	$62,682
Tuition and Fees	$11,964	$35,630
Other (includes living expenses)	$25,339	$25,339
Health Insurance (can be waived)	$1,713	$1,713

Average 2007 Graduate Indebtedness: $81,985
% of Enrolled Students Receiving Aid: 84%

Criminal Background Check

This medical school requires a criminal background check prior to matriculation.

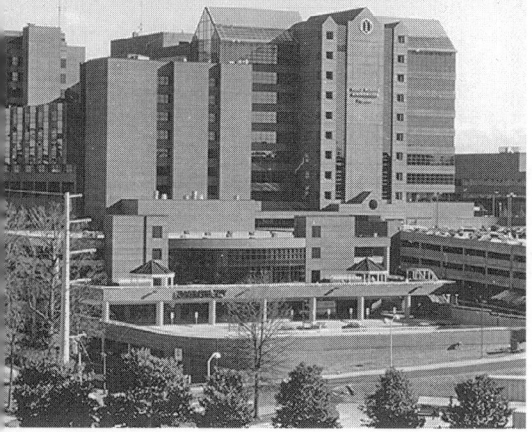

Wake Forest University School of Medicine
Winston-Salem, North Carolina

Office of Medical School Admissions
Wake Forest University School of Medicine
Medical Center Boulevard
Winston-Salem, North Carolina 27157-1090
T 336 716 4264   **F** 336 716 9593

Admissions www1.wfubmc.edu/MDProgram/Admissions
Main www.wfubmc.edu/school
Financial www1.wfubmc.edu/FinancialAid
Email medadmit@wfubmc.edu

Private Institution

Dr. William B. Applegate, Interim President and Dean

Dr. Lewis H. Nelson III, Associate Dean for Admissions

Dr. Brenda Latham-Sadler, Assistant Dean, Director Diversity Development Initiatives

Melissa Stevens, Financial Aid Director

Irene B. Tise, Coordinator, Student Admissions

General Information

The School of Medicine was established in 1902 at Wake Forest, North Carolina, and, of the existing 166 medical schools, it was one of 11 that required college preparation. Patient care, research, education, and community service remain the fourfold mission of the school as part of Wake Forest University. The name of the medical school was changed from The Bowman Gray School of Medicine to Wake Forest University School of Medicine, the Bowman Gray Campus, in 1997. The main teaching hospital of the medical school is the 880-bed North Carolina Baptist Hospital. Affiliated institutions include the 896-bed Forsyth Memorial Hospital, the Downtown Health Plaza of Baptist Hospital, and Northwest Area Health Education Center.

Mission Statement

The Medical Center is committed to serving society by providing a superior education; by rendering exemplary and efficient patient care; by fostering the discovery and application of new knowledge through research; and to improve the health and well-being of the nation.

Curricular Highlights

Community Service Requirement: Required.
Research/Thesis Requirement: Optional.

WFUSM provides excellence in teaching in a collegial atmosphere. The curriculum is organized to meet the seven goals of the undergraduate medical education program: self-directed learning and life-long learning skills, core biomedical science know-ledge, clinical skills, problem-solving/clinical-reasoning skills, interviewing and communication skills, information management skills, and professional attitudes and behavior. Students study the basic and clinical sciences in an integrated fashion throughout the four-year curriculum utilizing small-group problem-based learning, lectures, and labs which are closely integrated through the computer network. Early community-based clinical experience, as well as a focus on population health, are hallmarks of the curriculum. Professionalism issues are addressed longitudinally across the curriculum in formats designed to provide students with a clear understanding of the role and responsibilities of physicians within society. Information technology is integrated into the curriculum.

USMLE

Step 1: Required. Students must record a passing score for promotion.
Step 2: Clinical Skills (CS): Required. Students must record a passing total score to graduate.
Step 2: Clinical Knowledge (CK): Required. Students must record a passing total score to graduate.

Selection Factors

Candidates are selected on the basis of the quality of their academic records, MCAT® scores, and general qualifications. There are no restrictions because of race, creed, sex, religion, age, physical disadvantages, marital status, or national origin. The Committee on Admissions (CoA) and/or the Associate Dean for Admissions evaluate each application. Secondary applications are selectively sent and all other applicants notified of their status. Applicants who have completed secondaries are considered for local interviews. The School of Medicine may be able to accept an application for transfer from a student who is currently enrolled, and in good standing, in a medical school accredited by the Liaison Committee on Medical Education and who meets the prerequisite requirements. Early assurance of a place in medical school is offered to rising juniors who meet certain stringent requirements in an Early Assurance Program (EAP). More detailed information can be found on the Web site or by inquiry to the admissions office.

Financial Aid

Loans and scholarships are awarded to qualified applicants on the basis of financial need and academic standing. Applicants must complete required application forms prior to the April 1 deadline. Students receive a significant amount of their funding from federal student loan programs. Students should not work part-time because of the demands of medical study.

Information about Diversity Programs

The Office of Student Services/Diversity and Development Initiatives actively recruits students from groups underrepresented in medicine and has developed programs for academic enrichment, academic reinforcement, tutorial, and counseling services for enrolled students. Address inquiries to the Office of Diversity and Development Initiatives.

Campus Information
Setting

The school is located in a stable neighborhood near the heart of Winston-Salem, adjacent to hospital and medical facilities.

Enrollment

For 2007, total enrollment was: 441

Special Features

The Wake Forest University Health Sciences and the NC Baptist Hospital-associated medical center has more than 1,000 research studies and clinical trials underway, is home to NC's only Gamma Knife, and is establishing a 200 acre downtown research campus in biotechnology. One of the first tenants on the downtown campus is The Institute for Regenerative Medicine, where staff are working to grow 20 different organs and tissue types. The Anatomical Resource Clinical Training Center is a newly designed multidisciplinary learning center providing computational resources and both CT and MRI data acquired from actual cadavers dissected.

Housing

Available in the community surrounding the medical center. Listings are on Web site.

Application Process and Requirements 2009–2010

Primary Application Service: AMCAS
Earliest filing date: June 1, 2008
Latest filing date: November 1, 2008

Secondary Application Required?: Yes
Sent to: Screened applicants
Email: medadmit@wfubmc.edu
Fee: Yes, $55
Fee waiver available: Yes
Earliest filing date: July 15, 2008
Latest filing date: January 15, 2009

Latest MCAT® considered: September 2008
Oldest MCAT® considered: 2005

Early Decision Program
School does have EDP
Applicants notified: October 1, 2008
EDP available for: Both Residents
and Non-Residents

Regular Acceptance Notice
Earliest date: October 15, 2008
Latest date: Until class is full

**Applicant's Response to Acceptance
Offer – Maximum Time:** Two weeks

**Requests for Deferred
Entrance Considered:** Yes

Deposit to Hold Place in Class: Yes
Deposit (Resident): $100
Deposit (Non-Resident): $100
Deposit due: With response to acceptance offer
Applied to tuition: Yes
Deposit refundable: Yes
Refundable by: May 1, 2009

Estimated number of new entrants: 120
EDP: 2, special program: n/a

Start Month/Year: July 27, 2009

Interview Format: Three individual
20-minute interviews with faculty.
Regional interviews are not available.

Other Programs
PREPARATORY PROGRAMS
Postbaccalaureate Program: Yes
www1.wfubmc.edu/Minority+Programs
Summer Program: No
Two Week Pre-Matriculation Program:
medadmit@wfubmc.edu
MD/MS in Health Science Research
www1.wfubmc.edu/MDProgram/Admissions/
Joint+Degree.htm
COMBINED DEGREE PROGRAMS
Baccalaureate/MD: No
MD/MPH: No
MD/MBA: Yes,
www.mba.wfu.edu/default.aspx?id=141
MD/JD: No
MD/PhD: Yes,
www1.wfubmc.edu/MDProgram/Admissions/
Joint+Degree.htm

Premedical Coursework

Course	Req.	Rec.	Lab.	Hrs.	Course	Req.	Rec.	Lab.	Hrs.
Inorganic Chemistry	•			8	Computer Science				
Behavioral Sciences					Genetics				
Biochemistry					Humanities				
Biology	•			8	Organic Chemistry	•			8
Biology/Zoology					Physics	•			8
Calculus					Psychology				
College English					Social Sciences				
College Mathematics					Other				

Selection Factors: 2007 Accepted Applicants

Proportion of Accepted Applicants with Relevant Experience (Data Self-Reported to AMCAS®)		
Community Service/Volunteer		73%
Medically-Related Work		89%
Research		81%

Shaded bar represents accepted scores ranging from the 10th percentile to the 90th percentile. School Median ● National Median ●

Overall GPA	2.0	2.1	2.2	2.3	2.4	2.5	2.6	2.7	2.8	2.9	3.0	3.1	3.2	3.3	3.4	3.5	3.6	(3.7)	3.8 3.9 4.0
Science GPA	2.0	2.1	2.2	2.3	2.4	2.5	2.6	2.7	2.8	2.9	3.0	3.1	3.2	3.3	3.4	3.5	3.6	(3.7)	3.8 3.9 4.0

MCAT® required: Yes, 94% of 2007 accepted applicants took MCAT®

Verbal Reasoning	3	4	5	6	7	8	9	(10)	(11)	12	13	14	15
Physical Sciences	3	4	5	6	7	8	9	10	(11)	12	13	14	15
Biological Sciences	3	4	5	6	7	8	9	10	(11)	12	13	14	15
Writing Sample					J	K	L	M	N	O	(P)	(Q)	R	S	T

Acceptance & Matriculation Data for 2007–2008 First Year Class

	Resident	Non-Resident	International	Total
Applied	688	6392	405	7485
Interviewed	141	357	3	501
Deferred	2	5	1	8
Matriculants				
Early Assurance Program	2	8	0	10
Early Decision Program	0	0	0	0
Baccalaureate/MD	n/a	n/a	n/a	n/a
MD/PhD	0	2	0	2
Matriculated	47	70	3	**120**

Applications accepted from International Applicants: Yes

Specialty Choice

2003, 2004, 2005 Graduates, Specialty Choice (As reported by program directors to GME Track™)	
Anesthesiology	11%
Emergency Medicine	8%
Family Practice	10%
Internal Medicine	14%
Obstetrics/Gynecology	4%
Orthopaedic Surgery	2%
Pediatrics	10%
Psychiatry	3%
Radiology	5%
Surgery	8%

Matriculant Demographics: 2007–2008 First Year Class

Men: 61 **Women:** 59

Matriculants' Self-Reported Race/Ethnicity

Mexican American	3	Korean	1
Cuban	0	Vietnamese	0
Puerto Rican	1	Other Asian	4
Other Hispanic	1	Total Asian	16
Total Hispanic	5	Native American	1
Chinese	3	Black	9
Asian Indian	6	Native Hawaiian	0
Pakistani	2	White	90
Filipino	0	Unduplicated Number	
Japanese	1	of Matriculants	120

Science and Math Majors: 82%
Matriculants with:
   Baccalaureate degree: 100%
   Graduate degree(s): 8%

Financial Information
Source: 2006–2007 LCME I-B survey
and 2007–2008 AAMC TSF questionnaire

	Residents	Non-Residents
Total Cost of Attendance	$56,172	$56,172
Tuition and Fees	$37,134	$37,134
Other (includes living expenses)	$16,686	$16,686
Health Insurance (can be waived)	$2,352	$2,352

Average 2007 Graduate Indebtedness: $138,553
% of Enrolled Students Receiving Aid: 91%

Criminal Background Check

This medical school requires a criminal background check
prior to matriculation.

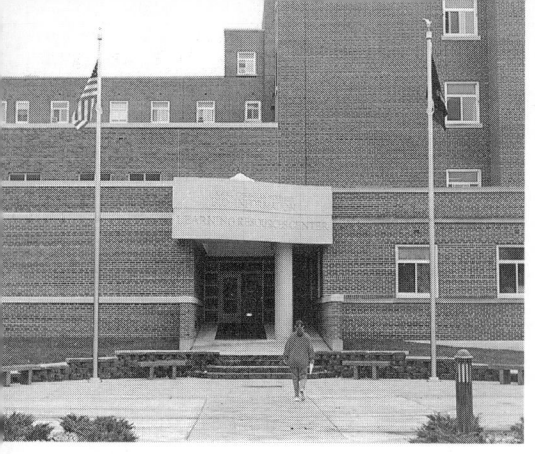

University of North Dakota
School of Medicine and Health Sciences
Grand Forks, North Dakota

Secretary, Committee on Admissions
University of North Dakota
School of Medicine and Health Sciences
501 North Columbia Road, Stop 9037
Grand Forks, North Dakota 58202-9037
T 701 777 4221   **F** 701 777 4942

Admissions http://smhs.med.und.nodak.edu/
UNDSMHS/admissions.html
Main www.med.und.nodak.edu
Financial www.med.und.edu/depts/saff/brochure.htm
Email jdheit@medicine.nodak.edu

Public Institution

Dr. H. David Wilson, Dean

Judy L. DeMers, Associate Dean, Student Affairs and Admissions

Eugene DeLorme, Director, INMED Program

Sandra K. Elshaug, Financial Aid Administrator

General Information

The School of Medicine was established in 1905 as a basic science public medical school. In 1973, legislative action created an expanded curriculum and, in 1981, a full four-year medical education program was instituted in the state. The school is university-based and community-integrated.

Mission Statement

The mission of the University of North Dakota School of Medicine and Health Sciences is to educate and prepare physicians, medical scientists, and other health professionals for service to North Dakota and the nation, and to advance medical and biomedical knowledge through research.

Curricular Highlights

Community Service Requirement: Optional. A variety of activities is available.
Research/Thesis Requirement: Required during third year.

The School of Medicine's renewed curriculum was initiated during the 1998-99 academic year. Utilizing a "patient-centered learning" (PCL) approach, the number of lecture hours was reduced significantly, and greater emphasis was placed on small-group teaching and learning, active student participation, and early clinical experience. The curriculum is integrated across disciplines, consisting of four 10-week blocks of instruction during each of the first two years. Students either complete six 8-week clerkships in year 3 or they participate in the ROME (Rural Opportunities in Medical Education) Program, completing 7 months of clinical experience in a rural community. The school emphasizes the training of primary care physicians, but also offers a MD-PhD program.

USMLE

Step 1: Required. Students must record a passing score for graduation, but not promotion.
Step 2: Clinical Skills (CS): Required. Students must record a passing total score to graduate.
Step 2: Clinical Knowledge (CK): Required. Students must record a passing total score to graduate.

Selection Factors

A student must maintain a GPA of 3.0 or better to be considered for admission. Selection is based upon the scholastic record, letters of recommendation, MCAT® scores, and a personal interview. Interviews are conducted only at the medical school. In addition to high academic achievement, selection is based on a number of factors, including the demonstration of motivation and commitment to a medical career, empathy, compassion in interpersonal relationships, problem-solving, and the ability to work well in small groups. Qualified North Dakota residents are given preference in admission. The only exceptions include a limited number of Minnesota residents or admission through WICHE participation. Only persons who are U.S. citizens or legal permanent residents of the United States are eligible for consideration for admission. The school participates in the Professional Student Exchange Program administered by WICHE, under which legal residents of western states without a medical school may receive preference in admission. WICHE students who are certified and supported by their home state pay resident tuition. The school does not utilize AMCAS. Applications are ranked based on a combination of state of residency, grade-point average, and MCAT® scores. The school is unable to accept transfer students from other medical schools except in very unique circumstances.

Financial Aid

The financial resources of applicants are not considered in the selection process. Immediately after acceptance into the School of Medicine, the applicant is sent all available financial aid information and is encouraged to apply. The awarding of financial aid is based on documented need. Loans and a limited number of scholarships and prizes are available. Some awards and scholarships are based on academics as well as need. Students are discouraged from working. The financial aid office may be reached at (701) 777-2849.

Information about Diversity Programs

The INMED (Indians into Medicine) Program is a recruitment and retention program for American Indian students. It is a federally funded program that provides educational opportunities for fully qualified enrolled members of U.S. recognized tribes. State residency is not a consideration for admission through the INMED Program.

Campus Information

Setting

The medical school is located on the University of North Dakota campus, a state-supported institution located in Grand Forks in the heart of the Red River Valley. The Grand Forks-East Grand Forks (MN) community has a total population of approximately 75,000. UND is a Carnegie Doctoral II institution, offering a wide diversity of educational programs.

Enrollment

For 2007, total enrollment was: 245

Special Features

The Center for Rural Health is a recognized leader nationally. The school also has a Center of Excellence in Women's Health and a Center for Excellence in Neurosciences. A medical student exchange program exists with two medical schools in Norway.

Housing

On-campus housing is available in the form of residence halls and apartments for families and single students. A shuttle service runs between the housing area and the main campus. Rental housing also is plentiful in the community.

Satellite Campuses/Facilities

Students are assigned to one of four regional campuses statewide in Bismarck, Fargo, Grand Forks, and Minot for third and fourth year clinical experiences.

Application Process and Requirements 2009–2010

Primary Application Service: School specific
Earliest filing date: July 1, 2008
Latest filing date: November 1, 2008

Secondary Application Required?: No
Sent to: All applicants
URL: www.med.und.nodak.edu/
Fee: Yes, $50
Fee waiver available: Yes
Earliest filing date: July 1, 2008
Latest filing date: November 1, 2008

Latest MCAT® considered: n/r
Oldest MCAT® considered: August 2005

Early Decision Program
School does not have EDP
Applicants notified: n/a
EDP available for: n/a

Regular Acceptance Notice
Earliest date: January 15, 2009
Latest date: Until class is full

Applicant's Response to Acceptance
Offer – Maximum Time: Four weeks

Requests for Deferred
Entrance Considered: Yes

Deposit to Hold Place in Class: Yes
Deposit (Resident): $100
Deposit (Non-Resident): $100
Deposit due: With response to acceptance offer
Applied to tuition: Yes
Deposit refundable: Yes
Refundable by: May 15, 2009

Estimated number of new entrants: 62
EDP: n/a, special program: n/a

Start Month/Year: August 2009

Interview Format: MD and PhD faculty members and medical students conduct one-hour interviews.

Other Programs

PREPARATORY PROGRAMS
Postbaccalaureate Program: No
Summer Program: Yes, INMED Program
(701) 777-3039, edelorme@medicine.nodak.edu

COMBINED DEGREE PROGRAMS
Baccalaureate/MD: No
MD/MPH: Yes, Robert Beattie, MD
(701) 777-3264, beattie@medicine.nodak.edu
MD/MBA: No
MD/JD: No
MD/PhD: Yes, Joshua Wynne, M.D.
(701) 777-2515, jwynne@medicine.nodak.edu

Premedical Coursework

Course	Req.	Rec.	Lab.	Hrs.
Inorganic Chemistry	•		•	8
Behavioral Sciences				
Biochemistry		•		
Biology				
Biology/Zoology	•		•	8
Calculus				
College English	•			6
College Mathematics	•			3

Course	Req.	Rec.	Lab.	Hrs.
Computer Science		•		
Genetics				
Humanities		•		
Organic Chemistry	•		•	8
Physics	•		•	8
Psychology	•			3
Social Sciences				
Other				

Selection Factors: 2007 Accepted Applicants

Proportion of Accepted Applicants with Relevant Experience (Data Self-Reported to AMCAS®)		
Community Service/Volunteer	66%
Medically-Related Work	78%
Research	61%

Shaded bar represents accepted scores ranging from the 10th percentile to the 90th percentile. **School Median** ● **National Median** ●

Overall GPA	2.0	2.1	2.2	2.3	2.4	2.5	2.6	2.7	2.8	2.9	3.0	3.1	3.2	3.3	3.4	3.5	3.6	3.7	(3.8)	3.9	4.0
Science GPA	2.0	2.1	2.2	2.3	2.4	2.5	2.6	2.7	2.8	2.9	3.0	3.1	3.2	3.3	3.4	3.5	3.6	(3.7)	3.8	3.9	4.0

MCAT® required: Yes, 100% of 2007 accepted applicants took MCAT®

Verbal Reasoning	3	4	5	6	7	8	(9)	(10)	11	12	13	14	15
Physical Sciences	3	4	5	6	7	8	(9)	10	(11)	12	13	14	15
Biological Sciences	3	4	5	6	7	8	(9)	10	(11)	12	13	14	15
Writing Sample			J	K	L	M	(N)	O	P	(Q)	R	S	T

Acceptance & Matriculation Data for 2007–2008 First Year Class

	Resident	Non-Resident	International	Total
Applied	142	159	0	301
Interviewed	100	49	0	149
Deferred	4	1	0	5
Matriculants				
Early Assurance Program	0	0	0	0
Early Decision Program	0	0	0	0
Baccalaureate/MD	n/a	n/a	n/a	n/a
MD/PhD	1	0	0	1
Matriculated	43	19	0	**62**

Applications accepted from International Applicants: No

Specialty Choice

2003, 2004, 2005 Graduates, Specialty Choice (As reported by program directors to GME Track™)	
Anesthesiology	4%
Emergency Medicine	11%
Family Practice	15%
Internal Medicine	10%
Obstetrics/Gynecology	11%
Orthopaedic Surgery	4%
Pediatrics	8%
Psychiatry	2%
Radiology	6%
Surgery	8%

Matriculant Demographics: 2007–2008 First Year Class

Men: 38   **Women:** 24

Matriculants' Self-Reported Race/Ethnicity

Mexican American	0	Korean	0
Cuban	0	Vietnamese	0
Puerto Rican	0	Other Asian	0
Other Hispanic	0	Total Asian	0
Total Hispanic	0	Native American	7
Chinese	0	Black	0
Asian Indian	0	Native Hawaiian	0
Pakistani	0	White	55
Filipino	0	Unduplicated Number	
Japanese	0	of Matriculants	62

Science and Math Majors: 65%
Matriculants with:
　　Baccalaureate degree: 100%
　　Graduate degree(s): 3%

Financial Information

Source: 2006–2007 LCME I-B survey and 2007–2008 AAMC TSF questionnaire

	Residents	Non-Residents
Total Cost of Attendance	$41,676	$59,920
Tuition and Fees	$22,873	$41,120
Other (includes living expenses)	$18,803	$18,800
Health Insurance (not applicable)	$0	$0

Average 2007 Graduate Indebtedness: $139,386
% of Enrolled Students Receiving Aid: 97%

Criminal Background Check

This medical school requires a criminal background check prior to matriculation.

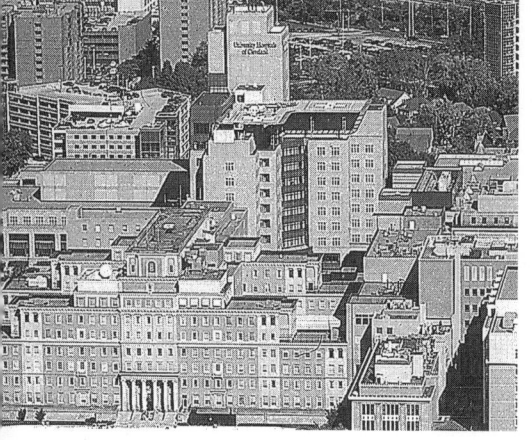

Case Western Reserve University School of Medicine

Cleveland, Ohio

Office of Admissions
Case Western Reserve University School Of Medicine
10900 Euclid Avenue
Cleveland, Ohio 44106-4920
T 216 368 3450   **F** 216 368 6011

Admissions http://casemed.case.edu/admissions
Main http://casemed.case.edu
Financial http://casemed.case.edu.edu/financial_aid
Email casemed-admissions@case.edu

Private Institution

Dr. Pamela B. Davis, Dean and Vice President for Medical Affairs

Dr. Lina Mehta, Associate Dean for Admissions

Joseph T. Williams, Director of Multicultural Programs

Wanda L. Rollins, Director of Financial Aid

Christian Essman, Director of Admissions

General Information

Since 1843, the Case Western Reserve University School of Medicine has been at the forefront of medical education and research. CWRU SOM is one of the nation's leaders in NIH funding. Current educational innovations include curricular reform within the University Program and partnership since 2002 with the Cleveland Clinic in the Cleveland Clinic Lerner College of Medicine (College Program), a distinct program to train physician-investigators.

Mission Statement

To advance the health of humankind through research, service and education.

Curricular Highlights

Community Service Requirement: Optional.
Research/Thesis Requirement: Required.

Case Western School of Medicine offers two types of MD programs, a Medical Scientist Training program (MSTP), and several dual-degree and masters programs. Applicants may choose one or more programs through AMCAS by applying to the CWRU School of Medicine, and must interview separately for each. The University Program (UP), a 4-year MD program designed to train physician-scholars, is based on four tenets: clinical mastery, research, leadership, and civic professionalism. The innovative curriculum integrates basic sciences, clinical medicine, and population health, focusing on the care of individual patients within social and environmental contexts. Students are introduced to basic sciences in a learner-centered environment which emphasizes small group and team-based learning.

Learning is interactive with faculty and students as partners. Independent learning and scholarship are emphasized. Material is organized in system-based blocks, with basic science and clinical integration throughout the four years. Early clinical experiences include rotating apprenticeships and a longitudinal outpatient preceptorship. A required, mentored research thesis is supported by the Office of Medical Student Research. Advising occurs in small groups by the Office of Student Affairs. The 5-year College Program (CP) admits 32 students, each of whom will graduate with an MD with Special Qualifications in Bio-medical Research. A student-centered approach fosters critical thinking and self-directed learning. Basic sciences are taught in small groups using problem-based learning, interactive seminars, journal clubs, and labs; there are no formal lectures. Early clinical experience includes a longitudinal outpatient preceptorship throughout the first two years. A core research curriculum focuses on basic and clinical research and includes hands-on research during the first two summers. A master's level thesis is required. Students document their progress using a portfolio that details skills and expertise they achieve. A physician adviser ensures students' mastery of required competencies. A college level biochemistry course and research experience is required of all applicants to the College Program. Neither program utilizes grades or class rank.

USMLE

Step 1: Required. Students must record a passing score for promotion.
Step 2: Clinical Skills (CS): Required. Students must record a passing total score to graduate.
Step 2: Clinical Knowledge (CK): Required. Students must record a passing total score to graduate.

Selection Factors

The School of Medicine seeks a diverse student body. Students are selected without regard to age, nationality, race, religion, sex, sexual orientation or state of residence. All candidates must have demonstrated exceptional academic strength and personal achievements. Written statements and letters of recommendation are also important. Transfer students are not accepted.

Financial Aid

Financial aid is based on demonstrated need. Merit scholarships may be awarded to some students with outstanding personal and academic achievement. The College Program also provides stipends for research. Accepted students receive financial aid applications in January; awards are made by April.

Information about Diversity Programs

The Office of Multicultural Affairs offers academic and personal support for all underrepresented medical students. This office also recruits students for all programs, sponsors a rigorous, six-week, summer premed/predental program for college freshmen and sophomores and has an NIH-funded summer research program for undergraduate and medical students. The office supports the Case Western Student National Medical Association chapter and the Minority Graduate Student Organization.

Campus Information

Setting

The School of Medicine sits within the heart of the university's 150-acre campus in the city's University Circle area, a cultural and educational hub. Teaching affiliates are adjacent or nearby.

Enrollment

For 2007, total enrollment was: 711

Special Features

The Center for Global Health and Diseases offers opportunities for students to study abroad. The Mt. Sinai Skills and Simulation Center offers a state-of-the-art clinical learning laboratory.

Housing

On campus housing is not available; however, ample housing exists within walking distance. Rents average $400-$600 month.

Satellite Campuses/Facilities

Affiliate hospitals include University Hospitals Case Medical Center (including Rainbow), the Cleveland Clinic, MetroHealth, and the VA Hospital.

Application Process and Requirements 2009–2010

Primary Application Service: AMCAS
Earliest filing date: June 1, 2008
Latest filing date: November 1, 2008

Secondary Application Required?: Yes
Sent to: All applicants
URL: Sent when verified AMCAS application is received.
Fee: Yes, $85
Fee waiver available: Yes
Earliest filing date: July 1, 2008
Latest filing date: December 15, 2008

Latest MCAT® considered: September 2008
Oldest MCAT® considered: 2005

Early Decision Program
School does not have EDP
Applicants notified: n/a
EDP available for: n/a

Regular Acceptance Notice
Earliest date: October 15, 2008
Latest date: Until class is full

Applicant's Response to Acceptance Offer – Maximum Time: Four weeks

Requests for Deferred Entrance Considered: Yes

Deposit to Hold Place in Class: No
Deposit (Resident): n/a
Deposit (Non-Resident): n/a
Deposit due: n/a
Applied to tuition: n/a
Deposit refundable: n/a
Refundable by: n/a

Estimated number of new entrants: 194
EDP: n/a, special program: 12

Start Month/Year: July 2009

Interview Format: UP: one faculty and one student. CP: two faculty interviews.

Other Program

PREPARATORY PROGRAMS
Postbaccalaureate Program: No
Summer Program: Yes, www.smdep.org
Joseph T. Williams, (216) 368-1914
joseph.williams@case.edu

COMBINED DEGREE PROGRAMS
Baccalaureate/MD: Yes, http://admission.
case.edu/admissions/application/ppsp.asp,
Christine DeSalvo Miller
(216) 368-5450, christine.desalvo@case.edu
MD/MPH: Yes, www.casemph.org
Kristina Knight, (216) 368-1967, info@casemph.org
MD/MBA: Yes, http://weatherhead.case.edu/mba/
jointDegree/joint_mbaMd.cfm, Deborah Bibb,
(216) 368-6702, deborah.bibb@case.edu
MD/JD: Yes, http://law.case.edu/curriculum/
content.asp?id=101
MD/PhD: Yes, http://mstp.cwru.edu
Donna McIllwain, (216) 368-3404, mstp@case.edu
Additional Program: Yes,
http://bme.case.edu/, Tiffany Thomas
216-368-4094, bmedept@case.edu

Premedical Coursework

Course	Req.	Rec.	Lab.	Sems.	Course	Req.	Rec.	Lab.	Sems.
Inorganic Chemistry	•		•	2	Computer Science				
Behavioral Sciences					Genetics				
Biochemistry		•		1	Humanities				
Biology	•		•	2	Organic Chemistry	•		•	2
Biology/Zoology					Physics	•		•	2
Calculus					Psychology				
College English	•			1	Social Sciences				
College Mathematics					Biochemistry for CP	•		•	1

Selection Factors: 2007 Accepted Applicants

Proportion of Accepted Applicants with Relevant Experience (Data Self-Reported to AMCAS®)		
Community Service/Volunteer		69%
Medically-Related Work		83%
Research		89%

Shaded bar represents accepted scores ranging from the 10th percentile to the 90th percentile   School Median ●   National Median ●

Overall GPA	2.0	2.1	2.2	2.3	2.4	2.5	2.6	2.7	2.8	2.9	3.0	3.1	3.2	3.3	3.4	3.5	3.6	③.7	3.8	3.9	4.0
Science GPA	2.0	2.1	2.2	2.3	2.4	2.5	2.6	2.7	2.8	2.9	3.0	3.1	3.2	3.3	3.4	3.5	3.6	③.7	3.8	3.9	4.0

MCAT® required: Yes, 97% of 2007 accepted applicants took MCAT®

Verbal Reasoning	3	4	5	6	7	8	9	⑩	⑪	12	13	14	15
Physical Sciences	3	4	5	6	7	8	9	10	⑪	⑫	13	14	15
Biological Sciences	3	4	5	6	7	8	9	10	⑪	⑫	13	14	15
Writing Sample					J	K	L	M	N	O	P	⑫ Q	R	S	T

Acceptance & Matriculation Data for 2007–2008 First Year Class

	Resident	Non-Resident	International	Total
Applied	783	4914	331	6028
Interviewed	194	1041	105	1340
Deferred	2	6	0	8
Matriculants				
Early Assurance Program	n/a	n/a	n/a	n/a
Early Decision Program	0	0	0	0
Baccalaureate/MD	4	9	0	13
MD/PhD	1	8	0	9
Matriculated	39	137	9	**185**

Applications accepted from International Applicants: Yes

Specialty Choice

2003, 2004, 2005 Graduates, Specialty Choice (As reported by program directors to GME Track™)	
Anesthesiology	4%
Emergency Medicine	6%
Family Practice	5%
Internal Medicine	18%
Obstetrics/Gynecology	4%
Orthopaedic Surgery	5%
Pediatrics	12%
Psychiatry	5%
Radiology	5%
Surgery	4%

Matriculant Demographics: 2007–2008 First Year Class

Men: 101   **Women:** 84

Matriculants' Self-Reported Race/Ethnicity

Mexican American	2	Korean	4
Cuban	1	Vietnamese	1
Puerto Rican	2	Other Asian	8
Other Hispanic	5	Total Asian	55
Total Hispanic	10	Native American	0
Chinese	20	Black	18
Asian Indian	21	Native Hawaiian	0
Pakistani	1	White	103
Filipino	1	Unduplicated Number	
Japanese	1	of Matriculants	185

Science and Math Majors: 67%
Matriculants with:
  Baccalaureate degree: 99%
  Graduate degree(s): 10%

Financial Information

Source: 2006–2007 LCME I-B survey and 2007–2008 AAMC TSF questionnaire

	Residents	Non-Residents
Total Cost of Attendance	$64,136	$64,136
Tuition and Fees	$41,966	$41,966
Other (includes living expenses)	$20,930	$20,930
Health Insurance (can be waived)	$1,240	$1,240

Average 2007 Graduate Indebtedness: $128,003
% of Enrolled Students Receiving Aid: 80%

Criminal Background Check

This medical school requires a criminal background check prior to matriculation.

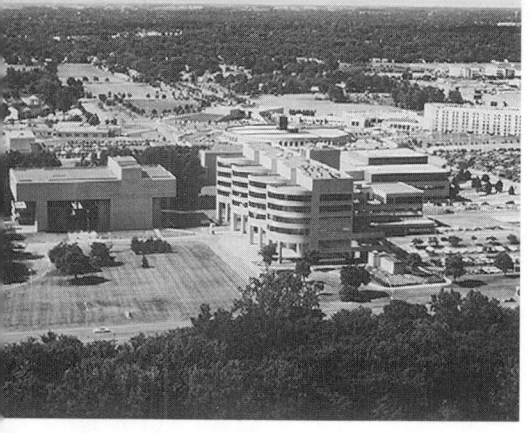

University of Toledo College of Medicine
(Formerly Medical University of Ohio)
Toledo, Ohio

Admissions Office
3045 Arlington Avenue, Mail Stop 1043
Toledo, Ohio 43614
T 419 383 4229   **F** 419 383 3322

Admissions www.hsc.utoledo/med/admissions/
application.html
Main www.hsc.utoledo.edu
Financial www.utoledo.edu/depts/stufnaid/
sfamed.html
Email medadmissions@utnet.utoledo.edu

Public Institution

Dr. Jeffrey P. Gold, Dean

Dr. James F. Kleshinski,
Associate Dean for Admissions

Dr. Samuel H. Hancock, Assistant to
the President for Institutional Diversity

Kathryn A. Coy, Director,
Office of Student Financial Aid

Dr. Robert S. Crissman, Assistant Dean
for Admissions

General Information
The Medical University of Ohio and the University of Toledo merged on July 1, 2006, thus creating the third largest university in Ohio, which is now known as the University of Toledo. Four health and research colleges are located on the Health Science Campus: the College of Medicine, the College of Health Science and Human Service, the College of Nursing, and the College of Graduate Studies.

Mission Statement
The mission of the University of Toledo College of Medicine is to improve the human condition. We do this by providing a world-class education for the next generation of physicians and scientists, by creating new knowledge that is translated into cutting edge clinical practice, and by providing the highest level of professionalism and compassion as we deliver university quality health care.

Curricular Highlights
Community Service Requirement: Optional.
Research/Thesis Requirement: Optional.

The preclinical years integrate the basic sciences into interdisciplinary blocks of Cellular and Molecular Biology, Human Structure and Development, Neuroscience/Behavioral Science, Immunity and Infection, and Organ Systems. Integrative Pathophysiology, which spans the first two years, uses a case-based format designed to help students develop clinical reasoning skills by applying principles learned in the basic sciences. Fundamentals of Clinical Practice also spans both preclinical years and includes medical

ethics, interviewing, physical diagnosis, and introduction to primary care. The third year of the curriculum is devoted to mandatory clerkships in internal medicine, surgery, pediatrics, obstetrics and gynecology, psychiatry, and family medicine. The fourth year includes required clerkships in neurology, an acting internship, and basic science, as well as 24 weeks of clinical electives. Most components of the curriculum are evaluated on an Honors, High Pass, Pass, Fail system.

USMLE
Step 1: Required. Students must record a passing score for promotion.
Step 2: Clinical Skills (CS): Required. Students must record a passing total score to graduate.
Step 2: Clinical Knowledge (CK): Required. Students must record a passing total score to graduate.

Selection Factors
Interviews are by invitation only. Re-applicants are not penalized. Preference is given to Ohio residents.

Financial Aid
Financial aid is awarded on the basis of demonstrated financial need according to federal methodology. Applicants for financial aid must file the FAFSA. Several full tuition Presidential Scholarships are available, as well as a number of both merit and need-based scholarships. Many students are employed during the academic year in the Federal Work-Study Program. Employment opportunities in research, community health, family practice, and acute care are also provided through the summer preceptorship programs.

Information about Diversity Programs
The University of Toledo is committed to increasing opportunities for individuals from traditionally underrepresented groups, as well as those from economically disadvantaged backgrounds. The Admissions Office works in cooperation with the Office for Institutional Diversity and the Office of Student Affairs and other campus departments in the recruitment, selection, and retention of qualified students.

Campus Information

Setting
The University of Toledo Health Science Campus is located on 475 acres in suburban south Toledo, approximately three miles south of the Main Campus. Toledo's many cultural attractions include the world famous Toledo Museum of Art, a symphony orchestra, opera company, zoological gardens, and an international institute serving the multicultural life of the city. Recreational activities include metroparks, boating, fishing, hiking, and cross-country skiing.

Enrollment
For 2007, total enrollment was: 612

Special Features
Four schools comprise the University of Toledo Health Science Campus: the College of Medicine, College of Nursing, College of Graduate Studies, and College of Health Science and Human Service. Researchers received more than $21 million in research grants and contracts in the 2007 fiscal year. Major areas of research include cellular and molecular neurobiology, molecular and cellular biology, and the molecular basis of diseases, covering such areas as cancer, diabetes, cardiovascular diseases, molecular and cellular immunology, and vaccine development.

Housing
On-campus housing is available on the main campus.

Satellite Campuses/Facilities
The clinical clerkships are completed at the University of Toledo Medical Center on the Health Science Campus, as well as at several other area teaching hospitals, including St. Vincent Mercy Medical Center, The Toledo Hospital, Mercy Children's Hospital, Toledo Children's Hospital, Flower Hospital, St. Charles Mercy Hospital and St. Luke's Hospital. All students complete a minimum of 8 weeks of clerkships in a rural Area Health Education Center. Opportunities are also available for students to do their required clerkships at Riverside Methodist Hospital in Columbus, Ohio, and at Henry Ford Health System in Detroit, Michigan. In the fourth-year, students are able to complete up to several months of elective rotations at other approved institutions.

Application Process and Requirements 2009–2010

Primary Application Service: AMCAS
Earliest filing date: June 1, 2008
Latest filing date: November 1, 2008

Secondary Application Required?: Yes
Sent to: Screened applicants
URL: http://hsc.utoledo.edu/med/admissions/
secondary.html
Fee: Yes, $80
Fee waiver available: Yes
Earliest filing date: June 15, 2008
Latest filing date: January 1, 2009

Latest MCAT® considered: September 2008
Oldest MCAT® considered: 2006

Early Decision Program
School does have EDP
Applicants notified: October 1, 2008
EDP available for: Residents only

Regular Acceptance Notice
Earliest date: October 16, 2008
Latest date: Until class is full

Applicant's Response to Acceptance
Offer – Maximum Time: Two weeks

Requests for Deferred
Entrance Considered: Yes

Deposit to Hold Place in Class: No
Deposit (Resident): n/a
Deposit (Non-Resident): n/a
Deposit due: n/a
Applied to tuition: n/a
Deposit refundable: n/a
Refundable by: n/a

Estimated number of new entrants: 165
EDP: 5, special program: 25

Start Month/Year: August 2009

Interview Format: Two, one-on-one interviews with faculty. Regional interviews are not available.

Other Programs

PREPARATORY PROGRAMS
Postbaccalaureate Program: Yes,
www.hsc.utoledo.edu/grad
Summer Program: Yes, www.hsc.utoledo.edu/
med/admissions/srp.html
Additional Program: Yes,
www.hsc.utoledo.edu/med/admissions.medstarz.html

COMBINED DEGREE PROGRAMS
Baccalaureate/MD: Yes, www.utoledo.edu/
colleges/as/index.asp?id=84
MD/MPH: Yes,
www.hsc.utoledo.edu/medpubhealth/index.html
MD/MBA: No
MD/JD: No
MD/PhD: Yes, www.hsc.utoledo.edu/grad/
mdphd/index.html

Premedical Coursework

Course	Req.	Rec.	Lab.	Sems.	Course	Req.	Rec.	Lab.	Sems.
Inorganic Chemistry	•		•	2	Computer Science				
Behavioral Sciences					Genetics				
Biochemistry					Humanities		•		
Biology	•		•	2	Organic Chemistry	•		•	2
Biology/Zoology					Physics	•		•	2
Calculus					Psychology				
College English	•			2	Social Sciences		•		
College Mathematics	•			2	Other		•		

Selection Factors: 2007 Accepted Applicants

Proportion of Accepted Applicants with Relevant Experience (Data Self-Reported to AMCAS®)		
Community Service/Volunteer		68%
Medically-Related Work		81%
Research		77%

Shaded bar represents accepted scores ranging from the 10th percentile to the 90th percentile.   School Median ●   National Median ●

Overall GPA	2.0	2.1	2.2	2.3	2.4	2.5	2.6	2.7	2.8	2.9	3.0	3.1	3.2	3.3	3.4	3.5	3.6	(3.7)	3.8	3.9	4.0
Science GPA	2.0	2.1	2.2	2.3	2.4	2.5	2.6	2.7	2.8	2.9	3.0	3.1	3.2	3.3	3.4	3.5	(3.6)	3.7	3.8	3.9	4.0

MCAT® required: Yes, 91% of 2007 accepted applicants took MCAT®

Verbal Reasoning	3	4	5	6	7	8	9	(10)	11	12	13	14	15
Physical Sciences	3	4	5	6	7	8	9	(10)	(11)	12	13	14	15
Biological Sciences	3	4	5	6	7	8	9	(10)	(11)	12	13	14	15
Writing Sample			J	K	L	M	N	O	(P)	(Q)	R	S	T

Acceptance & Matriculation Data for 2007–2008 First Year Class

	Resident	Non-Resident	International	Total
Applied	1032	2313	24	3369
Interviewed	257	191	0	448
Deferred	22	7	0	29
Matriculants				
Early Assurance Program	16	2	0	18
Early Decision Program	2	0	0	2
Baccalaureate/MD	n/a	n/a	n/a	n/a
MD/PhD	1	0	0	1
Matriculated	105	59	1	**165**

Applications accepted from International Applicants: No

Specialty Choice

2003, 2004, 2005 Graduates, Specialty Choice (As reported by program directors to GME Track™)

Anesthesiology	4%
Emergency Medicine	8%
Family Practice	11%
Internal Medicine	18%
Obstetrics/Gynecology	4%
Orthopaedic Surgery	4%
Pediatrics	10%
Psychiatry	4%
Radiology	6%
Surgery	6%

Matriculant Demographics: 2007–2008 First Year Class

Men: 97   **Women:** 68

Matriculants' Self-Reported Race/Ethnicity

Mexican American	2	Korean	3
Cuban	0	Vietnamese	3
Puerto Rican	0	Other Asian	7
Other Hispanic	0	Total Asian	41
Total Hispanic	2	Native American	1
Chinese	6	Black	8
Asian Indian	17	Native Hawaiian	0
Pakistani	5	White	114
Filipino	0	Unduplicated Number	
Japanese	0	of Matriculants	165

Science and Math Majors: 76%
Matriculants with:
    Baccalaureate degree: 100%
    Graduate degree(s): 24%

Financial Information

Source: 2006–2007 LCME I-B survey and 2007–2008 AAMC TSF questionnaire

	Residents	Non-Residents
Total Cost of Attendance	$39,232	$67,972
Tuition and Fees	$24,850	$53,590
Other (includes living expenses)	$12,270	$12,270
Health Insurance (can be waived)	$2,112	$2,112

Average 2007 Graduate Indebtedness: $135,543
% of Enrolled Students Receiving Aid: 90%

Criminal Background Check

This medical school requires a criminal background check prior to matriculation.

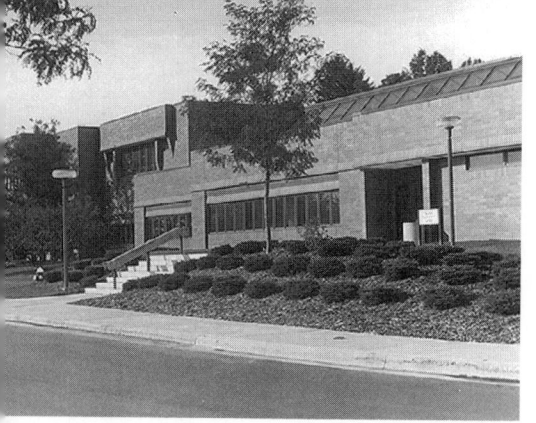

Northeastern Ohio Universities College of Medicine

Rootstown, Ohio

Office of Admissions
Northeastern Ohio Universities College of Medicine
P.O. Box 95
Rootstown, Ohio 44272-0095
T 330 325 6270   F 330 325 8372

Admissions www.neoucom.edu/audience/applicants
Main www.neoucom.edu
Financial www.neoucom.edu/audience/students
Email admission@neoucom.edu

Public Institution

Dr. Lois Margaret Nora, President and Dean

Yvonne Mathis, Director of Diversity Affairs

Michelle Cassetty, Director, Student Services and Registrar

Polly Moss, Assistant Dean, Student Affairs and Admissions

General Information

The Northeastern Ohio Universities College of Medicine (NEOUCOM) is a state (public) Community-based medical school consisting of a basic medical sciences campus in Rootstown, a consortium of three major public universities, 22 associated hospitals/health systems, including eight major teaching hospitals and two health departments in the greater Akron, Canton, and Youngstown areas.

Mission Statement

The mission of the Northeastern Ohio Universities College of Medicine (NEOUCOM) is to graduate qualified physicians oriented to the practice of medicine at the community level, with an emphasis on primary care: family medicine, internal medicine, pediatrics, and obstetrics/gynecology. NEOUCOM strives to improve the quality of health care in northeast Ohio.

Curricular Highlights

Community Service Requirement: Required.
Research/Thesis Requirement: Optional.

The integrated curriculum is offered in five steps during the four years. The four-year Doctoring course provides an understanding of professionalism, doctor-patient relationships, and community health. Step 1: Prologue addresses issues of professionalism, doctor-patient relationships, and community health; Human Development and Structure emphasizes human anatomy; Molecules to Cells addresses biochemistry, molecular pathology, and genetics. Step 2: Physiological Basis of Medicine emphasizes physiological concepts in the practice of internal medicine; Brain, Mind and Behavior includes anatomy, physiology, and chemistry of the nervous system with basic clinical concepts and pathologies. Step 3: instruction is centered on systems and application in clinical settings. Step 4: core clerkships – family medicine, internal medicine, obstetrics/gynecology, pediatrics, psychiatry, and surgery, an exploratory elective, and an Intersession. Step 5: electives and a Capstone focusing on professionalism, humanities, and social science disciplines. The Bridge to Residency provides vital skills needed as interns and residents.

USMLE

Step 1: Required. Students must record a passing score for promotion.
Step 2: Clinical Skills (CS): Required. Students must record a passing total score to graduate.
Step 2: Clinical Knowledge (CK): Required. Students must record a passing total score to graduate.

Selection Factors

Applicants must demonstrate strong academic preparation as measured by GPAs and MCAT scores, and show appropriate personal characteristics and motivation for the practice of medicine. Interviews are by invitation only. Admission preference is given to Ohio residents. All applicants are considered; no formulas are used for the selection process. Only those who complete supplementary applications are given full consideration. Early submission of application materials is strongly encouraged, particularly through the Early Decision Plan (EDP). NEOUCOM is an equal opportunity/affirmative action educator and employer, committed to preparing students for the practice of medicine in a multicultural environment by increasing the diversity of the student body, faculty, and staff and by enhancing policies, procedures, and practices that support a collaborative environment.

Financial Aid

Campus-based financial aid (grants and low interest loans) is awarded on the basis of need. Students apply for this aid by completing the FAFSA, the NEOUCOM financial aid application and submitting copies of federal tax returns. To be eligible for campus-based aid, students must submit parent information on the FAFSA and provide their federal tax returns. A limited number of grants are available for students who demonstrate need, are from a disadvantaged background or from groups underrepresented in medicine. Federal student loans are a major part of the financial aid award with 80 percent of students receiving some form of financial aid. Financial need is not a factor in admission considerations.

Information about Diversity Programs

One of the goals of the Admissions Committee is to seek out, recruit, and support qualified nontraditional applicants (members of groups underrepresented in medicine and disadvantaged rural students).

Campus Information

Setting

Rootstown is 20 minutes from Akron and 50 minutes from Cleveland. The 55-acre NEOUCOM complex, centrally located among the consortium universities and clinical campuses, houses the institution's administrative offices, the divisions of basic medical sciences and community health sciences, and the College of Pharmacy.

Enrollment

For 2007, total enrollment was: 455

Special Features

The state-of-the-art facilities on campus include the Wasson Center for Clinical Skills Training, Assessment, and Scholarship; newly renovated lecture halls; multidisciplinary labs; and the Regional Medical Informational Center, which houses more than 110,000 books and more than 725 journals. For relaxation, students can enjoy the workout room, student lounge, and basketball, tennis, and volleyball courts.

Housing

NEOUCOM maintains a listing of local housing options; no on-campus housing is available.

Satellite Campuses/Facilities

Rotations are completed among 22 associated hospitals, eight of which are major teaching facilities.

Application Process and Requirements 2009–2010

Primary Application Service: AMCAS
Earliest filing date: June 1, 2008
Latest filing date: November 1, 2008

Secondary Application Required?: Yes
Sent to: Screened applicants
URL: n/a
(330) 325-6274, admission@neoucom.edu
Fee: Yes, $50
Fee waiver available: Yes
Earliest filing date: July 1, 2008
Latest filing date: December 1, 2008

Latest MCAT® considered: January 2009
Oldest MCAT® considered: 2006

Early Decision Program
School does have EDP
Applicants notified: October 1, 2008
EDP available for: Both Residents and Non-Residents

Regular Acceptance Notice
Earliest date: October 16, 2008
Latest date: Until class is full

Applicant's Response to Acceptance Offer – Maximum Time: Two weeks

Requests for Deferred Entrance Considered: No

Deposit to Hold Place in Class: Yes
Deposit (Resident): $100
Deposit (Non-Resident): $100
Deposit due: Two weeks after offer of acceptance
Applied to tuition: Yes
Deposit refundable: Yes
Refundable by: May 15, 2009 (except for Early Decision Program)

Estimated number of new entrants: 30
EDP: 5, special program: 85

Start Month/Year: August 2009

Interview Format: Thirty-minute interviews with two faculty. Regional interviews are not available.

Other Programs

PREPARATORY PROGRAMS
Postbaccalaureate Program: Yes
www.neoucom.edu/audience/gradschool/
Summer Program: No
COMBINED DEGREE PROGRAMS
Baccalaureate/MD: Yes
www.neoucom.edu/audience/applicants
330-325-6270, admission@neoucom.edu
MD/MPH: Yes
MD/MBA: No
MD/JD: No
MD/PhD: Yes
Additional Program: Yes,
www.neoucom.edu/PharmD
330-325-6270, pharmacy@neoucom.edu

Premedical Coursework

Course	Req.	Rec.	Lab.	Sems.
Inorganic Chemistry		•		
Behavioral Sciences		•		
Biochemistry		•		
Biology	•			1
Biology/Zoology		•		
Calculus		•		
College English		•		
College Mathematics		•		

Course	Req.	Rec.	Lab.	Sems.
Computer Science				
Genetics		•		
Humanities		•		
Organic Chemistry	•			2
Physics	•			2
Psychology		•		
Social Sciences		•		
Other				

Selection Factors: 2007 Accepted Applicants

Proportion of Accepted Applicants with Relevant Experience (Data Self-Reported to AMCAS®)		
Community Service/Volunteer		51%
Medically-Related Work		49%
Research		45%

Shaded bar represents accepted scores ranging from the 10th percentile to the 90th percentile. School Median ● National Median ●

Overall GPA	2.0	2.1	2.2	2.3	2.4	2.5	2.6	2.7	2.8	2.9	3.0	3.1	3.2	3.3	3.4	3.5	3.6	3.7	(3.8)	3.9	4.0
Science GPA	2.0	2.1	2.2	2.3	2.4	2.5	2.6	2.7	2.8	2.9	3.0	3.1	3.2	3.3	3.4	3.5	3.6	(3.7)	3.8	3.9	4.0

MCAT® required: Yes, 100% of 2007 accepted applicants took MCAT®

Verbal Reasoning	3	4	5	6	7	8	9	(10)	11	12	13	14	15
Physical Sciences	3	4	5	6	7	8	(9)	10	(11)	12	13	14	15
Biological Sciences	3	4	5	6	7	8	9	(10)	(11)	12	13	14	15
Writing Sample			J	K	L	M	N	(O)	P	(Q)	R	S	T

Acceptance & Matriculation Data for 2007–2008 First Year Class

	Resident	Non-Resident	International	Total
Applied	823	1111	31	1965
Interviewed	136	2	0	138
Deferred	1	0	0	1
Matriculants				
Early Assurance Program	0	0	0	0
Early Decision Program	3	0	0	3
Baccalaureate/MD	72	2	0	74
MD/PhD	n/a	n/a	n/a	n/a
Matriculated	119	2	0	**121**

Applications accepted from International Applicants: No

Matriculant Demographics: 2007–2008 First Year Class

Men: 61   **Women:** 60

Matriculants' Self-Reported Race/Ethnicity

Mexican American	1	Korean	1
Cuban	1	Vietnamese	0
Puerto Rican	0	Other Asian	4
Other Hispanic	3	Total Asian	40
Total Hispanic	5	Native American	1
Chinese	7	Black	5
Asian Indian	25	Native Hawaiian	1
Pakistani	4	White	82
Filipino	0	**Unduplicated Number**	
Japanese	1	**of Matriculants**	121

Science and Math Majors: 69%
Matriculants with:
　　Baccalaureate degree: 100%
　　Graduate degree(s): 2%

Specialty Choice

2003, 2004, 2005 Graduates, Specialty Choice (As reported by program directors to GME Track™)

Anesthesiology	6%
Emergency Medicine	7%
Family Practice	10%
Internal Medicine	19%
Obstetrics/Gynecology	6%
Orthopaedic Surgery	5%
Pediatrics	10%
Psychiatry	3%
Radiology	4%
Surgery	5%

Financial Information

Source: 2006–2007 LCME I-B survey and 2007–2008 AAMC TSF questionnaire

	Residents	Non-Residents
Total Cost of Attendance	$51,885	$78,690
Tuition and Fees	$28,881	$55,686
Other (includes living expenses)	$21,850	$21,850
Health Insurance (can be waived)	$1,154	$1,154

Average 2007 Graduate Indebtedness: $118,112
% of Enrolled Students Receiving Aid: 83%

Criminal Background Check

This medical school requires a criminal background check prior to matriculation.

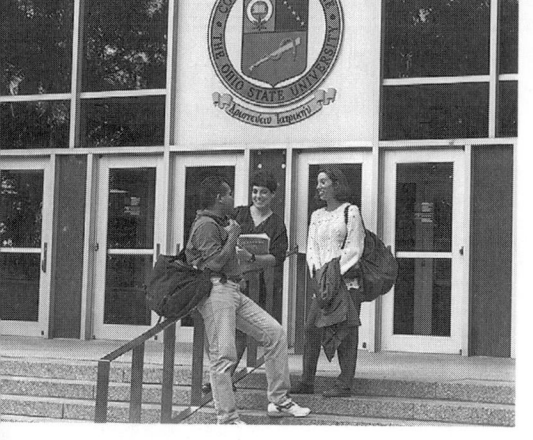

The Ohio State University College of Medicine

Columbus, Ohio

Admissions Committee, The Ohio State University
College of Medicine
I55D Meiling Hall, 370 West 9th Avenue
Columbus, Ohio 43210-1238
T 614 292 7137   **F** 614 247 7959

Admissions http://medicine.osu.edu/futurestudents/
admissions
Main http://medicine.osu.edu
Financial http://medicine.osu.edu/futurestudents/
financialaid
Email medicine@osu.edu

Public Institution

Dr. Wiley Chip Souba, Dean

Dr. Don Batisky, Associate Dean, Admissions

*Dr. Leon McDougle, Assistant Dean,
Minority Affairs*

Samuel Matheny, Director, Financial Services

Lorna Kenyon, Director, Admissions

General Information

Since 1914, The Ohio State University College of
Medicine has blended traditional medical education, innovative learning opportunities, and a
strong reputation in the preparation of students
for primary care and specialized residencies,
encouraging research interests and a strong
emphasis on a biopsychosocial approach to
patient care.

Mission Statement

To achieve distinction in education, scholarship
and public service; to educate skilled professionals
in the basic and clinical medical sciences, public
health, and allied medical professions; to create,
evaluate, and disseminate knowledge and technology; and, to provide innovative solutions for
improving the health of our people.

Curricular Highlights

Community Service Requirement: Required.
This is part of Patient Centered Medicine.
Research/Thesis Requirement: Optional.

Initial 14-week course in anatomy, histology, and
embryology, followed by choice of two preclinical pathways. Integrated Pathway features body
systems-oriented content that fuses the basic and
clinical sciences using methods of student-centered active learning, small-group case-based
discussion, and lectures. Independent Study
Pathway students use highly structured objectives, resource guides, and Web and computer-
based materials to read, review, and learn on
their own. Clinical experiences begin the first
year with Patient Centered Medicine and
Physician Development. In addition, standardized patients allow students to build clinical proficiency in a setting that includes patient actors.

Third-year clerkships include family medicine,
internal medicine, obstetrics and gynecology,
pediatrics, psychiatry, neurology, and surgery.
A clinical skills immersion experience ensures
that all students have an in-depth understanding
of a core set of procedurally based clinical skills.
Fourth-year selectives focus on the care of
patients at various stages of illness and wellness:
undifferentiated patient; patient with chronic
care needs; and a sub-internship. Students have
more flexibility in the fourth year, with 4 months
of elective rotations and 3 months of vacation.
There is a state-of-the-art Clinical Skills facility.

USMLE

Step 1: Required. Students must record a passing
score for promotion.
Step 2: Clinical Skills (CS): Required. Students
must record a passing total score to graduate.
Step 2: Clinical Knowledge (CK): Required. Students must record a passing total score to graduate.

Selection Factors

Completed applications are reviewed to ensure
that excellent candidates who do not fit the general profile are not overlooked. Factors considered
include clinical and shadowing experiences, community service and leadership activities, research
experience, recommendations, suitability for the
study of medicine, and personal information.

Financial Aid

There is need-based financial aid assistance.
Students participate in various scholarship
and low-interest loan programs. Accepted
candidates are mailed financial aid materials
prior to entering to be considered with students already in school. Financial need is not
a deterrent to acceptance. Every effort is made
to assist each student in securing sufficient
resources for continuing their education.

Information about Diversity Programs

Students whose previous educational and economic deprivation warrant special consideration are carefully evaluated and offered special
help in the acquisition of additional resources.
The Medpath Medical Careers Pathway is a
postbaccalaureate program aimed at develop

ing the academic knowledge base and skills of
students enhancing their preparation for medical school.

Campus Information

Setting

The Ohio State University has the nation's
largest single college campus enrollment and
the resources that go with it. Columbus offers
diversity in the arts, cultural events, festivals,
restaurants, sports, and nightlife.

Enrollment

For 2007, total enrollment was: 819

Special Features

The Ohio State University Medical Center is at
the center of cutting-edge developments in the
areas of clinical care, education, and research.
Ohio State was the first U.S. medical center to
perform a complete heart bypass using robotics. In 2003, an Ohio State faculty member
became the first physician in the U.S. to
implant a digital pacemaker in a patient. U.S.
News & World Report annually recognizes the
Ohio State Medical Center as being among the
nation's best hospitals. In 2004, the National
Cancer Institute awarded the University's cancer program a numerical score equivalent to
its highest possible rating—outstanding. The
Patient Centered Medicine course was recognized in 2004 by the Institute of Medicine of
the National Academies as one of four exemplary curricula for teaching social and behavioral science components of medicine.

Housing

The Neil Building and the Gateway Center offer
professional student housing. Victorian Village and
Grandview Heights are also popular. Rent: $400-
2000 monthly.

Satellite Campuses/Facilities

Clinical rotations occur within the Medical
Center, at community hospitals within Columbus,
in rural settings in Ohio, and at locations outside
of Ohio. About 35 percent of the fourth-year
class gains exposure to international health care
with the assistance of the College of Medicine
Office of Global Health.

Application Process and Requirements 2009–2010

Primary Application Service: AMCAS
Earliest filing date: June 1, 2008
Latest filing date: November 1, 2008

Secondary Application Required?: Yes
Sent to: All applicants
Contact: Admissions Office
(614) 292-7137, medicine@osu.edu
Fee: Yes, $60
Fee waiver available: Yes
Earliest filing date: July 1, 2008
Latest filing date: Varies

Latest MCAT® considered: September 2008
Oldest MCAT® considered: 2006

Early Decision Program
School does have EDP
Applicants notified: October 1, 2008
EDP available for: Both Residents
and Non-Residents

Regular Acceptance Notice
Earliest date: October 16, 2008
Latest date: Varies

Applicant's Response to Acceptance
Offer – Maximum Time: Two weeks

Requests for Deferred
Entrance Considered: Yes

Deposit to Hold Place in Class: No
Deposit (Resident): n/a
Deposit (Non-Resident): n/a
Deposit due: n/a
Applied to tuition: n/a
Deposit refundable: n/a
Refundable by: n/a

Estimated number of new entrants: 210
EDP: 10, special program: n/a

Start Month/Year: August 2009

Interview Format: Open-file conversation; one
faculty interview and one student interview.

Other Programs

PREPARATORY PROGRAMS
Postbaccalaureate Program: Yes,
http://medicine.osu.edu/odca/medpath.cfm
Kelly Price, (614) 292-3161
Summer Program: Yes,
Kelly Price, (614) 292-3161, kelly.price@osumc.edu
COMBINED DEGREE PROGRAMS
Baccalaureate/MD: Yes, www.medicine.osu.edu/
futurestudents/admissions/eap/index.cfm
MD/MPH: Yes, http://sph.osu.edu/
academicprograms/mph (614) 293-3907, sph@osu.edu
MD/MBA: Yes, http://fisher.osu.edu/
prospective/graduate/mba (614) 292-8511
fishergrad@cob.osu.edu
MD/JD: Yes, http://moritzlaw.osu.edu
(614)292-8810, lawadmit@osu.edu
MD/PhD: Yes, www.osumdphd.org, (614) 292-7790
Additional Program: Yes,
http://sph.osu.edu/mha, (614) 292-8193

Premedical Coursework

Course	Req.	Rec.	Lab.	Sems.
Inorganic Chemistry	•	•		2
Behavioral Sciences		•		
Biochemistry		•		
Biology	•			2
Biology/Zoology				
Calculus				
College English		•		
College Mathematics				

Course	Req.	Rec.	Lab.	Sems.
Computer Science				
Genetics		•		
Humanities				
Organic Chemistry	•		•	2
Physics	•			2
Psychology				
Social Sciences				
Diversity/Ethics				

Selection Factors: 2007 Accepted Applicants

Proportion of Accepted Applicants with Relevant Experience (Data Self-Reported to AMCAS®)		
Community Service/Volunteer		73%
Medically-Related Work		85%
Research		86%

Shaded bar represents accepted scores ranging from the 10th percentile to the 90th percentile ▬   **School Median** ●   **National Median** ●

Overall GPA	2.0	2.1	2.2	2.3	2.4	2.5	2.6	2.7	2.8	2.9	3.0	3.1	3.2	3.3	3.4	3.5	3.6	3.7	(3.8)	3.9	4.0
Science GPA	2.0	2.1	2.2	2.3	2.4	2.5	2.6	2.7	2.8	2.9	3.0	3.1	3.2	3.3	3.4	3.5	3.6	3.7	(3.8)	3.9	4.0

MCAT® required: Yes, 98% of 2007 accepted applicants took MCAT®

Verbal Reasoning	3	4	5	6	7	8	9	(10)	(11)	12	13	14	15
Physical Sciences	3	4	5	6	7	8	9	10	(11)	(12)	13	14	15
Biological Sciences	3	4	5	6	7	8	9	10	(11)	(12)	13	14	15
Writing Sample			J	K	L	M	N	O	P	(Q)	R	S	T

Acceptance & Matriculation Data for 2007–2008 First Year Class

	Resident	Non-Resident	International	Total
Applied	1158	3468	11	4637
Interviewed	279	429	0	708
Deferred	4	7	0	11
Matriculants				
Early Assurance Program	0	0	0	0
Early Decision Program	5	0	0	5
Baccalaureate/MD	9	1	0	10
MD/PhD	2	3	0	5
Matriculated	109	101	0	**210**

Applications accepted from International Applicants: No

Specialty Choice

2003, 2004, 2005 Graduates, Specialty Choice (As reported by program directors to GME Track™)	
Anesthesiology	5%
Emergency Medicine	6%
Family Practice	11%
Internal Medicine	19%
Obstetrics/Gynecology	4%
Orthopaedic Surgery	4%
Pediatrics	9%
Psychiatry	3%
Radiology	3%
Surgery	7%

Matriculant Demographics: 2007–2008 First Year Class

Men: 118   **Women:** 92

Matriculants' Self-Reported Race/Ethnicity

Mexican American	1	Korean	1
Cuban	0	Vietnamese	0
Puerto Rican	6	Other Asian	3
Other Hispanic	1	Total Asian	43
Total Hispanic	**8**	Native American	2
Chinese	20	Black	13
Asian Indian	16	Native Hawaiian	0
Pakistani	2	White	154
Filipino	3	**Unduplicated Number**	
Japanese	0	**of Matriculants**	**210**

Science and Math Majors: 76%
Matriculants with:
  Baccalaureate degree: 100%
  Graduate degree(s): 7%

Financial Information

Source: 2006–2007 LCME I-B survey
and 2007–2008 AAMC TSF questionnaire

	Residents	Non-Residents
Total Cost of Attendance	$48,305	$62,723
Tuition and Fees	$27,234	$41,652
Other (includes living expenses)	$19,477	$19,477
Health Insurance (can be waived)	$1,594	$1,594

Average 2007 Graduate Indebtedness: $141,220
% of Enrolled Students Receiving Aid: 91%

Criminal Background Check

This medical school requires a criminal background check prior to matriculation.

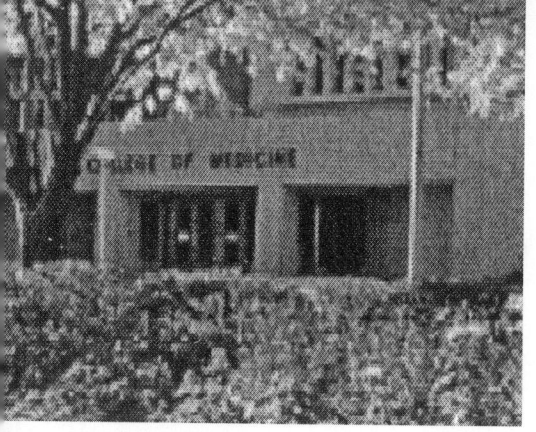

University of Cincinnati College of Medicine

Cincinnati, Ohio

Office of Student Affairs/Admissions
University of Cincinnati College of Medicine
P.O. Box 670552
Cincinnati, Ohio 45267-0552
T 513 5587314   **F** 513 558 1165

Admissions www.med.uc.edu/admissions/
Main www.med.uc.edu
Financial http://medonestop.uc.edu
Email comadmis@ucmail.uc.edu

Public Institution

Dr. David M. Stern, Dean

Dr. Laura Wexler, Associate Dean for Student Affairs/Admissions

Dr. R. Stephen Manuel, Assistant Dean for Admissions

Dr. Charles W. Collins, Associate Dean for Diversity and Community Affairs

Dr. Daniel Burr, Assistant Dean for Student Financial Planning

General Information

The UCCOM provides both outstanding research facilities and superb clinical and teaching experiences. Graduates, ranked as highly competitive by national residency program directors, choose careers in a broad range of specialty areas. Extensive research opportunities are available. UCCOM is ranked in the top third among all public medical schools in NIH research funding.

Mission Statement

The mission of the University of Cincinnati College of Medicine is to improve the health of the public by educating physicians and scientists and by producing new knowledge.

Curricular Highlights

Community Service Requirement: Optional.
Research/Thesis Requirement: Optional.

UCCOM provides a stimulating learning environment, creating the undifferentiated MD ready to excel in residency training and provide excellent patient care. Using an integrated curricular approach including lab, small-group discussion, and team-based learning and lectures, the first two years provide students with the scientific, clinical and humanistic principles of medicine. Year 1 focuses on the normal structure, function and development of the human body. Year 2 emphasizes the basis and mechanisms of human disease. During Year 3, students rotate through six core clerkships. Students also begin exploring career options by participating in three specialty clerkships of their choosing. In Year 4, students hone their clinical skills during

their Acting Internship and required Neuroscience selectives. Students can also choose from over 100 elective offerings.

USMLE

Step 1: Required. Students must record a passing score for promotion.
Step 2: Clinical Skills (CS): Required. Students must record a passing total score to graduate.
Step 2: Clinical Knowledge (CK): Required. Students must record a passing total score to graduate.

Selection Factors

After AMCAS, secondary applications and letters of recommendations are received, completed applicants are evaluated for interviews. The UCCOM Web site provides applicants with admissions progress information. The interview day consists of a brief description of the College and student services and includes: one interview; a presentation about the admissions process, curriculum and student services and financial aid; lunch; and tour. Acceptance offers are based upon the overall and holistic evaluation of academic and personal qualities. Postbaccalaureate and graduate coursework will be considered. Personal characteristics include demonstrated motivation, maturity, coping skills, interpersonal skills, sensitivity and tolerance toward others and communication and critical-thinking skills. Students are admitted on the basis of individual qualifications, regardless of age, religion, sex, sexual orientation, race, color, national origin or disability.

Financial Aid

The College provides counseling to help students fund their medical education and make sound financial decisions. Accepted applicants receive a financial aid packet in February. Applicants with complete files are sent estimated award letters by May 15. To be considered for need-based aid, applicants must submit the Need Access application, which includes parental information. Further information at *www.medonestop.uc.edu*.

Information about Diversity Programs

UCCOM Office of Diversity & Community Affairs works to increase diversity of the medical student body, residency training programs

and faculty through regional and national recruitment efforts of underrepresented groups. The Office retention activities include mentoring, connections with community physicians, academic support and career development. Collaboration with community partners is essential to the Office success.

Campus Information

Setting

The clinical facilities of University Hospital, VA Medical Center, Cincinnati Children's Hospital Medical Center and Shriners Hospital for Children, along with the Cardiovascular Research Center and Vontz Center for Molecular Studies, are all within walking distance of the college. Easily accessible by free shuttle service to the main campus are other dining options, a convenience store and top-of-the-line recreation facilities.

Enrollment

For 2007, total enrollment was: 634

Special Features

The Medical Scholars Program (MSSP) provides students with extracurricular clinical and didactic experiences throughout their education in topical areas such as Neuroscience; Geriatrics; the Art of Family Medicine; Child and Adolescent Health; Poverty, Justice and Health; and Nutrition. The "Shoulder to Shoulder" program explores international health and includes lectures, discussions, and an opportunity to visit Honduras with a medical team. Cincinnati Children's Hospital Medical Center is one of the top pediatric hospitals in the country, providing research and outstanding clinical opportunities. The Center for Surgical Intervention (CSI) bridges new technology in biomedical and surgical care. Using robotics, medical simulation, telecommunications, and medical informatics, the CSI uses new technology in surgical procedures.

Housing

While graduate housing is available on campus, most medical school students reside off campus. Housing information is provided, and students are encouraged to look for housing early.

Application Process and Requirements 2009–2010

Primary Application Service: AMCAS
Earliest filing date: June 1, 2008
Latest filing date: November 15, 2008

Secondary Application Required?: Yes
Sent to: All applicants
URL: www.MedOneStop.uc.edu
Fee: Yes, $25
Fee waiver available: Yes
Earliest filing date: July 15, 2008
Latest filing date: December 15, 2008

Latest MCAT® considered: September 2008
Oldest MCAT® considered: August 2006

Early Decision Program
School does have EDP
Applicants notified: October 1, 2008
EDP available for: Both Residents
and Non-Residents

Regular Acceptance Notice
Earliest date: October 15, 2008
Latest date: Until class is full

**Applicant's Response to Acceptance
Offer – Maximum Time:** Two weeks

**Requests for Deferred
Entrance Considered:** Yes

Deposit to Hold Place in Class: No
Deposit (Resident): n/a
Deposit (Non-Resident): n/a
Deposit due: n/a
Applied to tuition: n/a
Deposit refundable: n/a
Refundable by: n/a

Estimated number of new entrants: 160
EDP: 12, special program: n/a

Start Month/Year: August 2009

Interview Format: Interview with one
member of the Admissions Committee. Regional
interviews are not available.

Other Programs

PREPARATORY PROGRAMS
Postbaccalaureate Program: Yes,
www.mcp.uc.edu, Karen Coleman, (513) 558-3104,
Summer Program: Yes,
www.med.uc.edu/admissions/summerenrich.cfm
Lathel Bryant, MA, (513) 558-0693,
lathel.bryant@uc.edu
Summer Research Scholars (SRS):
www.med.uc.edu/admissions/summerenrich.cfm
COMBINED DEGREE PROGRAMS
Baccalaureate/MD: Yes,
www.med.uc.edu/HS2MD, Nikki Bibler
(513) 558-5581, DualAdmissionsProgram@uc.edu
MD/MPH: Yes, www.med.uc.edu/PublicHealth/
MPH.cfm, James Boex, Ph.D., MBA,
(513) 558-5613, james.boex@uc.edu
MD/MBA: Yes, www.business.uc.edu,
Dawn Owens, (513) 556-7024, dawn.owens@uc.edu
MD/PhD: Yes, www.med.uc.edu/pstp, Leslie Myatt,
PHD, (513) 558-2380, leslie.myatt@uc.edu

Premedical Coursework

Course	Req.	Rec.	Lab.	Sems.	Course	Req.	Rec.	Lab.	Sems.
Inorganic Chemistry		•			Computer Science		•		
Behavioral Sciences		•			Genetics		•		
Biochemistry		•			Humanities		•		
Biology		•			Organic Chemistry		•		
Biology/Zoology		•			Physics		•		
Calculus		•			Psychology		•		
College English		•			Social Sciences		•		
College Mathematics		•			Other				

Selection Factors: 2007 Accepted Applicants

Proportion of Accepted Applicants with Relevant Experience (Data Self-Reported to AMCAS®)			Community Service/Volunteer	67%
			Medically-Related Work	76%
			Research	77%

Shaded bar represents accepted scores ranging from the 10th percentile to the 90th percentile.   School Median ●   National Median ●

Overall GPA	2.0	2.1	2.2	2.3	2.4	2.5	2.6	2.7	2.8	2.9	3.0	3.1	3.2	3.3	3.4	3.5	3.6	(3.7)	3.8	3.9	4.0
Science GPA	2.0	2.1	2.2	2.3	2.4	2.5	2.6	2.7	2.8	2.9	3.0	3.1	3.2	3.3	3.4	3.5	3.6	(3.7)	3.8	3.9	4.0

MCAT® required: Yes, 100% of 2007 accepted applicants took MCAT®

Verbal Reasoning	3	4	5	6	7	8	9	(10)	(11)	12	13	14	15
Physical Sciences	3	4	5	6	7	8	9	10	(11)	12	13	14	15
Biological Sciences	3	4	5	6	7	8	9	10	(11)	12	13	14	15
Writing Sample			J	K	L	M	N	O	(P)	(Q)	R	S	T

Acceptance & Matriculation Data for 2007–2008 First Year Class

	Resident	Non-Resident	International	Total
Applied	1167	2947	41	4155
Interviewed	352	222	0	574
Deferred	3	0	0	3
Matriculants				
Early Assurance Program	20	4	0	24
Early Decision Program	10	2	0	12
Baccalaureate/MD	n/a	n/a	n/a	n/a
MD/PhD	1	5	0	6
Matriculated	121	39	1	**161**

Applications accepted from International Applicants: No

Specialty Choice

2003, 2004, 2005 Graduates, Specialty Choice (As reported by program directors to GME Track™)

Anesthesiology	8%
Emergency Medicine	8%
Family Practice	8%
Internal Medicine	16%
Obstetrics/Gynecology	3%
Orthopaedic Surgery	4%
Pediatrics	12%
Psychiatry	6%
Radiology	6%
Surgery	8%

Matriculant Demographics: 2007–2008 First Year Class

Men: 95   **Women:** 66

Matriculants' Self-Reported Race/Ethnicity

Mexican American	0	Korean	3
Cuban	0	Vietnamese	1
Puerto Rican	0	Other Asian	5
Other Hispanic	0	Total Asian	33
Total Hispanic	0	Native American	0
Chinese	11	Black	11
Asian Indian	11	Native Hawaiian	0
Pakistani	2	White	119
Filipino	0	**Unduplicated Number**	
Japanese	1	**of Matriculants**	161

Science and Math Majors: 83%
Matriculants with:
      Baccalaureate degree: 99%
      Graduate degree(s): 9%

Financial Information

Source: 2006–2007 LCME I-B survey
and 2007–2008 AAMC TSF questionnaire

	Residents	Non-Residents
Total Cost of Attendance	$47,430	$66,797
Tuition and Fees	$26,910	$46,077
Other (includes living expenses)	$19,284	$19,484
Health Insurance (can be waived)	$1,236	$1,236

Average 2007 Graduate Indebtedness: $139,091
% of Enrolled Students Receiving Aid: 88%

Criminal Background Check

This medical school requires a criminal background check
prior to matriculation.

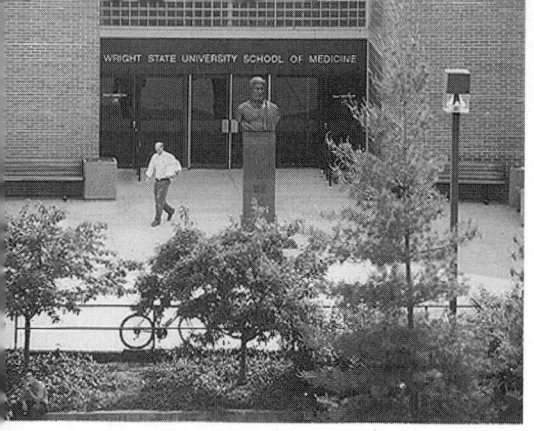

Wright State University School of Medicine
Dayton, Ohio

Office of Student Affairs/Admissions
Wright State University
Boonshoft School of Medicine
P.O. Box 1751
Dayton, Ohio 45401-1751
T 937 775 2934 **F** 937 775 3322

Admissions www.med.wright.edu/admiss
Main www.med.wright.edu
Financial www.med.wright.edu/students/financialaid.html
Email som_saa@wright.edu

Public Institution

Dr. Howard Part, Dean

Dr. Gary LeRoy, Associate Dean for Student Affairs/Admissions

Charlotta Taylor, Director of Recruitment

Dr. Gwen Sloas, Director of Financial Aid

Dr. Stephen Peterson, Assistant Dean for Student Affairs and Admissions

General Information
The Boonshoft School of Medicine is a community-based medical school. Clinical facilities include six major teaching hospitals with over 3,500 patient beds. A faculty of over 1,000 provides students with opportunities for individualized attention. The educational program emphasizes research, generalist training, community health care, community service, patient focused care, cultural competence, cultural diversity, health promotion, disease prevention, and the provision of care to underserved populations.

Mission Statement
The mission of the School is to educate culturally diverse students to become excellent physicians by focusing on generalist training that is integrated, supported, and strengthened by specialists and researchers. The faculty values patient-focused care, community service, research, and have passion for improving health in our communities. These goals and objectives are achieved through: opportunities to learn in clinical settings beginning in the first month; integration of basic and clinical science throughout four years; instruction in community-based, in-patient and outpatient settings; utilization of diverse learning strategies; interaction with faculty in an atmosphere that fosters teamwork, camaraderie, and collegiality; and diversity in the student body and patient population, reflecting many ethnic, racial, social, age, lifestyle, and gender differences.

Curricular Highlights
Community Service Requirement: Optional. Opportunities are Numerous
Research/Thesis Requirement: Optional.

Students are taught in an interdisciplinary fashion using diverse techniques. In the first year, basic principles, mechanisms of disease, social and ethical issues, and evidence-based medicine are taught. Throughout the first two years, students are instructed in medical history-taking, physical examination, and catastrophic illnesses. Each year includes a two-week clinical elective. In the second year, pathobiology, therapeutics and eight organ systems are taught. The year concludes with USMLE preparation and time for study. In the third year, students learn through six core clerkships. The fourth year includes two clerkships, six electives (some of which may be done away) and time for USMLE study.

USMLE
Step 1: Required. Students must record a passing score for promotion.
Step 2: Clinical Skills (CS): Required. Students must record a passing total score to graduate.
Step 2: Clinical Knowledge (CK): Required. Students must record a passing total score to graduate.

Selection Factors
The school seeks a student body of diverse social, ethnic, and educational backgrounds. Applicants are admitted solely on the basis of individual qualifications without regard to race, religion, gender, sexual orientation, disability, veteran status, national origin, age, or ancestry. Dedication to human concerns, compassion, intellectual capacity, and maturity are of greater importance than specific areas of preprofessional preparation. The School also values evidence of motivation, altruism, leadership, and communication skills. Also considered are one's academic record, MCAT® performance, letters of recommendation, history of service, and the results of a personal interview (by invitation). Ohio residents are given preference, but some non-residents are accepted.

Financial Aid
Scholarships, grants, and loans are available. The school offers financial counseling services and assists students in obtaining needed support. An emergency loan fund is available. Financial status has no effect on one's acceptance.

Information about Diversity Programs
The school and its faculty have a stated policy of providing educational opportunities to disadvantaged applicants and applicants from groups underrepresented in medicine. A pre-matriculation program, mentoring, big brother/big sister program, tutoring, USMLE preparation, and assistance in critical thinking and learning are available. The admissions process gives careful consideration to all applicants.

Campus Information

Setting
The first two years are spent primarily on the main campus in Fairborn, Ohio, a suburb of Dayton. The bucolic campus occupies 250 acres, with over half devoted to wooded acreage and preserve. Dayton is a mid-sized city within a metropolitan area of nearly one million residents.

Enrollment
For 2007, total enrollment was: 400

Special Features
The school's hallmarks include a focus on generalist physician training, dynamic partnerships with our community, community service, and collaborative research. Our curriculum niche puts us on the cutting edge of medical instruction, but retains the personal touch so important to our students' education.

Housing
Housing is readily available at reasonable costs adjacent to campus and throughout the Dayton area. The school assists students in finding housing and roommates.

Satellite Campuses/Facilities
The School partners with area hospitals, clinics, and other health care providers. Students spend time in federal hospitals, private hospitals, a children's hospital, neighborhood clinics, nursing homes, and private physician offices. Approximately 250 full time clinical faculty are located in affiliated health care institutions. Many of the School's outreach programs have received national recognition.

Application Process and Requirements 2009–2010

Primary Application Service: AMCAS
Earliest filing date: June 1, 2008
Latest filing date: November 15, 2008

Secondary Application Required?: Yes
Sent to: All applicants
URL: www.med.wright.edu/admiss/start.html
Fee: Yes, $45
Fee waiver available: Yes
Earliest filing date: June 15, 2008
Latest filing date: December 31, 2008

Latest MCAT® considered: September 2008
Oldest MCAT® considered: January 2005

Early Decision Program
School does have EDP
Applicants notified: October 1, 2008
EDP available for: Residents only

Regular Acceptance Notice
Earliest date: October 15, 2008
Latest date: Until class is full

Applicant's Response to Acceptance
Offer – Maximum Time: Two weeks

Requests for Deferred
Entrance Considered: Yes

Deposit to Hold Place in Class: No
Deposit (Resident): n/a
Deposit (Non-Resident): n/a
Deposit due: n/a
Applied to tuition: n/a
Deposit refundable: n/a
Refundable by: n/a

Estimated number of new entrants: 100
EDP: 5, special program: n/a

Start Month/Year: August 2009

Interview Format: Two one-on-one interviews, each lasting 30-40 minutes. Regional interviews are not available.

Other Programs

PREPARATORY PROGRAMS
Postbaccalaureate Program: No
Summer Program: No
Prematriculation Program:
(last 3 weeks of July) www.med.wright.edu

COMBINED DEGREE PROGRAMS
Baccalaureate/MD: No
MD/MPH: Yes
www.med.wright.edu/md-mph
MD/MBA: Yes
www.med.wright.edu/md-mba
MD/JD: No
MD/PhD: Yes
www.med.wright.edu/md-phd

Premedical Coursework

Course	Req.	Rec.	Lab.	Sems.	Course	Req.	Rec.	Lab.	Sems.
Inorganic Chemistry	•			2	Computer Science		•		
Behavioral Sciences					Genetics				
Biochemistry		•			Humanities		•		
Biology	•			2	Organic Chemistry	•			2
Biology/Zoology					Physics	•			2
Calculus		•			Psychology		•		
College English	•			2	Social Sciences		•		
College Mathematics	•			2	Other				

Selection Factors: 2007 Accepted Applicants

Proportion of Accepted Applicants with Relevant Experience (Data Self-Reported to AMCAS®)		Community Service/Volunteer	70%
		Medically-Related Work	83%
		Research	75%

Shaded bar represents accepted scores ranging from the 10th percentile to the 90th percentile. School Median ● National Median ●

Overall GPA	2.0	2.1	2.2	2.3	2.4	2.5	2.6	2.7	2.8	2.9	3.0	3.1	3.2	3.3	3.4	3.5	3.6	(3.7)	3.8	3.9	4.0
Science GPA	2.0	2.1	2.2	2.3	2.4	2.5	2.6	2.7	2.8	2.9	3.0	3.1	3.2	3.3	3.4	3.5	(3.6)	3.7	3.8	3.9	4.0

MCAT® required: Yes, 100% of 2007 accepted applicants took MCAT®

Verbal Reasoning	3	4	5	6	7	8	9	(10)	11	12	13	14	15
Physical Sciences	3	4	5	6	7	8	(9)	10	(11)	12	13	14	15
Biological Sciences	3	4	5	6	7	8	9	(10)	(11)	12	13	14	15
Writing Sample				J	K	L	M	N	O	(P)	(Q)	R	S	T

Acceptance & Matriculation Data for 2007–2008 First Year Class

	Resident	Non-Resident	International	Total
Applied	1061	2056	36	3153
Interviewed	399	48	0	447
Deferred	3	1	0	4
Matriculants				
Early Assurance Program	5	0	0	5
Early Decision Program	7	0	0	7
Baccalaureate/MD	n/a	n/a	n/a	n/a
MD/PhD	2	0	0	2
Matriculated	92	8	0	**100**

Applications accepted from International Applicants: No

Specialty Choice

2003, 2004, 2005 Graduates, Specialty Choice (As reported by program directors to GME Track™)	
Anesthesiology	4%
Emergency Medicine	8%
Family Practice	17%
Internal Medicine	15%
Obstetrics/Gynecology	9%
Orthopaedic Surgery	2%
Pediatrics	13%
Psychiatry	6%
Radiology	1%
Surgery	6%

Matriculant Demographics: 2007–2008 First Year Class

Men: 51   **Women:** 49

Matriculants' Self-Reported Race/Ethnicity

Mexican American	1	Korean	1
Cuban	0	Vietnamese	0
Puerto Rican	0	Other Asian	3
Other Hispanic	1	Total Asian	16
Total Hispanic	2	Native American	1
Chinese	4	Black	3
Asian Indian	7	Native Hawaiian	0
Pakistani	0	White	83
Filipino	1	Unduplicated Number	
Japanese	1	of Matriculants	100

Science and Math Majors: 72%
Matriculants with:
   Baccalaureate degree: 99%
   Graduate degree(s): 13%

Financial Information

Source: 2006–2007 LCME I-B survey and 2007–2008 AAMC TSF questionnaire

	Residents	Non-Residents
Total Cost of Attendance	$49,089	$59,157
Tuition and Fees	$26,280	$36,348
Other (includes living expenses)	$20,721	$20,721
Health Insurance (can be waived)	$2,088	$2,088

Average 2007 Graduate Indebtedness: $139,649
% of Enrolled Students Receiving Aid: 92%

Criminal Background Check

This medical school requires a criminal background check prior to matriculation.

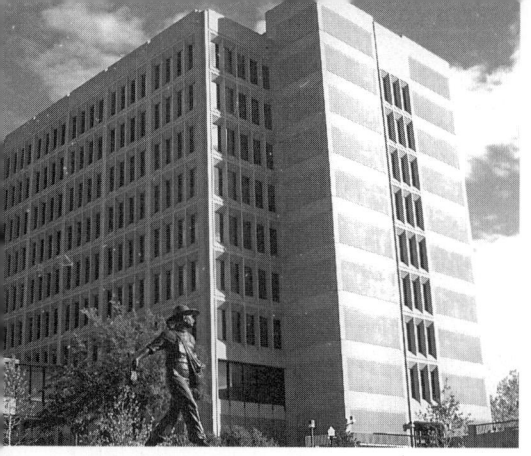

University of Oklahoma College of Medicine
Oklahoma City, Oklahoma

Dotty Shaw Killam
University of Oklahoma College of Medicine
P.O. Box 26901
Oklahoma City, Oklahoma 73126
T 405 271 2331   F 405 271 3032

Admissions www.medicine.ouhsc.edu/admissions
Main www.medicine.ouhsc.edu
Financial http://w3.ouhsc.edu/sfs/
Email AdminMed@ouhsc.edu

Public Institution

Dr. Nancy K. Hall, Associate Dean for Academic Affairs

Dotty Shaw Killam, Director of Admissions

James Albertson, Director of Student Services

Pamela Jordan, Director of Financial Aid

Kate Stanton, Director for Student Affairs

Dr. Sherri S. Baker, Assistant Dean for Admissions

General Information
The University of Oklahoma College of Medicine offers students a quality education with added advantages. Access to modern patient care facilities and an aggressive research program are provided at a reasonable cost with a proven record of choice residency placement. Students gain experience in a variety of settings. The college is part of a modern health sciences complex that serves as the state's principal education and research facility for physicians, dentists, nurses, biomedical scientists, pharmacists, public health administrators, and a wide range of allied health professionals.

Mission Statement
The mission of the University of Oklahoma is to provide the best educational experience for our students through excellence in teaching, research and creative activity, and service to the state and society. New structures, facilities, and technology — plus an internationally prominent faculty — will undoubtedly make the University of Oklahoma Health Sciences Center and the O.U. College of Medicine one of the next century's regional leaders in education, research, and patient care.

Curricular Highlights
Community Service Requirement: Optional.
Research/Thesis Requirement: Optional.

The four-year curriculum consists of two years of study in basic sciences and two in clinical sciences. Letter grades are awarded for all coursework on a course-hour basis rather than a credit-hour basis.

The first two years are complemented by a Web-based on-line curriculum. All students are required to have a computer. There are 17 required courses in the basic science portion of the curriculum. They account for 1,636 hours of instruction or 33 percent of the total. First-year courses provide a strong basic science foundation, and second-year classes form a bridge leading directly into the clinical portion of the curriculum. A significant feature of the curriculum is early exposure to patients through the continuum courses: Principles of Clinical Medicine I and II. Courses in bioethical and legal issues in medicine are also offered. The clinical program provides training at two sites.

USMLE
Step 1: Required. Students must record a passing score for promotion.
Step 2: Clinical Skills (CS): Required. Students must only record a score.
Step 2: Clinical Knowledge (CK): Required. Students must only record a score.

Selection Factors
Acceptance into the College of Medicine is based on GPA, MCAT® scores, letters of evaluation from faculty and premedical committees, and personal interviews conducted on campus by members of the Admissions Board. Emphasis is placed on self-awareness, self-discipline, empathy, personal competence, social competence, and an over-all evaluation of character. Non-residents can represent up to 15% of the student body. The University of Oklahoma College of Medicine does not discriminate on the basis of race, sex, creed, national origin, age, or handicap.

Financial Aid
The College of Medicine offers a number of financial assistance opportunities in addition to the federally sponsored programs. The most prominent scholarships are the Regents' Scholarship Fee Waiver, the Oklahoma Rural Medical Education Loan Scholarship Fund (designed for residents wishing to practice in rural communities). The loan funds established by the Shepherd Foundation, Inc., and the Lew Wentz Foundation, along with over 20 other scholarships, also aid many students

annually. Additional support for students from groups underrepresented in medicine is available through the State Regents for Higher Education, the Ungerman Trust, and the Belknap, Culpeper, Maurer, and Reid-Winnie scholarships. In a need or merit-based application process, the College of Medicine awards approximately $350,000.00 in scholarships to over 150 medical students.

Information about Diversity Programs
The University of Oklahoma has a strong commitment to identify, recruit, and educate qualified students from groups underrepresented in medicine. Applications are strongly encouraged from these groups, as well as from any candidate with a disadvantaged background.

Campus Information

Setting
The College of Medicine offers programs in Oklahoma City and Tulsa. The Health Sciences Center in Oklahoma City is part of a 200-acre complex of 28 public and private institutions known as the Oklahoma Health Center.

Enrollment
For 2007, total enrollment was: 599

Special Features
The OU College of Medicine and OU Medical Center operate the state's only American College of Surgeons Level-I Trauma Center. The Health Sciences Center also has an Oklahoma Diabetes Center and an Oklahoma Cancer Institute with new facilities being built.

Housing
The University of Oklahoma operates an on-campus apartment complex. Off-campus housing options are also available to students.

Satellite Campuses/Facilities
The College of Medicine's primary campus is in Oklahoma City, with a clinical campus in Tulsa.

Application Process and Requirements 2009–2010

Primary Application Service: AMCAS
Earliest filing date: June 1, 2008
Latest filing date: October 15, 2008

Secondary Application Required?: Yes
Sent to: All applicants
URL: www.medicine.ouhsc.edu/admissions/supplemental.asp
Fee: Yes, $65
Fee waiver available: No
Earliest filing date: June 1, 2008
Latest filing date: November 1, 2008

Latest MCAT® considered: August 2008
Oldest MCAT® considered: 2005

Early Decision Program
School does not have EDP
Applicants notified: n/a
EDP available for: n/a

Regular Acceptance Notice
Earliest date: November 1, 2008
Latest date: Until class is full

Applicant's Response to Acceptance
Offer – Maximum Time: Two weeks

Requests for Deferred
Entrance Considered: No

Deposit to Hold Place in Class: Yes
Deposit (Resident): $100
Deposit (Non-Resident): $100
Deposit due: Within two weeks with response to acceptance offer
Applied to tuition: Yes
Deposit refundable: Yes
Refundable by: May 15, 2009

Estimated number of new entrants: 162
EDP: n/a, special program: n/a

Start Month/Year: August 2009

Interview Format: Held October through February. Regional interviews are not available.

Other Programs

PREPARATORY PROGRAMS
Postbaccalaureate Program: No
Summer Program: No

COMBINED DEGREE PROGRAMS
Baccalaureate/MD: No
MD/MPH: Yes, www.medicine.ouhsc.edu/programs/mdmph.asp
MD/MBA: No
MD/JD: No
MD/PhD: Yes, http://mdphd.ouhsc.edu/
Melissa Beben, (405) 271-2503
mdphd-program@ouhsc.edu

Premedical Coursework

Course	Req.	Rec.	Lab.	Sems.
Inorganic Chemistry	•			2
Behavioral Sciences				
Biochemistry				
Biology				
Biology/Zoology	•		•	1
Calculus				
College English	•			3
College Mathematics				

Course	Req.	Rec.	Lab.	Sems.
Computer Science				
Genetics		•		1
Humanities		•		1
Organic Chemistry	•			2
Physics	•			2
Psychology			•	1
Social Sciences			•	1
Other				

Selection Factors: 2007 Accepted Applicants

Proportion of Accepted Applicants with Relevant Experience (Data Self-Reported to AMCAS)		
Community Service/Volunteer		72%
Medically-Related Work		81%
Research		59%

Shaded bar represents accepted scores ranging from the 10th percentile to the 90th percentile. School Median ● National Median ●

	2.0	2.1	2.2	2.3	2.4	2.5	2.6	2.7	2.8	2.9	3.0	3.1	3.2	3.3	3.4	3.5	3.6	3.7	3.8	3.9	4.0
Overall GPA	2.0	2.1	2.2	2.3	2.4	2.5	2.6	2.7	2.8	2.9	3.0	3.1	3.2	3.3	3.4	3.5	3.6	3.7	(3.8)	3.9	4.0
Science GPA	2.0	2.1	2.2	2.3	2.4	2.5	2.6	2.7	2.8	2.9	3.0	3.1	3.2	3.3	3.4	3.5	3.6	3.7	(3.8)	3.9	4.0

MCAT® required: Yes, 100% of 2007 accepted applicants took MCAT®

Verbal Reasoning	3	4	5	6	7	8	9	(10)	11	12	13	14	15
Physical Sciences	3	4	5	6	7	8	9	(10)	(11)	12	13	14	15
Biological Sciences	3	4	5	6	7	8	9	(10)	(11)	12	13	14	15
Writing Sample				J	K	L	M	N	(O)	P	(Q)	R	S	T

Acceptance & Matriculation Data for 2007–2008 First Year Class

	Resident	Non-Resident	International	Total
Applied	401	875	12	1288
Interviewed	237	62	0	299
Deferred	0	0	0	0
Matriculants				
Early Assurance Program	0	0	0	0
Early Decision Program	0	0	0	0
Baccalaureate/MD	n/a	n/a	n/a	n/a
MD/PhD	0	0	0	0
Matriculated	144	20	0	**164**

Applications accepted from International Applicants: No

Specialty Choice

2003, 2004, 2005 Graduates, Specialty Choice (As reported by program directors to GME Track™)	
Anesthesiology	7%
Emergency Medicine	5%
Family Practice	16%
Internal Medicine	14%
Obstetrics/Gynecology	4%
Orthopaedic Surgery	4%
Pediatrics	10%
Psychiatry	6%
Radiology	6%
Surgery	7%

Matriculant Demographics: 2007–2008 First Year Class

Men: 98   **Women:** 66

Matriculants' Self-Reported Race/Ethnicity

Mexican American	1	Korean	2
Cuban	0	Vietnamese	11
Puerto Rican	0	Other Asian	5
Other Hispanic	3	Total Asian	30
Total Hispanic	4	Native American	19
Chinese	5	Black	3
Asian Indian	10	Native Hawaiian	0
Pakistani	0	White	116
Filipino	1	Unduplicated Number	
Japanese	0	of Matriculants	164

Science and Math Majors: 84%
Matriculants with:
Baccalaureate degree: 100%
Graduate degree(s): 6%

Financial Information

Source: 2006–2007 LCME I-B survey and 2007–2008 AAMC TSF questionnaire

	Residents	Non-Residents
Total Cost of Attendance	$19,206	$42,176
Tuition and Fees	$19,078	$42,048
Other (includes living expenses)	$0	$0
Health Insurance (not applicable)	$128	$128

Average 2007 Graduate Indebtedness: $112,085
% of Enrolled Students Receiving Aid: 90%

Criminal Background Check

This medical school requires a criminal background check prior to matriculation.

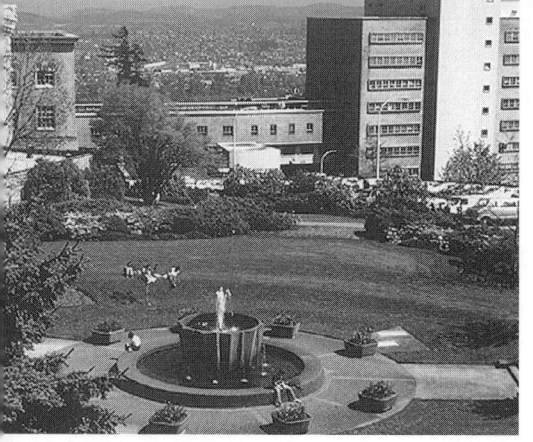

Oregon Health & Science University School of Medicine

Portland, Oregon

Oregon Health & Science University
Office of Education and Student Affairs, L102
3181 S.W. Sam Jackson Park Road
Portland, Oregon 97239-3098
T 503 494 2998   **F** 503 494 3400

Admissions www.ohsu.edu/som/dean/md/
admissions/index.shtml
Main www.ohsu.edu/som
Financial www.ohsu.edu/finaid
Email n/a

Public Institution

Dr. Mark Richardson, Dean

Dr. Cynthia Morris, Assistant Dean for Admissions

Dr. Ella Booth, Associate Dean for Diversity

Debbie Melton, Director of Admissions

General Information

Oregon Health & Science University (OHSU) occupies a 101-acre site and 31 buildings in Sam Jackson Park overlooking the city of Portland. Campus physical facilities include basic science, research, and laboratory buildings; two hospital units with a licensed capacity of 509 beds; and outpatient clinics. The 3rd and 4th year curriculum is already regionalized throughout Oregon. Plans are being developed to expand the first year curriculum to other major universities in Oregon.

Mission Statement

The mission of the School of Medicine is to enhance human health through programs of excellence in education, research, health care, and public service to the larger community including underserved populations. In achieving these goals, the Oregon Health & Science University School of Medicine seeks to establish an educational environment that challenges students to strive for academic excellence and fosters development of compassion, humanism, professionalism, and cultural competence in the care of patients from their first days in the classroom to their final rotation in the hospitals and clinics. A priority throughout OHSU is to enable each student to fulfill his or her potential as a human being and as a health care professional while effectively meeting the health-related needs of the multiple communities he or she will serve.

Curricular Highlights

Community Service Requirement: Optional.
Research/Thesis Requirement: Optional.

The preclincal integrated curriculum is devoted to the sciences basic to medicine, focusing on the normal structure and function of the body and continuing with the study of the pathophysiological basis of disease and its treatment. An early clinical experience is afforded through the Principles of Clinical Medicine, which teaches fundamental knowledge and skills in interviewing and physical diagnosis through a continuity clinical preceptorship experience. Clinical clerkships are undertaken at OHSU Hospital and Clinics and affiliated hospitals in the Portland area. OHSU offers regional clinical experiences throughout Oregon.

USMLE

Step 1: Required. Students must only record a score.
Step 2: Clinical Skills (CS): Required. Students must only record a score.
Step 2: Clinical Knowledge (CK): Required. Students must only record a score.

Selection Factors

The Admissions Committee seeks students who have demonstrated academic excellence and readiness for the profession of medicine and who will contribute to the diversity necessary to enhance the medical education of all students. Applicants are selected on the basis of demonstrated motivation for medicine, humanistic attitudes, and a realistic understanding of the role of the physician in providing excellent health care to all communities in need of care. The ideal student will demonstrate evidence of strong communication skills; altruism, empathy, and personal integrity; self-appraisal and emotional maturity; and an ability to make a positive contribution to society and the profession. Attention is paid to achievements that demonstrate applicants' breadth of interests and experiences, commitment to others, leadership among their peers, and the ability to contribute diverse and innovative perspectives to problem-solving in medicine and health care. Evaluation of applicants includes the academic record as demonstration of scholarship; the MCAT®; recommendations from undergraduate or graduate school faculty, employers, and those familiar with applicants' health care, volunteer, and community service experiences; and the personal interview. Preference is given to residents of Oregon, WICHE-certified residents of Montana and Wyoming, MD/PhD and

MD/MPH candidates, and non-resident applicants with superior achievements in academics and other related experiences. The School of Medicine Admissions Committee fully recognizes the importance of diversity in its student body and in the physician workforce in providing for effective delivery of health care. Accordingly, the OHSU School of Medicine strongly encourages applications from persons from all socioeconomic, racial, ethnic, religious, and educational backgrounds and persons from groups underrepresented in medicine. The committee adheres to a policy of equal opportunity and non-discrimination on the basis of sex, age, race, ethnic origin, religion, disability, or sexual orientation.

Financial Aid

Financial aid in the form of scholarships, grants, and loans is available based upon the demonstrated need of the student. For more information please review the web site at *www.ohsu.edu/finaid*.

Information about Diversity Programs

More information may be obtained by contacting the Office of Diversity, Dr. Ella Booth, Associate Dean, at (503) 494-1681.

Setting

University Hospital and the School of Medicine are located on a hilltop overlooking the city of Portland, Oregon. Students have easy access to the city center as well as the surrounding communities.

Campus Information

Enrollment

For 2007, total enrollment was: 512

Satellite Campuses/Facilities

Third and Fourth year students may participate in required and elective clinical experiences in Eugene, Bend and Medford, Oregon.

Application Process and Requirements 2009–2010

Primary Application Service: AMCAS
Earliest filing date: June 1, 2008
Latest filing date: October 15, 2008

Secondary Application Required?: Yes
Sent to: Screened applicants
URL: n/a
Fee: Yes, $100
Fee waiver available: Yes
Earliest filing date: July 1, 2008
Latest filing date: January 15, 2009

Latest MCAT® considered: September 2008
Oldest MCAT® considered: 2006

Early Decision Program
School does not have EDP
Applicants notified: n/a
EDP available for: n/a

Regular Acceptance Notice
Earliest date: October 15, 2008
Latest date: Until class is full

Applicant's Response to Acceptance
Offer – Maximum Time: Two weeks

Requests for Deferred
Entrance Considered: No

Deposit to Hold Place in Class: No
Deposit (Resident): n/a
Deposit (Non-Resident): n/a
Deposit due: n/a
Applied to tuition: n/a
Deposit refundable: n/a
Refundable by: n/a

Estimated number of new entrants: 115
EDP: n/a, special program: n/a

Start Month/Year: August 2009

Interview Format: Two, one-on-one 30-45 minute interviews. Regional interviews are not available.

Other Programs

PREPARATORY PROGRAMS
Health Careers Opportunity Program:
hcop@ohsu.edu
Postbaccalaureate Program: Yes,
www.ohsu.edu/ohsuedu/academic/som/diversity/diversity-achievement.cfm
Summer Program: No

COMBINED DEGREE PROGRAMS
Baccalaureate/MD: No
MD/MPH: Yes,
www.ohsu.edu/public-health
MD/MBA: No
MD/JD: No
MD/PhD: Yes,
www.ohsu.edu/mdphd

Premedical Coursework

Course	Req.	Rec.	Lab.	Qtrs.	Course	Req.	Rec.	Lab.	Qtrs.
Inorganic Chemistry	•		•	1	Computer Science				
Behavioral Sciences					Genetics		•		1
Biochemistry	•		•	1	Humanities				
Biology	•		•	3	Organic Chemistry	•		•	1
Biology/Zoology					Physics	•		•	3
Calculus		•		1	Psychology				
College English	•			1	Statistics		•		1
College Mathematics	•			1	Humanities/Social Sciences	•			6

Selection Factors: 2007 Accepted Applicants

Proportion of Accepted Applicants with Relevant Experience (Data Self-Reported to AMCAS®)		Community Service/Volunteer	77%
		Medically-Related Work	93%
		Research	71%

Shaded bar represents accepted scores ranging from the 10th percentile to the 90th percentile ▬   School Median ● National Median ●

Overall GPA	2.0	2.1	2.2	2.3	2.4	2.5	2.6	2.7	2.8	2.9	3.0	3.1	3.2	3.3	3.4	3.5	3.6	3.7	(3.8)	3.9	4.0
Science GPA	2.0	2.1	2.2	2.3	2.4	2.5	2.6	2.7	2.8	2.9	3.0	3.1	3.2	3.3	3.4	3.5	3.6	(3.7)	3.8	3.9	4.0

MCAT® required: Yes, 100% of 2007 accepted applicants took MCAT®

Verbal Reasoning	3	4	5	6	7	8	9	(10)	(11)	12	13	14	15
Physical Sciences	3	4	5	6	7	8	9	(10)	(11)	12	13	14	15
Biological Sciences	3	4	5	6	7	8	9	10	(11)	12	13	14	15
Writing Sample				J	K	L	M	N	O	P	(Q)	R	S	T

Acceptance & Matriculation Data for 2007–2008 First Year Class

	Resident	Non-Resident	International	Total
Applied	389	3955	27	4371
Interviewed	209	304	0	513
Deferred	0	0	0	0
Matriculants				
Early Assurance Program	0	0	0	0
Early Decision Program	0	0	0	0
Baccalaureate/MD	n/a	n/a	n/a	n/a
MD/PhD	1	4	0	5
Matriculated	81	37	0	**118**

Applications accepted from International Applicants: No

Matriculant Demographics: 2007–2008 First Year Class

Men: 56   **Women:** 62

Matriculants' Self-Reported Race/Ethnicity

Mexican American	2	**Korean**	2
Cuban	0	**Vietnamese**	4
Puerto Rican	0	**Other Asian**	4
Other Hispanic	2	**Total Asian**	18
Total Hispanic	4	**Native American**	1
Chinese	6	**Black**	3
Asian Indian	1	**Native Hawaiian**	0
Pakistani	0	**White**	95
Filipino	2	**Unduplicated Number**	
Japanese	0	**of Matriculants**	118

Science and Math Majors: 63%
Matriculants with:
Baccalaureate degree: 100%
Graduate degree(s): 12%

Specialty Choice

2003, 2004, 2005 Graduates, Specialty Choice
(As reported by program directors to GME Track™)

Anesthesiology	6%
Emergency Medicine	11%
Family Practice	12%
Internal Medicine	18%
Obstetrics/Gynecology	7%
Orthopaedic Surgery	1%
Pediatrics	10%
Psychiatry	4%
Radiology	6%
Surgery	6%

Financial Information

Source: 2006–2007 LCME I-B survey and 2007–2008 AAMC TSF questionnaire

	Residents	Non-Residents
Total Cost of Attendance	$51,012	$61,827
Tuition and Fees	$29,665	$40,480
Other (includes living expenses)	$19,474	$19,474
Health Insurance (can be waived)	$1,873	$1,873

Average 2007 Graduate Indebtedness: $153,826
% of Enrolled Students Receiving Aid: 91%

Criminal Background Check

This medical school requires a criminal background check prior to matriculation.

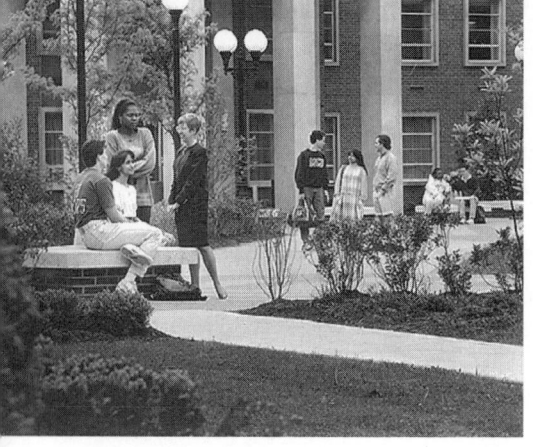

Drexel University College of Medicine

Philadelphia, Pennsylvania

Admissions Office
Drexel University College of Medicine
2900 Queen Lane
Philadelphia, Pennsylvania 19129
T 215 991 8202   **F** 215 843 1766

Admissions http://webcampus.drexelmed.
edu/admissions
Main www.drexelmed.edu
Financial www.drexel.edu/provost/financialaid
Email medadmis@drexel.edu

Private Institution

Dr. Richard V. Homan, Dean

*Dr. Cheryl A. Hanau, Associate Dean
for Admissions*

*Dr. Anthony Rodriguez, Associate Dean
of Student Affairs and Diversity*

Elreo Campbell, Director of Financial Aid

General Information

Drexel University College of Medicine was formed when two historic Philadelphia medical schools joined their rich histories and resources. The Medical College of Pennsylvania (MCP) was founded in 1850 as the first medical school for women. Hahnemann University, a private nondenominational institution, was founded in 1848. Drexel offers a medical education rich in history and diversity, while providing the foundational curriculum and learning environment necessary for the scientific, technological, and ethical decisions required of physicians in the 21st century.

Mission Statement

Drexel is committed to providing our students with the finest possible medical education. Academic instruction in basic and clinical sciences, utilizing state-of-the-art technology, is enriched by an emphasis on compassionate patient care and community service.

Curricular Highlights

Community Service Requirement:
Required. 16 hours is required in year one.
Research/Thesis Requirement:
Optional. Though optional, many students conduct research.

Medical students are trained to consider each patient in a comprehensive, integrated manner, taking into account more factors than the presenting physiological condition. The school is dedicated to preparing "physician healers," who practice the art, science, and skill of medicine. Drexel offers a choice between two innovative curricula for the first two years of study. Interdisciplinary Foundations of Medicine (IFM) integrates basic science courses and

presents them through symptom-based modules. Learning in IFM is faculty-driven; students learn in lectures, labs, and small groups. Learning in the Program for Integrated Learning (PIL), a problem-based curriculum, is student-driven, supervised and facilitated by faculty. Students learn in small groups, labs, and resource sessions by focusing on case studies. Both options stress problem-solving, lifelong learning, and the coordinated training of basic science with clinical medicine. Both include the introduction of clinical skills training very early in the first year. The Pathway Program in the fourth year includes a balance of four week-long required and elective clinical experiences selected with the pathway advisors to be consistent with general medical training and the students ultimate career goals.

USMLE

Step 1: Required. Students must record a passing score for promotion.
Step 2: Clinical Skills (CS): Required. Students must record a passing total score to graduate.
Step 2: Clinical Knowledge (CK): Required. Students must record a passing total score to graduate.

Selection Factors

Drexel seeks highly qualified, motivated students who demonstrate the desire, intelligence, integrity, and emotional maturity to become excellent physicians. We encourage nontraditional applicants and are committed to a diverse student body. We seek students who have a firm grasp of the biological and physical sciences as well as broad educational experiences in other areas. Students who demonstrate a commitment to the service of others are given strong consideration. All students must be able to meet the essential functions of the medical school. Applicants must be U.S. citizens or permanent residents. All aspects of an applicant's file are considered, including grades, MCATs®, experiences, letters of recommendation and essay. Interviews with a faculty member and student are important to an applicant's review at committee.

Financial Aid

In addition to the Stafford Student Loan Program, the Primary Care Loan Program, other federally funded programs, and assistance in obtaining

money from foundation sources, the Financial Affairs Office has at its disposal limited private grant and loan funds. A Work-Study Program for qualified students is available. Money allocated by the school is awarded on the basis of financial need. Fee waivers are only granted if approved by AMCAS.

Information about Diversity Programs

Applications are actively encouraged from groups underrepresented in medicine. Applications from women, those who come from Pennsylvania, and students interested in a career as a generalist physician are also encouraged.

Campus Information

Setting

Located in a largely residential section of Philadelphia, the college is only 15 minutes from Center City. Opened in 1992, this 15-acre site houses the education and research facility which is home for the first and second years of medical education. The campus features wireless internet access.

Enrollment

For 2007, total enrollment was: 1,056

Special Features

The medical school has a supportive environment that fosters a spirit of teamwork and personal interaction. Our state-of-the-art facility includes the CEAC Center with 10 exam rooms where students see standardized patients. Elective enrichment programs include Women's Health and Medical Humanities. Students in their clinical years use PDAs to record patient encounters and log procedures. The recently added 17,620 square-foot Student Activities Center greatly enhances the learning and living environment of the campus.

Housing

On-campus housing is not available. However, the college maintains an on-line list of rentals averaging $500 to $1,400 per month.

Satellite Campuses/Facilities

Students have the opportunity for clinical training in our extensive, integrated network of clinical campuses.

Application Process and Requirements 2009–2010

Primary Application Service: AMCAS
Earliest filing date: June 1, 2008
Latest filing date: December 15, 2008

Secondary Application Required?: Yes
Sent to: All applicants
URL: http://webcampus.drexelmed.edu/admissions
Kelli Kennedy, (215) 881-8220
kelli.kennedy@drexel.edu
Fee: Yes, $75
Fee waiver available: Yes
Earliest filing date: Upon receipt of application
Latest filing date: January 1, 2009

Latest MCAT® considered: September 2008
Oldest MCAT® considered: 2006

Early Decision Program
School does have EDP
Applicants notified: October 1, 2008
EDP available for: Both Residents
and Non-Residents

Regular Acceptance Notice
Earliest date: October 15, 2008
Latest date: Until class is full

Applicant's Response to Acceptance Offer – Maximum Time: 21 days

Requests for Deferred Entrance Considered: Yes

Deposit to Hold Place in Class: Yes
Deposit (Resident): $100
Deposit (Non-Resident): $100
Deposit due: 21 days from acceptance offer
Applied to tuition: Yes
Deposit refundable: Yes
Refundable by: May 15, 2009

Estimated number of new entrants: 255
EDP: n/a, special program: 80

Start Month/Year: August 2009

Interview Format: One faculty open-file, one student closed-file. Regional interviews are not available.

Other Programs

PREPARATORY PROGRAMS
Postbaccalaureate Program: Yes,
www.drexel.edu/med/ims
Summer Program: No
Drexel links with a number of post-baccalaureate programs:
http://webcampus.drexelmed.edu/admissions/linkage.asp
COMBINED DEGREE PROGRAMS
Baccalaureate/MD: Yes, http://webcampus.drexelmed.edu/admissions/linkage.asp
MD/MPH: Yes, publichealth.drexel.edu/1
MD/MBA: Yes,
www.lebow.drexel.edu/graduate/mba/md_mba.html
MD/JD: No
MD/PhD: Yes, www.drexelmed.edu/Graduate Studies/Programs/CombinedMDPhD/tabid/641/Default.aspx
Additional Program: Yes, http://webcampus.drexelmed.edu/admissions/linkage.asp

Premedical Coursework

Course	Req.	Rec.	Lab.	Sems.	Course	Req.	Rec.	Lab.	Sems.
Inorganic Chemistry	•		•	2	Computer Science				
Behavioral Sciences					Genetics		•		
Biochemistry		•			Humanities				
Biology	•		•	2	Organic Chemistry	•		•	2
Biology/Zoology					Physics	•		•	2
Calculus					Psychology				
College English	•			2	Social Sciences				
College Mathematics					Molecular Biology		•		

Selection Factors: 2007 Accepted Applicants

Proportion of Accepted Applicants with Relevant Experience (Data Self-Reported to AMCAS®)		
Community Service/Volunteer	63%
Medically-Related Work	84%
Research	82%

Shaded bar represents accepted scores ranging from the 10th percentile to the 90th percentile   School Median ● National Median ●

Overall GPA	2.0	2.1	2.2	2.3	2.4	2.5	2.6	2.7	2.8	2.9	3.0	3.1	3.2	3.3	3.4	3.5	(3.6)	3.7	3.8	3.9	4.0
Science GPA	2.0	2.1	2.2	2.3	2.4	2.5	2.6	2.7	2.8	2.9	3.0	3.1	3.2	3.3	3.4	3.5	(3.6)	3.7	3.8	3.9	4.0

MCAT® required: Yes, 100% of 2007 accepted applicants took MCAT®

Verbal Reasoning	3	4	5	6	7	8	9	(10)	11	12	13	14	15
Physical Sciences	3	4	5	6	7	8	9	(10)	(11)	12	13	14	15
Biological Sciences	3	4	5	6	7	8	9	10	(11)	12	13	14	15
Writing Sample			J	K	L	M	N	O	(P)	(Q)	R	S	T

Acceptance & Matriculation Data for 2007–2008 First Year Class

	Resident	Non-Resident	International	Total
Applied	1082	11025	67	12174
Interviewed	377	1173	0	1550
Deferred	2	4	0	6
Matriculants				
Early Assurance Program	3	6	0	9
Early Decision Program	0	0	0	0
Baccalaureate/MD	8	37	0	45
MD/PhD	0	3	0	3
Matriculated	93	188	0	**281**
Applications accepted from International Applicants: No				

Matriculant Demographics: 2007–2008 First Year Class

Men: 149   **Women:** 132

Matriculants' Self-Reported Race/Ethnicity

Mexican American	2	Korean	12
Cuban	0	Vietnamese	5
Puerto Rican	1	Other Asian	7
Other Hispanic	5	Total Asian	99
Total Hispanic	8	Native American	1
Chinese	22	Black	10
Asian Indian	53	Native Hawaiian	1
Pakistani	6	White	167
Filipino	1	Unduplicated Number	
Japanese	1	of Matriculants	281

Science and Math Majors: 74%
Matriculants with:
   Baccalaureate degree: 100%
   Graduate degree(s): 14%

Specialty Choice

2003, 2004, 2005 Graduates, Specialty Choice (As reported by program directors to GME Track™)	
Anesthesiology	5%
Emergency Medicine	8%
Family Practice	10%
Internal Medicine	20%
Obstetrics/Gynecology	5%
Orthopaedic Surgery	4%
Pediatrics	12%
Psychiatry	5%
Radiology	5%
Surgery	8%

Financial Information

Source: 2006–2007 LCME I-B survey and 2007–2008 AAMC TSF questionnaire

	Residents	Non-Residents
Total Cost of Attendance	$69,046	$69,046
Tuition and Fees	$42,130	$42,130
Other (includes living expenses)	$24,350	$24,350
Health Insurance (can be waived)	$2,566	$2,566

Average 2007 Graduate Indebtedness: $188,888
% of Enrolled Students Receiving Aid: 87%

Criminal Background Check

This medical school requires a criminal background check prior to matriculation.

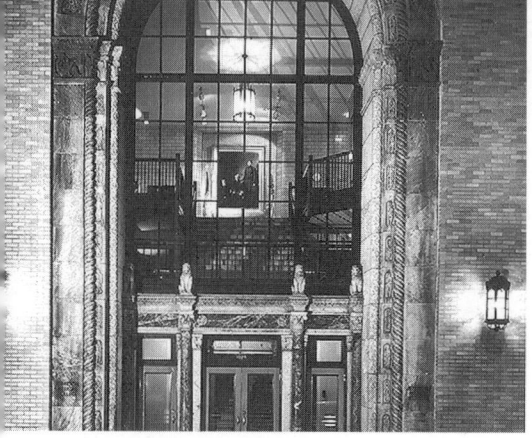

Jefferson Medical College
of Thomas Jefferson University

Philadelphia, Pennsylvania

Office of Admissions
Jefferson Medical College of Thomas Jefferson University
1015 Walnut Street, Suite 110
Philadelphia, Pennsylvania 19107-5099
T 215 955 6983   **F** 215 955 5151

Admissions www.jefferson.edu/jmc/admissions
Main www.jefferson.edu/jmc
Financial www.jefferson.edu/financialaid
Email jmc.admissions@jefferson.edu

Private Institution

Dr. Thomas J. Nasca, Senior Vice President and Dean

Dr. Clara Callahan, Dean of Students and Admissions

Dr. Edward Christian, Associate Dean for Diversity and Minority Affairs

Susan Batchelor, Director of Student Financial Aid

Dr. Elizabeth Brooks, Associate Director of Admissions

General Information

As one of the oldest institutions of higher education in the nation, Thomas Jefferson University has, since its founding as the Jefferson Medical College in 1824, emphasized the attainment of clinical excellence in its educational programs. A recent significant expansion of the research programs has created a balanced institutional mission and has enhanced the clinical instruction at Thomas Jefferson University Hospital and its 17 affiliated hospitals.

Mission Statement

Jefferson's teaching mission centers on the education of outstanding individuals in the art and science of medicine. By helping these individuals to develop their medical knowledge, clinical and research skills, and professional values, attitudes, and behaviors, we strive to provide outstanding physicians for the United States and the world.

Curricular Highlights

Community Service Requirement: Required.
Research/Thesis Requirement: Optional.

The curriculum has been developed to enable students to acquire basic knowledge and skills in the biomedical sciences and to develop appropriate professional behaviors. The curriculum also allows students to pursue some of their special interests throughout their medical training. The tradition of providing a clinically balanced medical education, encouraged by the faculty, is that students support and cooperate with each other. In the first year, students focus on the

function of human organism in its physical and psychosocial context. Clinical coursework focuses on the doctor-patient relationship, medical interviewing and history-taking, human development, behavioral science principles, and core clinical skills and reasoning. In addition to increasing emphasis on the study of clinical skills, the curriculum shifts in the second year to the study of pathophysioiogy and disease. The curriculum includes small-group sessions focusing on problem-solving, evidence-based medicine, and service-based learning. The clinical program consists of two 42-week phases. Phase I covers required clerkships. Advanced basic science, neurology/rehabilitation medicine, emergency medicine/advanced clinical skills, in- and outpatient subinternships, as well as 16 weeks of elective time, are included in Phase II.

USMLE

Step 1: Required. Students must record a passing score for promotion.
Step 2: Clinical Skills (CS): Required. Students must only record a score.
Step 2: Clinical Knowledge (CK): Required. Students must record a passing total score to graduate.

Selection Factors

Jefferson, in accordance with local, state, and federal law, is committed to providing equal educational and employment opportunities for all persons, without regard to race, color, national and ethnic origin, religion, sexual orientation, age, handicap, or veteran status. Jefferson complies with all relevant ordinances and state and federal statutes in the administration of its educational and employment policies and is an affirmative action employer. The selection of students is made after careful consideration of many factors, including the academic record, letters of recommendation, MCAT® scores (an average of 8 in each section), and interview results regarding the applicant's personal qualities, motivation, interpersonal skills, and achievement in nonacademic areas. Jefferson Medical College traditionally has given special consideration to the offspring of alumni and faculty, groups underrepresented in medicine, and applicants to Jefferson's special

programs. International applicants must have a baccalaureate degree from an accredited U.S. or Canadian college or university.

Financial Aid

Financial aid awards are based on need determined by a confidential analysis of information provided by the student and the student's family to the designated needs analysis service. If need is established, the student is directed to obtain a federally subsidized Stafford loan. If need exists beyond this loan program, Jefferson will try to meet a portion of this need from loan and grant funds. Applications for financial aid are available after December from the Office of Student Financial Aid. Completed financial aid applications for the next academic year must be submitted before April 1 or within two weeks of the date of acceptance.

Information about Diversity Programs

Applications from qualified students from groups underrepresented in medicine are encouraged.

Campus Information

Setting

The medical school is proud to be situated near the most historic square mile in America. The campus is 13 square acres in the heart of Center City Philadelphia.

Enrollment

For 2007, total enrollment was: 966

Special Features

Thomas Jefferson University Hospital is one of the area's largest medical centers and includes both a Level I regional resource trauma center and a Spinal Cord Injury Center (SCI).

Housing

On-campus housing is available.

Application Process and Requirements 2009–2010

Primary Application Service: AMCAS
Earliest filing date: June 1, 2008
Latest filing date: November 15, 2008

Secondary Application Required?: Yes
Sent to: All applicants
URL: www.jefferson.edu/jmc/admissions/appforms.cfm
Fee: Yes, $80
Fee waiver available: Yes
Earliest filing date: June 1, 2008
Latest filing date: January 15, 2009

Latest MCAT® considered: September 2008
Oldest MCAT® considered: 2005

Early Decision Program
School does have EDP
Applicants notified: October 1, 2008
EDP available for: Both Residents and Non-Residents

Regular Acceptance Notice
Earliest date: October 15, 2008
Latest date: Until class is full

Applicant's Response to Acceptance Offer – Maximum Time: Three weeks

Requests for Deferred Entrance Considered: Yes

Deposit to Hold Place in Class: Yes
Deposit (Resident): $100
Deposit (Non-Resident): $100
Deposit due: May 15, 2009
Applied to tuition: Yes
Deposit refundable: Yes
Refundable by: May 15, 2009

Estimated number of new entrants: 255
EDP: 6, special program: n/a

Start Month/Year: August 2009

Interview Format: One-on-one, open file (faculty) and closed file (student). Regional interview available on campus only.

Other Programs

PREPARATORY PROGRAMS
Postbaccalaureate Program: No
Summer Program: No

COMBINED DEGREE PROGRAMS
Baccalaureate/MD: Yes
www.science.psu.edu/premedmed/
MD/MPH: Yes, Rob Simmons, DrPh, (215) 955-7312, Rob.Simmins@jefferson.edu
MD/MBA: Yes, David Nash, MD, MBA, (215) 955-6969, David.Nash@jefferson.edu
MD/JD: No
MD/PhD: Yes, www.jefferson.edu/jcgs/mdphd

Premedical Coursework

Course	Req.	Rec.	Lab.	Sems.	Course	Req.	Rec.	Lab.	Sems.
Inorganic Chemistry	•		•	2	Computer Science				
Behavioral Sciences					Genetics				
Biochemistry		•		1	Humanities		•		
Biology	•		•	2	Organic Chemistry	•		•	2
Biology/Zoology					Physics	•		•	2
Calculus					Psychology				
College English		•			Social Sciences		•		
College Mathematics		•			Other				

Selection Factors: 2007 Accepted Applicants

Proportion of Accepted Applicants with Relevant Experience (Data Self-Reported to AMCAS®)		
Community Service/Volunteer		70%
Medically-Related Work		86%
Research		78%

Shaded bar represents accepted scores ranging from the 10th percentile to the 90th percentile. School Median ● National Median ●

Overall GPA	2.0	2.1	2.2	2.3	2.4	2.5	2.6	2.7	2.8	2.9	3.0	3.1	3.2	3.3	3.4	3.5	3.6	(3.7)	3.8	3.9	4.0
Science GPA	2.0	2.1	2.2	2.3	2.4	2.5	2.6	2.7	2.8	2.9	3.0	3.1	3.2	3.3	3.4	3.5	(3.6)	3.7	3.8	3.9	4.0

MCAT® required: Yes, 100% of 2007 accepted applicants took MCAT®

Verbal Reasoning	3	4	5	6	7	8	9	(10)	11	12	13	14	15
Physical Sciences	3	4	5	6	7	8	9	(10)	(11)	12	13	14	15
Biological Sciences	3	4	5	6	7	8	9	10	(11)	12	13	14	15
Writing Sample			J	K	L	M	N	O	P	(Q)	R	S	T

Acceptance & Matriculation Data for 2007–2008 First Year Class

	Resident	Non-Resident	International	Total
Applied	1068	7435	494	8997
Interviewed	207	578	20	805
Deferred	2	9	2	13
Matriculants				
Early Assurance Program	6	13	0	19
Early Decision Program	4	3	0	7
Baccalaureate/MD	6	22	2	30
MD/PhD	0	4	0	4
Matriculated	85	162	12	**259**
Applications accepted from International Applicants: Yes				

Matriculant Demographics: 2007–2008 First Year Class

Men: 140   **Women:** 119

Matriculants' Self-Reported Race/Ethnicity

Mexican American	1	Korean	9
Cuban	0	Vietnamese	8
Puerto Rican	0	Other Asian	7
Other Hispanic	3	Total Asian	77
Total Hispanic	4	Native American	2
Chinese	17	Black	9
Asian Indian	35	Native Hawaiian	1
Pakistani	4	White	168
Filipino	5	Unduplicated Number	
Japanese	3	of Matriculants	259

Science and Math Majors: 68%
Matriculants with:
      Baccalaureate degree: 100%
      Graduate degree(s): 5%

Specialty Choice

2003, 2004, 2005 Graduates, Specialty Choice (As reported by program directors to GME Track™)

Anesthesiology	6%
Emergency Medicine	9%
Family Practice	8%
Internal Medicine	20%
Obstetrics/Gynecology	3%
Orthopaedic Surgery	5%
Pediatrics	8%
Psychiatry	3%
Radiology	4%
Surgery	9%

Financial Information

Source: 2006–2007 LCME I-B survey and 2007–2008 AAMC TSF questionnaire

	Residents	Non-Residents
Total Cost of Attendance	$63,608	$63,608
Tuition and Fees	$41,101	$41,101
Other (includes living expenses)	$19,517	$19,517
Health Insurance (can be waived)	$2,990	$2,990

Average 2007 Graduate Indebtedness: $150,383
% of Enrolled Students Receiving Aid: 83%

Criminal Background Check

This medical school requires a criminal background check prior to matriculation.

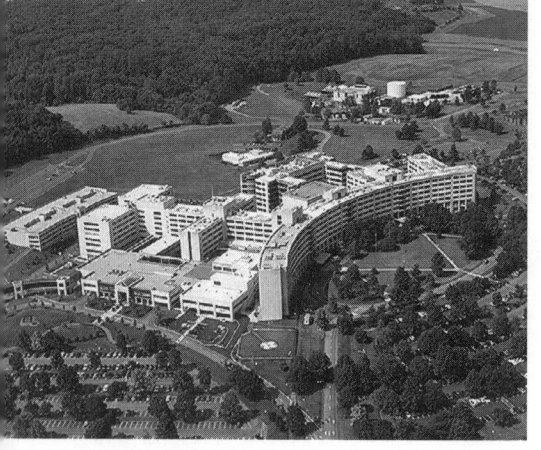

Pennsylvania State University College of Medicine

Hershey, Pennsylvania

Pennsylvania State University College of Medicine
Office of Medical Student Affairs, H060
500 University Drive; P.O. Box 850
Hershey, Pennsylvania 17033
T 717 531 8755   F 717 531 6225

Admissions www.hmc.psu.edu/md/admissions
Main www.hmc.psu.edu/md
Financial www.hmc.psu.edu/md/financialaid
Email studentadmissions@hmc.psu.edu

Public Institution

Dr. Harold L. Paz, Dean, Senior Vice President for Health Affairs

Dr. Dwight Davis, Associate Dean for Admissions and Student Affairs

Dr. Alphonse E. Leure-duPree, Associate Dean for Academic Achievement

Dr. Joetta Bradica, Assistant Director for Financial Aid

Marc Lubbers, Assistant Director for Admissions

General Information

Penn State's Milton S. Hershey Medical Center opened its doors to the first class of medical students in 1967 and became the first medical school in the nation to establish a Department of Humanities, introducing humanistic disciplines into the required medical curriculum. The College of Medicine was also the first to start an independent Department of Family and Community Medicine. From its beginning, medical education and patient care have been guided by the institution's commitment to provide humane, compassionate, and expert care.

Mission Statement

Penn State College of Medicine is dedicated to the education of physicians and scientists in all of the disciplines of medicine and biomedical investigation for careers in practice, teaching, and research. Necessary to this educational mission are the provision of outstanding medical care and services and the enhancement of new knowledge through clinical and basic biomedical research.

Curricular Highlights

Community Service Requirement: Optional.
www.hmc.psu.edu/md/studentlife/studentorgs.html
Research/Thesis Requirement: Required.
Full details at: *www.hmc.psu.edu/msr*

A single integrated curriculum for years one and two combines elements of traditional medical teaching and case-based learning. The first-year curriculum and courses are interdisciplinary, combining case-based, student-centered learning with strategic lectures, laboratories, and small-group discussions. The second-year curriculum is more

heavily oriented to case-based learning in an organ/organ system approach to human health, pathophysiology, and disease. Year three includes a sequence of required core clinical clerkships in internal medicine, general surgery, pediatrics, obstetrics and gynecology, psychiatry, family and community medicine, and primary care supplemented by available selectives. In addition, there are week-long sessions in Advanced Clinical Diagnostics and Therapeutics, Communications and Professionalism, and Improving Healthcare. Year four consists of four elective rotations and four required advanced experiences. The College of Medicine offers a wide variety of both clinical and research electives. Students may select outpatient clinical rotations at teaching hospitals or in university-affiliated physicians' offices located in a variety of rural and metropolitan communities nationwide and abroad. All students participate in an individualized research program.

USMLE

Step 1: Required. Students must record a passing score for promotion.
Step 2: Clinical Skills (CS): Required. Students must record a passing total score to graduate.
Step 2: Clinical Knowledge (CK): Required. Students must record a passing total score to graduate.

Selection Factors

Applicants must show evidence of superior undergraduate achievement and outstanding personal characteristics. Each application is considered individually. A decision is reached after thorough evaluation of the applicant's academic record, letters of assessment, extracurricular activities, MCAT® scores, and personal interviews. Since the practice of medicine requires a lifelong devotion to self-education, emphasis is placed on the excellence of the individual scholar no matter what the student's previous area of study.

Financial Aid

Financial aid is granted based upon need as determined by federal methodology. Parental income information is required for university scholarship and loan consideration, as well as some other financial assistance programs.

Additional financial aid information is available on the school's Web site.

Information about Diversity Programs

Students from groups underrepresented in medicine are encouraged to apply. Faculty members, with student support, are active in the recruitment of students from groups underrepresented in medicine.

Campus Information

Setting

The 550-acre campus is located in the rolling hills of southeastern Pennsylvania near the state capital, Harrisburg. The main facility houses the College of Medicine, the 500+ bed University Hospital and Children's Hospital, the Rehabilitation Center, the Biomedical Research Building, and the Emergency Medical Center. The hospital serves as the only regional Level I Trauma Center.

Enrollment

For 2007, total enrollment was: 566

Special Features

The College of Medicine has state-of-the art facilities, innovative programs, and an award-winning staff that combines medical expertise with compassionate patient care. Learn more at *www.hmc.psu.edu/md/admissions/eduexp.html*.

Housing

University Manor is a safe and affordable housing complex situated on campus with numerous ammenities. Learn more at *www.pennstatehersheyhousing.com*.

Satellite Campuses/Facilities

The College of Medicine has forged a large number of collaborations that provide extensive opportunities for its medical students. Students rotate at defined institutions that meet the College of Medicine's high standards of educational quality.

Application Process and Requirements 2009–2010

Primary Application Service: AMCAS
Earliest filing date: June 1, 2008
Latest filing date: November 15, 2008

Secondary Application Required?: Yes
Sent to: All applicants
Contact: Office of Medical Student Admissions,
(717) 531-8755, studentadmissions@hmc.psu.edu
Fee: Yes, $70
Fee waiver available: Yes
Earliest filing date: Based on email invitation
Latest filing date: January 15, 2009

Latest MCAT® considered: September 2008
Oldest MCAT® considered: 2006

Early Decision Program
School does have EDP
Applicants notified: October 1, 2008
EDP available for: Both Residents and Non-Residents

Regular Acceptance Notice
Earliest date: October 16, 2008
Latest date: Until class is full

Applicant's Response to Acceptance Offer – Maximum Time: Two weeks

Requests for Deferred Entrance Considered: Yes

Deposit to Hold Place in Class: Yes
Deposit (Resident): $100
Deposit (Non-Resident): $100
Deposit due: May 15, 2009
Applied to tuition: Yes
Deposit refundable: Yes
Refundable by: May 15, 2009

Estimated number of new entrants: 145
EDP: n/a, special program: n/a

Start Month/Year: August 2009

Interview Format: Interviews occur on campus by individual invitation. Regional interviews are not available.

Other Programs

PREPARATORY PROGRAMS
Postbaccalaureate Program: No
Summer Program: No
Early Assurance Program:
www.hmc.psu.edu/md/admissions/specialprog

COMBINED DEGREE PROGRAMS
Baccalaureate/MD: No
MD/MPH: No
MD/MBA: No
MD/JD: No
MD/PhD: Yes, www.hmc.psu.edu/mdphd

Premedical Coursework

Course	Req.	Rec.	Lab.	Sems.	Course	Req.	Rec.	Lab.	Sems.
Inorganic Chemistry	•		•	2	Computer Science				
Behavioral Sciences	•			1	Genetics		•		1
Biochemistry		•			Humanities		•		1
Biology	•		•	2	Organic Chemistry	•		•	2
Biology/Zoology					Physics	•		•	2
Calculus		•			Psychology		•		
College English		•			Social Sciences	•			
College Mathematics	•			2	Other				

Selection Factors: 2007 Accepted Applicants

Proportion of Accepted Applicants with Relevant Experience (Data Self-Reported to AMCAS)		
Community Service/Volunteer		71%
Medically-Related Work		88%
Research		86%

Shaded bar represents accepted scores ranging from the 10th percentile to the 90th percentile. School Median ● National Median ●

Overall GPA	2.0	2.1	2.2	2.3	2.4	2.5	2.6	2.7	2.8	2.9	3.0	3.1	3.2	3.3	3.4	3.5	3.6	(3.7)	3.8	3.9	4.0
Science GPA	2.0	2.1	2.2	2.3	2.4	2.5	2.6	2.7	2.8	2.9	3.0	3.1	3.2	3.3	3.4	3.5	3.6	(3.7)	3.8	3.9	4.0

MCAT® required: Yes, 100% of 2007 accepted applicants took MCAT®

Verbal Reasoning	3	4	5	6	7	8	9	(10)	11	12	13	14	15
Physical Sciences	3	4	5	6	7	8	9	(10)	(11)	12	13	14	15
Biological Sciences	3	4	5	6	7	8	9	10	(11)	12	13	14	15
Writing Sample			J	K	L	M	N	O	(P)	(Q)	R	S	T

Acceptance & Matriculation Data for 2007–2008 First Year Class

	Resident	Non-Resident	International	Total
Applied	1029	5204	458	6691
Interviewed	232	664	46	942
Deferred	2	2	1	5
Matriculants				
Early Assurance Program	4	0	0	4
Early Decision Program	0	0	0	0
Baccalaureate/MD	n/a	n/a	n/a	n/a
MD/PhD	2	4	0	6
Matriculated	58	81	15	**154**

Applications accepted from International Applicants: Yes

Matriculant Demographics: 2007–2008 First Year Class

Men: 77   **Women:** 77

Matriculants' Self-Reported Race/Ethnicity

Mexican American	2	Korean	3
Cuban	2	Vietnamese	0
Puerto Rican	1	Other Asian	3
Other Hispanic	0	Total Asian	22
Total Hispanic	4	Native American	0
Chinese	6	Black	10
Asian Indian	6	Native Hawaiian	2
Pakistani	1	White	109
Filipino	2	Unduplicated Number	
Japanese	1	of Matriculants	154

Science and Math Majors: 76%
Matriculants with:
Baccalaureate degree: 100%
Graduate degree(s): 10%

Specialty Choice

2003, 2004, 2005 Graduates, Specialty Choice
(As reported by program directors to GME Track™)

Anesthesiology	6%
Emergency Medicine	8%
Family Practice	14%
Internal Medicine	16%
Obstetrics/Gynecology	5%
Orthopaedic Surgery	4%
Pediatrics	15%
Psychiatry	5%
Radiology	4%
Surgery	6%

Financial Information

Source: 2006–2007 LCME I-B survey and 2007–2008 AAMC TSF questionnaire

	Residents	Non-Residents
Total Cost of Attendance	$47,866	$59,728
Tuition and Fees	$33,058	$44,920
Other (includes living expenses)	$13,620	$13,620
Health Insurance (can be waived)	$1,188	$1,188

Average 2007 Graduate Indebtedness: $155,099
% of Enrolled Students Receiving Aid: 93%

Criminal Background Check

This medical school requires a criminal background check prior to matriculation.

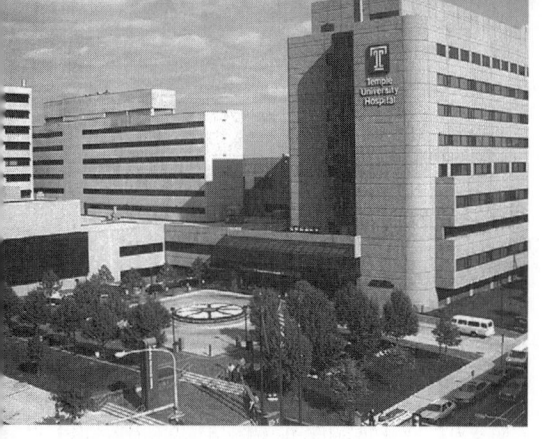

Temple University
School of Medicine
Philadelphia, Pennsylvania

Office of Admissions
Temple University School of Medicine
3340 N. Broad Street, SFC, Suite 305
Philadelphia, Pennsylvania 19140
T 215 707 3656   F 215 707 6932

Admissions www.temple.edu/medicine/admissions
Main www.temple.edu/medicine
Financial www.temple.edu/sfs/med
Email medadmissions@temple.edu

Private Institution

Dr. John M. Daly, Dean

Dr. Audrey B. Uknis, Associate Dean for Admissions

Dr. Raul De La Cadena, Assistant Dean for Recruitment, Admissions, and Retention

General Information

A new 480,000 square foot 11-story medical school building will open in June 2009. This state of the art teaching and collaborative research space will transform the medical school campus and allow its continued growth as one of the nation's premier urban academic medical centers.

Mission Statement

A center of humanistic medicine, Temple University School of Medicine is known for its culture of service, diversity and collaboration. The School's tripartite mission is to: 1) Prepare students for careers as clinicians, researchers, and/or educators, instilling in them an ethic of human service and life long learning; 2) Advance medical science and clinical care; 3) Provide superb healthcare in our communities and beyond.

Curricular Highlights

Community Service Requirement: Optional.
Research/Thesis Requirement: Optional.

In fall 2005, Temple introduced an Integrated Curriculum (IC), which provides integration among basic science disciplines and between basic science and clinical disciplines. The IC is competency-based, providing students with the opportunities to learn and practice the basic knowledge, clinical skills, and attitudes/behaviors essential to the medical profession. The curriculum incorporates state-of-the-art teaching technologies, including patient simulation. The IC is divided into a number of interdisciplinary blocks, each organized according to body or organ systems and taught by faculty from several basic science and clinical academic departments. The clerkships in years 3 and 4 will continue to provide exposure to a unique variety of clinical experiences, both inpatient and ambulatory. The IC facilitates the acquisition of an

increasingly large body of biomedical information through the integration of basic science and medical information and places both in relevant clinical contexts.

USMLE

Step 1: Required. Students must record a passing score for promotion.
Step 2: Clinical Skills (CS): Required. Students must only record a score.
Step 2: Clinical Knowledge (CK): Required. Students must record a passing total score to graduate.

Selection Factors

A variety of objective and subjective factors are considered in making decisions. These include: the academic record, the college attended, MCAT® scores, recommendations, extracurricular activities, work experience, medically related experience, and community service activities. While not required, many students have participated in research activities. While about half of matriculants are Pennsylvania residents, non-residents with a particular interest in Temple and strong credentials are encouraged to apply.

Financial Aid

Temple offers a variety of both merit and need-based scholarships. Students are encouraged to complete a FAFSA by March 1, including the parental section and submit tax returns to be considered for need-based University funds.

Information about Diversity Programs

The School of Medicine is committed to diversity in the faculty and student body. The Recruitment, Admissions, & Retention (RAR) program provides exceptional resources for professional academic guidance and counseling for applicants and students who are from disadvantaged backgrounds or groups underrepresented in medicine.

Campus Information

Setting

An urban institution, Temple serves a diverse population, drawing patients from the North Philadelphia community and from the greater Philadelphia region for specialized care. The School of Medicine shares a campus with Temple

University Hospital and other health-related schools of the University. The campus is easily accessible by public transportation.

Enrollment

For 2007, total enrollment was: 707

Special Features

The Institute for Clinical Simulation and Patient Safety is a 10,000 sq foot learning laboratory which provides excellence in clinical skills training utilizing a combination of high-tech and traditional methods. The Clinical Simulation Center houses the programmable, anatomically detailed, and physiologically functional mannequins that are used to present a variety of clinical scenarios. The Clinical Skills Center houses the standardized patient program, which helps students learn to take histories, conduct physical examinations, make diagnoses, and communicate in a caring manner.

Housing

Students live about 20 minutes by car, in neighborhoods northwest of the campus or in downtown Philadelphia. The university provides housing and roommate lists to assist students.

Satellite Campuses/Facilities

Clinical experience and instruction are provided at Temple University Hospital, St. Christopher's Hospital for Children, Crozer-Chester Medical Center, Fox Chase Cancer Center, Abington Memorial Hospital, and 15 other affiliated hospitals located throughout Pennsylvania. Clinical campuses have been established at the Western Pennsylvania Hospital in Pittsburgh, Geisinger Medical Center in Danville, and St. Luke's Hospital in Bethlehem. Students may elect to do all of the third and fourth-year rotations at one of the clinical campuses.

Application Process and Requirements 2009–2010

Primary Application Service: AMCAS
Earliest filing date: June 1, 2008
Latest filing date: December 15, 2008

Secondary Application Required?: Yes
Sent to: U.S. citizens, permanent residents or applicants who have refugee/asylee status.
URL: Sent when verified AMCAS application is received
Fee: Yes, $70
Fee waiver available: Yes
Earliest filing date: July 15, 2008
Latest filing date: January 15, 2009

Latest MCAT® considered: September 2008
Oldest MCAT® considered: 2006

Early Decision Program
School does have EDP
Applicants notified: October 1, 2008
EDP available for: Both Residents and Non-Residents

Regular Acceptance Notice
Earliest date: October 15, 2008
Latest date: Varies

Applicant's Response to Acceptance Offer – Maximum Time: Two weeks

Requests for Deferred Entrance Considered: Yes

Deposit to Hold Place in Class: Yes
Deposit (Resident): $100
Deposit (Non-Resident): $100
Deposit due: Within two weeks of acceptance
Applied to tuition: Yes
Deposit refundable: Yes
Refundable by: May 15, 2009

Estimated number of new entrants: 200
EDP: 5, special program: 20

Start Month/Year: August 2009

Interview Format: Interviews are conducted with a faculty member. Regional interviews are not available.

Other Programs

PREPARATORY PROGRAMS
Postbaccalaureate Program: Yes, www.temple.edu/medicine/postbac
Summer Program: Yes, www.temple.edu/medicine/ departments_centers/ research/center_minority_health_recruitment_ retention.htm
Early Assurance: Yes, www.temple.edu/ medicine/admissions/special_admissions.htm
COMBINED DEGREE PROGRAMS
Baccalaureate/MD: Yes, www.temple.edu/medicine/admissions/ special_admissions.htm
MD/MPH: Yes, www.temple.edu/medicine/ education/dualdegree
MD/MBA: No
MD/JD: No
MD/PhD: Yes, www.temple.edu/medicine/ education/dualdegree/mdphd.htm

Premedical Coursework

Course	Req.	Rec.	Lab.	Hrs.
Inorganic Chemistry	•		•	8
Behavioral Sciences				
Biochemistry				
Biology	•	•		8
Biology/Zoology				
Calculus				
College English				
College Mathematics				

Course	Req.	Rec.	Lab.	Hrs.
Computer Science				
Genetics				
Humanities	•			6
Organic Chemistry	•		•	8
Physics	•		•	8
Psychology				
Social Sciences				
Other				

Selection Factors: 2007 Accepted Applicants

Proportion of Accepted Applicants with Relevant Experience (Data Self-Reported to AMCAS®)		
Community Service/Volunteer		67%
Medically-Related Work		88%
Research		82%

Shaded bar represents accepted scores ranging from the 10th percentile to the 90th percentile. School Median ● National Median ●

Overall GPA	2.0	2.1	2.2	2.3	2.4	2.5	2.6	2.7	2.8	2.9	3.0	3.1	3.2	3.3	3.4	3.5	3.6	(3.7)	3.8	3.9	4.0
Science GPA	2.0	2.1	2.2	2.3	2.4	2.5	2.6	2.7	2.8	2.9	3.0	3.1	3.2	3.3	3.4	3.5	3.6	(3.7)	3.8	3.9	4.0

MCAT® required: Yes, 100% of 2007 accepted applicants took MCAT®

Verbal Reasoning	3	4	5	6	7	8	9	(10)	11	12	13	14	15
Physical Sciences	3	4	5	6	7	8	9	(10)	(11)	12	13	14	15
Biological Sciences	3	4	5	6	7	8	9	10	(11)	12	13	14	15
Writing Sample			J	K	L	M	N	O	(P)	(Q)	R	S	T

Acceptance & Matriculation Data for 2007–2008 First Year Class

	Resident	Non-Resident	International	Total
Applied	1090	8545	80	9715
Interviewed	218	599	0	817
Deferred	3	3	0	6
Matriculants				
Early Assurance Program	0	0	0	0
Early Decision Program	1	1	0	2
Baccalaureate/MD	5	2	0	7
MD/PhD	2	1	0	3
Matriculated	77	101	0	**178**

Applications accepted from International Applicants: No

Matriculant Demographics: 2007–2008 First Year Class

Men: 95 **Women:** 83

Matriculants' Self-Reported Race/Ethnicity

Mexican American	3	**Korean**	6
Cuban	6	**Vietnamese**	1
Puerto Rican	6	**Other Asian**	2
Other Hispanic	6	**Total Asian**	31
Total Hispanic	20	**Native American**	2
Chinese	9	**Black**	13
Asian Indian	13	**Native Hawaiian**	1
Pakistani	0	**White**	128
Filipino	2	**Unduplicated Number**	
Japanese	0	**of Matriculants**	178

Science and Math Majors: 75%
Matriculants with:
    Baccalaureate degree: 99%
    Graduate degree(s): 5%

Specialty Choice

2003, 2004, 2005 Graduates, Specialty Choice (As reported by program directors to GME Track™)	
Anesthesiology	4%
Emergency Medicine	8%
Family Practice	6%
Internal Medicine	31%
Obstetrics/Gynecology	3%
Orthopaedic Surgery	4%
Pediatrics	8%
Psychiatry	3%
Radiology	4%
Surgery	9%

Financial Information

Source: 2006–2007 LCME I-B survey and 2007–2008 AAMC TSF questionnaire

	Residents	Non-Residents
Total Cost of Attendance	$58,958	$67,460
Tuition and Fees	$38,502	$47,004
Other (includes living expenses)	$18,301	$18,301
Health Insurance (can be waived)	$2,155	$2,155

Average 2007 Graduate Indebtedness: $154,340
% of Enrolled Students Receiving Aid: 88%

Criminal Background Check

This medical school requires a criminal background check prior to matriculation.

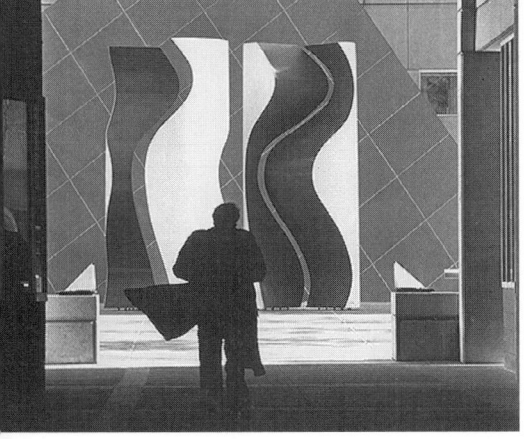

University of Pennsylvania
School of Medicine
Philadelphia, Pennsylvania

Office of Admissions and Financial Aid
Suite 100, Edward J. Stemmler Hall
University of Pennsylvania School of Medicine
3450 Hamilton Walk
Philadelphia, Pennsylvania 19104-6056

T 215 898 8001   **F** 215 573 6645
Admissions www.med.upenn.edu/admiss
Main www.med.upenn.edu
Financial www.med.upenn.edu/financialaid/
Email admiss@mail.med.upenn.edu

Private Institution

Dr. Arthur H. Rubenstein, Dean

Dr. Gail Morrison, Vice Dean for Education

Gaye W. Sheffler, Director of Admissions and Financial Aid

Dr. Karen Hamilton, Assistant Dean for Diversity and Community Outreach in Undergraduate Medical Education

General Information
The School of Medicine, the first in the United States, was founded in 1765 and is a private, nondenominational school on the urban campus of the University of Pennsylvania. The one university concept enrolls medical students as members of the university as well as the School of Medicine community. Clinical education occurs in the Hospital of the University of Pennsylvania, Children's Hospital of Philadelphia, Veterans Administration Hospital of Philadelphia, Presbyterian Medical Center, and Pennsylvania Hospital.

Mission Statement
Our mission is to create the future of medicine through: Patient Care and Service Excellence, Educational Pre-eminence, New Knowledge and Innovation, and National and International Leadership.

Curricular Highlights
Community Service Requirement: Required. Three-year patient-centered experience.
Research/Thesis Requirement: Required. Three month scholarly pursuit and/or dual degree.

The four-year curriculum has three themes: Science of Medicine, Technology and Practice of Medicine, and Professionalism and Humanism. Module 1 (four months) provides the foundation of basic sciences and is divided into four blocks: Developmental and Molecular Biology; Cell Physiology and Metabolism: Human Body, Structure, and Function; and Host Defenses and Responses. Grades are pass/fail. Module 2 (40 weeks) integrates basic science across organ

systems and ends in December of Year 2. Topics are organized by: Normal Development, Normal Processes, Abnormal Processes, Therapeutics and Disease Management, Epidemiology/Evidenced-based Medicine, Prevention, and Nutrition. Grades are honors/pass/fail. Module 3, Technology and Practice of Medicine, runs concurrent with modules 1 and 2 and promotes competency in epidemiology and biostatistics, decision-making, health care economics, population-based medicine, managed care and quality assurance, and basic clinical medicine. Grades are pass/fail. Module 4, (clinical clerkships), runs from January of Year 2 through December of Year 3 and is composed of 48 weeks of required clinical clerkships divided into four three-month cross-disciplinary experiences. Basic science concepts are reinforced weekly in didactic sessions. Module 5 (16 months) begins in January of Year 3 and continues until graduation. It provides students flexibility in their elective/selective and scholarly pursuit experiences and exposure to upper level electives and mentors prior to residency selection. Grades are honors/high pass/pass/fail. Module 6, Professionalism and Humanism, runs concurrently throughout the curriculum and covers bioethics, multiculturalism, spirituality, research, ethics, and confidentiality. Grades are pass/fail. Detailed curriculum information can be found at *www.med.upenn. edu/admiss/curriculum.*

USMLE
Step 1: Required. Students must only record a score.
Step 2: Clinical Skills (CS): Required. Students must only record a score.
Step 2: Clinical Knowledge (CK): Required. Students must only record a score.

Selection Factors
Selection factors include academic excellence, out-of-classroom activities, and life experience, as well as community service, research, letters of recommendation, and leadership potential. Personal qualities of maturity, integrity, the ability to work with others, and humanistic interests are sought. The entering class of 2007 has representation from 54 undergraduate colleges.

Applicants from all states are welcome, but some preference is given to PA residents. Penn does not discriminate on the basis of race, sex, sexual orientation, age, religion, national or ethnic origin, or physical handicap. There is no transfer admission program.

Financial Aid
Students come from all social, economic, and cultural backgrounds. Financial aid includes: need-based scholarship and loans restricted to U.S. citizens or permanent residents and 11-12 full-tuition merit scholarships awarded annually regardless of citizenship. Approximately 20 students annually are fully funded in the MD/PHD program.

Information about Diversity Programs
Penn values diversity in the student body, faculty, and health system. Its goal is to recruit, admit, and graduate students from groups underrepresented in medicine. The Office of Diversity and Community Outreach has programs and pipelines to assist in meeting the objectives of a diverse student body. There is a curriculum focus on cultural competency.

Campus Information

Setting
Penn's urban campus is located in Philadelphia, one of America's most historic and livable cities. The fact that all 12 of Penn's graduate schools are located within walking distance of one another supports and fosters Penn's interdisciplinary approach to education, scholarship, and research. The city is a vibrant cultural center of urban life.

Enrollment
For 2007, total enrollment was: 706

Special Features
Global health experiences throughout the world. Pediatrics at Children's Hospital of Philadelphia, a world-renowned pediatric center.

Housing
Housing is affordable. Campus resources help students find housing. University transit is available within boundaries.

Application Process and Requirements 2009–2010

Primary Application Service: AMCAS
Earliest filing date: June 1, 2008
Latest filing date: October 15, 2008, 12:00 a.m., EST

Secondary Application Required?: Yes
Sent to: All applicants
URL: n/a
Fee: Yes, $80
Fee waiver available: Yes
Earliest filing date: July 1, 2008
Latest filing date: November 15, 2008, 12:00 a.m. EST

Latest MCAT® considered: September 2008
Oldest MCAT® considered: 2005

Early Decision Program
School does have EDP
Applicants notified: October 1, 2008
EDP available for: Both Residents and Non-Residents

Regular Acceptance Notice
Earliest date: March 30, 2009
Latest date: Until class is full

Applicant's Response to Acceptance
Offer – Latest Date: May 15, 2009, 5 p.m., EST

Requests for Deferred
Entrance Considered: Yes
Deposit to Hold Place in Class: Yes
Deposit (Resident): $100
Deposit (Non-Resident): $100
Deposit due: May 15, 2009 5 p.m. EST
Applied to tuition: Yes
Deposit refundable: Yes
Refundable by: May 15, 2009 5 p.m. EST

Estimated number of new entrants: 155
EDP: 5, special program: n/a

Start Month/Year: August 2009

Interview Format: Two individual interviews/faculty and student. Regional interviews are not available.

Other Programs

PREPARATORY PROGRAMS
Postbaccalaureate Program: Yes, www.sas.upenn.edu/CGS/postbac/premed
Summer Program: Yes, www.med.upenn.edu/bgs/
Clinical Epidemiology Program: www.cceb.upenn.edu/education/
COMBINED DEGREE PROGRAMS
Baccalaureate/MD: No
MD/MPH: Yes, www.publichealth.med.upenn.edu
MD/MBA: Yes, www.med.upenn.edu/educ_combdeg/mdmba.html
MD/JD: Yes, www.med.upenn.edu/educ_combdeg/mdjd.html
MD/PhD: Yes, www.med.upenn.edu/mstp/
Additional Program: Yes, www.med.upenn.edu/mbe/

Premedical Coursework

Course	Req.	Rec.	Lab.	Hrs.	Course	Req.	Rec.	Lab.	Hrs.
Inorganic Chemistry		•			Computer Science		•		
Behavioral Sciences		•			Genetics		•		
Biochemistry		•			Humanities		•		
Biology		•	•		Organic Chemistry		•	•	
Biology/Zoology					Physics		•	•	
Calculus		•			Psychology		•		
College English		•			Social Sciences		•		
College Mathematics		•			Statistics		•		

Selection Factors: 2007 Accepted Applicants

Proportion of Accepted Applicants with Relevant Experience (Data Self-Reported to AMCAS®)			Community Service/Volunteer	67%
			Medically-Related Work	88%
			Research	90%

Shaded bar represents accepted scores ranging from the 10th percentile to the 90th percentile School Median ● National Median ●

Overall GPA	2.0	2.1	2.2	2.3	2.4	2.5	2.6	2.7	2.8	2.9	3.0	3.1	3.2	3.3	3.4	3.5	3.6	3.7	(3.8)	3.9	4.0
Science GPA	2.0	2.1	2.2	2.3	2.4	2.5	2.6	2.7	2.8	2.9	3.0	3.1	3.2	3.3	3.4	3.5	3.6	3.7	(3.8)	3.9	4.0

MCAT® required: Yes, 100% of 2007 accepted applicants took MCAT®

Verbal Reasoning	3	4	5	6	7	8	9	(10)	(11)	12	13	14	15
Physical Sciences	3	4	5	6	7	8	9	10	(11)	(12)	13	14	15
Biological Sciences	3	4	5	6	7	8	9	10	(11)	(12)	13	14	15
Writing Sample				J	K	L	M	N	O	P	(Q)	R	S	T

Acceptance & Matriculation Data for 2007–2008 First Year Class

	Resident	Non-Resident	International	Total
Applied	668	5384	292	6344
Interviewed	140	784	14	938
Deferred	3	5	0	8
Matriculants				
Early Assurance Program	0	0	0	0
Early Decision Program	0	2	1	3
Baccalaureate/MD	n/a	n/a	n/a	n/a
MD/PhD	5	15	4	24
Matriculated	37	111	5	**153**
Applications accepted from International Applicants: Yes				

Specialty Choice

2003, 2004, 2005 Graduates, Specialty Choice (As reported by program directors to GME Track™)

Anesthesiology	2%
Emergency Medicine	4%
Family Practice	2%
Internal Medicine	19%
Obstetrics/Gynecology	2%
Orthopaedic Surgery	6%
Pediatrics	13%
Psychiatry	5%
Radiology	8%
Surgery	6%

Matriculant Demographics: 2007–2008 First Year Class

Men: 74 **Women:** 79

Matriculants' Self-Reported Race/Ethnicity

Mexican American	0	Korean	3
Cuban	1	Vietnamese	0
Puerto Rican	3	Other Asian	2
Other Hispanic	3	Total Asian	28
Total Hispanic	7	Native American	0
Chinese	12	Black	16
Asian Indian	10	Native Hawaiian	0
Pakistani	1	White	106
Filipino	1	Unduplicated Number	
Japanese	0	of Matriculants	153

Science and Math Majors: 61%
Matriculants with:
Baccalaureate degree: 100%
Graduate degree(s): 6%

Financial Information

Source: 2006–2007 LCME I-B survey and 2007–2008 AAMC TSF questionnaire

	Residents	Non-Residents
Total Cost of Attendance	$63,533	$63,533
Tuition and Fees	$42,873	$42,873
Other (includes living expenses)	$18,060	$18,060
Health Insurance (can be waived)	$2,600	$2,600

Average 2007 Graduate Indebtedness: $107,538
% of Enrolled Students Receiving Aid: 83%

Criminal Background Check

This medical school requires a criminal background check prior to matriculation.

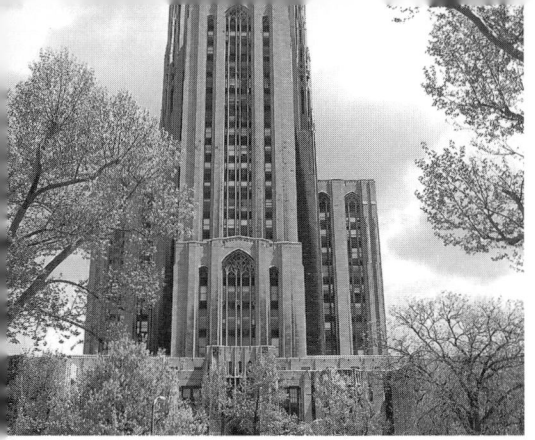

University of Pittsburgh School of Medicine
Pittsburgh, Pennsylvania

Office of Admissions and Financial Aid
3550 Terrace Street, 518 Scaife Hall
University of Pittsburgh School of Medicine
Pittsburgh, Pennsylvania 15261
T 412 648 9891   F 412 648 8768

Admissions www.medschool.pitt.edu/
future/future_02.asp
Main www.medschool.pitt.edu
Financial www.medschool.pitt.edu/future/future_04.asp
Email admissions@medschool.pitt.edu

Private Institution

Dr. Arthur S. Levine, Dean, Senior Vice Chancellor for Health Sciences

Dr. Beth Piraino, Associate Dean for Admissions and Financial Aid

Dr. Chenits Pettigrew, Jr. Assistant Dean for Student Affairs and Diversity Programs

Pamela Rikstad, Director of Financial Aid

Cynthia M. Bonetti, Executive Director of Admissions and Financial Aid

Lisa T. Wick, Assistant Director for Admissions and Financial Aid

General Information

Drawing patients from all over the nation and from more than 30 foreign countries, the University of Pittsburgh Medical Center (UPMC) is one of the largest non-profit academic health systems in the nation. UPMC sites and affiliates on the main campus in Oakland, or nearby, include Western Psychiatric Institute and Clinic, the University of Pittsburgh Cancer Institute, UPMC Presbyterian Hospital, UPMC Shadyside Hospital, Magee Women's Hospital, Eye and Ear Institute, the Benedum Geriatric Center, Children's Hospital of Pittsburgh, and the University Drive and Highland Drive VA Medical Centers.

Mission Statement

The principal goal of the University of Pittsburgh School of Medicine remains the education of scholarly physicians. This goal is achieved by emphasizing the centrality of the patient, by providing a firm understanding of the sciences basic to medicine, and by fostering the application of principles of biomedical problem-solving to the care of patients. We feel that students must develop an understanding of ethical principles in medicine and the application of these principles to specific problems. Development, early in the student's career, of habits of self-education by methods that include problem-based and self-directed learning, communication skills, and computer-assisted education is critical to the learning process, which must occur throughout the professional life of a physician.

Curricular Highlights

Community Service Requirement: Optional. Participation in multiple activities possible.
Research/Thesis Requirement: Required. Performance of a longitudinal scholarly project.

Our multidisciplinary curriculum is organized by organ systems rather than by individual disciplines (e.g., physiology and biochemistry). It emphasizes problem-solving and learning in small groups. It also introduces students to clinical medicine in the first year. All students have required rotations in family medicine, internal medicine, obstetrics-gynecology, pediatrics, psychiatry, and surgery, as well as in ambulatory subspecialties. All fourth-year students rotate through both neurology and diagnostic imaging clerkships. Students may have some electives scheduled during the third year, and extensive elective time during the fourth year. All students complete a mentored scholarly project using the scientific method to examine a clinical, basic science or community-based problem. An Honors/Pass/Fail system is used for grading.

USMLE

Step 1: Required. Students must record a passing score for graduation, but not promotion.
Step 2: Clinical Skills (CS): Required. Students must record a passing total score to graduate.
Step 2: Clinical Knowledge (CK): Required. Students must record a passing total score to graduate.

Selection Factors

Applicants are chosen on the basis of intellect, integrity, maturity, and the ability to interact sensitively with people. Consideration is given to the past academic record and MCAT® scores; evaluations of college preprofessional committees; letters of recommendation, preferably from faculty members with whom the student has interacted in scholarly pursuits; extracurricular activities; and personal interviews. Interviews are required and are conducted only at the medical school campus. All applicants are considered without regard to race, color, religion, ethnicity, national origin, age, sex, sexual orientation, marital, veteran, or handicap status.

Financial Aid

Most loans and scholarships are awarded on the basis of financial need as documented by information on the FAFSA. Parental income information is required to be considered for University need-based resources. Students are considered for academic scholarships during the admissions process. Additional financial aid information is available on the school's website.

Information about Diversity Programs

The School of Medicine is committed to maintaining a diverse student body; in the application process, students are asked how they might contribute to this diversity. The school hosts premedical summer enrichment programs, as well as a prematriculation program for all admitted students. Following admission, a broad range of support services are available to ensure retention. Specific information on the services provided to applicants from groups underrepresented in medicine can be obtained by contacting the Office of Student Affairs and Diversity Programs at (412) 648-8987.

Campus Information
Setting
Urban setting on the University of Pittsburgh campus; within a five-block radius of five UPMC hospitals and the Graduate School of Public Health.

Enrollment
For 2007, total enrollment was: 580

Special Features
The School of Medicine has implemented extensive curricular revisions. The goal-oriented, integrated, and centrally governed new curriculum emphasizes general principles and encourages student self-learning based on actual clinical cases.

Housing
New housing is available on campus specifically for medical students. See: *www.ocl.pitt.edu/apartments/darragh.html.*

Satellite Campuses/Facilities
The University of Pittsburgh Medical Center has 20 hospitals, 19 of which are in the Western Pennsylvania region. In addition, UPMC Palermo is a transplant hospital located in Sicily at which students may do a senior elective.

Application Process and Requirements 2009–2010

Primary Application Service: AMCAS
Earliest filing date: June 1, 2008
Latest filing date: November 15, 2008

Secondary Application Required?: Yes
Sent to: All applicants
URL: https://admissions.medschool.pitt.edu
Fee: Yes, $75
Fee waiver available: Yes
Earliest filing date: July 1, 2008
Latest filing date: December 15, 2008

Latest MCAT® considered: September 2008
Oldest MCAT® considered: 2005

Early Decision Program
School does not have EDP
Applicants notified: n/a
EDP available for: n/a

Regular Acceptance Notice
Earliest date: October 15, 2008
Latest date: Until class is full

Applicant's Response to Acceptance Offer – Maximum Time: Two weeks

Requests for Deferred Entrance Considered: Yes

Deposit to Hold Place in Class: Yes
Deposit (Resident): $100
Deposit (Non-Resident): $100
Deposit due: May 18-22, 2009
Applied to tuition: Yes
Deposit refundable: No
Refundable by: n/a

Estimated number of new entrants: 148
EDP: n/a, special program: n/a

Start Month/Year: August 2009

Interview Format: A faculty and student interview are required. Regional interviews are not available.

Other Programs

PREPARATORY PROGRAMS
Postbaccalaureate Program: No
Summer Program: Yes, www.medschool.pitt.edu/future/future_03.asp

COMBINED DEGREE PROGRAMS
Baccalaureate/MD: No
MD/MPH: Yes, www.publichealth.pitt.edu/interior.php?pageID=203
MD/MBA: No
MD/JD: No
MD/PhD: Yes, www.mdphd.pitt.edu
Additional Program: Yes, www.icre.pitt.edu/cstp-m/index.aspx; www.pstp.pitt.edu

Premedical Coursework

Course	Req.	Rec.	Lab.	Sems.	Course	Req.	Rec.	Lab.	Sems.
Inorganic Chemistry	•		•	2	Computer Science				
Behavioral Sciences					Genetics				
Biochemistry					Humanities				
Biology	•		•	2	Organic Chemistry	•		•	2
Biology/Zoology					Physics	•		•	2
Calculus					Psychology				
College English	•			2	Social Sciences				
College Mathematics					Other				

Selection Factors: 2007 Accepted Applicants

Proportion of Accepted Applicants with Relevant Experience (Data Self-Reported to AMCAS®)		
Community Service/Volunteer	72%
Medically-Related Work	88%
Research	89%

Shaded bar represents accepted scores ranging from the 10th percentile to the 90th percentile. School Median ● National Median ●

Overall GPA	2.0	2.1	2.2	2.3	2.4	2.5	2.6	2.7	2.8	2.9	3.0	3.1	3.2	3.3	3.4	3.5	3.6	3.7	(3.8)	3.9	4.0
Science GPA	2.0	2.1	2.2	2.3	2.4	2.5	2.6	2.7	2.8	2.9	3.0	3.1	3.2	3.3	3.4	3.5	3.6	3.7	(3.8)	3.9	4.0

MCAT® required: Yes, 99% of 2007 accepted applicants took MCAT®

Verbal Reasoning	3	4	5	6	7	8	9	(10)	(11)	12	13	14	15
Physical Sciences	3	4	5	6	7	8	9	10	(11)	(12)	13	14	15
Biological Sciences	3	4	5	6	7	8	9	10	(11)	(12)	13	14	15
Writing Sample			J	K	L	M	N	O	P	(Q)	R	S	T

Acceptance & Matriculation Data for 2007–2008 First Year Class

	Resident	Non-Resident	International	Total
Applied	840	4705	71	5616
Interviewed	220	1009	0	1229
Deferred	0	9	0	9
Matriculants				
Early Assurance Program	2	1	0	3
Early Decision Program	0	0	0	0
Baccalaureate/MD	n/a	n/a	n/a	n/a
MD/PhD	1	8	0	9
Matriculated	49	97	0	**146**

Applications accepted from International Applicants: No

Matriculant Demographics: 2007–2008 First Year Class

Men: 70   **Women:** 76

Matriculants' Self-Reported Race/Ethnicity

Mexican American	0	Korean	6
Cuban	1	Vietnamese	3
Puerto Rican	2	Other Asian	6
Other Hispanic	6	Total Asian	40
Total Hispanic	9	Native American	0
Chinese	13	Black	18
Asian Indian	12	Native Hawaiian	1
Pakistani	0	White	92
Filipino	0	Unduplicated Number	
Japanese	0	of Matriculants	146

Science and Math Majors: 73%
Matriculants with:
Baccalaureate degree: 99%
Graduate degree(s): 14%

Specialty Choice

2003, 2004, 2005 Graduates, Specialty Choice (As reported by program directors to GME Track™)	
Anesthesiology	5%
Emergency Medicine	11%
Family Practice	8%
Internal Medicine	14%
Obstetrics/Gynecology	6%
Orthopaedic Surgery	5%
Pediatrics	13%
Psychiatry	7%
Radiology Diagnostic	3%
Surgery General	6%

Financial Information

Source: 2006–2007 LCME I-B survey and 2007–2008 AAMC TSF questionnaire

	Residents	Non-Residents
Total Cost of Attendance	$55,256	$59,122
Tuition and Fees	$35,990	$39,856
Other (includes living expenses)	$16,500	$16,500
Health Insurance (can be waived)	$2,766	$2,766

Average 2007 Graduate Indebtedness: $138,632
% of Enrolled Students Receiving Aid: 89%

Criminal Background Check

This medical school requires a criminal background check prior to matriculation.

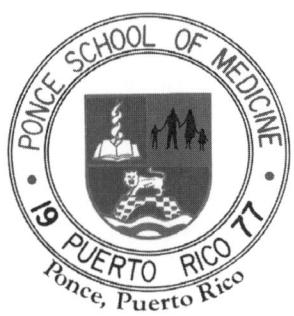

Ponce School of Medicine
Ponce, Puerto Rico

Admissions Office
Ponce School of Medicine
P.O. Box 7004
Ponce, Puerto Rico 00732
T 787 840 2575   **F** 787 842 0461

Admissions www.psm.edu/Student_Affairs/
Admissions/about_department.htm
Main www.psm.edu
Financial www.psm.edu/Student_Affairs/
Financial_Aid/fin_aid_about_department.htm
Email admissions@psm.edu

Private Institution

Dr. Raúl Armstrong, President and Dean

Dr. Carmen M. Mercado,
Assistant Dean for Admissions

Pedro Barnés, Financial Aid Director

Arvin Báez, Assistant Dean for Student Affairs

General Information
The Ponce School of Medicine of the Ponce Medical School Foundation, Inc. (formerly the Catholic University of Puerto Rico School of Medicine) took over the school's operations on July 1, 1980, under the governance of a board of trustees. The school graduated its first class in June 1981. Clinical training is offered at the following facilities in Ponce: Damas Hospital, a private institution with 356 beds; La Playa Diagnostic Center, which serves as the main training area for community and family practice; Dr. Pila Hospital, with 160 beds; and St. Luke's Hospital, with 550 beds. Clinical training is also offered at the Concepcion Hospital, with 188 beds, located in San German, and at Yauco Regional Hospital, with 140 beds.

Mission Statement
Ponce School of Medicine has as its mission the provision of high quality education and graduate training, which shall strengthen students' character, moral fiber, and ethics, and prepare physicians and scientists for a fast-changing world in the area of healthcare delivery and research.

Curricular Highlights
Community Service Requirement: Optional.
Research/Thesis Requirement: Optional.

The medical program's basic objective is to provide the Commonwealth of Puerto Rico, especially the southern region of the island, with ethically motivated, professionally competent primary care physicians. The curriculum provides students with an early experience in family and community health needs. During the first two years, the basic medical sciences are thoroughly emphasized. Clinical experience takes precedence during the third and fourth years.

The correlation between the basic and clinical sciences is achieved in a multidisciplinary program. Throughout the four-year program great emphasis is placed on the student's contact with patients and their families as a complement to the student's academic-hospital experience. Every academic semester contains, in addition to the regular curriculum, a series of supplementary seminars dealing with the ethical and social components of medical practice, as well as with additional specific subjects that are incidental and relevant to the profession. A problem-based learning program has been introduced in clinical correlation sessions in the first year of medical studies and in the Pathophysiology course, where it is presented as a student-centered integrative exercise. Subject-oriented small-group discussions are included in basic sciences courses. The program seeks to develop well-balanced, mature general practitioners, equally well qualified in the professional and ethical aspects of medicine. Students' work is graded according to an Honor/Pass/Fail system.

USMLE
Step 1: Required. Students must record a passing score for promotion.
Step 2: Clinical Skills (CS): Required. Students must only record a score.
Step 2: Clinical Knowledge (CK): Required. Students must record a passing total score to graduate.

Selection Factors
Selection of applicants is made by the Admissions Committee on the basis of academic achievement, MCAT® scores, evaluation letters, and personal interviews. The interviews are used to determine the motivation and character of the applicants. Only those who pass a preliminary screening, based on MCAT® scores and college grades, are interviewed. Careful consideration is given to all applicants regardless of racial or ethnic background, religious affiliation, sex, or national origin. Residents of Puerto Rico are given preference, although a limited number of applicants who live in the United States are accepted. Candidates who do not have a functional knowledge of both English and Spanish are not encouraged to apply, since instruction is given in both languages. In the 2007 entering class, 66 percent of students were from Puerto Rico and 34 percent were from the continental United States.

Financial Aid
Students are admitted to Ponce School of Medicine without regard to financial circumstances. After acceptance, prospective students are informed of the necessary forms they must submit in order to complete the financial aid process.

Campus Information

Setting
Our medical school is located in Ponce Puerto Rico, the second largest city in Puerto Rico. It is on the south side of the island.

Enrollment
For 2007, total enrollment was: 66

Housing
On-campus housing is not available. The university does maintain a list of affordable apartments within a 10-mile radius. Rents average $400-$800 per month.

Application Process and Requirements 2009–2010

Primary Application Service: AMCAS
Earliest filing date: June 1, 2008
Latest filing date: December 15, 2008

Secondary Application Required?: Yes
Sent to: All applicants
URL: Yes
Fee: $100
Fee waiver available: No
Earliest filing date: n/a
Latest filing date: n/a

Latest MCAT® considered: 2008
Oldest MCAT® considered: 2006

Early Decision Program
School does have EDP
Applicants notified: October 1, 2008
EDP available for: Both Residents and Non-Residents

Regular Acceptance Notice
Earliest date: November 15, 2008
Latest date: Until class is full

Applicant's Response to Acceptance Offer – Maximum Time: Twenty days

Requests for Deferred Entrance Considered: No

Deposit to Hold Place in Class: Yes
Deposit (Resident): $1,000
Deposit (Non-Resident): $1,000
Deposit due: With response to acceptance offer
Applied to tuition: Yes
Deposit refundable: No
Refundable by: n/a

Estimated number of new entrants: 65
EDP: 3, special program: n/a

Start Month/Year: July 2009

Interview Format: Interviews are in groups or individually. Regional interviews are not available.

Other Programs

PREPARATORY PROGRAMS
Postbaccalaureate Program: No
Summer Program: No

COMBINED DEGREE PROGRAMS
Baccalaureate/MD: Yes
MD/MPH: No
MD/MBA: No
MD/JD: No
MD/PhD: No

Premedical Coursework

Course	Req.	Rec.	Lab.	Hrs.	Course	Req.	Rec.	Lab.	Hrs.
Inorganic Chemistry	•		•	8	Computer Science				
Behavioral Sciences	•			12	Genetics				
Biochemistry		•			Humanities				
Biology	•			8	Organic Chemistry	•		•	8
Biology/Zoology			•		Physics	•		•	8
Calculus					Psychology				
College English	•			12	Social Sciences				
College Mathematics	•			6	Spanish	•			6

Selection Factors: 2007 Accepted Applicants

Proportion of Accepted Applicants with Relevant Experience (Data Self-Reported to AMCAS®)		
Community Service/Volunteer		52%
Medically-Related Work		53%
Research		61%

Shaded bar represents accepted scores ranging from the 10th percentile to the 90th percentile.   School Median ○   National Median ○

| Overall GPA | 2.0 | 2.1 | 2.2 | 2.3 | 2.4 | 2.5 | 2.6 | 2.7 | 2.8 | 2.9 | 3.0 | 3.1 | 3.2 | 3.3 | 3.4 | (3.5) | 3.6 | 3.7 | 3.8 | 3.9 | 4.0 |
| Science GPA | 2.0 | 2.1 | 2.2 | 2.3 | 2.4 | 2.5 | 2.6 | 2.7 | 2.8 | 2.9 | 3.0 | 3.1 | 3.2 | (3.3) | 3.4 | 3.5 | 3.6 | 3.7 | 3.8 | 3.9 | 4.0 |

MCAT® required: Yes, 100% of 2007 accepted applicants took MCAT®

Verbal Reasoning	3	4	5	6	(7)	8	9	(10)	11	12	13	14	15
Physical Sciences	3	4	5	6	(7)	8	9	10	(11)	12	13	14	15
Biological Sciences	3	4	5	6	7	(8)	9	10	(11)	12	13	14	15
Writing Sample		J	K	L	(M)	N	O	P	(Q)	R	S	T

Acceptance & Matriculation Data for 2007–2008 First Year Class

	Resident	Non-Resident	International	Total
Applied	340	905	35	1280
Interviewed	155	26	0	193
Deferred	0	0	0	0
Matriculants				
Early Assurance Program	0	0	0	0
Early Decision Program	0	0	0	0
Baccalaureate/MD	1	0	0	1
MD/PhD	n/a	n/a	n/a	n/a
Matriculated	39	24	0	**63**

Applications accepted from International Applicants: Yes

Matriculant Demographics: 2007–2008 First Year Class

Men: 28   **Women:** 35

Matriculants' Self-Reported Race/Ethnicity

Mexican American	0	Korean	0
Cuban	6	Vietnamese	0
Puerto Rican	47	Other Asian	0
Other Hispanic	7	Total Asian	1
Total Hispanic	57	Native American	0
Chinese	0	Black	2
Asian Indian	1	Native Hawaiian	2
Pakistani	0	White	47
Filipino	0	**Unduplicated Number**	
Japanese	0	**of Matriculants**	63

Science and Math Majors: 70%
Matriculants with:
Baccalaureate degree: 98%
Graduate degree(s): 13%

Specialty Choice

2003, 2004, 2005 Graduates, Specialty Choice (As reported by program directors to GME Track™)	
Anesthesiology	4%
Emergency Medicine	7%
Family Practice	3%
Internal Medicine	21%
Obstetrics/Gynecology	9%
Orthopaedic Surgery	4%
Pediatrics	10%
Psychiatry	4%
Radiology	5%
Surgery	9%

Financial Information

Source: 2006–2007 LCME I-B survey and 2007–2008 AAMC TSF questionnaire

	Residents	Non-Residents
Total Cost of Attendance	$33,861	$47,445
Tuition and Fees	$20,199	$28,953
Other (includes living expenses)	$12,400	$17,230
Health Insurance (can be waived)	$1,262	$1,262

Average 2007 Graduate Indebtedness: $151,119
% of Enrolled Students Receiving Aid: 85%

Criminal Background Check

This medical school requires a criminal background check prior to matriculation.

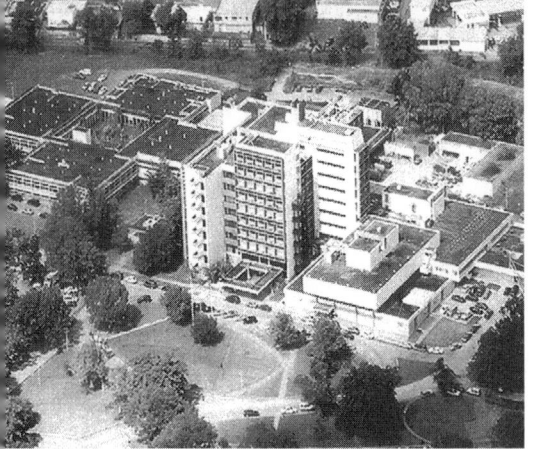

San Juan Bautista School of Medicine
Caguas, Puerto Rico

Admissions Office
P.O. Box 4968
Caguas, Puerto Rico 00726-4968
T 787 743 3038 x236   F 787 746 3093

Admissions www.sanjuanbautista.edu/Admissions.aspx
Main www.sanjuanbautista.edu
Financial www.sanjuanbautista.edu/Admissions.aspx
Email admissions@sanjuanbautista.edu

Private Institution

Dr. Yocasta Brugal-Mena, President/Dean of Medicine

Dr. Myraida Rivera-Colon, Director of Admissions

Dr. Myraida Rivera-Colon, Minority Affairs Officer

Ms. Beatriz De Leon-Rivera, Financial Aid Officer

Dr. Lourdes M. Pérez-De Alejo, Associate Dean for Student Affairs

Ms. Jaymi Sanchez-Cruz, Admissions Officer

General Information

The School of Medicine was founded in 1978 in San Juan, Puerto Rico, as a not-for-profit corporation, incorporated under the laws of the Commonwealth of Puerto Rico. It is located in Caguas, Puerto Rico, one of the most important urban centers. It is authorized by the Puerto Rico Council on Higher Education to offer studies leading to the M.D. degree. The MSCHE granted accreditation to the School in 2004. The next evaluation visit is scheduled for 2009. The LCME granted accreditation to the academic program on 2007. The next evaluation visit will be on 2011. Up to June 30, 2007, the School of Medicine has graduated a total of 864 medical doctors who have been successfully integrated in their communities as competent and caring health providers, both in Puerto Rico and abroad.

Mission Statement

The Mission of the School is to teach and train students to become primary care physicians that can provide holistic diagnosis and treatment to communities in need of health services in Puerto Rico. The School is committed to provide high quality medical education, service, and research, that will foster student's comprehensive development, so that they can become capable, competent, skilled, and honest professionals.

Curricular Highlights

Community Service Requirement: Required. 155 hrs required during the first three years
Research/Thesis Requirement: n/a

SJBSM had defined its curriculum within a student-centered approach, highlighting the values, attitudes, and social responsibility of the practice of medicine. It facilitates active learning and integration, offering early exposure to clinical scenarios and technological experiences in the learning process and using diverse assessment methodologies. The curriculum is structured in five emphases: medical knowledge, clinical skills, research and information literacy, professionalism and community awareness. These emphases are incorporated throughout the four years. The preclinical courses are offered during the first two years. The third year is devoted to core clinical clerkships, both inpatient and outpatient scenarios, including a research clerkship. The fourth year reinforces the practice of medicine with core and electives clinical clerkships, and a sub-specialties clerkship. Several curricular innovations strengthen the learning process: multidisciplinary exercises that promote vertical and horizontal integration, development of a research proposal throughout the four years, and different levels/types of community experiences, according to the School's mission.

USMLE

Step 1: Required. Students must record a passing score for promotion.
Step 2: Clinical Skills (CS): Required. Students must record a passing total score to graduate.
Step 2: Clinical Knowledge (CK): Student must record a passing total score to graduate.

Selection Factors

The Admissions office evaluates all applications, taking into consideration academic and personal qualifications. The analysis includes academic achievement, premedical studies required for admission to the program, and MCAT® scores. The motivations to study medicine, leadership qualities, ability to relate to other people and deal with problems, and participation in community/scientific activities, are also taken into consideration by the Admission's Committee. Qualified applicants are required to appear for an interview.

Financial Aid

The Financial Aid Office counsels students regarding the availability of economic aid and the procedure to file up applications. For further information, please refer to: *http://sanjuanbautista.edu/Admissions.asp*.

Information about Diversity Programs

The School of Medicine is committed to diversity in the faculty and the student body. Its goal is to recruit, admit and graduate students that are underrepresented in medicine. The office of Minority Affairs has programs to assist to help meeting the objectives of a diverse student body.

Campus Information

Setting

The School's facilities are located on the grounds of the San Juan Bautista Medical Center. The 52 acre campus is the location for the Hospital and the School, which houses administrative offices, the biomedical sciences faculty, and the Library/Learning Resources Center, as well as the classrooms and laboratories for teaching and research. Clinical training at the SJBMC brings students into contact with a patient population drawn from many different socio-economic groups. The SJBMC is the principal clinical training facility for third and fourth year students.

Enrollment

For 2007, total enrollment was: 234

Special Features

Our School is a community-based institution, in which community service is a curricular axis. Courses and activities are patient-focused throughout the program.

Housing

On-campus housing is not available. However, the School provides information about available housing facilities in Caguas.

Satellite Campuses/Facilities

The School of Medicine has established several collaborations that provide opportunities for its students. Students rotate at hospitals and ambulatory health care systems that met the school's high standards of educational quality.

Application Process and Requirements 2009–2010

Primary Application Service: AMCAS
Earliest filing date: June 1, 2008
Latest filing date: December 15, 2008

Secondary Application
URL: http://www.sanjuanbautista.edu/Admissions.aspx
Jaymi Sanchez-Cruz, (787) 743-3038 x236
admissions@sanjuanbautista.edu
Sent to: All applicants
Fee: Yes, $75
Fee Waiver Available: No
Earliest filing date: July 1, 2008
Latest filing date: April 15, 2009

Latest MCAT® considered: January 2009
Oldest MCAT® considered: January 2006

Early Decision Program
School does not have EDP
Applicants notified: n/a
EDP available for: n/a

Regular Acceptance Notice
Earliest date: April 2009
Latest date: Until Class is Full

Applicant's Response to Acceptance Offer – Maximum Time: Two weeks

Requests for deferred entrance considered: No

Deposit to Hold Place in Class: Yes,
Deposit (Resident): Yes, $1,000
Deposit (Non-Resident): Yes, $1,000
Deposit due: Two weeks
Applied to tuition: Yes
Deposit refundable: No
Refundable by: n/a

Estimated number of new entrants: 60
EDP: n/a, special program: n/a

Start month/year: August 2009

Interview format: Interviews occur individually or in groups on campus. Regional interviews are not available.

Other Programs

PREPARATORY PROGRAMS
Postbaccalaureate Program: No
Summer Program: No

COMBINED DEGREE PROGRAMS
Baccalaureate/MD: No
MD/MPH: No
MD/MBA: No
MD/JD: No
MD/PhD: No

Premedical Coursework

Course	Req.	Rec.	Lab.	Sems.	Course	Req.	Rec.	Lab.	Sems.
Inorganic Chemistry	•			2	Computer Science				
Behavioral Sciences	•			4	Genetics				
Biochemistry		•			Humanities				
Biology	•			2	Organic Chemistry	•			2
Biology/Zoology					Physics	•			2
Calculus					Psychology				
College English	•			4	Social Sciences				
College Mathematics					Spanish		•		2

Selection Factors: 2007 Accepted Applicants

Proportion of Accepted Applicants with Relevant Experience (Data Self-Reported to AMCAS®)		
Community Service/Volunteer		80%
Medically-Related Work		30%
Research		53%

Shaded bar represents accepted scores ranging from the 10th percentile to the 90th percentile   School Median ●   National Median ●

Overall GPA	2.0 2.1 2.2 2.3 2.4 2.5 2.6 2.7 2.8 2.9 3.0 3.1 ⟨3.2⟩ 3.3 3.4 3.5 3.6 3.7 3.8 3.9 4.0
Science GPA	2.0 2.1 2.2 2.3 2.4 2.5 2.6 2.7 2.8 2.9 3.0 ⟨3.1⟩ 3.2 3.3 3.4 3.5 3.6 3.7 3.8 3.9 4.0

MCAT® required: Yes, n/a of 2007 accepted applicants took MCAT®

Verbal Reasoning	2 3 4 ⑤ 6 7 8 9 ⑩ 11 12 13 14 15
Physical Sciences	3 4 5 ⑥ 7 8 9 10 ⑪ 12 13 14 15
Biological Sciences	3 4 5 ⑥ 7 8 9 10 ⑪ 12 13 14 15
Writing Sample	J ⑭ L M N O P ⑯ R S T

Acceptance & Matriculation Data for 2007–2008 First Year Class

	Resident	Non-Resident	International	Total
Applied	174	30	0	204
Interviewed	100	24	0	124
Deferred	n/r	n/r	n/r	n/r
Matriculants				
Early Assurance Program	n/r	n/r	n/r	n/r
Early Decision Program	n/r	n/r	n/r	n/r
Baccalaureate/MD Program	n/r	n/r	n/r	n/r
MD/PhD Program	n/r	n/r	n/r	n/r
Matriculated	51	9	0	**60**

Applications accepted from International Applicants: Yes

Specialty Choice

2003, 2004, 2005 Graduates, Specialty Choice (As reported by program directors to GME Track™)

Anesthesiology
Emergency Medicine
Family Practice
Int
Ot   **DATA NOT AVAILABLE**
Or
Pediatrics
Psychiatry
Radiology
Surgery

Matriculant Demographics: 2007–2008 First Year Class

Men: 22   **Women:** 38

Matriculants' Self-Reported Race/Ethnicity

Mexican American	0	Korean	0
Cuban	0	Vietnamese	0
Puerto Rican	51	Other Asian	2
Other Hispanic	6	Total Asian	0
Total Hispanic	0	Native American	0
Chinese	0	Black	0
Asian Indian	0	Native Hawaiian	0
Pakistani	1	White	0
Filipino	0	Unduplicated Number	
Japanese	0	of Matriculants	60

Science Majors: 100%
Matriculants with:
Baccalaureate Degree: 80%
Graduate Degree(s): 21%

Financial Information

Source: 2006–2007 LCME I-B survey and 2007–2008 AAMC TSF questionnaire

	Residents	Non-Residents
Total Cost of Attendance	$31,801	$34,801
Tuition and Fees	$18,770	$21,770
Other (includes living expenses)	$11,650	$11,650
Health Insurance (can be waived)	$1,381	$1,381

Average 2007 Graduate Indebtedness: $0
% of Enrolled Students Receiving Aid: 92%

Criminal Background Check

This medical school requires a criminal background check prior to matriculation.

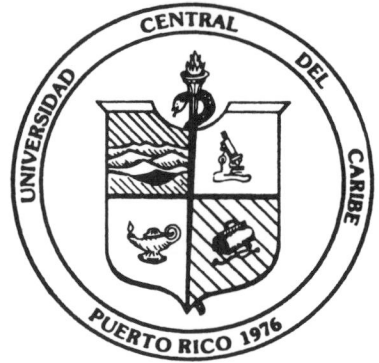

Universidad Central del Caribe
School of Medicine

Bayamón, Puerto Rico

Office of Admissions
Universidad Central del Caribe
School of Medicine, P.O. Box 60-327
Bayamon, Puerto Rico 00960-6032
T 787 798 3001   F 787 269 7550

Admissions www.uccaribe.edu
Main www.uccaribe.edu
Financial www.uccaribe.edu
Email icordero@uccaribe.edu
edlopez@uccaribe.edu

Private Institution

Dr. Jose Ginel Rodriguez, Dean of Medicine

Dr. Nereida Diaz-Rodriguez, Dean of Admissions and Student Affairs

Ana M. Galan, Financial Aid Director

Irma L. Cordero, Admissions Officer

General Information

The Universidad Central del Caribe School of Medicine was founded in 1976 as a nonprofit private institution chartered under the laws of the Commonwealth of Puerto Rico. The new building for the basic sciences, library, animal house, and central administration was inaugurated in 1990 adjacent to Dr. Ramon Ruiz Arnau University Hospital, which serves as the principal teaching hospital. The school facilities are located in a 56-acre academic health center in the city of Bayamon.

Mission Statement

The mission of the School of Medicine is to develop competent physicians with an outstanding academic preparation within a humanistic and holistic framework. A guiding principle of our mission is to ensure that our graduates possess a strong sense of professionalism and commitment to social duties and service to Puerto Rico and Hispanic communities throughout the U.S. mainland.

Curricular Highlights

Community Service Requirement: Optional.
Research/Thesis Requirement: Optional.

The medical curriculum is organized in two years of preclinical and two years of clinical experiences. A longitudinal curriculum in bioethics and humanities in medicine characterizes the medical education program. Clinical correlations are included in the basic science courses. Exposure to real and standardized patients is provided beginning with the first year. Introduction to clinical medicine has as its foundation the biopsychosocial model. A

problem-based course is structured around prevalent problems encountered in primary care. The third-year learning experience revolves around required clerkships in internal medicine, pediatrics, obstetrics-gynecology, general surgery, and family medicine. The latter takes place in the ambulatory setting. Also, during the third year, students enroll in the surgical subspecialties and psychiatry clerkships. Eighteen weeks of electives are provided in the fourth year, plus three months in required courses in neurology, ambulatory medicine, selected topics, and bioethics and humanities in medicine. Individual student evaluation in all requisite basic science and clinical science courses is based on letter grade and Pass/Fail systems. Student evaluation in all elective courses is based on an Honors/Pass/Fail system.

USMLE

Step 1: Required. Students must record a passing score for promotion.
Step 2: Clinical Skills (CS): Required. Students must record a passing total score to graduate.
Step 2: Clinical Knowledge (CK): Required. Students must record a passing total score to graduate.

Selection Factors

The selection of candidates for admission is made exclusively by the Admissions Committee. The admission process does not discriminate against any individual on the basis of sex, age, race, religion, economic status, political ideology, or national origin. Applicants must demonstrate proficiency in both Spanish and English. Lectures may be in either language. Spanish is the predominant language of the institution. Major factors considered in the selection of candidates for admission include undergraduate academic record, overall GPA and science GPA, performance in all areas of the MCAT®, results of a personal interview, and letters of recommendation. A personal interview is required prior to consideration for admission. All interviews are arranged by the Office of Admissions and are conducted at the medical school facilities in Bayamon. Rejected applicants are given the opportunity to reapply for admission.

Financial Aid

The Office of the Dean for Student Affairs provides financial aid counseling to all prospective students. Incoming students qualify for application to all pertinent federal and commonwealth scholarship and loan programs. Economic status of the applicant is not a consideration during the selection of candidates for admission.

Campus Information

Enrollment

For 2007, total enrollment was: 243

Housing

On-campus housing is not available. However, the dean for student affairs maintains a list of affordable apartments in the vicinity.

Satellite Campuses/Facilities

Student rotations are divided between the University Hospital and a rich network of clinical settings in the metro area.

Application Process and Requirements 2009–2010

Primary Application Service: AMCAS
Earliest filing date: June 1, 2008
Latest filing date: December 15, 2008

Secondary Application Required?: No
Sent to: Several documents must be submitted.
Irma L. Cordero, (787) 798-3001 x 2403
icordero@uccaribe.edu
Fee: Yes, $100
Fee waiver available: No
Earliest filing date: n/a
Latest filing date: n/a

Latest MCAT® considered: September 2008
Oldest MCAT® considered: 2006

**Early Decision Program
School does not have EDP
Applicants notified:** n/a
EDP available for: n/a

**Regular Acceptance Notice
Earliest date:** January 2009
Latest date: Until class is full

**Applicant's Response to Acceptance
Offer – Maximum Time:** Two weeks

**Requests for Deferred
Entrance Considered:** No

Deposit to Hold Place in Class: Yes
Deposit (Resident): $100
Deposit (Non-Resident): $100
Deposit due: 15 days after notification
Applied to tuition: No
Deposit refundable: No
Refundable by: n/a

Estimated number of new entrants: 60
EDP: n/a, special program: n/a

Start Month/Year: August 2009

Interview Format: Group interviews.
Regional interviews are not available.

Other Programs

**PREPARATORY PROGRAMS
Postbaccalaureate Program:** No
Summer Program: No

**COMBINED DEGREE PROGRAMS
Baccalaureate/MD:** No
MD/MPH: No
MD/MBA: No
MD/JD: No
MD/PhD: No

Premedical Coursework

Course	Req.	Rec.	Lab.	Hrs.
Inorganic Chemistry	•		•	8
Behavioral Sciences		•		
Biochemistry		•		
Biology		•		8
Biology/Zoology	•		•	8
Calculus				
College English	•			12
College Mathematics	•			6
Computer Science		•		

Course	Req.	Rec.	Lab.	Hrs.
Genetics		•		
Humanities				
Organic Chemistry	•		•	8
Physics	•		•	8
Psychology		•		
Social Sciences		•		
Behavioral/Social Sciences	•			12
Spanish	•			6

Selection Factors: 2007 Accepted Applicants

Proportion of Accepted Applicants with Relevant Experience (Data Self-Reported to AMCAS°)		
Community Service/Volunteer		43%
Medically-Related Work		50%
Research		59%

Shaded bar represents accepted scores ranging from the 10th percentile to the 90th percentile   **School Median** ●   **National Median** ●

Overall GPA	2.0	2.1	2.2	2.3	2.4	2.5	2.6	2.7	2.8	2.9	3.0	3.1	3.2	3.3	3.4	(3.5)	3.6	3.7	3.8	3.9	4.0
Science GPA	2.0	2.1	2.2	2.3	2.4	2.5	2.6	2.7	2.8	2.9	3.0	3.1	3.2	(3.3)	3.4	3.5	3.6	3.7	3.8	3.9	4.0

MCAT® required: Yes, 100% of 2007 accepted applicants took MCAT®

Verbal Reasoning	3	4	5	(6)	7	8	9	(10)	11	12	13	14	15
Physical Sciences	3	4	5	6	(7)	8	9	10	(11)	12	13	14	15
Biological Sciences	3	4	5	6	7	(8)	9	10	(11)	12	13	14	15
Writing Sample			J	K	L	(M)	N	O	P	(Q)	R	S	T

Acceptance & Matriculation Data for 2007–2008 First Year Class

	Resident	Non-Resident	International	Total
Applied	309	604	27	940
Interviewed	101	20	1	122
Deferred	0	0	0	0
Matriculants				
Early Assurance Program	0	0	0	0
Early Decision Program	0	0	0	0
Baccalaureate/MD	n/a	n/a	n/a	n/a
MD/PhD	n/a	n/a	n/a	n/a
Matriculated	50	15	1	**66**

Applications accepted from International Applicants: Yes

Specialty Choice

2003, 2004, 2005 Graduates, Specialty Choice (As reported by program directors to GME Track™)	
Anesthesiology	0%
Emergency Medicine	4%
Family Practice	6%
Internal Medicine	31%
Obstetrics/Gynecology	3%
Orthopaedic Surgery	1%
Pediatrics	8%
Psychiatry	10%
Radiology	4%
Surgery	3%

Matriculant Demographics: 2007–2008 First Year Class

Men: 33   **Women:** 33

Matriculants' Self-Reported Race/Ethnicity

Mexican American	3	**Korean**	0
Cuban	5	**Vietnamese**	0
Puerto Rican	50	**Other Asian**	0
Other Hispanic	6	**Total Asian**	0
Total Hispanic	61	**Native American**	0
Chinese	0	**Black**	3
Asian Indian	0	**Native Hawaiian**	0
Pakistani	0	**White**	50
Filipino	0	**Unduplicated Number**	
Japanese	0	**of Matriculants**	66

Science and Math Majors: 68%
Matriculants with:
          Baccalaureate degree: 97%
          Graduate degree(s): 2%

Financial Information

Source: 2006–2007 LCME I-B survey
and 2007–2008 AAMC TSF questionnaire

	Residents	Non-Residents
Total Cost of Attendance	$41,525	$48,525
Tuition and Fees	$24,890	$31,890
Other (includes living expenses)	$15,255	$15,255
Health Insurance (can be waived)	$1,380	$1,380

Average 2007 Graduate Indebtedness: $6,164
% of Enrolled Students Receiving Aid: 87%

Criminal Background Check

This medical school requires a criminal background check prior to matriculation.

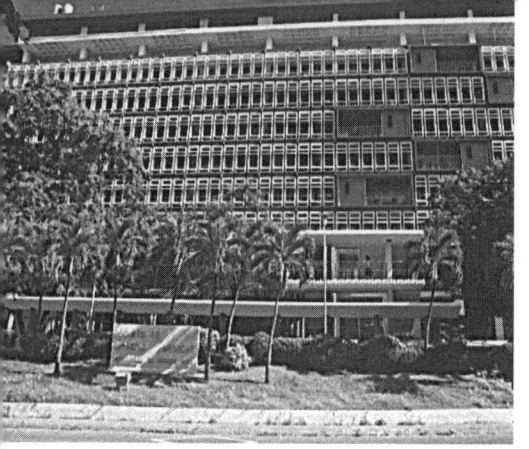

University of Puerto Rico School of Medicine

San Juan, Puerto Rico

Central Admissions Office
School of Medicine, Medical Sciences Campus
University of Puerto Rico, P.O. Box 365067
San Juan, Puerto Rico 00936-5067
T 787 758 2525 x 5215   **F** 787 282 7117

Admissions www.md.rcm.upr.edu
Main www.md.rcm.upr.edu
Financial www.upr.edu/Asistencia%20
Economica/asisecon.htm
Email marrivera@rcm.upr.edu

Public Institution

Dr. Walter Frontera, Dean

Dr. Gladys Gonzalez-Navarrete, Assistant Dean for Student Affairs

Margarita Rivera, Admissions Officer

Zoraida Cruz, Director, Financial Aid Office

General Information

The UPR-SOM was established in 1949. The affiliated hospitals of the P.R. Medical Center and the Hospital Consortium, which include the main health care facilities in other cities, serve the medical school for teaching purposes. On the Medical Sciences Campus, the School of Medicine works in close relation with the School of Dentistry, the College of Allied Health Professions, the Faculty of Biosocial Sciences and Graduate School of Public Health, the School of Nursing, and the School of Pharmacy in an interdisciplinary team approach. Its location, adjacent to the University District Hospital, permits integration of basic and clinical departments and an improved utilization of all Medical Sciences Campus resources.

Mission Statement

The mission of the UPR-SOM is to transmit, enrich, and increase knowledge in the medical sciences through teaching, research, and clinical service. The school is committed to achieve the ideals of personal and academic excellence through the interdisciplinary model for providing education and health services, especially at the primary level. The school will provide an academic and institutional environment conducive to the personal and professional development of both students and faculty.

Curricular Highlights

Community Service Requirement: Optional.
Research/Thesis Requirement: Optional.

The new curriculum is four academic years in length. The first two years include the fundamentals of biological, behavioral, and clinical sciences and are mostly handled by the basic sciences departments. Part of the sophomore year is dedicated to pathophysiology, physical diagnosis, and basic clerkship, which are offered by a multidisciplinary faculty. Small-group sessions utilizing the problem-based learning approach are introduced at the beginning of the medical studies. Human behavior, environmental factors, and public health concepts are integrated into the curriculum. The third and fourth years are dedicated to required clinical experiences and elective courses. Through the Hispanic Center of Excellence, the curriculum has been focused on community-oriented primary care exposure. Support services, counseling, tutorials, and other services are provided to students to assist in retention. Students are graded on a letter grade system during all four years.

USMLE

Step 1: Required. Students must record a passing score for promotion.
Step 2: Clinical Skills (CS): Optional.
Step 2: Clinical Knowledge (CK): Required. Students must record a passing total score to graduate.

Selection Factors

Since the UPR-SOM is a state-supported institution, preference will be given to qualified applicants who are legal residents of Puerto Rico. Foreign national applicants with an established residence in P.R. will be considered only if, at the time of application, they are either U.S. citizens or have been granted a permanent resident visa in the United States. In selecting students, the Admissions Committee considers the candidate's academic performance, MCAT® scores, recommendations of instructors, attitudinal and other personality factors assessed in personal interviews, extracurricular activities, and any other pertinent information. Personal interviews are conducted only by invitation from the Admissions Committee for those students with high numerical ranks according to the admission formula. The admission formula gives equal weight to academic indices and MCAT® scores, with somewhat less weight given to ratings derived from evaluations by premedical committees and interviewers. Rejected applicants are given the opportunity to reapply for admission.

Applicants, without exception, must submit all application material and supporting documents by December 1 of the year preceding the school year for which they request admission. The UPR-SOM has the policy of giving equal opportunity for education and training in the practice of the health professions without regard to race, creed, sex, national origin, age, or handicap.

Financial Aid

Financial aid is available to students. Awards are made on the basis of confidential applications submitted by students. Financial need is the major criterion. Applicants who require scholarship assistance may make application in conjunction with the application for admission or before April 30. Financial need will not influence the selection process. Forms are available from the Financial Aid Office upon request. We do not offer financial assistance to foreign students.

Campus Information

Enrollment

For 2007, total enrollment was: 108

Application Process and Requirements 2009–2010

Primary Application Service: AMCAS
Earliest filing date: June 1, 2008
Latest filing date: December 1, 2008

Secondary Application Required?: Yes
Sent to: All applicants
URL: www.md.rcm.upr.edu
Fee: Yes, $20
Fee waiver available: No
Earliest filing date: June 1, 2008
Latest filing date: December 1, 2008

Latest MCAT® considered: September 2008
Oldest MCAT® considered: August 2006

Early Decision Program
School does not have EDP
Applicants notified: n/a
EDP available for: n/a

Regular Acceptance Notice
Earliest date: December 2008
Latest date: Varies

Applicant's Response to Acceptance
Offer – Maximum Time: Two weeks

Requests for Deferred
Entrance Considered: No

Deposit to Hold Place in Class: Yes
Deposit (Resident): $100
Deposit (Non-Resident): n/a
Deposit due: With response to acceptance offer
Applied to tuition: Yes
Deposit refundable: No
Refundable by: n/a

Estimated number of new entrants: 110
EDP: n/a, special program: n/a

Start Month/Year: August 2009

Interview Format:
Regional interviews are not available.

Other Programs

PREPARATORY PROGRAMS
Postbaccalaureate Program: No
Summer Program: No

COMBINED DEGREE PROGRAMS
Baccalaureate/MD: No
MD/MPH: No
MD/MBA: No
MD/JD: Yes, www.md.rcm.upr.edu
http://medweb.rcm.upr.edu
MD/PhD: Yes, www.md.rcm.upr.edu

Premedical Coursework

Course	Req.	Rec.	Lab.	Hrs.
Inorganic Chemistry	•	•		8
Behavioral Sciences	•			6
Biochemistry		•		
Biology	•			8
Biology/Zoology				
Calculus				
College English	•			12
College Mathematics				

Course	Req.	Rec.	Lab.	Hrs.
Computer Science		•		
Genetics				
Humanities		•		
Organic Chemistry	•		•	8
Physics	•		•	8
Psychology				
Social Sciences	•			6
Spanish				12

Selection Factors: 2007 Accepted Applicants

Proportion of Accepted Applicants with Relevant Experience (Data Self-Reported to AMCAS®)		
Community Service/Volunteer	50%	
Medically-Related Work	47%	
Research	75%	

Shaded bar represents accepted scores ranging from the 10th percentile to the 90th percentile.   School Median ●   National Median ●

Overall GPA	2.0	2.1	2.2	2.3	2.4	2.5	2.6	2.7	2.8	2.9	3.0	3.1	3.2	3.3	3.4	3.5	3.6	(3.7)	3.8	3.9	4.0
Science GPA	2.0	2.1	2.2	2.3	2.4	2.5	2.6	2.7	2.8	2.9	3.0	3.1	3.2	3.3	3.4	3.5	(3.6)	3.7	3.8	3.9	4.0

MCAT® required: Yes, 100% of 2007 accepted applicants took MCAT®

Verbal Reasoning	3	4	5	6	(7)	8	9	(10)	11	12	13	14	15
Physical Sciences	3	4	5	6	(7)	8	9	10	(11)	12	13	14	15
Biological Sciences	3	4	5	6	7	8	(9)	10	(11)	12	13	14	15
Writing Sample			J	K	L	(M)	N	O	P	(Q)	R	S	T

Acceptance & Matriculation Data for 2007–2008 First Year Class

	Resident	Non-Resident	International	Total
Applied	293	569	13	875
Interviewed	138	0	0	138
Deferred	0	0	0	0
Matriculants				
Early Assurance Program	n/a	n/a	n/a	n/a
Early Decision Program	0	0	0	0
Baccalaureate/MD	n/a	n/a	n/a	n/a
MD/PhD	n/a	n/a	n/a	n/a
Matriculated	102	3	0	**105**

Applications accepted from International Applicants: No

Matriculant Demographics: 2007–2008 First Year Class

Men: 54   **Women:** 51

Matriculants' Self-Reported Race/Ethnicity

Mexican American	1	Korean	0
Cuban	1	Vietnamese	0
Puerto Rican	100	Other Asian	0
Other Hispanic	3	Total Asian	0
Total Hispanic	103	Native American	1
Chinese	0	Black	11
Asian Indian	0	Native Hawaiian	0
Pakistani	0	White	73
Filipino	0	Unduplicated Number	
Japanese	0	of Matriculants	105

Science and Math Majors: 84%
Matriculants with:
Baccalaureate degree: 98%
Graduate degree(s): 4%

Specialty Choice

2003, 2004, 2005 Graduates, Specialty Choice (As reported by program directors to GME Track™)	
Anesthesiology	0%
Emergency Medicine	5%
Family Practice	4%
Internal Medicine	22%
Obstetrics/Gynecology	3%
Orthopaedic Surgery	2%
Pediatrics	12%
Psychiatry	8%
Radiology	5%
Surgery	4%

Financial Information

Source: 2006–2007 LCME I-B survey and 2007–2008 AAMC TSF questionnaire

	Residents	Non-Residents
Total Cost of Attendance	$29,683	$37,911
Tuition and Fees	$9,081	$17,309
Other (includes living expenses)	$20,602	$20,602
Health Insurance (can be waived)	$0	$0

Average 2007 Graduate Indebtedness: $20,079
% of Enrolled Students Receiving Aid: 66%

Criminal Background Check

This medical school does not require a criminal background check prior to matriculation.

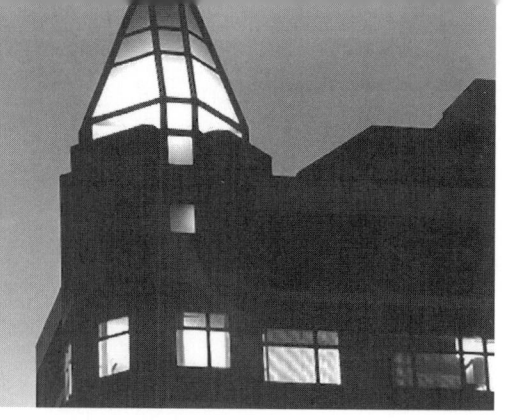

The Warren Alpert Medical School of Brown University

Providence, Rhode Island

Office of Admissions and Financial Aid
Alpert Medical School
97 Waterman Street, Box G-A213
Providence, Rhode Island
T 401 863 2149   F 401 863 2660

Admissions http://med.brown.edu/admissions
Main http://med.brown.edu
Financial http://med.brown.edu/financialaid/
Email MedSchool_Admissions@brown.edu

Private Institution

Dr. Eli Y. Adashi, Dean of Medicine and Biological Sciences

Kathleen A. Baer, Director of Admissions and Financial Aid

Dr. Alicia D. Monroe, Associate Dean for Diversity

Linda A. Gillette, Assistant Director of Admissions and Financial Aid

Dr. Philip Gruppuso, Associate Dean for Medical Education

John Deeley, Executive Dean for Administration

General Information

Since its accreditation in 1975, Alpert Medical School has become a national leader in medical education and biomedical research. The medical school and its eight affiliated hospitals receive $200 million annually in research funding. Brown is home to the state's only Master of Public Health degree program and to nine public health research centers. Entry into Alpert Medical School is possible through many admission routes, including a combined Bachelor's/Medical degree program, standard AMCAS admission, and an Early Identification Program for students from Tougaloo College (MS) and for Rhode Island residents enrolled at three Rhode Island Institutions of higher education.

Mission Statement

Our mission is to educate physicians in the scientific, ethical, and humanistic dimensions of medicine and to advance our ability to diagnose, treat, and prevent human illness.

Curricular Highlights

Community Service Requirement: Optional.
Research/Thesis Requirement: Optional.

The medical curriculum is demanding, yet flexible. The first year is devoted to core basic sciences in the form of two semester-length, integrated medical sciences courses and Doctoring, in which students encounter individual, community-based clinical skills teaching with group sessions on ethics, patient interviewing, and professional development topics. The second year consists of organ- or system-based pathophysiology with integrated pharmacology, pathology, neurologic pathophysiology, epidemiology, and Doctoring. Students in the third and fourth years are required to complete 50 weeks of clinical clerkships and 30 weeks of electives. Clinical clerkships include internal medicine, surgery, psychiatry, obstetrics and gynecology, pediatrics, family medicine, and community health. Elective requirements include an advanced clinical clerkship in medicine, surgery, or pediatrics, and an ambulatory longitudinal clerkship.

USMLE

Step 1: Required. Students must only record a score.
Step 2: Clinical Skills (CS): Required. Students must record a passing total score to graduate.
Step 2: Clinical Knowledge (CK): Required. Students must only record a score.

Selection Factors

Selection criteria are academic achievement, faculty evaluations, and evidence of maturity, leadership, integrity, and compassion. Applicants to the MD/PhD program are evaluated on the basis of their research accomplishment and potential. Eligible candidates generally must present a minimum cumulative grade point average of 3.00 (4.00 scale) in undergraduate courses. Applicants who have attended graduate school must achieve a cumulative grade point average of 3.00 (4.00 scale). Applicants must complete baccalaureate degree requirements before entry into medical school. Brown University adheres to a policy of equal opportunity in medical education and considers applicants without regard to sex, race, religion, age, disability, status as a veteran, national or ethnic origin, sexual orientation, or gender identity. An affirmative action program is maintained in all admission entry routes.

Financial Aid

Brown assists students in meeting their educational costs through low-interest loans and scholarships. Forty-five percent of students received need-based scholarships in 2007-08. MD/PhD students are eligible for a graduate fellowship during the PhD portion of their studies and a full tuition grant during the last two years of medical school.

Information about Diversity Programs

Alpert Medical School invites applications from members of ethnic and racial groups underrepresented in medicine. The objective of the Office of Minority Medical Affairs (OMMA) is the recruitment, retention, and graduation of students from groups underrepresented in medicine. The OMMA provides academic and personal counseling, workshops, information on scholarship awards, and a program linking students from groups underrepresented in medicine with alumni/ae from such groups.

Campus Information

Setting

The medical school is located on the main campus of Brown University in an historic residential area of Providence. The revitalized downtown center, with its riverfront park, shopping mall, restaurants, train station, and arts and theater district, is within walking distance of the campus.

Enrollment

For 2007, total enrollment was: 372

Special Features

Alpert Medical School is affiliated with eight hospitals within a five-mile radius, including a Level I trauma center, a children's hospital, two community hospitals, two psychiatric hospitals, a Veterans Medical Center, and a women's hospital with the largest neonatal intensive care unit in the Northeast. Students may experience clinical electives in exchange programs in Germany, Kenya, Sweden, and Israel.

Housing

Affordable housing options are available in several neighborhoods within walking distance of campus. Students have an on-campus dorm option. The university leases and manages about 100 apartments and homes in the vicinity. Monthly rents range from $700 to $1,150 in Brown-owned housing.

Satellite Campuses/Facilities

Clinical training in all four years occurs in a variety of settings, from the affiliated hospitals to diverse community-based sites.

Application Process and Requirements 2009–2010

Primary Application Service: AMCAS
Earliest filing date: June 1, 2008
Latest filing date: November 1, 2008

Secondary Application Required?: Yes
Sent to: All verified AMCAS applicants
URL: http://bms.brown.edu/admissions/applications
Fee: Yes, $95
Fee waiver available: Yes
Earliest filing date: July 1, 2008
Latest filing date: December 15, 2008

Latest MCAT® considered: September 2008
Oldest MCAT® considered: 2004

Early Decision Program
School does not have EDP
Applicants notified: n/a
EDP available for: n/a

Regular Acceptance Notice
Earliest date: December 2008
Latest date: Until Class is Full

Applicant's Response to Acceptance
Offer – Maximum Time: Three weeks

Requests for Deferred
Entrance Considered: Yes

Deposit to Hold Place in Class: No
Deposit (Resident): n/a
Deposit (Non-Resident): n/a
Deposit due: n/a
Applied to tuition: n/a
Deposit refundable: n/a
Refundable by: n/a

Estimated number of new entrants: 40
EDP: n/a, special program: 56

Start Month/Year: August 2009

Interview Format: Group session and
two individual meetings.
All interviews are at Alpert Medical School.

Other Programs

PREPARATORY PROGRAMS
Postbaccalaureate Program: No
Summer Program: No
Scholarly Concentrations Program: Yes,
http://med.brown.edu/students/curriculum/
concentrations/sc_program
Program for Academic Enhancement: Yes,
http://med.brown.edu/students/asp

COMBINED DEGREE PROGRAMS
Baccalaureate/MD: Yes,
http://bms.brown.edu/plme/
MD/MPH: Yes,
http://bms.brown.edu/pubhealth
MD/MBA: No
MD/JD: No
MD/PhD: Yes,
http://bms.brown.edu/mdphd/

Premedical Coursework

Course	Req.	Rec.	Lab.	Sems.
Inorganic Chemistry	•			2
Behavioral Sciences	•			1
Biochemistry		•		
Biology	•			1
Biology/Zoology				
Calculus	•			1
College English				
College Mathematics				

Course	Req.	Rec.	Lab.	Sems.
Computer Science				
Genetics				
Humanities				
Organic Chemistry	•			1
Physics	•			2
Psychology				
Social Sciences	•			1
Other				

Selection Factors: 2007 Accepted Applicants

Proportion of Accepted Applicants with Relevant Experience (Data Self-Reported to AMCAS®)		
Community Service/Volunteer		59%
Medically-Related Work		67%
Research		83%

Shaded bar represents accepted scores ranging from the 10th percentile to the 90th percentile   **School Median** ●   **National Median** ●

Overall GPA	2.0	2.1	2.2	2.3	2.4	2.5	2.6	2.7	2.8	2.9	3.0	3.1	3.2	3.3	3.4	3.5	3.6	3.7	(3.8)	3.9	4.0
Science GPA	2.0	2.1	2.2	2.3	2.4	2.5	2.6	2.7	2.8	2.9	3.0	3.1	3.2	3.3	3.4	3.5	3.6	3.7	(3.8)	3.9	4.0

MCAT® required: No, 63% of 2007 accepted applicants took MCAT®

Verbal Reasoning	3	4	5	6	7	8	9	(10)	(11)	12	13	14	15
Physical Sciences	3	4	5	6	7	8	9	10	(11)	(12)	13	14	15
Biological Sciences	3	4	5	6	7	8	9	10	(11)	(12)	13	14	15
Writing Sample		J	K	L	M	N	O	P	(Q)	R	S	T	

Acceptance & Matriculation Data for 2007–2008 First Year Class

	Resident	Non-Resident	International	Total
Applied	89	5428	499	6016
Interviewed	17	202	10	229
Deferred	0	1	0	1
Matriculants				
Early Assurance Program	0	2	0	2
Early Decision Program	n/a	n/a	n/a	n/a
Baccalaureate/MD	3	51	0	54
MD/PhD	0	1	0	1
Matriculated	7	86	2	**95**

Applications accepted from International Applicants: Yes

Specialty Choice

2003, 2004, 2005 Graduates, Specialty Choice (As reported by program directors to GME Track™)	
Anesthesiology	2%
Emergency Medicine	5%
Family Practice	11%
Internal Medicine	21%
Obstetrics/Gynecology	6%
Orthopaedic Surgery	4%
Pediatrics	9%
Psychiatry	4%
Radiology	6%
Surgery	5%

Matriculant Demographics: 2007–2008 First Year Class

Men: 42   **Women:** 53

Matriculants' Self-Reported Race/Ethnicity

Mexican American	5	**Korean**	4
Cuban	1	**Vietnamese**	0
Puerto Rican	1	**Other Asian**	4
Other Hispanic	2	**Total Asian**	25
Total Hispanic	9	**Native American**	0
Chinese	8	**Black**	7
Asian Indian	8	**Native Hawaiian**	0
Pakistani	0	**White**	46
Filipino	0	**Unduplicated Number**	
Japanese	1	**of Matriculants**	95

Science and Math Majors: 44%
Matriculants with:
  Baccalaureate degree: 100%
  Graduate degree(s): 5%

Financial Information

Source: 2006–2007 LCME I-B survey
and 2007–2008 AAMC TSF questionnaire

	Residents	Non-Residents
Total Cost of Attendance	$57,980	57,980
Tuition and Fees	$38,672	$38,672
Other (includes living expenses)	$16,796	$16,796
Health Insurance (can be waived)	$2,512	$2,512

Average 2007 Graduate Indebtedness: $128,216
% of Enrolled Students Receiving Aid: 73%

Criminal Background Check

This medical school does not require a criminal background check prior to matriculation.

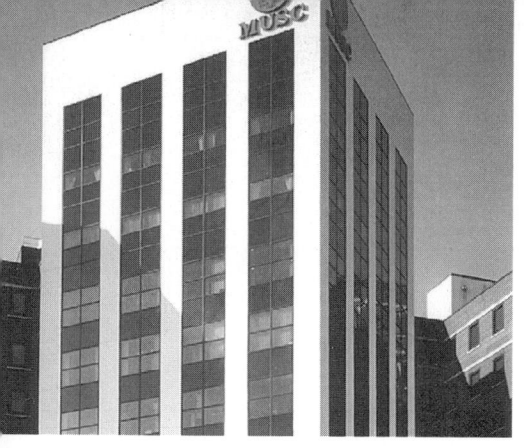

Medical University of South Carolina
College of Medicine

Charleston, South Carolina

College of Medicine Dean's Office
Medical University of South Carolina
96 Jonathan Lucas Street, Suite 601
PO Box 250617, Charleston, South Carolina 29425
T 843 792 3283   F 843 792 0204

Admissions www.musc.edu/es/
Main www2.musc.edu/COM/COM1.shtml
Financial www.musc.edu/financialmanagement/
Email taylorwl@musc.edu

Public Institution

Dr. Jerry Reves, Dean

*Dr. Paul B. Underwood,
Associate Dean for Admissions*

*Dr. Deborah Deas,
Associate Dean for Admissions*

Wanda Taylor, Director of Admissions

General Information

The College of Medicine at MUSC was founded in Charleston in 1824 and is the South's oldest medical school. MUSC's Medical Center is comprised of the MU Hospital, the Ashley River Tower, the Children's Hospital, the Storm Eye Institute, the Psychiatric Institute, the Hollings Cancer Center, and the Gazes/Strom Thurmond Research Bldg. The adjacent VA Hospital and Charleston Memorial Hospital, with consortium/community hospitals in Greenville, Spartanburg, Columbia, and Florence, supply additional facilities for clinical teaching. The Department of Family Medicine conducts a model program in the clinical area.

Mission Statement

The COM is committed to maintaining an educational environment for all students which prepares them for a career of excellence in the practice of medicine and service. It ensures optimal opportunities for all students, faculty, and administration, including all backgrounds and levels of diversity, to achieve full potential.

Curricular Highlights

Community Service Requirement: Required.
Research/Thesis Requirement: Optional.

The goal of the COM is to produce caring and competent physicians capable of choosing any postgraduate career. The curriculum in the first two years provides basic science concepts and problem-solving strategies, develops skills for taking histories and physical examinations, and introduces students to the role of the physician in society. Emphasis is placed on small-group instruction and independent, self-directed learning. The 3rd year consists of clerkships in medicine, ob/gyn, pediatrics, family medicine, surgery,and psychiatry. Selectives in multiple disciplines are also provided for students to gain exposure to major specialty areas. Emphasis is placed on the development of clinical, interpersonal, and professional competence. In the 4th year, students are required to take additional training in surgery and internal medicine and up to seven elective rotations in a wide variety of subspecialties.

USMLE

Step 1: Required. Students must record a passing score for promotion.
Step 2: Clinical Skills (CS): Required. Students Must only record a score.
Step 2: Clinical Knowledge (CK): Required. Students must record a passing total score to graduate.

Selection Factors

Selection is based on a total evaluation of the student. Initial screening is based on the cumulative undergraduate GPA and MCAT. Students passing this screening are invited for interviews. Noncognitive traits, accomplishments, and criteria for added value are evaluated during interviews. Personality, motivation, judgment, and integrity are important – as well as the quality of letters of recommendation, leadership, and volunteer/work experiences. Applicants with unique qualities may be considered for added value. Early Decision is encouraged for SC applicants with competitive grades and MCAT® scores. SC residency is a primary admission consideration. Foreign students without a permanent resident visa are ineligible.

Financial Aid

Financial need is not a factor in the selection process. Loan programs and scholarships are available for entering students. A financial aid counselor advises new and current students on loan opportunities and debt management. Merit scholarships are awarded by the Scholarship Board and are based on outstanding academic and personal achievement.

Information about Diversity Programs

Students from groups underrepresented in medicine are encouraged to apply. An active recruitment program is in place. PREP is an individually tailored undergraduate course of study prescribed for under-prepared, but promising SC students who seek admission through AMCAS. The program is full time; the curriculum is 12 months. No separate application is required. Students who apply through AMCAS and are denied admission are considered. Two students are selected annually; stipends are provided. A Summer Institute, devoted to underrepresented students, focuses on test-taking skills. The COM and the Center for Academic Excellence provide counseling and support services. Academic assistance is provided to students through tutorial programs and test-taking skill development.

Campus Information

Setting

MUSC's 67-acre campus is located in historic Charleston, SC. Charleston combines the best that life has to offer: historic homes, art, music, museums, libraries, restaurants, beaches, and some of the country's finest golf courses. Within a short walk from the city's main street are all the hospitals, research centers, clinical, and basic science buildings that make up the MUSC complex.

Enrollment

For 2007, total enrollment was: 620

Special Features

Ashley River Tower, a Digestive Disease/Cardiology hospital has opened recently. This is Phase I of a 20-year plan to update facilities and expand capacity at the MUSC complex. The MUSC Children's Research Institute, which opened in early 2006, is the state's largest research center dedicated to treating and exploring childhood diseases.

Housing

On-campus housing is not available. The MUSC Office of Student Programs maintains an online listing of affordable apartments near the MUSC campus. Rents average $600-$800 per month.

Application Process and Requirements 2009–2010

Primary Application Service: AMCAS
Earliest filing date: June 1, 2008
Latest filing date: December 1, 2008

Secondary Application Required?: Yes
Sent to: All applicants
URL: www.musc.edu/em/admissions/apply.html
Fee: Yes, $75
Fee waiver available: No
Earliest filing date: July 14, 2008
Latest filing date: January 15, 2009

Latest MCAT® considered: September 2008
Oldest MCAT® considered: August 2004

Early Decision Program
School does have EDP
Applicants notified: October 1, 2008
EDP available for: Residents only

Regular Acceptance Notice
Earliest date: November 1, 2008
Latest date: Until class is full

Applicant's Response to Acceptance
Offer – Maximum Time: Four weeks

Requests for Deferred
Entrance Considered: Yes

Deposit to Hold Place in Class: Yes
Deposit (Resident): $359
Deposit (Non-Resident): $359
Deposit due: Within four weeks of response to acceptance offer
Applied to tuition: No
Deposit refundable: Yes
Refundable by: May 15, 2009

Estimated number of new entrants: 150
EDP: 30, special program: n/a

Start Month/Year: August 2009

Interview Format: Three one-on-one interviews are required. Regional physicians assist with interviews.

Other Programs

PREPARATORY PROGRAMS
Postbaccalaureate Program: No
Summer Program: No

COMBINED DEGREE PROGRAMS
Baccalaureate/MD: No
MD/MPH: Yes, Dr. Amy Blue,
(843) 792-3409, blueav@musc.edu
MD/MBA: Yes, Dr. Amy Blue,
(843) 792-3409, blueav@musc.edu
MD/JD: No
MD/PhD: Yes,
www.musc.edu/grad/mstp/
Dr. Perry Halushka, (843) 792-3012,
halushpv@musc.edu
Additional Program: Yes, Dr. Amy Blue,
(843) 792-3409, blueav@musc.edu

Premedical Coursework

Course	Req.	Rec.	Lab.	Sems.	Course	Req.	Rec.	Lab.	Sems.
Inorganic Chemistry		•	•	8	Humanities				
Behavioral Sciences					Organic Chemistry		•	•	8
Biochemistry		•		4	Physics		•		8
Biology		•	•	8	Psychology				
Biology/Zoology					Social Sciences				
Calculus					Other				
College English		•		6	Cell Biology				4
College Mathematics					Physiology				4
Computer Science					Anatomy				4
Genetics									

Selection Factors: 2007 Accepted Applicants

Proportion of Accepted Applicants with Relevant Experience (Data Self-Reported to AMCAS®)	Community Service/Volunteer	62%
	Medically-Related Work	74%
	Research	65%

Shaded bar represents accepted scores ranging from the 10th percentile to the 90th percentile. School Median ● National Median ●

Overall GPA	2.0	2.1	2.2	2.3	2.4	2.5	2.6	2.7	2.8	2.9	3.0	3.1	3.2	3.3	3.4	3.5	3.6	(3.7)	3.8	3.9	4.0
Science GPA	2.0	2.1	2.2	2.3	2.4	2.5	2.6	2.7	2.8	2.9	3.0	3.1	3.2	3.3	3.4	3.5	(3.6)	3.7	3.8	3.9	4.0

MCAT® required: Yes, 100% of 2007 accepted applicants took MCAT®

Verbal Reasoning	3	4	5	6	7	8	9	(10)	11	12	13	14	15
Physical Sciences	3	4	5	6	7	8	9	(10)	(11)	12	13	14	15
Biological Sciences	3	4	5	6	7	8	9	(10)	(11)	12	13	14	15
Writing Sample				J	K	L	M	N	(O)	P	(Q)	R	S	T

Acceptance & Matriculation Data for 2007–2008 First Year Class

	Resident	Non-Resident	International	Total
Applied	513	1504	26	2043
Interviewed	337	44	0	381
Deferred	2	0	0	2
Matriculants				
Early Assurance Program	0	0	0	0
Early Decision Program	36	0	0	36
Baccalaureate/MD	n/a	n/a	n/a	n/a
MD/PhD	2	3	1	6
Matriculated	143	14	1	**158**

Applications accepted from International Applicants: No

Matriculant Demographics: 2007–2008 First Year Class

Men: 97   **Women:** 61

Matriculants' Self-Reported Race/Ethnicity

Mexican American	2	Korean	1
Cuban	0	Vietnamese	2
Puerto Rican	0	Other Asian	2
Other Hispanic	3	Total Asian	11
Total Hispanic	5	Native American	3
Chinese	1	Black	20
Asian Indian	7	Native Hawaiian	1
Pakistani	2	White	127
Filipino	1	Unduplicated Number	
Japanese	2	of Matriculants	158

Science and Math Majors: 70%
Matriculants with:
  Baccalaureate degree: 100%
  Graduate degree(s): 8%

Specialty Choice

2003, 2004, 2005 Graduates, Specialty Choice (As reported by program directors to GME Track™)	
Anesthesiology	5%
Emergency Medicine	4%
Family Practice	11%
Internal Medicine	15%
Obstetrics/Gynecology	10%
Orthopaedic Surgery	4%
Pediatrics	12%
Psychiatry	3%
Radiology	6%
Surgery	7%

Financial Information

Source: 2006–2007 LCME I-B survey and 2007–2008 AAMC TSF questionnaire

	Residents	Non-Residents
Total Cost of Attendance	$45,090	$87,619
Tuition and Fees	$24,637	$67,166
Other (includes living expenses)	$19,508	$19,508
Health Insurance (can be waived)	$945	$945

Average 2007 Graduate Indebtedness: $131,521
% of Enrolled Students Receiving Aid: 88%

Criminal Background Check

This medical school requires a criminal background check prior to matriculation.

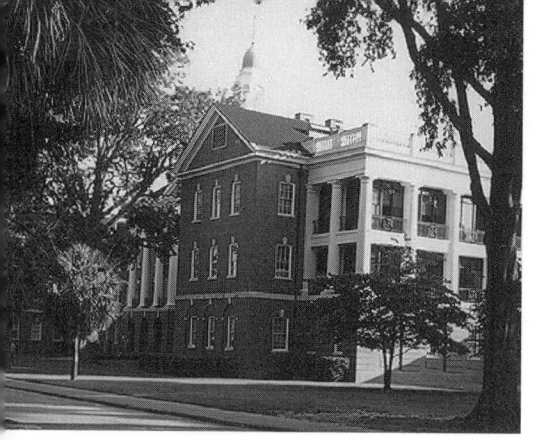

University of South Carolina School of Medicine
Columbia, South Carolina

Associate Dean for Medical Education
and Academic Affairs
University of South Carolina School of Medicine
Columbia, South Carolina 29208
T 803 733 3325   F 803 733 3328

Admissions http://medicaleducationoffice.med.sc.edu/
AdmissionsHomePage.htm
Main www.med.sc.edu
Financial www.sc.edu/financialaid
Email jeanette@gw.med.sc.edu

Public Institution

Dr. Donald J. DiPette, Dean

*Dr. Jeanette H. Ford, Registrar, Administrator,
Office of Admissions*

*Dr. Carol L. McMahon, Assistant Dean
for Minority Affairs*

*Dr. Richard A. Hoppmann, Associate Dean
for Medical Education and Academic Affairs*

Dr. Donald J. Kenney, Director, Student Services

General Information

The USC SOM was established in 1974 by the SC General Assembly in conjunction with the VA. The charter class matriculated in 1977 and graduated in 1981. Clinical instruction takes place in a variety of area hospitals that provide an ample number of teaching beds and extensive outpatient facilities. Elective opportunities are available throughout SC at community hospitals affiliated with the Area Health Education Consortium (AHEC), at other medical centers in the United States, and abroad.

Mission Statement

The mission of the USC SOM is to improve the health of the people of the state of SC through the development and implementation of programs for medical education, research, and the delivery of health care. Programs will be developed in collaboration with affiliated institutions, and allocation of resources will be based upon the physician manpower and health care needs of SC, the effectiveness and efficiency of specific programs, and the accreditation requirements of all appropriate organizations. Medical education and graduate education at all levels are conducted in a highly personal atmosphere that emphasizes a balance among scientific disciplines, humanistic concerns, and societal needs.

Curricular Highlights

Community Service Requirement: Optional.
Research/Thesis Requirement: Optional.

The SOM offers a program of study designed to provide education and training in the art and science of medicine and to prepare students for a wide variety of medical career choices. Each of the first two years consists of two academic semesters of both basic science and clinically relevant coursework in which students are exposed to patients in various inpatient, outpatient, community, and rural settings. The correlation between basic and clinical science information in the first two years is emphasized by means of an interdisciplinary, four-semester Introduction to Clinical Medicine course continuum. The third year consists of required clinical clerkships in medicine, surgery, pediatrics, obstetrics-gynecology, family medicine, and psychiatry. The fourth year is devoted to advanced clinical work, including 20 weeks each of required and elective rotations, during which students have the opportunity to strengthen their clinical skills and pursue individual academic interests and career goals in preparation for the lifelong study of medicine. A vertical curriculum in ultrasonography has been introduced in both the basic science and clinical years.

USMLE

Step 1: Required. Students must record a passing score for promotion.
Step 2: Clinical Skills (CS): Required. Students must record a passing total score to graduate.
Step 2: Clinical Knowledge (CK): Required. Students must record a passing total score to graduate.

Selection Factors

The selection process involves the comparative evaluation and review of all available application data, including MCAT® scores, undergraduate academic performance, comments contained in letters of evaluation, and the results of personal interviews with Admissions Committee members. The opportunity for admission is greatest for legal residents of South Carolina. Applications are only accepted from permanent residents or US citizens. The ultimate selection of a student is based upon a total and comparative appraisal of the applicant's suitability for the successful practice of medicine. The AMCAS application is used for preliminary screening. After this initial review, the Admissions Committee may extend an invitation for personal interviews. Each applicant is evaluated on the basis of individual qualifications without regard to age, race, creed, national origin, sex, or disability.

Financial Aid

The SOM participates in all federally funded loan and scholarship programs. A SOM-sponsored low-interest loan program is available to students with proven need. Every effort is made to provide information and assistance to help students meet their financial obligations. Students seeking part-time employment during medical school should have the prior approval of the director of student services.

Information about Diversity Programs

The SOM actively encourages applications from members of groups underrepresented in the medical profession. There is diverse membership on the Admissions Committee. For additional information, contact the assistant dean for minority affairs at (803) 733-3319.

Campus Information
Setting

The USC SOM campus, with its spacious lawns and trees, is located four miles east of the USC Columbia campus and adjacent to the Dorn V.A. Medical Center.

Enrollment

For 2007, total enrollment was: 315

Special Features

Students enjoy 24-hour secure access to USC SOM laboratories and library facilities. They participate in the extensive intramural athletic and recreational sports programs. The fitness center is located on-campus. USC SOM students also have access to all facilities and programs available to USC students.

Housing

The majority of USC SOM students choose housing in the area adjacent to the campus. Housing information can be obtained from the Student Services Office.

Satellite Campuses/Facilities

Students have the option of completing core clinical training in the third and fourth years at the Greenville Hospital System; 24 positions are available.

Application Process and Requirements 2009–2010

Primary Application Service: AMCAS
Earliest filing date: June 1, 2008
Latest filing date: December 1, 2008

Secondary Application Required?: Yes
Sent to: All applicants
URL: n/a
Fee: Yes, $75
Fee waiver available: Yes
Earliest filing date: June 1, 2008
Latest filing date: January 15, 2009

Latest MCAT® considered: September 2008
Oldest MCAT® considered: 2003

Early Decision Program
School does have EDP
Applicants notified: October 1, 2008
EDP available for: Residents only

Regular Acceptance Notice
Earliest date: October 15, 2008
Latest date: Until class is full

Applicant's Response to Acceptance
Offer – Maximum Time: Two weeks

Requests for Deferred
Entrance Considered: Yes

Deposit to Hold Place in Class: Yes
Deposit (Resident): $100
Deposit (Non-Resident): $100
Deposit due: With response within two weeks
Applied to tuition: Yes
Deposit refundable: Yes
Refundable by: May 15, 2009 with written request

Estimated number of new entrants: 85
EDP: 5, special program: n/a

Start Month/Year: August 2009

Interview Format: Two 30-minute interviews
Regional interviews are not available.

Other Programs

PREPARATORY PROGRAMS
Postbaccalaureate Program: No
Summer Program: No

COMBINED DEGREE PROGRAMS
Baccalaureate/MD: No
MD/MPH: Yes, www.sc.edu/bulletin/SOM/admissions.html
MD/MBA: No
MD/JD: No
MD/PhD: Yes, www.sc.edu/bulletin/SOM/admissions.html

Premedical Coursework

Course	Req.	Rec.	Lab.	Hrs.
Inorganic Chemistry	•		•	8
Behavioral Sciences				
Biochemistry		•		
Biology				
Biology/Zoology	•		•	8
Calculus				
College English	•			6
College Mathematics				

Course	Req.	Rec.	Lab.	Hrs.
Computer Science				
Genetics				
Humanities				
Organic Chemistry	•		•	8
Physics		•		
Psychology				
Social Sciences				
Other				

Selection Factors: 2007 Accepted Applicants

Proportion of Accepted Applicants with Relevant Experience (Data Self-Reported to AMCAS®)		
Community Service/Volunteer		64%
Medically-Related Work		83%
Research		69%

Shaded bar represents accepted scores ranging from the 10th percentile to the 90th percentile. School Median ● National Median ●

Overall GPA	2.0	2.1	2.2	2.3	2.4	2.5	2.6	2.7	2.8	2.9	3.0	3.1	3.2	3.3	3.4	3.5	3.6	(3.7)	3.8	3.9	4.0
Science GPA	2.0	2.1	2.2	2.3	2.4	2.5	2.6	2.7	2.8	2.9	3.0	3.1	3.2	3.3	3.4	3.5	3.6	(3.7)	3.8	3.9	4.0

MCAT® required: Yes, 100% of 2007 accepted applicants took MCAT®

Verbal Reasoning	3	4	5	6	7	8	9	(10)	11	12	13	14	15
Physical Sciences	3	4	5	6	7	8	9	(10)	(11)	12	13	14	15
Biological Sciences	3	4	5	6	7	8	9	(10)	(11)	12	13	14	15
Writing Sample			J	K	L	M	N	(O)	P	(Q)	R	S	T

Acceptance & Matriculation Data for 2007–2008 First Year Class

	Resident	Non-Resident	International	Total
Applied	434	1467	39	1940
Interviewed	237	99	0	336
Deferred	2	0	0	2
Matriculants				
Early Assurance Program	n/a	n/a	n/a	n/a
Early Decision Program	1	0	0	1
Baccalaureate/MD	n/a	n/a	n/a	n/a
MD/PhD	0	0	0	0
Matriculated	67	17	0	**84**

Applications accepted from International Applicants: No

Specialty Choice

2003, 2004, 2005 Graduates, Specialty Choice
(As reported by program directors to GME Track™)

Anesthesiology	4%
Emergency Medicine	10%
Family Practice	9%
Internal Medicine	20%
Obstetrics/Gynecology	6%
Orthopaedic Surgery	1%
Pediatrics	17%
Psychiatry	9%
Radiology	1%
Surgery	7%

Matriculant Demographics: 2007–2008 First Year Class

Men: 42   **Women:** 42

Matriculants' Self-Reported Race/Ethnicity

Mexican American	0	Korean	0
Cuban	0	Vietnamese	2
Puerto Rican	0	Other Asian	2
Other Hispanic	0	Total Asian	15
Total Hispanic	0	Native American	0
Chinese	0	Black	6
Asian Indian	10	Native Hawaiian	0
Pakistani	0	White	65
Filipino	1	Unduplicated Number	
Japanese	0	of Matriculants	84

Science and Math Majors: 80%
Matriculants with:
Baccalaureate degree: 99%
Graduate degree(s): 8%

Financial Information

Source: 2006–2007 LCME I-B survey and 2007–2008 AAMC TSF questionnaire

	Residents	Non-Residents
Total Cost of Attendance	$50,495	$87,811
Tuition and Fees	$22,594	$59,910
Other (includes living expenses)	$26,956	$26,956
Health Insurance (can be waived)	$945	$945

Average 2007 Graduate Indebtedness: $125,521
% of Enrolled Students Receiving Aid: 90%

Criminal Background Check

This medical school requires a criminal background check prior to matriculation.

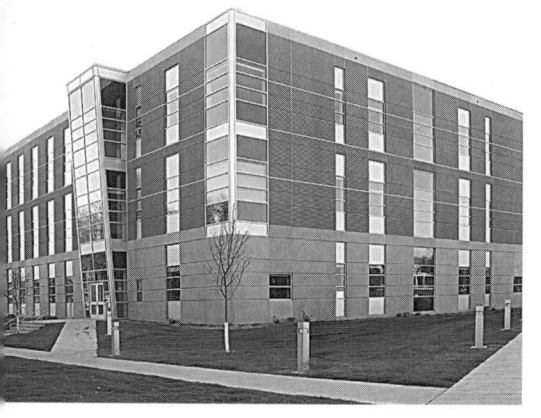

Sanford School of Medicine of the University of South Dakota

Vermillion, South Dakota

Medical School Admissions
Sanford School of Medicine
University of South Dakota
414 East Clark Street
Vermillion, South Dakota 57069
T 605 677 6886   **F** 605 677 5109

Admissions www.usd.edu/med/md/prospectivestudents/admissions.cfm
Main http://www.usd.edu/med/md
Financial http://www.usd.edu.med/md/prospectivestudents/tuition.cfm
Email usdsmsa@usd.edu

Public Institution

Dr. Rodney R. Parry, Dean

Dr. Paul C. Bunger, Dean, Medical Student Affairs

Dr. Gerald J. Yutrzenka, Director, Minority Affairs

Carol Hemmingson, Program Assistant, Financial Aid

Jill Christopherson, Program Assistant – Admissions

General Information

The School of Medicine was established in 1907 as a two-year school for the basic sciences and in 1974 became a four-year, MD degree program with the first class of graduates in 1977. The first two years are located in Vermillion, with years three and four available on campuses in Sioux Falls, Yankton or Rapid City. In 2005, the name was changed to Sanford School of Medicine of the University of South Dakota.

Mission Statement

The mission of the Sanford School of Medicine of the University of South Dakota is to provide the opportunity for South Dakota residents to receive a quality, broad-based medical education with an emphasis on family practice. The curriculum is to be established to encourage graduates to serve people living in medically underserved areas of South Dakota and to require excellence in the basic sciences and in all clinical disciplines. The School of Medicine is to provide to its students and to the people of South Dakota excellence in education, research, and service. (For complete mission statement, see Web site.)

Curricular Highlights

Community Service Requirement: Required. A community based, cultural diversity program.
Research/Thesis Requirement: Optional.

The first two years use traditional courses, problem/case-based teaching, and clinical experiences. To cap year two, students spend four weeks with a physician in a primary care setting in a South Dakota community. At the Sioux Falls and Rapid City sites, the third year is hospital-based, with clerkships in family medicine, internal medicine, pediatrics, ob/gyn, psychiatry, neurology, and surgery. Students also take clinical colloquium, ambulatory program and radiology. At the Yankton site, the third year is a clinic-based program, with students rotating through all six of the clerkships throughout the year. Year four requirements are rural family medicine, emergency medicine, surgical subspecialties and a sub-internship. Students also have 22 weeks of electives; many take 4-8 weeks outside of South Dakota. Grading is A-B-C-D-F. Students must pass USMLE Step 1 for promotion, and Step 2-CK and a School OSCE to graduate. They must also take Step 2-CS.

USMLE

Step 1: Required. Students must record a passing score for promotion.
Step 2: Clinical Skills (CS) Required. Students must only record a score.
Step 2: Clinical Knowledge (CK): Required. Students must record a passing total score to graduate.

Selection Factors

Applicants are chosen on the basis of intellect, character, and motivation. The Admissions Committee considers: academic achievement as indicated by scholastic records; recall, reading comprehension, and ability to perform within time constraints as reflected by MCAT® scores; intellectual curiosity, work ethic, and fitness for a career in medicine as viewed by the applicant's former instructors; assessments of personal factors of the applicant as determined by interviews conducted by the committee. Applicants invited to interview must meet in person with at least two committee members. Interviews are conducted at the office or clinic of the interviewer or at the Vermillion campus. The school does not discriminate on the basis of race, color, creed, national origin, ancestry, citizenship, gender, sexual orientation, religion, age, or disability. Priority for supplemental applications and interviews is given to legal residents of South Dakota, non-residents with strong ties to South Dakota, and Native Americans affiliated with federally recognized tribes in the region. The School of Medicine does not sponsor an Early Decision Program. An Alumni Student Scholars Program (ASSP) offers a limited number of provisional acceptances to South Dakota high school seniors who meet strict criteria. The School of Medicine will consider applications for transfer only into Year 2 or Year 3 and only from students who are currently in good standing at an LCME-accredited medical school. Transfer opportunities are limited, with priority given to South Dakota residents.

Financial Aid

Financial aid is administered through the office of Medical Student Affairs. Loans are available to matriculated students on the basis of demonstrated financial need.

Information about Diversity Programs

The Sanford School of Medicine is committed to training a diverse group of students to meet the needs of the diverse population of the state. Interested applicants may contact the Director of Minority Affairs for information about programs for premedical and medical students.

Campus Information

Setting

The first two years are based in Vermillion. The clinical years are based in Sioux Falls (1/2 of the class), Yankton (1/4 of the class), and Rapid City (1/4 of the class).

Enrollment

For 2007, total enrollment was: 210

Special Features

Students have significant one-on-one teaching from clinical faculty, numerous experiences in clinical and surgical procedures and many options for cultural immersion experiences.

Housing

See University Web site at *www.usd.edu.*

Satellite Campuses/Facilities

In addition to the the four primary campuses, there are many other hospitals and clinics throughout the state where students rotate for their many clinical experiences and fourth-year electives.

Application Process and Requirements 2009–2010

Primary Application Service: AMCAS
Earliest filing date: June 1, 2008
Latest filing date: November 15, 2008

Secondary Application Required?: Yes
Sent to: Screened applicants
Name: Jill Christopherson
Phone: (605) 677-6886
Email: Jill.Christopherson@usd.edu
Fee: Yes, $35
Fee waiver available: No
Earliest filing date: July 15, 2008
Latest filing date: Two weeks following invitation to submit Secondary Application

Latest MCAT® considered: September 2008
Oldest MCAT® considered: April 2006

Early Decision Program
School does not have EDP
Applicants notified: n/a
EDP available for: n/a

Regular Acceptance Notice
Earliest date: November 18, 2008
Latest date: Until class is full

Applicant's Response to Acceptance Offer – Maximum Time: Two weeks

Requests for Deferred Entrance Considered: Yes

Deposit to Hold Place in Class: Yes
Deposit (Resident): $100
Deposit (Non-Resident): $100
Deposit due: With response to acceptance offer
Applied to tuition: Yes
Deposit refundable: Yes
Refundable by: June 1, 2009

Estimated number of new entrants: 47
EDP: n/a, special program: 7

Start Month/Year: August 3, 2009

Interview Format: Open file, two individual face-to-face interviews. Regional interviews are not available.

Other Programs

PREPARATORY PROGRAMS
Postbaccalaureate Program: No
Summer Program: No

COMBINED DEGREE PROGRAMS
Baccalaureate/MD: No
MD/MPH: No
MD/MBA: No
MD/JD: No
MD/PhD: Yes, www.usd.edu/mdphd
Jill Christopherson (605) 677-6886
Jill.Christopherson@usd.edu

Premedical Coursework

Course	Req.	Rec.	Lab.	Sems.	Course	Req.	Rec.	Lab.	Sems.
Inorganic Chemistry	•		•	2	Computer Science				
Behavioral Sciences		•			Genetics		•		
Biochemistry		•			Humanities		•		
Biology					Organic Chemistry	•		•	2
Biology/Zoology	•		•	2	Physics	•		•	2
Calculus		•			Psychology				
College English		•			Social Sciences				
College Mathematics	•			2	Other				

Selection Factors: 2007 Accepted Applicants

Proportion of Accepted Applicants with Relevant Experience (Data Self-Reported to AMCAS®)		
Community Service/Volunteer		78%
Medically-Related Work		57%
Research		78%

Shaded bar represents accepted scores ranging from the 10th percentile to the 90th percentile   **School Median ●**   **National Median ●**

Overall GPA	2.0	2.1	2.2	2.3	2.4	2.5	2.6	2.7	2.8	2.9	3.0	3.1	3.2	3.3	3.4	3.5	3.6	3.7	3.8	(3.9)	4.0
Science GPA	2.0	2.1	2.2	2.3	2.4	2.5	2.6	2.7	2.8	2.9	3.0	3.1	3.2	3.3	3.4	3.5	3.6	3.7	(3.8)	3.9	4.0

MCAT® required: Yes, 95% of 2007 accepted applicants took MCAT®

Verbal Reasoning	3	4	5	6	7	8	9	(10)	11	12	13	14	15
Physical Sciences	3	4	5	6	7	8	9	(10)	(11)	12	13	14	15
Biological Sciences	3	4	5	6	7	8	9	(10)	(11)	12	13	14	15
Writing Sample			J	K	L	M	N	(O)	P	(Q)	R	S	T

Acceptance & Matriculation Data for 2007–2008 First Year Class

	Resident	Non-Resident	International	Total
Applied	139	572	33	744
Interviewed	129	40	0	169
Deferred	1	0	0	1
Matriculants				
Early Assurance Program	4	0	0	4
Early Decision Program	0	0	0	0
Baccalaureate/MD	n/a	n/a	n/a	n/a
MD/PhD	4	0	0	4
Matriculated	50	4	0	**54**

Applications accepted from International Applicants: Can be Accepted from among South Dakota residents only

Matriculant Demographics: 2007–2008 First Year Class

Men: 25   **Women:** 29

Matriculants' Self-Reported Race/Ethnicity

Mexican American	0	**Korean**	0
Cuban	0	**Vietnamese**	0
Puerto Rican	0	**Other Asian**	0
Other Hispanic	0	**Total Asian**	1
Total Hispanic	0	**Native American**	0
Chinese	1	**Black**	0
Asian Indian	0	**Native Hawaiian**	0
Pakistani	0	**White**	53
Filipino	0	**Unduplicated Number**	
Japanese	0	**of Matriculants**	54

Science and Math Majors: 89%
Matriculants with:
> **Baccalaureate degree:** 100%
> **Graduate degree(s):** 6%

Specialty Choice

2003, 2004, 2005 Graduates, Specialty Choice (As reported by program directors to GME Track™)	
Anesthesiology	9%
Emergency Medicine	9%
Family Practice	14%
Internal Medicine	10%
Obstetrics/Gynecology	9%
Orthopaedic Surgery	5%
Pediatrics	7%
Psychiatry	7%
Radiology	5%
Surgery	9%

Financial Information

Source: 2006–2007 LCME I-B survey and 2007–2008 AAMC TSF questionnaire

	Residents	Non-Residents
Total Cost of Attendance	$38,466	$58,439
Tuition and Fees	$18,436	$38,409
Other (includes living expenses)	$17,858	$17,858
Health Insurance (can be waived)	$2,172	$2,172

Average 2007 Graduate Indebtedness: $129,457
% of Enrolled Students Receiving Aid: 94%

Criminal Background Check

This medical school requires a criminal background check prior to matriculation.

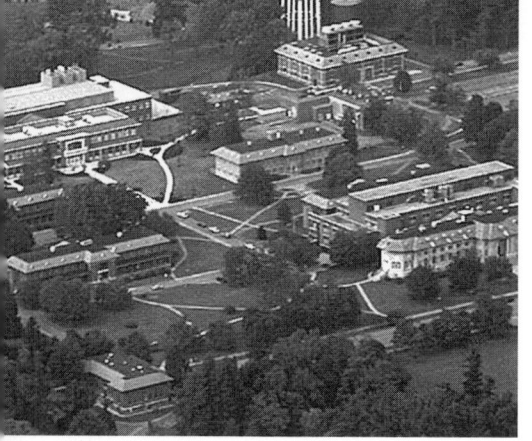

East Tennessee State University
James H. Quillen College of Medicine

Johnson City, Tennessee

Assistant Dean for Admissions and Records
East Tennessee State University
James H. Quillen College of Medicine
P.O. Box 70580, Johnson City, Tennessee 37614-1708
T 423 439 2033   F 423 439 2110

Admissions http://com.etsu.edu/default.asp?V_Site_ID=12
Main http://com.etsu.edu
Financial http://com.etsu.edu/default.asp?V_site_iD=5
Email sacom@etsu.edu

Public Institution

Dr. Philip C. Bagnell, Dean of Medicine

Edwin D. Taylor, Assistant Dean for Admissions and Records

Linda Embree, Director, Financial Services

Dr. Thomas Kwasigroch, Associate Dean for Student Affairs

General Information

Since its beginning in 1978, ETSU's Quillen College of Medicine has established itself as a national leader in its programs in primary care and especially rural medicine. ETSU students enjoy an exceptional success rate in the national residency match, and over 60 percent of graduates choose a career in primary care. ETSU's Community Partnerships Program is nationally recognized, and the Rural Primary Care Track has exceeded all expectations. Student input and participation are encouraged in all facets of their medical education. A collegial atmosphere is encouraged at all levels. The campus is unified on the grounds of the VA Medical Center pictured above. The school is located in Tennessee's fourth largest metropolitan area (population 1.2 million) and on the campus of the state's fourth largest university (enrollment 12,000 plus). It is supported by modern and convenient medical centers and clinics throughout the Tri-Cities area, as well as by hospitals and clinics located in small, rural communities such as Rogersville and Mountain City. The school enrolls one class of 60 new students in August of each year.

Mission Statement

The primary mission of Quillen College of Medicine is to educate future physicians, especially those with an interest in primary care, to practice in underserved rural communities. In addition, the college is committed to excellence in biomedical research and is dedicated to the improvement of health care in Northeast Tennessee and the surrounding Appalachian Region.

Curricular Highlights

Community Service Requirement: Optional.
Research/Thesis Requirement: Optional.

Quillen College of Medicine enjoys a dynamic and ever-changing curriculum. The curriculum includes a mix of traditional, systems-based, and case-based learning, as well as a wide range of educational experiences, patient populations, and hospitals. The highly diversified faculty considers students as colleagues. Patient contact comes early in the curriculum and continues throughout. Flexibility is allowed for students to decelerate a portion of the curriculum for elective courses, including research and advanced clinical studies. Student input is a key component in curricular change, along with the rapidly changing body of knowledge and the needs of the profession. The goals of the curriculum are to prepare students to be well-grounded in the science and art of medicine, capable practitioners of their profession, and self-directed, lifelong learners.

USMLE

Step 1: Required. Students must record a passing score for promotion.
Step 2: Clinical Skills (CS): Required. Students must record a passing total score to graduate.
Step 2: Clinical Knowledge (CK): Required. Students must record a passing total score to graduate.

Selection Factors

To be admitted, an applicant must be a U.S. or Canadian citizen or possess a U.S. permanent resident visa. Admission is based upon a competitive selection process involving those applicants who meet the minimum requirements for admission. The Admissions Committee selects students who give the promise of being not merely satisfactory medical students, but also capable, responsible physicians of high ethical standards. The Admissions Committee screens applicants on the basis of academic achievement, MCAT® scores, letters of recommendation, pertinent extracurricular research and work experiences, and evidence of non-scholastic accomplishments.

After a general screening, the Admissions Committee may request supplementary information and a personal interview with the applicant. Interviews are held only on the campus and are at the applicant's expense. Admission preferences are for residents of the state of Tennessee who are U.S. citizens, veterans of U.S. military service, and recipients of baccalaureate degrees prior to enrollment. Marginally qualified non-residents should not apply.

Financial Aid

The need for student financial assistance is not a consideration in the selection process. Scholarships, grants, and loans are available for students who demonstrate need as defined by a federal needs analysis and who meet the specific criteria set forth by the various agencies. Additional information may be obtained by writing directly to the medical school director for financial services.

Information about Diversity Programs

The College of Medicine actively seeks applicants of both sexes and members of groups underrepresented in medicine. African-American matriculants may be eligible for financial awards from the state of Tennessee. Support services are available to matriculants to assist in the timely completion of the medical curriculum. ETSU does not discriminate on the basis of race, sex, creed, national origin, age, or disability. The university is an equal opportunity/affirmative action employer.

Campus Information

Enrollment

For 2007, total enrollment was: 240

Application Process and Requirements 2009–2010

Primary Application Service: AMCAS
Earliest filing date: June 1, 2008
Latest filing date: November 15, 2008

Secondary Application Required?: Yes
Sent to: Selected applicants
URL: n/a
Fee: Yes, $50
Fee waiver available: Yes
Earliest filing date: June 1, 2008
Latest filing date: January 1, 2009

Latest MCAT® considered: September 2008
Oldest MCAT® considered: 2006

Early Decision Program
School does have EDP
Applicants notified: October 1, 2008
EDP available for: Both Residents and Non-Residents

Regular Acceptance Notice
Earliest date: October 16, 2008
Latest date: Until class is full

Applicant's Response to Acceptance Offer – Maximum Time: Two weeks

Requests for Deferred Entrance Considered: Yes

Deposit to Hold Place in Class: Yes
Deposit (Resident): $100
Deposit (Non-Resident): $100
Deposit due: With response to acceptance offer
Applied to tuition: Yes
Deposit refundable: Yes
Refundable by: May 15, 2009

Estimated number of new entrants: 60
EDP: 3, special program: n/a

Start Month/Year: August 2009

Interview Format: Two, one-hour interviews with an admissions committee member. Regional interviews are not available.

Other Programs

PREPARATORY PROGRAMS
Postbaccalaureate Program: No
Summer Program: No

COMBINED DEGREE PROGRAMS
Baccalaureate/MD: No
MD/MPH: No
MD/MBA: No
MD/JD: No
MD/PhD: No

Premedical Coursework

Course	Req.	Rec.	Lab.	Hrs.	Course	Req.	Rec.	Lab.	Hrs.
Inorganic Chemistry	•		•	8	Computer Science				
Behavioral Sciences					Genetics				
Biochemistry		•			Humanities				
Biology	•		•	8	Organic Chemistry	•		•	8
Biology/Zoology					Physics	•		•	8
Calculus					Psychology				
College English					Comm. Skills Courses	•			9
College Mathematics					Electives	•			49

Selection Factors: 2007 Accepted Applicants

Proportion of Accepted Applicants with Relevant Experience (Data Self-Reported to AMCAS®)		
Community Service/Volunteer		67%
Medically-Related Work		83%
Research		69%

Shaded bar represents accepted scores ranging from the 10th percentile to the 90th percentile   School Median ●   National Median ●

Overall GPA	2.0	2.1	2.2	2.3	2.4	2.5	2.6	2.7	2.8	2.9	3.0	3.1	3.2	3.3	3.4	3.5	3.6	(3.7)	3.8	3.9	4.0
Science GPA	2.0	2.1	2.2	2.3	2.4	2.5	2.6	2.7	2.8	2.9	3.0	3.1	3.2	3.3	3.4	3.5	3.6	(3.7)	3.8	3.9	4.0

MCAT® required: Yes, 100% of 2007 accepted applicants took MCAT®

Verbal Reasoning	3	4	5	6	7	8	9	(10)	11	12	13	14	15
Physical Sciences	3	4	5	6	7	8	9	(10)	(11)	12	13	14	15
Biological Sciences	3	4	5	6	7	8	9	(10)	(11)	12	13	14	15
Writing Sample				J	K	L	M	N	(O)	P	(Q)	R	S	T

Acceptance & Matriculation Data for 2007–2008 First Year Class

	Resident	Non-Resident	International	Total
Applied	546	869	34	1449
Interviewed	196	57	0	253
Deferred	0	1	0	1
Matriculants				
Early Assurance Program	0	0	0	0
Early Decision Program	3	0	0	3
Baccalaureate/MD	n/a	n/a	n/a	n/a
MD/PhD	n/a	n/a	n/a	n/a
Matriculated	53	7	0	**60**

Applications accepted from International Applicants: Canadian only

Specialty Choice

2003, 2004, 2005 Graduates, Specialty Choice (As reported by program directors to GME Track™)	
Anesthesiology	1%
Emergency Medicine	5%
Family Practice	16%
Internal Medicine	15%
Obstetrics/Gynecology	9%
Orthopaedic Surgery	2%
Pediatrics	12%
Psychiatry	8%
Radiology	2%
Surgery	10%

Matriculant Demographics: 2007–2008 First Year Class

Men: 27   **Women:** 33

Matriculants' Self-Reported Race/Ethnicity

Mexican American	0	Korean	0
Cuban	0	Vietnamese	0
Puerto Rican	1	Other Asian	1
Other Hispanic	0	Total Asian	6
Total Hispanic	1	Native American	0
Chinese	1	Black	3
Asian Indian	2	Native Hawaiian	0
Pakistani	0	White	52
Filipino	2	Unduplicated Number	
Japanese	0	of Matriculants	60

Science and Math Majors: 73%
Matriculants with:
Baccalaureate degree: 100%
Graduate degree(s): 3%

Financial Information

Source: 2006–2007 LCME I-B survey and 2007–2008 AAMC TSF questionnaire

	Residents	Non-Residents
Total Cost of Attendance	$39,668	$60,618
Tuition and Fees	$21,043	$41,993
Other (includes living expenses)	$17,635	$17,635
Health Insurance (can be waived)	$990	$990

Average 2007 Graduate Indebtedness: $120,894
% of Enrolled Students Receiving Aid: 90%

Criminal Background Check

This medical school does not require a criminal background check prior to matriculation.

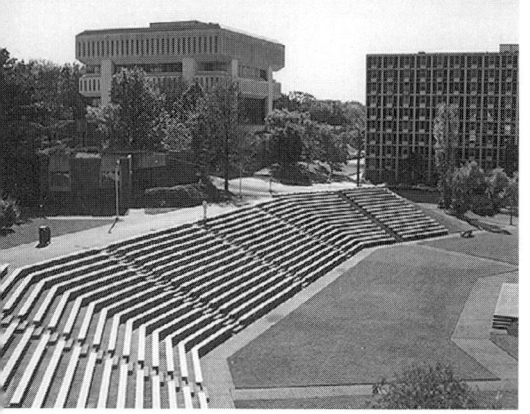

Meharry Medical College School of Medicine

Nashville, Tennessee

Director, Admissions and Recruitment
Meharry Medical College
1005 Dr. D. B. Todd Boulevard
Nashville, Tennessee 37208
T 615 327 6223   F 615 327 6228

Admissions www.mmc.edu/admissions/index.html
Main www.mmc.edu
Financial www.mmc.edu/students/student
financialaid.html
Email admissions@mmc.edu

Private Institution

Dr. Valerie Montgomery-Rice, Dean, Senior Vice President for Health Affairs

Allen D. Mosley, Director, Admissions and Recruitment

Vickie L. Johnson, Director, Student Financial Aid

Dr. Pamela Williams, Executive Vice Dean

Deborah Davis, Admissions Manager

General Information

In 1876, Meharry Medical College was founded and established as the Meharry Medical Department of Central Tennessee College by the Freedmen's Aid Society of the Methodist Episcopal Church. Meharry's inception was part of the society's continuing effort to educate freed slaves and to provide health care services for the poor and underserved. Today, the School of Medicine continues to provide excellent educational opportunities to promising students from groups underrepresented in medicine. Clinical teaching facilities include the Metropolitan Nashville General Hospital; Blanchfield Army Hospital; Veterans Affairs Tennessee Valley Health Care System, Nashville Campus and the Alvin C. York Murfreesboro Campus; Vanderbilt's Monroe Carrell Children's Hospital; and a number of affiliated hospitals and clinics. The provision of primary care, particularly in medically underserved areas, is a special emphasis, as is health disparities research.

Mission Statement

Meharry Medical College exists to improve the health and health care of minority and underserved communities by offering excellent educational and training programs in the health sciences, placing special emphasis on providing opportunities to people of color and individuals from disadvantaged backgrounds, regardless of race or ethnicity; delivering high quality health services; and conducting research that fosters the elimination of health disparities.

Curricular Highlights

Community Service Requirement: Optional.
Research/Thesis Requirement: Required. Encouraged in areas of health disparities.

The school has an integrated curriculum for the freshman year in which instruction is organized into modules that include basic, clinical, and social sciences. The modules include Principles and Practice Of Medicine, Molecular Cell Biology, Genetics, Gross Anatomy, and Embryology; also included are Integrated Neuroscience, Immunology, Principles of Infectious Disease, and Foundations in Human Disease and Treatment. The sophomore year is organized around a series of organ systems. The clinical years consist of the following blocks: family medicine, psychiatry, obstetrics and gynecology, pediatrics, internal medicine, surgery, an ambulatory rotation served in an urban or rural underserved area, and radiology, as well as guided electives.

USMLE

Step 1: Required. Students must record a passing score for promotion.
Step 2: Clinical Skills (CS): Required. Students must record a passing total score to graduate.
Step 2: Clinical Knowledge (CK): Required. Students must record a passing total score to graduate.

Selection Factors

Applicants are selected on a competitive basis with regard to cognitive and non-cognitive skills that denote probable success in medical school. Performance in the basic science prerequisite subjects and MCAT® scores form the basis for screening for the interview process in which the non-cognitive aspects of the applicant are assessed. While special empathy is held for minority and disadvantaged applicants of all origins, Meharry Medical College seeks to attract a wide demographic, cultural, and educational population to reflect the caliber of social interchange in which the eventual practice of medicine will occur. Meharry Medical College does not discriminate on the basis of race, sex, creed, national origin, age, or handicap.

Financial Aid

Financial aid awards are based on analyses of student needs and academic achievement. The limited financial aid program includes scholarships, grants-in-aid, and loans. Because of fluctuations in federal and private support for financial aid programs, the types and amounts of awards are revised and adjusted on a continuing basis. Therefore, it is necessary that applicants plan their financial program as carefully as their academic program.

Information about Diversity Programs

For over 130 years, Meharry has produced a large percentage of the minority health professionals in the United States and abroad.

Campus Information

Setting

Its campus in North Nashville places Meharry at the epicenter of Middle Tennessee's most vulnerable citizens. As such, Meharry students, faculty, staff, and residents provide services where they are most needed. Located off Nashville's historic Jefferson Street, nestled between two neighboring historically black universities and near Nashville's thriving downtown, Meharry provides students with a full-range of auxiliary services to make their experience intellectually stimulating and socially comfortable and enjoyable.

Enrollment

For 2007, total enrollment was: 422

Special Features

Through several Centers of Excellence, the college and its faculty are working to unlock the mysteries behind health disparities in a variety of areas, most notably in women's health, cancer, and HIV/AIDS.

Housing

On campus there is the Meharry Towers, a 10-story residential complex which contains 156 apartments and Dorothy Brown Hall, which houses 70 female students. The college also maintains a list of available off-campus accommodations in the Nashville area.

Application Process and Requirements 2009–2010

Primary Application Service: AMCAS
Earliest filing date: June 1, 2008
Latest filing date: December 15, 2008

Secondary Application Required?: Yes
Sent to: All applicants
Contact: Deborah Davis
(615) 327-6223, ddavis@mmc.edu
Fee: Yes, $60
Fee waiver available: Yes
Earliest filing date: August 1, 2008
Latest filing date: February 15, 2009

Latest MCAT® considered: January 2009
Oldest MCAT® considered: April 2006

Early Decision Program
School does have EDP
Applicants notified: October 1, 2008
EDP available for: Both Residents
and Non-Residents

Regular Acceptance Notice
Earliest date: November 1, 2008
Latest date: Until class is full

Applicant's Response to Acceptance
Offer – Maximum Time: Four weeks

Requests for Deferred
Entrance Considered: Yes

Deposit to Hold Place in Class: Yes
Deposit (Resident): $300
Deposit (Non-Resident): $300
Deposit due: With response to acceptance offer
Applied to tuition: Yes
Deposit refundable: Yes
Refundable by: $200 refundable prior
to April 15, 2009

Estimated number of new entrants: 70
EDP: 1, special program: 25

Start Month/Year: June 2009

Interview Format: Two 30-minute interviews.
Regional interviews are available.

Other Programs

PREPARATORY PROGRAMS
Postbaccalaureate Program: Yes,
By invitation only (25 places)
Summer Program: No

COMBINED DEGREE PROGRAMS
Baccalaureate/MD: Yes,
Allen Mosley, (615) 327-6223, amosley@mmc.edu
MD/MPH: No
MD/MBA: No
MD/JD: No
MD/PhD: Yes, Dr. Fatima Lima
(615) 327-6533, admissions@mmc.edu

Premedical Coursework

Course	Req.	Rec.	Lab.	Hrs.
Inorganic Chemistry	•		•	8
Behavioral Sciences				
Biochemistry		•		4
Biology				
Biology/Zoology	•		•	8
Calculus				
College English	•			6
College Mathematics	•			3

Course	Req.	Rec.	Lab.	Hrs.
Computer Science				
Genetics				
Humanities				
Organic Chemistry	•		•	8
Physics	•		•	8
Psychology				
Social Sciences				
Other				

Selection Factors: 2007 Accepted Applicants

Proportion of Accepted Applicants with Relevant Experience (Data Self-Reported to AMCAS®)		
Community Service/Volunteer		75%
Medically-Related Work		72%
Research		71%

Shaded bar represents accepted scores ranging from the 10th percentile to the 90th percentile. School Median ● National Median ●

Overall GPA	2.0	2.1	2.2	2.3	2.4	2.5	2.6	2.7	2.8	2.9	3.0	3.1	3.2	3.3	③.4	3.5	3.6	3.7	3.8	3.9	4.0
Science GPA	2.0	2.1	2.2	2.3	2.4	2.5	2.6	2.7	2.8	2.9	3.0	3.1	③.2	3.3	3.4	3.5	3.6	3.7	3.8	3.9	4.0

MCAT® required: Yes, 100% of 2007 accepted applicants took MCAT®

Verbal Reasoning	3	4	5	6	7	⑧	9	⑩	11	12	13	14	15
Physical Sciences	3	4	5	6	7	⑧	9	⑩	11	12	13	14	15
Biological Sciences	3	4	5	6	7	8	⑨	10	⑪	12	13	14	15
Writing Sample			J	K	L	M	N	⑩	P	⑩	R	S	T

Acceptance & Matriculation Data for 2007–2008 First Year Class

	Resident	Non-Resident	International	Total
Applied	231	4010	336	4577
Interviewed	54	341	10	405
Deferred	1	1	0	2
Matriculants				
Early Assurance Program	0	0	0	0
Early Decision Program	0	0	0	0
Baccalaureate/MD	0	0	0	0
MD/PhD	0	0	0	0
Matriculated	9	86	1	**96**

Applications accepted from International Applicants: Canadian Only

Specialty Choice

2003, 2004, 2005 Graduates, Specialty Choice (As reported by program directors to GME Track™)	
Anesthesiology	4%
Emergency Medicine	4%
Family Practice	11%
Internal Medicine	16%
Obstetrics/Gynecology	11%
Orthopaedic Surgery	2%
Pediatrics	10%
Psychiatry	6%
Radiology	2%
Surgery	7%

Matriculant Demographics: 2007–2008 First Year Class

Men: 31   **Women:** 65

Matriculants' Self-Reported Race/Ethnicity

Mexican American	0	**Korean**	1
Cuban	2	**Vietnamese**	0
Puerto Rican	1	**Other Asian**	1
Other Hispanic	4	**Total Asian**	6
Total Hispanic	7	**Native American**	1
Chinese	1	**Black**	80
Asian Indian	2	**Native Hawaiian**	0
Pakistani	0	**White**	9
Filipino	2	**Unduplicated Number**	
Japanese	0	**of Matriculants**	96

Science and Math Majors: 77%

Matriculants with:
    Baccalaureate degree: 100%
    Graduate degree(s): 17%

Financial Information

Source: 2006–2007 LCME I-B survey
and 2007–2008 AAMC TSF questionnaire

	Residents	Non-Residents
Total Cost of Attendance	$55,345	$55,345
Tuition and Fees	$32,336	$32,336
Other (includes living expenses)	$20,411	$20,411
Health Insurance (can be waived)	$2,598	$2,598

Average 2007 Graduate Indebtedness: $136,429
% of Enrolled Students Receiving Aid: 93%

Criminal Background Check

This medical school does not require a criminal background check prior to matriculation.

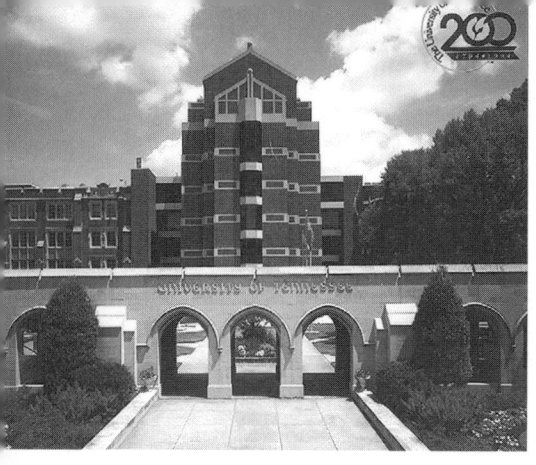

University of Tennessee Health Science Center College of Medicine
Memphis, Tennessee

University of Tennessee,
Health Science Center College of Medicine
910 Madison Avenue, Suite 500
Memphis, Tennessee 38163
T 901 448 5559 F 901 448 1740

Admissions www.utmem.edu/Medicine/Admissions
Main www.utmem.edu/Medicine
Financial www.utmem.edu/finaid
Email nstrother@utmem.edu

Public Institution

Dr. Steve J. Schwab, Executive Dean

E. Nelson Strother Jr., Assistant Dean for Admissions and Student Affairs

Dr. Gerald J. Presbury, Representative to Minority Affairs Section

Matthew Sanchez, Assistant Vice Chancellor, Student Affairs

General Information

The UTHSC College of Medicine traces its origin to 1851 as the Medical Department of the University of Nashville. Today, the college utilizes over 20 facilities statewide for its training programs, including the Boston-Baskin Cancer Group, Campbell Orthopaedic Clinic, LeBonheur Children's Medical Center, Methodist University Hospital, Regional Medical Center, Semmes-Murphy Clinic, St. Jude Children's Research Hospital, UT Medical Group, VA Medical Center, Baptist Hospital-Memphis, St. Francis Hospital, UT Knoxville Medical Center, Erlanger Medical Center-Chattanooga, Baptist Hospital-Nashville, and Family Practice Center-Jackson.

Mission Statement

The Faculty of the College of Medicine is committed to educating physicians whose primary responsibilities will be evaluating, treating and preventing disease. The educational program is designed to prepare students to become knowledgeable, skillful, and compassionate physicians. Students are imbued with both the ideal that the study of medicine is a lifelong process and the sense of a physician's deep commitment to high moral and ethical standards regarding patients, colleagues, and society.

Curricular Highlights

Community Service Requirement: Required. Community service project.
Research/Thesis Requirement: Optional.

Year 1 of the curriculum begins in August with Gross Anatomy; Prevention, Community and Culture (PCC); Doctoring: Recognizing Signs and Symptoms (DRS); Molecular Basis of Disease; and Physiology, and runs through March. In April and May of year 1, some concepts from the Pathophysiology, Microbiology, Pathology, and Pharmacology courses are presented. Year 2 begins in August with Pharmacology, Microbiology, Pathology, Pathophysiology, Neurosciences, PCC and DRS. Students are introduced to clinical medicine in their first semester through PCC and DRS. These courses expose students to the practice of medicine by placing them in a community physician's office and emphasizing professionalism. The third-year clerkships focus on patient problem-solving with an increasing level of responsibility. The fourth year is composed of six 4-week clerkships and four 4-week electives.

USMLE

Step 1: Required. Students must record a passing score for promotion.
Step 2: Clinical Skills (CS): Required. Students must record a passing total score to graduate.
Step 2: Clinical Knowledge (CK): Required. Students must record a passing total score to graduate.

Selection Factors

The criteria the Committee on Admissions uses in the selection process are the academic record, MCAT scores, preprofessional evaluations, and personal interviews. Personal interviews by members of the committee provide candidates with an opportunity to review their curricular and extracurricular activities. More important, the interviewers gain insight into the character of the applicants, as well as how they have formulated their plans for the study and practice of medicine. Applicants must be citizens or permanent residents of the U.S. at the time of application. Applications are considered from Tennessee and its contiguous states (Mississippi, Arkansas, Missouri, Kentucky, Virginia, North Carolina, Georgia, and Alabama). Children of UT alumni may also be considered, regardless of their state of residence. Since priority is given to qualified Tennesseans, non-residents must possess superior qualifications to be considered by the committee. Only 10 percent of the entering class may be non-residents. Upon initial review of the AMCAS application, a supplemental application will be sent to applicants considered competitive for further review. Advanced standing applications will be considered for year 3 only. Applicants for transfer must be residents of Tennessee, be attending LCME-accredited schools, have successfully completed the basic science curriculum, and have passed USMLE Step 1. Applicants must also provide evidence of circumstances necessitating a transfer. Deadline for transfer applications is April 1.

Financial Aid

Aid consists of loans, scholarships, and work-study. Merit-based scholarships are available to highly qualified students.

Information about Diversity Programs

The College of Medicine actively encourages applications from members of groups underrepresented in medicine. The Committee on Admissions evaluates both academic and non-academic factors in the selection process, with consideration given to the unique backgrounds and challenges of these applicants. Among American medical schools, the college is a national leader in the admission, matriculation, and graduation of students from groups underrepresented in medicine.

Campus Information

Setting

UTHSC is located near vibrant downtown Memphis, home of NBA basketball, AAA baseball, the Symphony, Broadway plays, legendary barbecue, and Beale Street blues.

Enrollment

For 2007, total enrollment was: 605

Special Features

Please go to *www.utmem.edu/Medicine*.

Housing

UTHSC has one dormitory. An abundance of affordable off-campus housing is available in the Memphis area.

Satellite Campuses/Facilities

Rotations are also available at the UT College of Medicine campuses in Knoxville and Chattanooga.

Application Process and Requirements 2009–2010

Primary Application Service: AMCAS
Earliest filing date: June 1, 2008
Latest filing date: November 15, 2008

Secondary Application Required?: Yes
Sent to: Screened applicants
Contact: Nelson Strother
(901) 448-5561
nstrother@utmem.edu
Fee: Yes, $50
Fee waiver available: Yes
Earliest filing date: July 2008
Latest filing date: February 2009

Latest MCAT® considered: September 2008
Oldest MCAT® considered: 2004

Early Decision Program
School does not have EDP
Applicants notified: n/a
EDP available for: n/a

Regular Acceptance Notice
Earliest date: October 15, 2008
Latest date: Varies

Applicant's Response to Acceptance
Offer – Maximum Time: Two weeks

Requests for Deferred
Entrance Considered: Yes

Deposit to Hold Place in Class: No
Deposit (Resident): n/a
Deposit (Non-Resident): n/a
Deposit due: n/a
Applied to tuition: n/a
Deposit refundable: n/a
Refundable by: n/a

Estimated number of new entrants: 150
EDP: 0, special program: n/a

Start Month/Year: August 2009

Interview Format: Two individual interviews with admissions committee members. May have 1 in Memphis and 1 regional.

Other Programs

PREPARATORY PROGRAMS
Postbaccalaureate Program: No
Summer Program: Yes
www.utmem.edu/HCP

COMBINED DEGREE PROGRAMS
Baccalaureate/MD: No
MD/MPH: No
MD/MBA: No
MD/JD: No
MD/PhD: Yes,
Dr. Don Thomason, (901) 448-7224
thomason@physio1.utmem.edu

Premedical Coursework

Course	Req.	Rec.	Lab.	Hrs.
Inorganic Chemistry	•		•	8
Behavioral Sciences				
Biochemistry				
Biology	•		•	8
Biology/Zoology				
Calculus				
College English	•			6
College Mathematics				

Course	Req.	Rec.	Lab.	Hrs.
Computer Science				
Genetics				
Humanities				
Organic Chemistry	•		•	8
Physics	•		•	8
Psychology				
Social Sciences				
Other				

Selection Factors: 2007 Accepted Applicants

Proportion of Accepted Applicants with Relevant Experience (Data Self-Reported to AMCAS")		
Community Service/Volunteer	68%
Medically-Related Work	80%
Research	75%

Shaded bar represents accepted scores ranging from the 10th percentile to the 90th percentile. School Median ● National Median ●

Overall GPA	2.0	2.1	2.2	2.3	2.4	2.5	2.6	2.7	2.8	2.9	3.0	3.1	3.2	3.3	3.4	3.5	3.6	(3.7)	3.8	3.9	4.0
Science GPA	2.0	2.1	2.2	2.3	2.4	2.5	2.6	2.7	2.8	2.9	3.0	3.1	3.2	3.3	3.4	3.5	3.6	(3.7)	3.8	3.9	4.0

MCAT® required: Yes, 100% of 2007 accepted applicants took MCAT®

Verbal Reasoning	3	4	5	6	7	8	9	(10)	11	12	13	14	15
Physical Sciences	3	4	5	6	7	8	9	(10)	(11)	12	13	14	15
Biological Sciences	3	4	5	6	7	8	9	(10)	(11)	12	13	14	15
Writing Sample			J	K	L	M	N	O	(P)	(Q)	R	S	T

Acceptance & Matriculation Data for 2007–2008 First Year Class

	Resident	Non-Resident	International	Total
Applied	638	776	10	1424
Interviewed	429	59	0	488
Deferred	7	1	0	8
Matriculants				
Early Assurance Program	n/a	n/a	n/a	n/a
Early Decision Program	0	0	0	0
Baccalaureate/MD	n/a	n/a	n/a	n/a
MD/PhD	0	0	0	0
Matriculated	143	7	0	**150**

Applications accepted from International Applicants: No

Specialty Choice

2003, 2004, 2005 Graduates, Specialty Choice (As reported by program directors to GME Track™)	
Anesthesiology	7%
Emergency Medicine	4%
Family Practice	6%
Internal Medicine	15%
Obstetrics/Gynecology	7%
Orthopaedic Surgery	4%
Pediatrics	10%
Psychiatry	5%
Radiology	7%
Surgery	10%

Matriculant Demographics: 2007–2008 First Year Class

Men: 88   **Women:** 62

Matriculants' Self-Reported Race/Ethnicity

Mexican American	0	Korean	1
Cuban	0	Vietnamese	2
Puerto Rican	1	Other Asian	4
Other Hispanic	2	Total Asian	18
Total Hispanic	2	Native American	1
Chinese	4	Black	19
Asian Indian	7	Native Hawaiian	0
Pakistani	0	White	113
Filipino	0	**Unduplicated Number**	
Japanese	0	**of Matriculants**	150

Science and Math Majors: 71%
Matriculants with:
   Baccalaureate degree: 100%
   Graduate degree(s): 9%

Financial Information

Source: 2006–2007 LCME I-B survey and 2007–2008 AAMC TSF questionnaire

	Residents	Non-Residents
Total Cost of Attendance	$47,245	$65,157
Tuition and Fees	$19,385	$37,297
Other (includes living expenses)	$26,132	$26,132
Health Insurance (can be waived)	$1,728	$1,728

Average 2007 Graduate Indebtedness: $116,936
% of Enrolled Students Receiving Aid: 90%

Criminal Background Check

This medical school requires a criminal background check prior to matriculation.

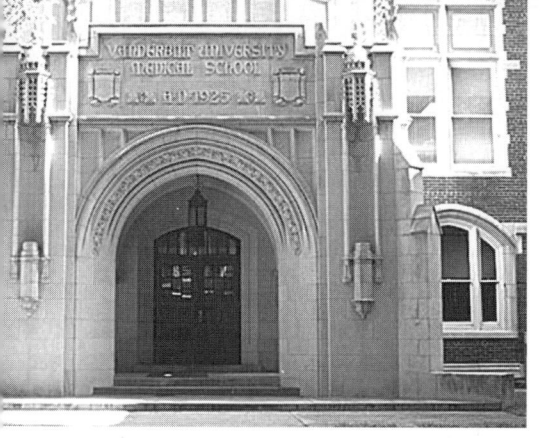

Vanderbilt University School of Medicine

Nashville, Tennessee

Office of Admissions
215 Light Hall
Vanderbilt University School of Medicine
Nashville, Tennessee 37232-0685
T 615 322 2145   **F** 615 343 8397

Admissions www.mc.vanderbilt.edu/medschool/admissions
Main www.mc.vanderbilt.edu/medschool
Financial www.mc.vanderbilt.edu/medschool/
finaid/finaid1.php
Email pat.sagen@vanderbilt.edu

Private Institution

Dr. Steven G. Gabbe, Dean

Dr. John A. Zic, Associate Dean for Admissions

*Dr. George C. Hill, Associate Dean
for Diversity in Medical Education*

*Vicky L. Cagle, Director of Student
Financial Services*

Dr. Patricia Sagen, Director of Admissions

General Information

Vanderbilt University School of Medicine is a private medical school located on the campus of Vanderbilt University. The Vanderbilt University Medical Center and affiliated hospitals provide a total of over 5,000 beds for diversified, comprehensive clinical experience. These hospitals share common goals of education, research, patient care, and community service.

Mission Statement

VUSM seeks to matriculate a diverse group of academically exceptional students whose attributes and accomplishments suggest that they will be future leaders and/or scholars in medicine to begin the process of lifelong learning in the science and practice of medicine.

Curricular Highlights

Community Service Requirement: Optional.
Research/Thesis Requirement: Optional.

Medical education at Vanderbilt is oriented toward promoting the intellectual development of students and equipping them with the disciplined approach, knowledge, and skills required of both a physician and scientist. The curriculum provides the student with a fundamental knowledge of basic medical principles, but flexibility is stressed. Changes in curriculum content and teaching methods continually evolve from Vanderbilt's focus upon new ways to assist students in their preparation for a lifetime of learning. The curriculum offers a productive blend of required and elective courses throughout all four years of the program. The Emphasis Program whose primary goal is to develop leadership potential is scheduled for the first two years of the curriculum, including eight weeks during the intervening summer. Areas of focus include: laboratory-based research, patient-oriented research, healthcare research, community health initiatives, international medicine, biomedical informatics, medical education, law and medicine, and medical humanities.

USMLE

Step 1: Optional.
Step 2: Clinical Skills (CS): Optional.
Step 2: Clinical Knowledge (CK): Optional.

Selection Factors

Applicants are invited without regard to race, sex, religion, national origin, sexual orientation, or state of residence. Applicants must possess sufficient intellectual ability, emotional stability, and sensory and motor functions to meet the academic requirements of the school of medicine without fundamental alteration in the nature of this program. Applications are reviewed in two stages. The initial review is made from material provided through AMCAS. Competitive strength of credentials reflecting preparation for medical studies, motivation, personal qualities, and educational background are evaluated by the Admissions Committee and determine the recipients of secondary applications and invitations to interview. There is a holistic review of academic performance and non-academic factors. Interviews are held at Vanderbilt. AP credit, CLEP credit, and PASS/FAIL credit are not accepted for any required courses. Vanderbilt undergraduates with at least a 3.5 GPA are eligible to apply for the binding Early Acceptance Program during the spring of the sophomore year. Those accepted are encouraged to broaden their curricular experiences. Acceptance for transfer is limited to third year with places made available by attrition only. Those students who have completed the second year in good standing at an LCME-accredited U.S. or Canadian medical school are eligible to apply. The deadline for applying is March 1.

Financial Aid

Every effort is made to see that each student who applies has sufficient funds to meet the total estimated cost of attendance by utilizing a variety of loans and scholarships. Thirty-two percent of the class receives full tuition scholarships on merit or through the MST program.

Information about Diversity Programs

Matriculation of a diverse student body is a central goal of VUSM. Diversity is defined in the broadest sense (gender, race, ethnicity, sexual preference, socio-economic background, geographic origin).

Campus Information

Setting

The medical school is part of a 323-acre campus that also serves as a national arboretum. Located southwest of downtown Nashville, the campus is a park-like setting on which are found the undergraduate and all professional schools.

Enrollment

For 2007, total enrollment was: 434

Special Features

The Monroe Carell, Jr. Children's Hospital at Vanderbilt is a state-of-the-art pediatric facility. VUSM has the only NIH-sponsored Comprehensive Cancer in the mid-South. The new Center for Experiential Learning and Assessment describes state of the art simulation technologies and standardized patient learning environments to master clinical skills. The new anatomy lab features plasma screen computers to enhance learning.

Housing

There is limited on-campus housing. The university does maintain a list of affordable apartments within a 10-mile radius. Rents average $500-$900 per month.

Satellite Campuses/Facilities

Student rotations are divided between Vanderbilt Hospital and the Nashville VA Hospital. Clinical opportunities also exist at Meharry Medical School as part of a formal collaboration.

Application Process and Requirements 2009–2010

Primary Application Service: AMCAS

Earliest filing date: June 1, 2008
Latest filing date: November 15, 2008

Secondary Application Required?: Yes
Sent to: Screened applicants invited to interview
URL: www.mc.vanderbilt.edu/medschool/admissions
Fee: Yes, $50
Fee waiver available: Yes
Earliest filing date: August 1, 2008
Latest filing date: December 31, 2008

Latest MCAT® considered: September 2008
Oldest MCAT® considered: 2005

Early Decision Program
School does have EDP
Applicants notified: October 1, 2008
EDP available for: Both Residents
and Non-Residents

Regular Acceptance Notice
Earliest date: October 15, 2008
Latest date: Until class is full

Applicant's Response to Acceptance
Offer – Maximum Time: Two weeks

Requests for Deferred
Entrance Considered: Yes

Deposit to Hold Place in Class: No
Deposit (Resident): n/a
Deposit (Non-Resident): n/a
Deposit due: n/a
Applied to tuition: n/a
Deposit refundable: n/a
Refundable by: n/a

Estimated number of new entrants: 104
EDP: 2, special program: 6

Start Month/Year: August 2009

Interview Format: Individual interview
with faculty member. Regional interviews
are not available.

Other Programs

PREPARATORY PROGRAMS
Postbaccalaureate Program: No
Summer Program: No

COMBINED DEGREE PROGRAMS
Baccalaureate/MD: No
MD/MPH: Yes, Wayne A. Ray, M.D.
(615) 322-2017, wayne.ray@vanderbilt.edu
MD/MBA: Yes, Nancy L. Hyer
(615) 322-2530, nancy.l.hyer.2@vanderbilt.edu
MD/JD: Yes, Nancy J. King
(615) 343-9836, nancy.king@vanderbilt.edu
MD/PhD: Yes, Michelle S. Grundy, Ph.D.
(615) 343-2573, michelle.grundy@vanderbilt.edu
Additional Program: Yes, MD/MDiv.,
Rev. Angela D. Davis, (615) 343-3963,
angela.d.davis@vanderbilt.edu

Premedical Coursework

Course	Req.	Rec.	Lab.	Hrs.
Inorganic Chemistry	•		•	8
Behavioral Sciences				
Biochemistry				
Biology				
Biology/Zoology	•		•	8
Calculus				
College English	•			6
College Mathematics				

Course	Req.	Rec.	Lab.	Hrs.
Computer Science				
Genetics				
Humanities				
Organic Chemistry	•		•	8
Physics	•		•	8
Psychology				
Social Sciences				
Other				

Selection Factors: 2007 Accepted Applicants

Proportion of Accepted Applicants with Relevant Experience (Data Self-Reported to AMCAS®)		
Community Service/Volunteer		72%
Medically-Related Work		88%
Research		96%

Shaded bar represents accepted scores ranging from the 10th percentile to the 90th percentile. School Median ● National Median ●

Overall GPA	2.0	2.1	2.2	2.3	2.4	2.5	2.6	2.7	2.8	2.9	3.0	3.1	3.2	3.3	3.4	3.5	3.6	3.7	(3.8)	3.9	4.0
Science GPA	2.0	2.1	2.2	2.3	2.4	2.5	2.6	2.7	2.8	2.9	3.0	3.1	3.2	3.3	3.4	3.5	3.6	3.7	(3.8)	3.9	4.0

MCAT® required: Yes, 100% of 2007 accepted applicants took MCAT®

Verbal Reasoning	3	4	5	6	7	8	9	(10)	(11)	12	13	14	15
Physical Sciences	3	4	5	6	7	8	9	10	(11)	(12)	13	14	15
Biological Sciences	3	4	5	6	7	8	9	10	(11)	(12)	13	14	15
Writing Sample				J	K	L	M	N	O	P	(Q)	R	S	T

Acceptance & Matriculation Data for 2007–2008 First Year Class

	Resident	Non-Resident	International	Total
Applied	342	4179	266	4787
Interviewed	54	844	68	966
Deferred	1	1	0	2
Matriculants				
Early Assurance Program	3	4	0	7
Early Decision Program	0	0	0	0
Baccalaureate/MD	n/a	n/a	n/a	n/a
MD/PhD	0	9	1	10
Matriculated	20	76	9	**105**

Applications accepted from International Applicants: Yes

Specialty Choice

2003, 2004, 2005 Graduates, Specialty Choice (As reported by program directors to GME Track™)	
Anesthesiology	2%
Emergency Medicine	6%
Family Practice	1%
Internal Medicine	22%
Obstetrics/Gynecology	3%
Orthopaedic Surgery	5%
Pediatrics	12%
Psychiatry	6%
Radiology	6%
Surgery	8%

Matriculant Demographics: 2007–2008 First Year Class

Men: 55   **Women:** 50

Matriculants' Self-Reported Race/Ethnicity

Mexican American	1	Korean	1
Cuban	1	Vietnamese	1
Puerto Rican	0	Other Asian	3
Other Hispanic	2	Total Asian	24
Total Hispanic	4	Native American	1
Chinese	7	Black	7
Asian Indian	10	Native Hawaiian	0
Pakistani	1	White	65
Filipino	0	Unduplicated Number	
Japanese	2	of Matriculants	105

Science and Math Majors: 79%
Matriculants with:
    Baccalaureate degree: 99%
    Graduate degree(s): 5%

Financial Information

Source: 2006–2007 LCME I-B survey
and 2007–2008 AAMC TSF questionnaire

	Residents	Non-Residents
Total Cost of Attendance	$56,090	$56,090
Tuition and Fees	$37,573	$37,573
Other (includes living expenses)	$16,579	$16,579
Health Insurance (can be waived)	$1,938	$1,938

Average 2007 Graduate Indebtedness: $111,313
% of Enrolled Students Receiving Aid: 84%

Criminal Background Check

This medical school requires a criminal background check
prior to matriculation.

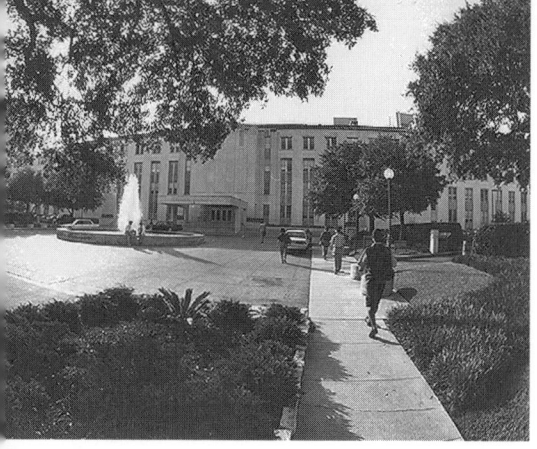

Baylor College of Medicine
Houston, Texas

Office of Admissions
Baylor College of Medicine
One Baylor Plaza
Houston, Texas 77030
T 713 798 4842 **F** 713 798 5563

Admissions www.bcm.edu/admissions
Main www.bcm.edu
Financial www.bcm.edu/osa/osa-financial.html
Email admissions@bcm.edu

Private Institution

Dr. Peter G. Traber, President

Dr. Lloyd H. Michael, Senior Associate Dean, Admissions

Dr. Stephen B. Greenberg, Senior Vice President and Dean of Education

Dr. Graciela B. Villarreal, Assistant Dean

General Information

Baylor College of Medicine (BCM) is a private, nonsectarian institution governed by an independent Board of Trustees composed of community leaders. BCM is the academic center around which the 1000-acre Texas Medical Center was developed. The Baylor faculty currently is composed of 1,700 full-time members and 1244 voluntary members. Facilities include teaching and research buildings and seven affiliated teaching hospitals (including private, county, and Veterans Affairs hospitals).

Mission Statement

The mission of BCM is to promote health for all people through education, research, and public service. The college pursues this mission by sustaining excellence in educating medical and graduate students, primary care and specialty physicians, biomedical scientists and allied health professionals; by advancing basic and clinical biomedical research; by fostering public awareness of health and the prevention of disease; and by promoting patient care of the highest standard.

Curricular Highlights

Community Service Requirement: Required.
Research/Thesis Requirement: Required.

The educational program is structured to prepare graduates to pursue careers as primary care physicians, specialists, research scientists, academic physicians, or physicians involved in public health policy. The integration of basic and clinical sciences includes direct patient-care experiences early in the first year and a focus on core basic science topics prior to graduation. This integration also includes special courses featuring integrated problem-solving and clinical skills

training that encourages application of content learned in lectures and labs. The BCM curriculum is unique in that the basic sciences are taught in slightly less than one and a half years, giving students more time to take advantage of a wealth of clinical experiences. During the clinical curriculum, students have flexibility in organizing their schedules to complete 56 weeks of required clinical clerkships, four weeks of selectives, and 20 weeks of elective experiences. All students will be expected to develop and execute with faculty mentorship a scholarly project of their choice during their medical education. Interested students are given the opportunity to do research or to apply for a combined M.D./Ph.D. program. Students with an interest in ethics, research, international health, or geriatrics may participate in tracks designed for the specific topic. There are several joint degree programs: a 5 year M.D./M.B.A. program with a health care focus with the Jones School of Management at Rice University; a six year M.D./J.D. program with the University of Houston Law Center and a 5 year M.D./M.P.H. with the University of Texas School of Public Health.

USMLE
Step 1: Required. Students must only record a score.
Step 2: Clinical Skills (CS): Required. Students must only record a score.
Step 2: Clinical Knowledge (CK): Required. Students must only record a score.

Selection Factors

All applicants offered places in the class are interviewed at BCM. All available information is utilized in the selection process. Attention is paid to course selections and the academic challenge imposed by the student's curriculum. Intellectual ability and academic achievement alone are not sufficient to support the development of the ideal physician. To work effectively in a profession dependent upon interpersonal relationships, physicians should possess those traits of personality and character which permit them to communicate effectively with warmth and compassion. Written requests for deferred

matriculation from accepted students will be reviewed on an individual basis. BCM does not discriminate on the basis of race, sex, marital status, creed, national origin, age, or disability.

Financial Aid

Financial need is not a factor in the selection of students. Aid funds are provided by private donors, the Board of Trustees, and various state and federal loan, scholarship, and work-study programs. Financial aid information and application materials are sent to all accepted applicants, and a financial aid officer is available for consultation with students and parents.

Information about Diversity Programs

BCM encourages applications from members of groups underrepresented in medicine. Students from these groups comprise a substantial portion of the student body; they also serve as Admissions Committee members. For additional information, contact Dr. Graciela Villarreal, Assistant Dean for Admissions, at 713-798-4842, or Dr. James L. Phillips, Senior Associate Dean.

Campus Information

Setting

BCM is located at the center of the Texas Medical Center, next door to Hermann Park, the zoo, and a public golf course. To the west is Rice University and the Village Shopping Center. The Museum District is to the north and offers more than 16 art organizations.

Enrollment

For 2007, total enrollment was: 681

Housing

There are many homes, apartments, townhouses, and condominiums for lease or purchase near the Texas Medical Center. Many of these living options are close to a light rail system that provides access to TMC at little or no cost to BCM students.

Application Process and Requirements 2009–2010

Primary Application Service: AMCAS
Earliest filing date: June 1, 2008
Latest filing date: November 1, 2008

Secondary Application Required?: Yes
Sent to: All applicants
URL: www.bcm.edu/admissions/?PMID=1776
Fee: Yes, $80
Fee waiver available: Yes
Earliest filing date: July 1, 2008
Latest filing date: December 1, 2008

Latest MCAT® considered: September 2008
Oldest MCAT® considered: 2004

Early Decision Program
School does have EDP
Applicants notified: October 1, 2008
EDP available for: Both Residents and Non-Residents

Regular Acceptance Notice
Earliest date: October 15, 2008
Latest date: Until class is full

Applicant's Response to Acceptance Offer – Maximum Time: n/a

Requests for Deferred Entrance Considered: Yes

Deposit to Hold Place in Class: Yes
Deposit (Resident): $300
Deposit (Non-Resident): $300
Deposit due: May 15, 2009
Applied to tuition: Yes
Deposit refundable: Yes
Refundable by: April 15, 2009

Estimated number of new entrants: 176
EDP: 5, special program: 40

Start Month/Year: July 2009

Interview Format: Two 30-minute one-on-one interviews. Regional interviews are not available.

Other Programs

PREPARATORY PROGRAMS
Postbaccalaureate Program: No
Summer Program: No
Additional Programs: Yes, www.bcm.edu/smart www.debakeydepartmentofsurgery.org/home/content.cfm?menu_id=17

COMBINED DEGREE PROGRAMS
Baccalaureate/MD: Yes, www.bcm.edu/medschool/baccmd.htm
MD/MPH: Yes, admissions@bcm.tmc.edu
MD/MBA: Yes, admissions@bcm.tmc.edu, www.bcm.edu/education/dual_programs.cfm#MD_MBA
MD/JD: Yes, admissions@bcm.tmc.edu
MD/PhD: Yes, www.bcm.edu/mstp

Premedical Coursework

Course	Req.	Rec.	Lab.	Sems.	Course	Req.	Rec.	Lab.	Sems.
Inorganic Chemistry	•		•	2	Computer Science				
Behavioral Sciences					Genetics				
Biochemistry					Humanities				
Biology	•		•	2	Organic Chemistry	•		•	2
Biology/Zoology					Physics				
Calculus					Psychology				
College English	•			2	Social Sciences				
College Mathematics					Other				

Selection Factors: 2007 Accepted Applicants

Proportion of Accepted Applicants with Relevant Experience (Data Self-Reported to AMCAS®)		
Community Service/Volunteer		68%
Medically-Related Work		83%
Research		88%

Shaded bar represents accepted scores ranging from the 10th percentile to the 90th percentile. School Median ● National Median ●

	2.0	2.1	2.2	2.3	2.4	2.5	2.6	2.7	2.8	2.9	3.0	3.1	3.2	3.3	3.4	3.5	3.6	3.7	3.8	3.9	4.0
Overall GPA																	3.6	3.7	3.8	(3.9)	4.0
Science GPA															3.5	3.6	3.7	3.8	(3.9)	4.0

MCAT® required: Yes, 96% of 2007 accepted applicants took MCAT®

	3	4	5	6	7	8	9	10	11	12	13	14	15
Verbal Reasoning	3	4	5	6	7	8	9	(10)	(11)	12	13	14	15
Physical Sciences	3	4	5	6	7	8	9	10	(11)	(12)	13	14	15
Biological Sciences	3	4	5	6	7	8	9	10	(11)	(12)	13	14	15
Writing Sample			J	K	L	M	N	O	P	(Q)	R	S	T

Acceptance & Matriculation Data for 2007–2008 First Year Class

	Resident	Non-Resident	International	Total
Applied	1534	3168	220	4922
Interviewed	394	345	12	751
Deferred	5	4	0	9
Matriculants				
Early Assurance Program	n/a	n/a	n/a	n/a
Early Decision Program	2	1	0	3
Baccalaureate/MD	38	4	1	43
MD/PhD	4	4	1	9
Matriculated	130	40	2	**172**

Applications accepted from International Applicants: Yes

Specialty Choice

2003, 2004, 2005 Graduates, Specialty Choice (As reported by program directors to GME Track™)	
Anesthesiology	8%
Emergency Medicine	2%
Family Practice	4%
Internal Medicine	18%
Obstetrics/Gynecology	3%
Orthopaedic Surgery	4%
Pediatrics	15%
Psychiatry	4%
Radiology	6%
Surgery	6%

Matriculant Demographics: 2007–2008 First Year Class

Men: 82   **Women:** 90

Matriculants' Self-Reported Race/Ethnicity

Mexican American	24	Korean	1
Cuban	2	Vietnamese	8
Puerto Rican	1	Other Asian	6
Other Hispanic	7	Total Asian	50
Total Hispanic	31	Native American	4
Chinese	16	Black	4
Asian Indian	17	Native Hawaiian	0
Pakistani	2	White	109
Filipino	3	Unduplicated Number	
Japanese	0	of Matriculants	172

Science and Math Majors: 75%
Matriculants with:
   Baccalaureate degree: 100%
   Graduate degree(s): 5%

Financial Information

Source: 2006–2007 LCME I-B survey and 2007–2008 AAMC TSF questionnaire

	Residents	Non-Residents
Total Cost of Attendance	$33,704	$46,804
Tuition and Fees	$12,782	$25,882
Other (includes living expenses)	$18,590	$18,590
Health Insurance (can be waived)	$2,332	$2,332

Average 2007 Graduate Indebtedness: $80,645
% of Enrolled Students Receiving Aid: 69%

Criminal Background Check

This medical school requires a criminal background check prior to matriculation.

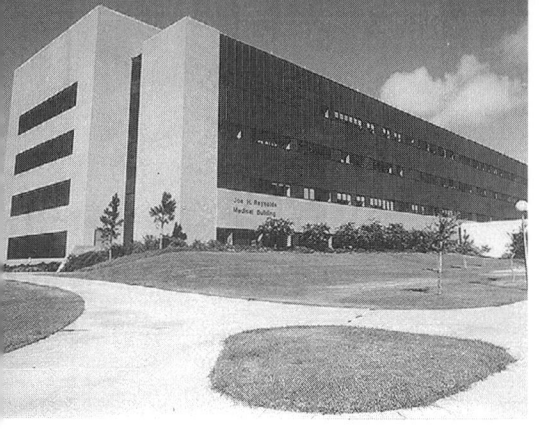

Texas A&M University System Health Science Center College of Medicine

College Station, Texas

Office of Student Affairs and Admissions
The Texas A&M Health Science Center
College of Medicine, 159 Joe Reynolds Medical Bldg.
College Station, Texas 77843-1114
T 979 845 7743 **F** 979 845 5533

Admissions http://medicine.tamhsc.edu/
admissions/index.htm
Main http://medicine.tamhsc.edu/
Financial http://tamhsc.edu/academics/finaid
Email admissions@medicine.tamhsc.edu

Public Institution

Dr. Christopher C. Colenda, Dean

*Filomeno G. Maldonado,
Assistant Dean for Admissions*

*Wanda J. Watson, Director of Recruitment
and Special Programs*

*Dr. Kathleen F. Fallon, Associate Dean
for Student Affairs and Admissions*

*Dr. Gary McCord, Assistant Dean
for Student Affairs*

General Information

Established in 1973, the College of Medicine is part of The Texas A&M Health Science Center, a public health sciences university. The college is affiliated with Scott & White Hospital and Clinic and the Olin E. Teague Veterans Center of the Central Texas Health Care System in Temple Texas. Combined, these clinical facilities provide 1,976 teaching beds and treat approximately 2,389,000 outpatients and another 45,500 inpatients each year.

Mission Statement

The College of Medicine is dedicated to the education of humane and highly skilled physicians and to the development of knowledge in the biomedical and clinical sciences. In order to improve the quality and efficacy of medical care through its programs of medical education and research, the College of Medicine maintains a personalized educational experience for medical students. The College's overarching goals are building signature research and clinical programs and reaffirming its land grant heritage of community outreach and service.

Curricular Highlights

Community Service Requirement: Optional.
Research/Thesis Requirement: Optional.

The goal of the curriculum is to produce undifferentiated physicians of the highest caliber. Years 1 and 2 taught at both the College Station and Temple campuses include an organ systems curriculum, which integrates the traditional basic sciences along with instruction in

behavioral science, working with patients, physical diagnosis, humanities in medicine, community medicine, leadership in medicine, evidence-based medicine, and epidemiology. Correlation of the basic sciences with clinical medicine is achieved from the start, with clinical instruction in both years 1 and 2. Years 3 and 4 consist of traditional clerkships and a mixed rotation of ambulatory care experiences.

USMLE

Step 1: Required. Students must record a passing score for graduation, but not promotion.
Step 2: Clinical Skills (CS): Required. Students must record a passing total score to graduate.
Step 2: Clinical Knowledge (CK): Required. Students must record a passing total score to graduate.

Selection Factors

Academic ability, grades in college courses, and performance on the MCAT® are important selection criteria. Equally important are interpersonal and communication skills, maturity, motivation, and compassion. Careful consideration is given to other factors such as dedication to service, disadvantaged circumstances, socioeconomic background, race/ethnicity, faculty support, primary care interest, and/or service in a rural/underserved area. Knowledge of and experiences in the medical profession are important. Admission is open to qualified individuals regardless of race, color, religion, gender, age, national origin, or disability. Applicants are invited for personal interviews based upon their competiveness in the review process.

Financial Aid

Scholarship and loan funds are available to students with financial need from local, state, and national sources. Financial needs of the applicant are not a consideration in the admission process.

Information about Diversity Programs

The college believes that diversity enhances its ability to provide care and to serve communities across a broad range of racial and ethnic groups. As part of its commitment to this effort, the college administers several programs for students who are disadvantaged or from groups underrepresented in medicine. The Joint Admissions

Medical Program is open to economically disadvantaged students, and the Partnership for Primary Care Program is open to students from rural/underserved communities in Texas. Also, the adjustment and retention of minority students is facilitated through the college's chapter of the Student National Medical Association (SNMA).

Campus Information

Setting

The college is located on the west campus of Texas A&M University in College Station, Texas. College Station and Bryan, its neighboring city to the north, are home to 124,493 people. College Station-Bryan is located in East-Central Texas between the Brazos and Navasota Rivers and 100 miles northwest of Houston.

Enrollment

For 2007, total enrollment was: 354

Special Features

The College of Medicine's primary clinical partner, Scott & White Hospital and Clinic, is one of the largest integrated multi-specialty health care systems in the U.S. and ranked for the third straight year among the Solucient 100 Top Hospitals in the country and the 15 Top Teaching Hospitals in the country.

Housing

Although on-campus housing is not available, the Coordinator of Student Services provides access to apartment listings and roommate search options. Rents for unfurnished apartments range from $290 to $1,200 per month.

Satellite Campuses/Facilities

Traditional clerkships and ambulatory care experiences are conducted predominantly at Scott & White and the Teague Veterans Center. The college is also affiliated with four other hospitals and clinics in College Station, Round Rock, Corpus Christi, Fort Worth, Waco, Austin, and Fort Hood, Texas.

Application Process and Requirements 2009–2010

Primary Application Service: TMDSAS
Earliest filing date: May 1, 2008
Latest filing date: October 1, 2008

Secondary Application Required?: Yes
Sent to: All applicants
URL: http://medicine.tamhsc.edu/
admissions/index.htm
Fee: Yes, $50
Fee waiver available: Yes
Earliest filing date: May 1, 2008
Latest filing date: October 1, 2008

Latest MCAT® considered: September 2008
Oldest MCAT® considered: August 2004

Early Decision Program
School does not have EDP
Applicants notified: n/a
EDP available for: n/a

Regular Acceptance Notice
Earliest date: November 15, 2008 for Texas residents; October 15 for non-residents
Latest date: Until class is full

Applicant's Response to Acceptance Offer – Maximum Time: Two weeks

Requests for Deferred Entrance Considered: Yes

Deposit to Hold Place in Class: No
Deposit (Resident): n/a
Deposit (Non-Resident): n/a
Deposit due: n/a
Applied to tuition: n/a
Deposit refundable: n/a
Refundable by: n/a

Estimated number of new entrants: 170
EDP: n/a, special program: n/a

Start Month/Year: July 2009

Interview Format: Two individual 30-minute interviews. Regional interviews are not available.

Other Programs

PREPARATORY PROGRAMS
Postbaccalaureate Program: No
Summer Program: Yes,
www.utsystem.edu/jamp/
Partnership for Primary Care: Yes,
http://medicine.tamhsc.edu/admissions/ppc/index.html
Summer Research Program: Yes,
http://medicine.tamhsc.edu/student-affairs/research/
summer-program.html
COMBINED DEGREE PROGRAMS
Baccalaureate/MD: No
MD/MPH: No
MD/MBA: Yes, http://medicine.tamhsc.edu/
admissions/dualdegree.htm, Dr. Kathleen Fallon,
(979) 845-7743 or (254) 724-0242
Fallon@medicine.tamhsc.edu
MD/JD: No
MD/PhD: Yes, http://medicine.tamhsc.edu/
admissions/dualdegree.htm

Premedical Coursework

Course	Req.	Rec.	Lab.	Hrs.
Inorganic Chemistry	•		•	8
Behavioral Sciences				
Biochemistry		•		3
Biology	•		•	14
Biology/Zoology				
Calculus	•			3
College English	•			6
College Mathematics				

Course	Req.	Rec.	Lab.	Hrs.
Computer Science				
Genetics				
Humanities				
Organic Chemistry	•		•	8
Physics	•		•	8
Psychology				
Social Sciences				
Math-based Statistics	•			3

Selection Factors: 2007 Accepted Applicants

Proportion of Accepted Applicants with Relevant Experience (Data Self-Reported to AMCAS®)		
Community Service/Volunteer		92%
Medically-Related Work		98%
Research		70%

Shaded bar represents accepted scores ranging from the 10th percentile to the 90th percentile ▬ School Median ● National Median ●

Overall GPA	2.0	2.1	2.2	2.3	2.4	2.5	2.6	2.7	2.8	2.9	3.0	3.1	3.2	3.3	3.4	3.5	3.6	3.7	(3.8)	3.9	4.0
Science GPA	2.0	2.1	2.2	2.3	2.4	2.5	2.6	2.7	2.8	2.9	3.0	3.1	3.2	3.3	3.4	3.5	3.6	3.7	(3.8)	3.9	4.0

MCAT® required: Yes, 96% of 2007 accepted applicants took MCAT®

Verbal Reasoning	3	4	5	6	7	8	9	(10)	11	12	13	14	15
Physical Sciences	3	4	5	6	7	8	9	(10)	(11)	12	13	14	15
Biological Sciences	3	4	5	6	7	8	9	(10)	(11)	12	13	14	15
Writing Sample			J	K	L	M	N	O	(P)	(Q)	R	S	T

Acceptance & Matriculation Data for 2007–2008 First Year Class

	Resident	Non-Resident	International	Total
Applied	2649	408	76	3133
Interviewed	674	52	1	727
Deferred	2	0	0	2
Matriculants				
Early Assurance Program	16	0	0	16
Early Decision Program	0	0	0	0
Baccalaureate/MD	n/a	n/a	n/a	n/a
MD/PhD	4	1	0	5
Matriculated	96	8	1	**105**

Applications accepted from International Applicants: Yes

Specialty Choice

2003, 2004, 2005 Graduates, Specialty Choice (As reported by program directors to GME Track™)	
Anesthesiology	7%
Emergency Medicine	7%
Family Practice	10%
Internal Medicine	17%
Obstetrics/Gynecology	8%
Orthopaedic Surgery	3%
Pediatrics	12%
Psychiatry	4%
Radiology	5%
Surgery	12%

Matriculant Demographics: 2007–2008 First Year Class

Men: 45 **Women:** 60

Matriculants' Self-Reported Race/Ethnicity

Mexican American	8	Korean	2
Cuban	0	Vietnamese	7
Puerto Rican	0	Other Asian	10
Other Hispanic	3	Total Asian	36
Total Hispanic	11	Native American	1
Chinese	8	Black	4
Asian Indian	7	Native Hawaiian	0
Pakistani	3	White	60
Filipino	0	**Unduplicated Number**	
Japanese	0	**of Matriculants**	105

Science and Math Majors: 83%
Matriculants with:
    Baccalaureate degree: 100%
    Graduate degree(s): 3%

Financial Information

Source: 2006–2007 LCME I-B survey and 2007–2008 AAMC TSF questionnaire

	Residents	Non-Residents
Total Cost of Attendance	$10,682	$23,782
Tuition and Fees	$10,682	$23,782
Other (includes living expenses)	$0	$0
Health Insurance (can be waived)	$0	$0

Average 2007 Graduate Indebtedness: $87,961
% of Enrolled Students Receiving Aid: 92%

Criminal Background Check

This medical school requires a criminal background check prior to matriculation.

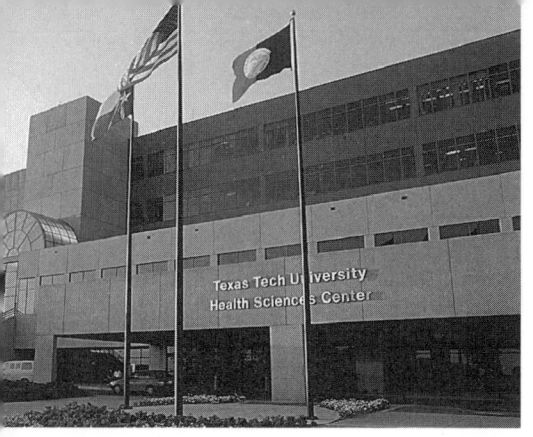

Texas Tech University Health Sciences Center School of Medicine

Lubbock, Texas

Texas Tech University Health Sciences Center
School of Medicine
Office of Admissions, Room 2B116
3601 4th Street
Lubbock, Texas 79430
T 806 743 2297   F 806 743 2725

Admissions www.ttuhsc.edu/som/admissions
Main www.ttuhsc.edu
Financial www.ttuhsc.edu/FinancialAid/
Email somadm@ttuhsc.edu

Public Institution

Dr. Steven L. Berk, Dean

Dr. Bernell K. Dalley, Associate Dean, Admissions and Minority Affairs

Dr. German Nunez, Vice President for Diversity and Multicultural Affairs

E. Marcus Wilson, Director, Financial Aid

Linda Prado, Director, Office of Admissions

General Information

The TTUHSC School of Medicine was established in 1969. All medical students spend the first two years at the Lubbock campus; third and fourth year students receive their clinical training in Lubbock, Amarillo, or Midland/Odessa (Permian Basin). Affiliations with teaching hospitals provide over 2,900 beds for clinical teaching. The medical school has 553 full-time and 48 part-time faculty members and more than 902 volunteer clinical faculty members. Agreements have been developed with four area universities to provide early acceptance of qualified students into TTUHSC School of Medicine. Applicants must be academically talented. Following satisfactory interview, the Admissions Committee recommends acceptance of the applicant. Applicants who continue to maintain the required GPA are guaranteed admission to Texas Tech School of Medicine in the fall following graduation. The MCAT is waived for these applicants.

Mission Statement

TTUHSC School of Medicine provides the highest standard of excellence in higher education, while pursuing continuous quality improvement. The school is committed to health care delivery for its 135,000 square mile service area. At the same time and as part of improvement of health care, its efforts include support of meaningful academic research for the betterment of future health care.

Curricular Highlights

Community Service Requirement: Optional.
Research/Thesis Requirement: Optional.

The new four-year curriculum provides a broad innovative integration of basic and clinical care, with emphasis on developing the student's analytical problem-solving skills. The first two years blend core concepts of basic sciences with early clinical experience. Introduction to patience care skills begins in the first month. The second year now follows an overall systems approach, again aligned with supervised patient care experiences. Teaching formats include small group discussions, PBL, and team learning. Summer preceptorships are also available. The third and fourth years include clerkships in family medicine, internal medicine, neurology, obstetric-gynecology, pediatrics, psychiatry, and surgery. The fourth year combines required and elective rotations. Research opportunities include summer preceptorships, a Research Honors Program, and an integrated M.D.-Ph.D. program. Joint degree programs in the M.B.A./M.D. and J.D./M.D. are also offered. Students are graded using a categorical grading system: Honors, Pass, and Fail.

USMLE

Step 1: Required. Students must record a passing score for promotion.
Step 2: Clinical Skills (CS): Required. Students must only record a score.
Step 2: Clinical Knowledge (CK): Required. Students must only record a score.

Selection Factors

Applications are invited from qualified Texas residents and service area counties of New Mexico and Oklahoma. Only U.S. citizens or applicants with permanent resident visas are considered. Application forms and procedural information may be obtained from the Texas Medical and Dental Schools Application Service (www.utsystem.edu/tmdsas). A secondary application to TTUHSC School of Medicine is also required. The Admissions Committee carefully reviews all applications. Evidence of high intellectual ability and a record of strong academic achievement are essential for success in the study of medicine. Qualities such as compassion, motivation, the ability to communicate with people, maturity, and personal integrity are also important. There is no discrimination on the basis of race, sex, creed, national origin, age, or disability. It is the goal of the institution to recruit a diverse medical class exhibiting the qualities promising academic success and to meet the needs of an increasingly diverse population. Personal interviews are offered to those candidates deemed competitive for admission. Interviews are conducted on the Lubbock campus.

Financial Aid

After a applicant has been accepted, financial aid assistance can be obtained from the Office of Student Financial Aid. Employment, other than during the summer, is discouraged.

Information about Diversity Programs

In an effort to recruit a highly qualified and diverse student body, which reflects the demographics of the West Texas region, race/ethnicity as well as a socioeconomically disadvantaged background are among the many factors considered in the admission process.

Campus Information

Setting

The medical school is situated at the north edge of the city of Lubbock. It is adjacent to Texas Tech University, which makes it one of the few medical schools in the country to be on or adjacent to a major undergraduate campus and law school. The Lubbock campus is across the street from a number of apartment complexes and is within easy driving distance of shopping, recreational and cultural areas.

Enrollment

For 2007, total enrollment was: 571

Satellite Campuses/Facilities

All students spend the first two years of medical school on the Lubbock campus. The in-depth clinical training for medical students is divided among three campuses: to Lubbock, Amarillo, or Midland/Odessa (Permian Basin).

Application Process and Requirements 2009–2010

Primary Application Service: TMDSAS
Earliest filing date: May 1, 2008
Latest filing date: October 1, 2008

Secondary Application Required?: Yes
Sent to: Required of all applicants
URL: www.ttuhsc.edu/som/admissions
Fee: Yes, $50
Fee waiver available: No
Earliest filing date: May 1, 2008
Latest filing date: October 1, 2008

Latest MCAT® considered: September 2008
Oldest MCAT® considered: 2004

Early Decision Program
School does have EDP
Applicants notified: October 1, 2008
EDP available for: Residents only

Regular Acceptance Notice
Earliest date: November 15, 2008
Latest date: Until class is full

Applicant's Response to Acceptance
Offer – Maximum Time: Two weeks

Requests for Deferred
Entrance Considered: Yes

Deposit to Hold Place in Class: Yes
Deposit (Resident): $100
Deposit (Non-Resident): $100
Deposit due: May 15, 2009
Applied to tuition: No
Deposit refundable: Yes
Refundable by: May 15, 2009

Estimated number of new entrants: 140
EDP: 3, special program: n/a

Start Month/Year: August 2009

Interview Format: Two individual thirty-minute interviews. Regional interviews are not available.

Other Programs

PREPARATORY PROGRAMS
Postbaccalaureate Program: No
Summer Program: Yes
www.ttuhsc.edu/som/admissions
Joint Admission to Medicine Program (JAMP):
www.utsystem.edu/jamp

COMBINED DEGREE PROGRAMS
Baccalaureate/MD: No
MD/MPH: No
MD/MBA: Yes,
www.ttuhsc.edu/som/admissions
MD/JD: Yes
MD/PhD: Yes,
www.ttuhsc.edu/som/admissions

Premedical Coursework

Course	Req.	Rec.	Lab.	Hrs.	Course	Req.	Rec.	Lab.	Hrs.
Inorganic Chemistry	•		•	8	Computer Science				
Behavioral Sciences					Genetics				
Biochemistry					Humanities				
Biology					Organic Chemistry	•		•	8
Biology/Zoology	•		•	14	Physics	•		•	8
Calculus					Psychology				
College English	•			6	Social Sciences				
College Mathematics					Statistics		•		3

Selection Factors: 2007 Accepted Applicants

Proportion of Accepted Applicants with Relevant Experience (Data Self-Reported to AMCAS®)		Community Service/Volunteer	88%
		Medically-Related Work	96%
		Research	61%

Shaded bar represents accepted scores ranging from the 10th percentile to the 90th percentile ▪ **School Median** ● **National Median** ●

Overall GPA	2.0	2.1	2.2	2.3	2.4	2.5	2.6	2.7	2.8	2.9	3.0	3.1	3.2	3.3	3.4	3.5	3.6	(3.7)	3.8	3.9	4.0
Science GPA	2.0	2.1	2.2	2.3	2.4	2.5	2.6	2.7	2.8	2.9	3.0	3.1	3.2	3.3	3.4	3.5	(3.6)	3.7	3.8	3.9	4.0

MCAT® required: Yes, 96% of 2007 accepted applicants took MCAT®

Verbal Reasoning	3	4	5	6	7	8	9	(10)	11	12	13	14	15
Physical Sciences	3	4	5	6	7	8	9	(10)	(11)	12	13	14	15
Biological Sciences	3	4	5	6	7	8	9	(10)	(11)	12	13	14	15
Writing Sample				J	K	L	M	N	O	(P)	(Q)	R	S	T

Acceptance & Matriculation Data for 2007–2008 First Year Class

	Resident	Non-Resident	International	Total
Applied	2599	392	57	3048
Interviewed	705	38	0	743
Deferred	7	0	0	7
Matriculants				
Early Assurance Program	3	0	0	3
Early Decision Program	5	0	0	5
Baccalaureate/MD	n/a	n/a	n/a	n/a
MD/PhD	0	1	0	1
Matriculated	130	9	1	**140**

Applications accepted from International Applicants: No

Specialty Choice

2003, 2004, 2005 Graduates, Specialty Choice (As reported by program directors to GME Track™)

Anesthesiology	9%
Emergency Medicine	5%
Family Practice	11%
Internal Medicine	14%
Obstetrics/Gynecology	9%
Orthopaedic Surgery	3%
Pediatrics	12%
Psychiatry	4%
Radiology Diagnostic	5%
Surgery General	10%

Matriculant Demographics: 2007–2008 First Year Class

Men: 84 **Women:** 56

Matriculants' Self-Reported Race/Ethnicity

Mexican American	11	**Korean**	0
Cuban	0	**Vietnamese**	3
Puerto Rican	0	**Other Asian**	18
Other Hispanic	5	**Total Asian**	34
Total Hispanic	18	**Native American**	2
Chinese	4	**Black**	1
Asian Indian	7	**Native Hawaiian**	0
Pakistani	3	**White**	82
Filipino	0	**Unduplicated Number**	
Japanese	0	**of Matriculants**	140

Science and Math Majors: 67%
Matriculants with:
Baccalaureate degree: 100%
Graduate degree(s): 6%

Financial Information

Source: 2006–2007 LCME I-B survey and 2007–2008 AAMC TSF questionnaire

	Residents	Non-Residents
Total Cost of Attendance	$32,898	$45,998
Tuition and Fees	$11,816	$24,916
Other (includes living expenses)	$20,182	$20,182
Health Insurance (not applicable)	$900	$900

Average 2007 Graduate Indebtedness: $122,818
% of Enrolled Students Receiving Aid: 89%

Criminal Background Check

This medical school requires a criminal background check prior to matriculation.

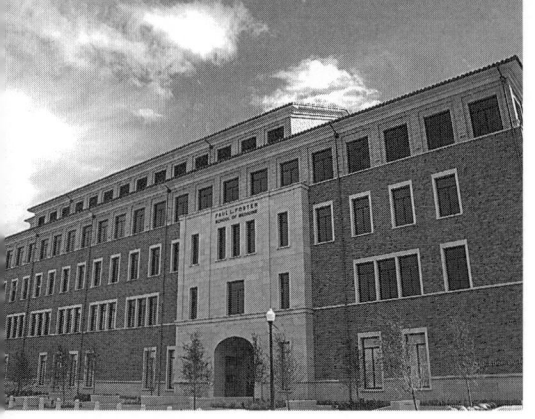

Paul L. Foster School of Medicine at Texas Tech University Health Sciences Center at El Paso

El Paso, Texas

4800 Alberta Avenue
El Paso, Texas 79905
T 915 545 6551   **F** 915 545 6548

Admissions www.ttuhsc.edu/fostersom/
Main www.ttuhsc.edu/fostersom/
Financial www.ttuhsc.edu/financialaid/

Public Institution

Dr. Jose Manuel de la Rosa, Dean

Dr. Manuel Schydlower, Associate Dean for Admissions

Dr. German R. Nunez, Vice President for Diversity and Multicultural Affairs

E. Marcus Wilson, Director, Financial Aid

John Snelling, Director of Admissions

Lorraine James, M.B.A., Assistant Director of Admissions

General Information

In 1999, then Texas Tech System Chancellor John T. Montford shared with the Board of Regents a vision for a full-fledged four-year medical school in El Paso by expanding the existing third and fourth year clinical program. The addition of the first two years of the medical school would allow students from El Paso and nearby regions to complete their education near home and help retain doctors in the area. On December 9, 2003, the ground breaking for El Paso Medical Science Building I took place and two years later, on January 31, 2006, a ribbon cutting followed. This $38 million, 93,000 square-foot facility houses research on diabetes, cancer, environmental health and infectious diseases, as well as a repository dedicated to data on Hispanic health and a genomic facility to link hereditary diseases in families. The medical classroom building was completed in November 2007. This $48 million 125,000 square-foot building has four floors and a partial penthouse. Included in the building are classrooms, library, small group rooms, a clinical skills area for students, faculty and administrative areas, basic science labs, gross anatomy lab, a student services area, and food services. The School of Medicine's graduates will have seen diseases that only a small fraction of medical students ever come across in their medical school clinical learning experiences. El Paso students may encounter diseases and other ailments that have virtually been wiped out in the United States, but flourish in many emerging nations. The variety and diversity of patients that our students see allow our future doctors to learn so much more than classic "text book" cases.

Mission Statement

The school's mission is to provide exceptional opportunities for students, trainees, and physicians; to advance knowledge through innovative scholarship and research in medicine with a focus on international health and health care disparities; and to provide exemplary patient care and service to the entire El Paso community and beyond.

General Information

Curricular Highlights

Community Service Requirement: Required. In years 1 and 2 all students take Society, Community and the Individual, which has a community service component.

Research/Thesis Requirement: Optional. Among the goals of the Paul L. Foster School of Medicine is the provision of a medical education that is consistent with modern scientific principles, supportive of strong ethical principles, sensitive to the needs of the community, and committed to excellence. The school offers an integrated curriculum that is permeated with clinical presentations assigned to organ-system based courses. Clinical presentations are the ways in which a patient presents to a physician. Students learn anatomy, biochemistry, physiology and other basic science concepts and content needed to understand specific clinical presentations at the time that the presentation is being addressed. This approach enhances knowledge comprehension and has been shown to improve retention of the basic sciences and to promote the acquisition of diagnostic reasoning skills that are more like those of the expert practicing physician. During the clinical science years students participate in a unique and rich variety of clinical patient-care learning experiences that include not only traditional medicine, but also international, bi-national, bicultural, and border health medicine.

USMLE

Step 1: Required. Students must record a passing score for promotion.

Step 2: Clinical Skills (CS): Required. Students must record a passing score for graduation, but not promotion.

Step 2: Clinical Knowledge (CK): Required. Students must record a passing score for graduation, but not promotion.

Selection Factors

Applications will be processed through the Texas Medical and Dental Schools Application Service (TMDSAS). Candidates who are considered to be competitive for admission, based on criteria established by the school, will be invited to interview. These criteria include scores from the MCAT®; academic performance as reflected by the science and overall GPA; rigor of the undergraduate curriculum, extracurricular activities (medical and non-medical) and employment and their impact on performance and maturation; recommendations from premedical advisors or faculty; socioeconomic and disadvantaged background; personal statement and its reflection of communication skills, personal qualities, leadership, maturity, determination, and motivation for a career in medicine; and regional origin. The interview evaluates the applicant's interest and knowledge of the health care field and motivation for a medical career; personal characteristics; and problem solving skills.

Financial Aid

Once accepted, financial aid assistance can be obtained from the Office of Student Financial Aid. Employment is discouraged, except in summer.

Information about Diversity Programs

In an effort to recruit a qualified and diverse student body that reflects the demographics of the West Texas region, ethnicity, as well as socioeconomically disadvantaged background are among the many factors considered in the admissions process.

Campus Information

Setting

The Paul L. Foster School of Medicine is located in South Central El Paso just a few hundred yards north of the international border with Mexico.

Enrollment

For 2007, total enrollment was: 115

Application Process and Requirements 2009–2010

Primary Application Service: TMDSAS
Earliest filing date: May 1, 2008
Latest filing date: October 1, 2008

Secondary Application
URL: n/a
Sent to: n/a
Fee: n/a
Fee Waiver Available: n/a
Earliest filing date: n/a
Latest filing date: n/a

Latest MCAT® considered: September 2008
Oldest MCAT® considered: 2004

Early Decision Program
School does not have EDP
Applicants notified: n/a
EDP available for: n/a

Regular Acceptance Notice
Earliest date: November 15, 2008
Latest date: Until class is full

Applicant's Response to Acceptance Offer – Maximum Time: Two weeks

Requests for deferred entrance considered: Yes

Deposit to Hold Place in Class: Yes,
Deposit (Resident): Yes, $100
Deposit (Non-Resident): Yes, $100
Deposit due: May 15, 2009
Applied to tuition: No
Deposit refundable: Yes
Refundable by: May 15, 2009

Estimated number of new entrants: 40
EDP: n/a, special program: n/a

Start month/year: August 2009

Interview format: Two individual 30 minute interviews. Regional interviews are not available.

Other Programs

PREPARATORY PROGRAMS
Postbaccalaureate Program: No
Summer Program: No

COMBINED DEGREE PROGRAMS
Baccalaureate/MD: No
MD/MPH: No
MD/MBA: No
MD/JD: No
MD/PhD: No

Premedical Coursework

Course	Req.	Rec.	Lab.	Hrs.
Inorganic Chemistry	•		•	8
Behavioral Sciences		•		
Biochemistry		•		
Biology	•		•	14
Biology/Zoology				
Calculus	•			3
College English	•			6
College Mathematics				

Course	Req.	Rec.	Lab.	Hrs.
Computer Science				
Genetics				
Humanities		•		
Organic Chemistry	•		•	8
Physics	•		•	8
Psychology				
Social Sciences		•		

Selection Factors: 2007 Accepted Applicants

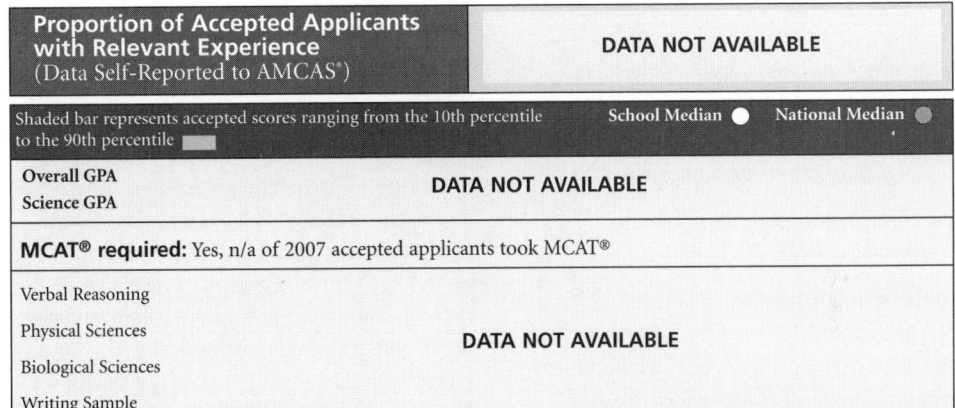

Proportion of Accepted Applicants with Relevant Experience (Data Self-Reported to AMCAS®)	DATA NOT AVAILABLE

Shaded bar represents accepted scores ranging from the 10th percentile to the 90th percentile ■ — School Median ● — National Median ●

Overall GPA	DATA NOT AVAILABLE
Science GPA	

MCAT® required: Yes, n/a of 2007 accepted applicants took MCAT®

Verbal Reasoning	DATA NOT AVAILABLE
Physical Sciences	
Biological Sciences	
Writing Sample	

Acceptance & Matriculation Data for 2007–2008 First Year Class

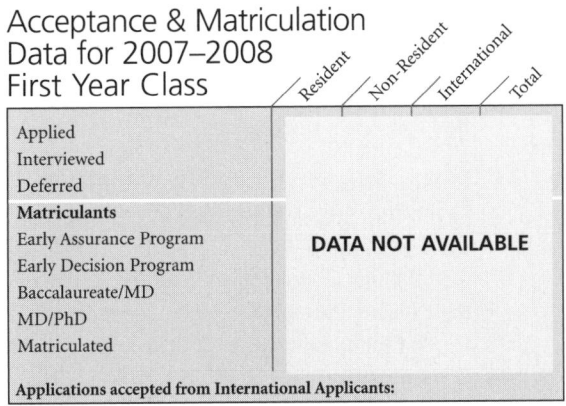

	Resident	Non-Resident	International	Total
Applied				
Interviewed				
Deferred				
Matriculants				
Early Assurance Program				
Early Decision Program		DATA NOT AVAILABLE		
Baccalaureate/MD				
MD/PhD				
Matriculated				

Applications accepted from International Applicants:

Specialty Choice

2003, 2004, 2005 Graduates, Specialty Choice (As reported by program directors to GME Track™)
Anesthesiology
Emergency Medicine
Family Practice
Int...
Ob... DATA NOT AVAILABLE
Or...
Pediatrics
Psychiatry
Radiology
Surgery

Matriculant Demographics: 2007–2008 First Year Class

Men: n/a   **Women:** n/a

Matriculants' Self-Reported Race/Ethnicity

Mexican American	Korean
Cuban	Vietnamese
Puerto Rican	Other Asian
Othe...	
Total	
Chine...	DATA NOT AVAILABLE
Asian	
Pakis...	
Filipino	**Unduplicated Number**
Japanese	**of Matriculants**

Science Majors: n/a
Matriculants with:
    Baccalaureate Degree: n/a
    Graduate Degree(s): n/a

Financial Information

Source: 2006–2007 LCME I-B survey and 2007–2008 AAMC TSF questionnaire

	Residents	Non-Residents
Total Cost of Attendance	$32,700	$45,800
Tuition and Fees	$11,700	$24,800
Other (includes living expenses)		
Health Insurance (can be waived)	$1,190	$1,190

Average 2007 Graduate Indebtedness: n/a
% of Enrolled Students Receiving Aid: n/a

Criminal Background Check

This medical school requires a criminal background check prior to matriculation.

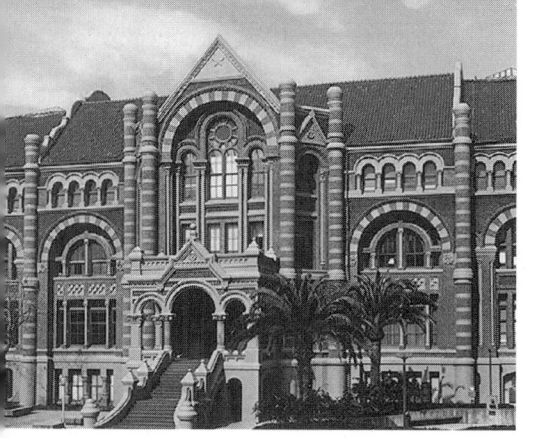

University of Texas Medical School at Galveston

Galveston, Texas

Office of Student Affairs & Admissions
University of Texas Medical Branch
301 University Boulevard
Galveston, Texas 77555-1317
T 409 772 6958 **F** 409 747 2909

Admissions www.utmb.edu/somstudentaffairs
Main www.som.utmb.edu
Financial www.utmb.edu/enrollmentservices
Email tsilva@utmb.edu

Public Institution

Dr. Garland Anderson, IV Dean

Dr. Lauree Thomas, Associate Dean for Student Affairs and Admissions

Melvin Williams, Director, Equal Opportunity and Diversity

Carl Gordon, Associate Director, Enrollment Services and University Financial Aid

Dr. Jeffrey Rabek, Assistant Dean for Student Affairs and Admissions

General Information

The University of Texas Medical Branch (UTMB), established in 1891, is a state-owned academic health center with seven hospitals, 797 teaching beds, and 147 specialty and subspecialty clinics directed by UTMB's administration. It is comprised of four schools (Medicine, Graduate School of Biomedical Sciences, Nursing, and Allied Health Sciences) and three institutes (Marine Biomedical, Medical Humanities, and Human Infections and Immunity).

Mission Statement

The mission of UTMB is to provide scholarly teaching, innovative scientific investigation, and state-of-the-art patient care in a learning environment to better the health of society. UTMB's education programs enable the state's talented individuals to become outstanding practitioners, teachers, and investigators in the health care sciences. Its comprehensive primary, specialty, and sub-specialty clinics support the educational mission of the SOM, which is committed to the healthcare of all Texans through the delivery of state-of-the-art preventive, diagnostic, and treatment services.

Curricular Highlights

Community Service Requirement: Optional.
Research/Thesis Requirement: Optional.

The Integrated Medical Curriculum (IMC) is a four-year program that emphasizes continuous integration of the basic medical sciences with clinical medicine, early clinical skills and clinical experiences, and professionalism. In this student-centered curriculum, which utilizes small-group problem-based learning, computer-assisted instruction, lectures, and labs, the basic medical sciences are learned in clinical contexts. Its organ system-based approach and clinical science contexts promote basic science integration across disciplines. The third and fourth years of the IMC are centered on ambulatory and inpatient experiences in emergency medicine, family medicine, internal medicine, neurology, obstetrics and gynecology, pediatrics, psychiatry, and surgery. A unique feature of the third-year curriculum is an elective month, which allows students to expand their experience in a primary care field or explore potential career interests in a medical specialty. The fourth year also includes an acting internship, community-based ambulatory medicine, and a scholarly project in which a basic science or medical humanities topic is explored in depth. UTMB employs a grading system of Honors, High Pass, Pass, and Fail for required core courses and Pass/Fail for elective courses.

USMLE

Step 1: Required. Students must record a passing score for promotion.
Step 2: Clinical Skills (CS): Required. Students must record a passing total score to graduate.
Step 2: Clinical Knowledge (CK): Required. Students must record a passing total score to graduate.

Selection Factors

In a new admissions policy authorized by the Board of Regents and approved by the U. T. System, UTMB has added race and ethnicity to the broad range of criteria considered for student admission and for scholarship awards. All information available is utilized in the selection process such as intellect, achievement, character, interpersonal skills, and motivation. In evaluating candidates, consideration is given to the total academic record, the results of aptitude and achievement tests, college preprofessional committee evaluations, and the personal interview.

Financial Aid

Long-term, low-interest and short-term loans are available to students with financial need. In addition, a number of scholarships are available which are based on need, disadvantaged status and academic merit.

Information about Diversity Programs

UTMB is committed to increasing the number of disadvantaged students in medicine. Each applicant is reviewed holistically and individually by experienced members of the Admissions Committee with particular emphasis on the applicant's potential. Both cognitive and non-cognitive factors are considered. Following admission, a broad range of support services are available to assist students in completing the medical curriculum. UTMB does not discriminate on the basis of race, sex, creed, national origin, age, or handicap.

Campus Information

Setting

UTMB is located on an island in the Gulf of Mexico, 50 miles south of Houston. It is a 99-acre campus with 77 major modern buildings, including the state-of-the-art Truman Blocker, Jr. Medical Research Building, Trauma Center, and Shriners Burns Hospital. Clinical training takes place in seven teaching hospitals; UTMB owns and operates all of the facilities, and they are physically located on the campus.

Enrollment

For 2007, total enrollment was: 880

Special Features

UTMB is one of two medical schools that received NIH funding for a Biosafety Level 4 Laboratory, which is currently under construction. The Galveston National Laboratory will house the new Institute for Human Infections and Immunity.

Housing

Student housing is available on campus and in the surrounding Galveston community.

Satellite Campuses/Facilities

A limited number of clerkship positions are available for third year students to spend their entire year in Austin, Texas. However, all third and fourth year students can choose to do a portion of their clerkships at this additional training site.

Application Process and Requirements 2009–2010

Primary Application Service: TMDSAS
Earliest filing date: May 1, 2008
Latest filing date: October 1, 2008

Secondary Application Required?: No
Sent to: n/a
URL: n/a
Fee: No
Fee waiver available: No
Earliest filing date: n/a
Latest filing date: n/a

Latest MCAT® considered: September 2008
Oldest MCAT® considered: 2004

Early Decision Program
School does not have EDP
Applicants notified: n/a
EDP available for: n/a

Regular Acceptance Notice
Earliest date: November 15, 2008
Latest date: Until class is full

Applicant's Response to Acceptance Offer – Maximum Time: varies

Requests for Deferred Entrance Considered: Yes

Deposit to Hold Place in Class: No
Deposit (Resident): n/a
Deposit (Non-Resident): n/a
Deposit due: n/a
Applied to tuition: n/a
Deposit refundable: n/a
Refundable by: n/a

Estimated number of new entrants: 230
EDP: n/a, special program: n/a

Start Month/Year: August 2009

Interview Format: Two interviews, presentation, and tour. Regional interviews are not available.

Other Programs

PREPARATORY PROGRAMS
Postbaccalaureate Program: No
Summer Program: Yes, www.utmb.edu/somstudentaffairs/specialprograms
Lisa Cain, Ph.D., (409) 772-5397, ldcain@utmb.edu
Early Medical School Acceptance Program (EMSAP) www.utmb.edu/somstudentaffairs/specialprograms
Prematriculation Reinforcement & Enrichment Program:
www.utmb.edu/somstudentaffairs/specialprograms
COMBINED DEGREE PROGRAMS
Baccalaureate/MD: No
MD/MPH: No
MD/MBA: No
MD/JD: No
MD/PhD: Yes, www.utmb.edu/mdphd
Shannol Carroll, (409) 772-8145
smcarrol@utmb.edu
Additional Program: Yes, www.mdphd.utexas.edu, Robin Dusek
(512) 471-0934, mdphd@austin.utexas.edu

Premedical Coursework

Course	Req.	Rec.	Lab.	Sems.
Inorganic Chemistry	•		•	2
Behavioral Sciences				
Biochemistry		•		4
Biology	•		•	4
Biology/Zoology				
Calculus	•			1
College English	•			2
College Mathematics				

Course	Req.	Rec.	Lab.	Sems.
Computer Science				
Genetics		•		
Humanities				
Organic Chemistry	•		•	2
Physics	•		•	2
Psychology				
Social Sciences				
Other				

Selection Factors: 2007 Accepted Applicants

Proportion of Accepted Applicants with Relevant Experience (Data Self-Reported to AMCAS®)		
Community Service/Volunteer		89%
Medically-Related Work		92%
Research		57%

Shaded bar represents accepted scores ranging from the 10th percentile to the 90th percentile   ○ School Median   ○ National Median

Overall GPA	2.0	2.1	2.2	2.3	2.4	2.5	2.6	2.7	2.8	2.9	3.0	3.1	3.2	3.3	3.4	3.5	3.6	3.7	(3.8)	3.9	4.0
Science GPA	2.0	2.1	2.2	2.3	2.4	2.5	2.6	2.7	2.8	2.9	3.0	3.1	3.2	3.3	3.4	3.5	3.6	3.7	(3.8)	3.9	4.0

MCAT® required: Yes, 100% of 2007 accepted applicants took MCAT®

Verbal Reasoning	3	4	5	6	7	8	9	(10)	11	12	13	14	15
Physical Sciences	3	4	5	6	7	8	9	(10)	(11)	12	13	14	15
Biological Sciences	3	4	5	6	7	8	9	10	(11)	12	13	14	15
Writing Sample				J	K	L	M	N	O	(P)	(Q)	R	S	T

Acceptance & Matriculation Data for 2007–2008 First Year Class

	Resident	Non-Resident	International	Total
Applied	2998	597	47	3642
Interviewed	916	70	4	990
Deferred	8	0	0	8
Matriculants				
Early Assurance Program	0	0	0	0
Early Decision Program	0	0	0	0
Baccalaureate/MD	n/a	n/a	n/a	n/a
MD/PhD	6	0	0	6
Matriculated	218	9	0	**227**

Applications accepted from International Applicants: Yes

Specialty Choice

2003, 2004, 2005 Graduates, Specialty Choice
(As reported by program directors to GME Track™)

Anesthesiology	8%
Emergency Medicine	7%
Family Practice	12%
Internal Medicine	14%
Obstetrics/Gynecology	4%
Orthopaedic Surgery	3%
Pediatrics	10%
Psychiatry	6%
Radiology	6%
Surgery	7%

Matriculant Demographics: 2007–2008 First Year Class

Men: 122   **Women:** 105

Matriculants' Self-Reported Race/Ethnicity

Mexican American	27	Korean	2
Cuban	0	Vietnamese	4
Puerto Rican	2	Other Asian	10
Other Hispanic	8	Total Asian	33
Total Hispanic	37	Native American	2
Chinese	9	Black	23
Asian Indian	8	Native Hawaiian	0
Pakistani	0	White	150
Filipino	0	Unduplicated Number	
Japanese	1	of Matriculants	227

Science and Math Majors: 48%
Matriculants with:
Baccalaureate degree: 100%
Graduate degree(s): 4%

Financial Information

Source: 2006–2007 LCME I-B survey and 2007–2008 AAMC TSF questionnaire

	Residents	Non-Residents
Total Cost of Attendance	$35,950	$49,050
Tuition and Fees	$12,230	$25,330
Other (includes living expenses)	$23,720	$23,720
Health Insurance (not applicable)	$0	$0

Average 2007 Graduate Indebtedness: $123,960
% of Enrolled Students Receiving Aid: 83%

Criminal Background Check

This medical school requires a criminal background check prior to matriculation.

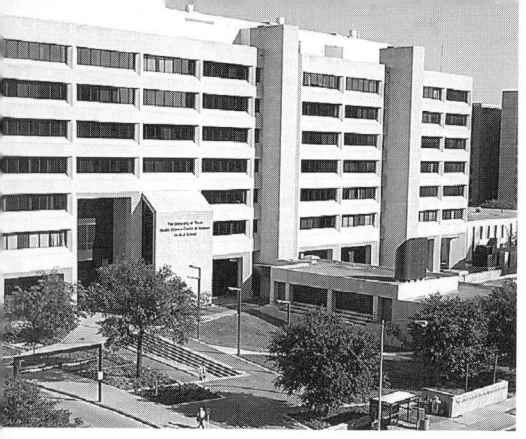

University of Texas
Medical School at Houston

Houston, Texas

Office of Admissions—Room G.420
University of Texas Medical School at Houston
6431 Fannin, MSB G.420
Houston, Texas 77030
T 713 500 5116   F 713 500 0604

Admissions http://med.uth.tmc.edu/administration/admissions/
Main http://med.uth.tmc.edu
Financial http://sfa.uth.tmc.edu
Email msadmissions@uth.tmc.edu

Public Institution

Dr. Giuseppe N. Colasurdo, Dean

Dr. Margaret McNeese, Associate Dean of Admissions and Student Affairs

Dr. Judianne Kellaway, Assistant Dean for Admissions

Tiffany Reyes, Coordinator of Admissions

General Information

The University of Texas Medical School at Houston is located in the Texas Medical Center in Houston in order to take advantage of the many other medical institutions in the area. Memorial Hermann Hospital, a 650-bed general medical and surgical hospital, is adjacent to the school. Other major teaching hospitals include the University of Texas M.D. Anderson Cancer Center, Southwest Memorial Hospital, and the Lyndon Baines Johnson Hospital of the Harris County Hospital District.

Mission Statement

The mission of the University of Texas Medical School at Houston is to provide the highest quality of education and training of future physicians for the state of Texas, in harmony with the state's diverse population, and to conduct the highest caliber of research in the biomedical and health sciences.

Curricular Highlights

Community Service Requirement: Optional. Endless opportunities
Research/Thesis Requirement: Optional.

The first two academic years are divided into four semesters, with three months of vacation between the first and second years. The initial four semesters are devoted to preparing the student for clerkship experiences in the clinical years. During the first two years the student becomes familiar with the basic and applied biomedical sciences. The student progresses from a study of the morphology of the human body and the fundamentals of molecular and cellular biology to that of the normal and abnormal structure and function of the various organ systems. Taking a history and conducting a physical examination are emphasized. After completion of this sequence, the student progresses through a series of clinical clerkships in the major disciplines for the next 12 months. In the remaining year, there are four months of required clerkships and five to seven months of electives. Medical jurisprudence and technical skills are taught. In consultation with faculty, each student devises an educational sequence that relates specifically to ultimate career goals and postgraduate educational plans.

USMLE

Step 1: Required. Students must only record a score.
Step 2: Clinical Skills (CS): Required. Students must only record a score.
Step 2: Clinical Knowledge (CK): Required. Students must only record a score.

Selection Factors

Applicants are selected with an emphasis on motivation and potential for service, especially in the state of Texas. Academic ability is evaluated to ensure that those who are accepted can complete medical studies. Emphasis is given to students who have a broad education and who display intellectual interest. A command of the English language with ability to write and speak well is essential. The applicant's academic record is evaluated with special attention to the subjects taken and the demonstration of a broadly based comprehensive educational experience. The overall philosophy is that knowledge is an end in itself; while vocational-type curricula are not ruled out, liberal arts are preferred. Universities with core curricula generally provide the type of diversity sought in subject distribution. Significant attention is given to humanitarian endeavors, achievement in a nonacademic field of activity, and the applicant's specific interest in the University of Texas Medical School at Houston. Admission decisions are made in light of the school's mission, with preference given to Texas residents and those who will practice in shortage areas and specialties in the state. Veteran status is also considered. The University of Texas Medical School at Houston does not discriminate on the basis of race, sex, creed, national origin, age, or handicap. For additional information, go to *med.uth.tmc.edu*.

Financial Aid

Scholarship and loan funds are available to students with financial need from local, state, federal, and national sources. Financial independence is not a criterion for admission.

Information about Diversity Programs

The primary goal of the Program of Equal Opportunity and Diversity is to develop a supportive environment that is based on equity (equal opportunity) and diversity for our faculty, staff, and student body.

Campus Information

Setting

The Medical School Building, located in the Texas Medical Center, was built in 1976 and, at 875,365 gross square feet, comprises the schools largest facility. The building houses approximately 2,300 faculty, staff, and students. The structure has ten levels and was partially renovated in 1989, 1994, and 2005.

Enrollment

For 2007, total enrollment was: 877

Housing

Apartment living is available to UTHSC-H students at two facilities. Floor plans range from a one bedroom efficiency to an apartment home with three bedrooms and two baths.

Satellite Campuses/Facilities

Student rotations are completed at several hospitals and clinics in the Texas Medical Center (TMC) and surrounding areas. While Memorial Hermann Hospital is the chief teaching hospital, students also complete rotations at other hospitals and clinics in the TMC and Houston area.

Application Process and Requirements 2009–2010

Primary Application Service: TMDSAS
Earliest filing date: May 1, 2008
Latest filing date: October 1, 2008

Secondary Application Required?: No
Sent to: n/a
URL: n/a
Fee: No
Fee waiver available: n/a
Earliest filing date: n/a
Latest filing date: n/a

Latest MCAT® considered: September 2008
Oldest MCAT® considered: 2003 or 5 years prior to application

Early Decision Program
School does not have EDP
Applicants notified: October 15/November 15
EDP available for: Both Residents and Non-Residents

Regular Acceptance Notice
Earliest date: October 15, 2008
Latest date: Until class is full

Applicant's Response to Acceptance Offer – Maximum Time: Two weeks

Requests for Deferred Entrance Considered: No

Deposit to Hold Place in Class: No
Deposit (Resident): n/a
Deposit (Non-Resident): n/a
Deposit due: n/a
Applied to tuition: n/a
Deposit refundable: n/a
Refundable by: n/a

Estimated number of new entrants: 230
EDP: n/a, special program: n/a

Start Month/Year: August 2009

Interview Format: Personal interview with two faculty members. Regional interviews are not available.

Other Programs

PREPARATORY PROGRAMS
Postbaccalaureate Program: No
Summer Program: Yes, http://med.uth.tmc.edu/administration/admissions/
Pre-Entry Program: http://med.uth.tmc.edu/administration/edu_programs/ep/summer_programs.htm, Elizabeth Green, (713) 500-7130

COMBINED DEGREE PROGRAMS
Baccalaureate/MD: No
MD/MPH: Yes, http://med.uth.tmc.edu/administration/admissions/MDMPH.html
MD/MBA: No
MD/JD: No
MD/PhD: Yes, http://med.uth.tmc.edu/www.uth.tmc.edu/gsbs/programs/mdphd/

Premedical Coursework

Course	Req.	Rec.	Lab.	Hrs.	Course	Req.	Rec.	Lab.	Hrs.
Inorganic Chemistry	•		•	8	Computer Science				
Behavioral Sciences					Genetics				
Biochemistry					Humanities		•		
Biology	•		•	14	Organic Chemistry	•		•	8
Biology/Zoology					Physics	•		•	8
Calculus					Psychology				
College English	•			6	Social Sciences				
College Mathematics					Other				

Selection Factors: 2007 Accepted Applicants

Proportion of Accepted Applicants with Relevant Experience (Data Self-Reported to AMCAS®)		
Community Service/Volunteer	89%
Medically-Related Work	96%
Research	70%

Shaded bar represents accepted scores ranging from the 10th percentile to the 90th percentile. **School Median** ● **National Median** ●

| Overall GPA | 2.0 2.1 2.2 2.3 2.4 2.5 2.6 2.7 2.8 2.9 3.0 3.1 3.2 3.3 **3.4 3.5 3.6 3.7** (3.8) 3.9 4.0 |
| Science GPA | 2.0 2.1 2.2 2.3 2.4 2.5 2.6 2.7 2.8 2.9 3.0 3.1 3.2 **3.3 3.4 3.5 3.6** (3.7) 3.8 3.9 4.0 |

MCAT® required: Yes, 100% of 2007 accepted applicants took MCAT®

Verbal Reasoning	3 4 5 6 7 **8 9** (10) 11 12 13 14 15
Physical Sciences	3 4 5 6 7 **8 9** (10) (11) 12 13 14 15
Biological Sciences	3 4 5 6 7 8 **9 10** (11) 12 13 14 15
Writing Sample	J K L **M N O** (P) (Q) R S T

Acceptance & Matriculation Data for 2007–2008 First Year Class

	Resident	Non-Resident	International	Total
Applied	3070	613	224	3907
Interviewed	1041	98	2	1141
Deferred	0	0	0	0
Matriculants				
Early Assurance Program	0	0	0	0
Early Decision Program	0	0	0	0
Baccalaureate/MD	n/a	n/a	n/a	n/a
MD/PhD	0	0	0	0
Matriculated	221	9	0	**230**

Applications accepted from International Applicants: Yes

Specialty Choice

2003, 2004, 2005 Graduates, Specialty Choice (As reported by program directors to GME Track™)	
Anesthesiology	9%
Emergency Medicine	6%
Family Practice	9%
Internal Medicine	16%
Obstetrics/Gynecology	6%
Orthopaedic Surgery	5%
Pediatrics	9%
Psychiatry	5%
Radiology	3%
Surgery	9%

Matriculant Demographics: 2007–2008 First Year Class

Men: 127 **Women:** 103

Matriculants' Self-Reported Race/Ethnicity

Mexican American	23	Korean	0
Cuban	2	Vietnamese	7
Puerto Rican	2	Other Asian	9
Other Hispanic	7	Total Asian	39
Total Hispanic	34	Native American	0
Chinese	12	Black	15
Asian Indian	10	Native Hawaiian	1
Pakistani	1	White	163
Filipino	1	Unduplicated Number	
Japanese	2	of Matriculants	230

Science and Math Majors: 55%
Matriculants with:
Baccalaureate degree: 100%
Graduate degree(s): 2%

Financial Information

Source: 2006–2007 LCME I-B survey and 2007–2008 AAMC TSF questionnaire

	Residents	Non-Residents
Total Cost of Attendance	$34,634	$47,734
Tuition and Fees	$10,769	$23,869
Other (includes living expenses)	$22,746	$22,746
Health Insurance (can be waived)	$1,119	$1,119

Average 2007 Graduate Indebtedness: $110,253
% of Enrolled Students Receiving Aid: 83%

Criminal Background Check

This medical school requires a criminal background check prior to matriculation.

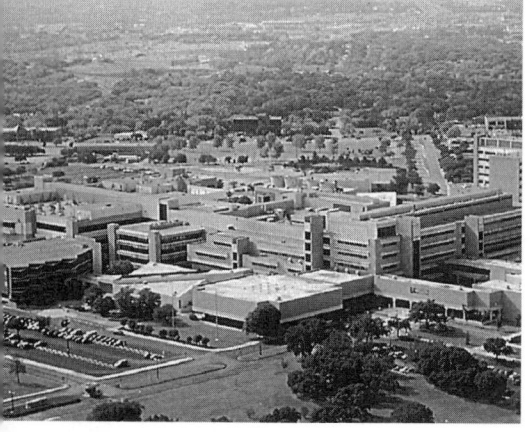

University of Texas
School of Medicine at San Antonio
San Antonio, Texas

Medical School Admissions, Office of the Dean
Univ. of Texas School of Medicine at San Antonio
7703 Floyd Curl Drive
San Antonio, Texas 78229-3900
T 210 567 6080   F 210 567 6962

Admissions som.uthscsa.edu/admissions/index.asp
Main som.uthscsa.edu
Financial studentservices.uthscsa.edu/
financialinfo/financialaid2.html
Email msprospect@uthscsa.edu

Public Institution

Dr. William L. Henrich, Dean

Dr. David J. Jones,
Associate Dean for Admissions

Belinda Chapa, Director of Admissions and
Special Programs

General Information
The University of Texas School of Medicine at San Antonio graduated its first class in 1970.The main campus is located at the South Texas Medical Center in NW San Antonio. Clinical instruction is carried out at the University Hospital, University Health Center, Audie Murphy Veterans Hospital, Santa Rosa Children's Hospital, and affiliated hospitals including Wilford Hall USAF Hospital and Brooke Army Hospital.

Mission Statement
The mission of the University of Texas School of Medicine at San Antonio is to serve the needs of the citizens of Texas by providing medical education and training to medical students and physicians at all career levels, with special commitment to the preparation of physicians for careers in the practice of primary health care; conducting biomedical and other health-related research; delivering exemplary quality health care; and providing a responsive resource in health-related affairs for the nation and the state, with particular emphasis on South Texas.

Curricular Highlights
Community Service Requirement: Optional.
Research/Thesis Requirement: Optional.

A four-year curriculum is offered. The first year is devoted to an organ systems-based presentation of anatomy, histology, biochemistry, physiology, and microbiology. The second year is anchored by the pathology course, and it incorporates pharmacology, medicine, pediatrics, obstetrics and gynecology, and surgery coordinated by organ systems. Behavioral sciences and an introduction to psychiatry are also included. Throughout the first two years, one-half day per week is devoted to clinical integration activities.

The third academic year is spent entirely in the clinical setting in eight consecutive assignments of six weeks each in family practice, medicine, the medical specialties, surgery, the surgical specialties, obstetrics and gynecology, psychiatry, and pediatrics. The senior year includes a didactic period of two months, with the rest of the academic year consisting of elective courses. A letter grading system is used.

USMLE
Step 1: Required. Students must record a passing score for promotion.
Step 2: Clinical Skills (CS): Required. Students must only record a score.
Step 2: Clinical Knowledge (CK): Required. Students must only record a score.

Selection Factors
Ranking of applicants considers GPA, MCAT® section scores, evaluation by premedical advisors, and judgment by the Committee on Admissions of the candidate's nonacademic achievements and personal qualifications, such as responsibility, integrity, maturity, and motivation. In addition, bilingual language ability, hometown or county of residence that has been designated a medically underserved area, socioeconomic history, positions of responsibility held, communication skills, experience with diverse populations, and clinical/volunteer experiences are considered. No person shall be excluded from participation in, denied the benefits of, or subject to discrimination under any program or activity sponsored or conducted by the University of Texas System on the basis of age, race, national origin, religion, or sex. Two hundred thirty five acceptances were offered to obtain a class of 200 first-year students. All procedural information including electronic submission of applications is available through the Texas Medical and Dental Schools Application Service. Questions related to completeness of an application or other information should be directed to the Admissions Office at the medical school (msprospect@uthscsa.edu). Additional information is available at 210-567-6080.

Financial Aid
Financial assistance for students in need is available in the form of loans and scholarships. Accepted applicants can obtain complete information regarding financial assistance from the financial aid administrator in the Office of Student Services (*http://studentservices.uthscsa. edu/financialinfo/financialaid2.html*).

Information about Diversity Programs
Diversity of the student body is a compelling interest of the University of Texas School of Medicine at San Antonio. With this in mind, race and ethnicity is among the factors considered for acceptance of students.

Campus Information

Setting
The University of Texas School of Medicine at San Antonio is located in the South Texas Medical Center in northwest San Antonio.

Enrollment
For 2007, total enrollment was: 852

Special Features
The newly completed Clinical Skills Center offers students 20 state-of-the-art examination rooms to develop patient examination skills.

Housing
On campus housing is not available. Homes, apartments, and condominiums are available within walking distance of the school of medicine and teaching hospitals.

Satellite Campuses/Facilities
The Regional Academic Health Center located in the Rio Grande Valley in Harlingen, Texas, is a second clinical education campus. At the end of their second year, 24 students move to Harlingen to complete their third and fourth years of medical school. Third-year clerkships are completed at Valley Baptist Hospital and Su Clinica Familiar. Fourth-year students participate in the same didactic and externship opportunities available at the San Antonio campus.

Application Process and Requirements 2009–2010

Primary Application Service: TMDSAS
Earliest filing date: May 1, 2008
Latest filing date: October 1, 2008

Secondary Application Required?: No
Sent to: All applicants
URL: http://som.uthscsa.edu/Images/
SecondaryApp05.doc
David J. Jones, Ph.D., (210) 567-6080
jonesd@uthscsa.edu

Fee: No
Fee waiver available: n/a
Earliest filing date: May 1, 2008
Latest filing date: October 15, 2008

Latest MCAT® considered: September 2008
Oldest MCAT® considered: 2005

Early Decision Program
School does not have EDP
Applicants notified: n/a
EDP available for: n/a

Regular Acceptance Notice
Earliest date: October 15, 2008 (non-residents)
November 15, 2008 (residents)
Latest date: Until class is full

Applicant's Response to Acceptance
Offer – Maximum Time: Two weeks

Requests for Deferred
Entrance Considered: Yes

Deposit to Hold Place in Class: No
Deposit (Resident): n/a
Deposit (Non-Resident): n/a
Deposit due: n/a
Applied to tuition: n/a
Deposit refundable: n/a
Refundable by: n/a

Estimated number of new entrants: 220
EDP: 0, special program: 5

Start Month/Year: July 28, 2009

Interview Format: Two 30-minute interviews;
interviewers have only personal essays.

Other Programs

PREPARATORY PROGRAMS
Postbaccalaureate Program: No
Summer Program: No

COMBINED DEGREE PROGRAMS
Baccalaureate/MD: Yes, http://som.uthscsa.edu/
Images/Application.doc
Belinda Chapa, (210) 567-6080,
chapab@uthscsa.edu
MD/MPH: No
MD/MBA: No
MD/JD: No
MD/PhD: Yes, http://som.uthscsa.edu/
admissions/MD_PhD.asp
Dr. Martin Adamo, (210) 567-3742
adamo@uthscsa.edu

Premedical Coursework

Course	Req.	Rec.	Lab.	Hrs.	Course	Req.	Rec.	Lab.	Hrs.
Inorganic Chemistry	•		•	8	Computer Science				
Behavioral Sciences					Genetics				
Biochemistry	•			3	Humanities				
Biology	•		•	11	Organic Chemistry	•		•	8
Biology/Zoology					Physics	•		•	8
Calculus	•			3	Psychology				
College English	•			6	Social Sciences				
College Mathematics					Other				

Selection Factors: 2007 Accepted Applicants

Proportion of Accepted Applicants with Relevant Experience (Data Self-Reported to AMCAS®)		
Community Service/Volunteer		77%
Medically-Related Work		87%
Research		72%

Shaded bar represents accepted scores ranging from the 10th percentile to the 90th percentile   **School Median** ●   **National Median** ●

Overall GPA	2.0	2.1	2.2	2.3	2.4	2.5	2.6	2.7	2.8	2.9	3.0	3.1	3.2	3.3	3.4	3.5	3.6	(3.7)	3.8	3.9	4.0
Science GPA	2.0	2.1	2.2	2.3	2.4	2.5	2.6	2.7	2.8	2.9	3.0	3.1	3.2	3.3	3.4	3.5	(3.6)	3.7	3.8	3.9	4.0

MCAT® required: Yes, 100% of 2007 accepted applicants took MCAT®

Verbal Reasoning	3	4	5	6	7	8	9	(10)	11	12	13	14	15
Physical Sciences	3	4	5	6	7	8	9	(10)	(11)	12	13	14	15
Biological Sciences	3	4	5	6	7	8	9	(10)	(11)	12	13	14	15
Writing Sample			J	K	L	M	N	O	(P)	(Q)	R	S	T

Acceptance & Matriculation Data for 2007–2008 First Year Class

	Resident	Non-Resident	International	Total
Applied	2961	590	66	3617
Interviewed	926	100	0	1026
Deferred	1	0	0	1
Matriculants				
Early Assurance Program	2	0	0	2
Early Decision Program	0	0	0	0
Baccalaureate/MD	2	0	0	2
MD/PhD	5	0	0	5
Matriculated	197	22	1	**220**

Applications accepted from International Applicants: No

Specialty Choice

2003, 2004, 2005 Graduates, Specialty Choice (As reported by program directors to GME Track™)	
Anesthesiology	10%
Emergency Medicine	4%
Family Practice	10%
Internal Medicine	16%
Obstetrics/Gynecology	7%
Orthopedic Surgery	4%
Pediatrics	11%
Psychiatry	3%
Radiology	4%
Surgery	10%

Matriculant Demographics: 2007–2008 First Year Class

Men: 111   **Women:** 109

Matriculants' Self-Reported Race/Ethnicity

Mexican American	28	Korean	4
Cuban	0	Vietnamese	4
Puerto Rican	1	Other Asian	16
Other Hispanic	7	**Total Asian**	44
Total Hispanic	36	Native American	3
Chinese	10	Black	12
Asian Indian	8	Native Hawaiian	0
Pakistani	1	White	152
Filipino	2	**Unduplicated Number**	
Japanese	0	**of Matriculants**	220

Science and Math Majors: 43%
Matriculants with:
       Baccalaureate degree: 70%
       Graduate degree(s): 8%

Financial Information

Source: 2006–2007 LCME I-B survey
and 2007–2008 AAMC TSF questionnaire

	Residents	Non-Residents
Total Cost of Attendance	$13,482	$28,666
Tuition and Fees	$12,443	$27,627
Other (includes living expenses)	$0	$0
Health Insurance (can be waived)	$1,039	$1,039

Average 2007 Graduate Indebtedness: $137,399
% of Enrolled Students Receiving Aid: 91%

Criminal Background Check

This medical school requires a criminal background check prior to matriculation.

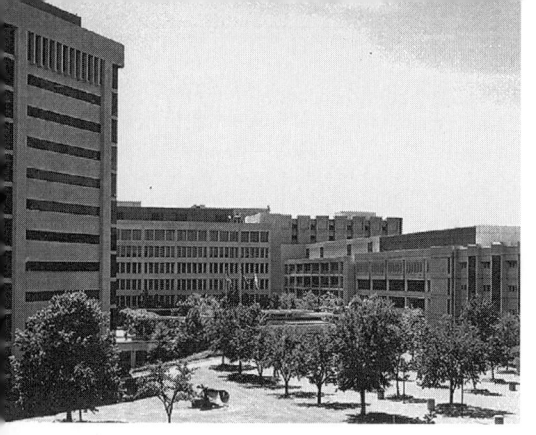

University of Texas Southwestern Medical Center at Dallas Southwestern Medical School

Dallas, Texas

University of Texas
Southwestern Medical Center at Dallas
5323 Harry Hines Boulevard
Dallas, Texas 75390-9162
T 214 648 5617   F 214 648 3289

Admissions www.utsouthwestern.edu/admissions
Main www.utsouthwestern.edu
Financial www.utsouthwestern.edu
Email admissions@utsouthwestern.edu

Public Institution

Dr. Alfred G. Gilman, Dean

Anne P. McLane, Associate Director of Admissions

Dr. Byron Cryer, Associate Dean for Minority Student Affairs

Charles L. Kettlewell, Director of Student Financial Aid

Dr. James Wagner, Associate Dean for Student Affairs

Dr. Angela Mihalic, Associate Dean for Student Affairs

General Information

Founded in 1943, UT Southwestern is a multi-faceted academic health science center nationally recognized for its excellence in educating physicians, biomedical scientists, and other health care professionals.

Mission Statement

UT Southwestern is dedicated to educating physicians who are thoroughly grounded in the scientific basis of modern medicine, who are inspired to maintain lifelong medical scholarship, and who care for patients in a responsible and compassionate manner. Southwestern Medical School's mission emphasizes the importance of training primary care physicians, educating doctors who will practice in under-served areas of Texas, and preparing physician-scientists who seek careers in academic medicine and research.

Curricular Highlights

Community Service Requirement: Optional.
Research/Thesis Requirement: Optional.

UT Southwestern offers a four-year curriculum based on departmental as well as interdisciplinary teaching. The purpose of the first two years is to provide a strong background in the basic sciences as well as an introduction to clinical medicine. The first-year curriculum is designed to begin the study of the normal human body and its processes at the molecular and cellular levels. The second year is an organ system-based curriculum that integrates pharmacology, microbiology, pathology, and clinical medicine.

Contact with patients begins early in the second year with history-taking and physical examination, as well as visits to outpatient clinics. The third and fourth years provide intense clinical experiences involving the student in direct inpatient and outpatient care in a variety of clinical settings. Specific information about the UT Southwestern medical curriculum is available on the curriculum Web site at *http://medschool.swmed.edu/*.

USMLE

Step 1: Required. Students must record a passing score for graduation, but not promotion.
Step 2: Clinical Skills (CS): Required. Students must record a passing total score to graduate.
Step 2: Clinical Knowledge (CK): Required. Students must record a passing total score to graduate.

Selection Factors

The following factors are considered in evaluating each applicant's acceptability: MCAT® scores; undergraduate GPA; the rigor of the undergraduate curriculum; letters of recommendation; extracurricular activities; socioeconomic background; time spent in outside employment; personal integrity and compassion for others; race/ethnicity; the ability to communicate in English; other personal qualities and individual factors such as leadership, social/family support, self-appraisal, maturity/coping skills, and determination; and motivation for a career in medicine. In addition, applicants are evaluated with regard to the mission of Southwestern Medical School. State law requires that at least 90 percent of the class be residents of Texas. Therefore, the minimum credentials for non-residents are more stringent than are those for Texas residents. Early application is strongly advised. A personal on-campus interview is required; interviews are held on Saturdays between early September and early January.

Financial Aid

UT Southwestern works directly with students to obtain funding for their medical education. Most of the financial aid available is obtained through federal and state loan programs. However, a limited number of scholarships from private sources is available. Non-residents are eligible to pay resident tuition on receipt of a competitive

academic scholarship. Students rarely discontinue school for financial reasons.

Information about Diversity Programs

The Admissions Committee at Southwestern Medical School recognizes the need for increased numbers of physicians from groups underrepresented in medicine and encourages applications from Texas residents who are members of these groups. UT Southwestern uses race/ethnicity as one of the criteria for evaluating applicants in an effort to provide a diverse educational environment.

Campus Information

Setting

Just located north of downtown Dallas, the 150-acre campus includes an extensive medical library, 45,000 square foot student recreation center, tennis and outdoor basketball courts, jogging paths, and a 6-acre wooded bird sanctuary. Four hospitals are adjacent to the campus: Parkland Hospital, Childrens Medical Center Dallas, University Hospital-Zale Lipshy, and University Hospital-St. Paul.

Enrollment

For 2007, total enrollment was: 925

Special Features

UT Southwestern Medical School offers an M.D. with Research Distinction program to recognize students who distinguish themselves in the conduct of meaningful clinical or basic research activities.

Housing

Ample and affordable housing opportunities are available within 5 to 10 miles of the campus. Additionally, UT Southwestern's Medical Park Apartments is a gated community with one and two-bedroom units with individually monitored security, clubhouse, study center, exercise room, and pool.

Satellite Campuses/Facilities

Clinical training takes place at university sites and affiliated hospitals and clinics throughout the North Texas area, including Parkland Memorial Hospital, Children's Medical Center Dallas, the Dallas VA Medical Center, and the two University Hospitals, Zale Lipshy and St. Paul.

Application Process and Requirements 2009–2010

Primary Application Service: TMDSAS
Earliest filing date: May 1, 2008
Latest filing date: October 1, 2008

Secondary Application Required?: Yes
Sent to: All applicants
URL: www.utsouthwestern.edu/admissions
Fee: No
Fee waiver available: n/a
Earliest filing date: May 1, 2008
Latest filing date: October 1, 2008

Latest MCAT® considered: August 2008
Oldest MCAT® considered: 2004

Early Decision Program
School does not have EDP
Applicants notified: n/a
EDP available for: n/a

Regular Acceptance Notice
Earliest date: November 1, 2008
Latest date: Varies

Applicant's Response to Acceptance
Offer – Maximum Time: Three weeks

Requests for Deferred
Entrance Considered: Yes

Deposit to Hold Place in Class: No
Deposit (Resident): n/a
Deposit (Non-Resident): n/a
Deposit due: n/a
Applied to tuition: n/a
Deposit refundable: n/a
Refundable by: n/a

Estimated number of new entrants: 230
EDP: n/a, special program: n/a

Start Month/Year: August 2009

Interview Format: Two 25-minute faculty interviews. Regional interviews are not available.

Other Programs

PREPARATORY PROGRAMS
Postbaccalaureate Program: No
Summer Program: No

COMBINED DEGREE PROGRAMS
Baccalaureate/MD: No
MD/MPH: Yes, www.sph.uth.tmc.edu
MD/MBA: Yes,
www.utsouthwestern.edu/md-mba
MD/JD: No
MD/PhD: Yes,
www.utsouthwestern.edu/md-phd
Dr. Dennis McKearin, (800) 633-6787
dennis.mckearin@utsouthwestern.edu
Additional Program: Yes,
www.utsouthwestern.edu/md-ms
Dr. Michael McPhaul, (214) 648-3685
michael.mcphaul@utsouthwestern.edu

Premedical Coursework

Course	Req.	Rec.	Lab.	Sems.	Course	Req.	Rec.	Lab.	Sems.
Inorganic Chemistry	•		•	2	Computer Science				
Behavioral Sciences					Genetics				
Biochemistry		•		1	Humanities				
Biology	•		•	4	Organic Chemistry	•		•	2
Biology/Zoology					Physics	•		•	2
Calculus	•			1	Psychology				
College English	•			2	Social Sciences				
College Mathematics					Other				

Selection Factors: 2007 Accepted Applicants

Proportion of Accepted Applicants with Relevant Experience (Data Self-Reported to AMCAS®)		Community Service/Volunteer	70%
		Medically-Related Work	84%
		Research	80%

Shaded bar represents accepted scores ranging from the 10th percentile to the 90th percentile. School Median ● National Median ●

Overall GPA 2.0 2.1 2.2 2.3 2.4 2.5 2.6 2.7 2.8 2.9 3.0 3.1 3.2 3.3 3.4 **3.5 3.6 3.7 (3.8)** 3.9 4.0
Science GPA 2.0 2.1 2.2 2.3 2.4 2.5 2.6 2.7 2.8 2.9 3.0 3.1 3.2 **3.3 3.4 3.5 3.6 3.7 (3.8)** 3.9 4.0

MCAT® required: Yes, 100% of 2007 accepted applicants took MCAT®

Verbal Reasoning 3 4 5 6 7 8 9 (10) 11 12 13 14 15
Physical Sciences 3 4 5 6 7 8 9 10 (11) 12 13 14 15
Biological Sciences 3 4 5 6 7 8 9 10 (11) (12) 13 14 15
Writing Sample J K L M N O P (Q) R S T

Acceptance & Matriculation Data for 2007–2008 First Year Class

	Resident	Non-Resident	International	Total
Applied	2780	608	102	3490
Interviewed	715	69	29	813
Deferred	9	1	1	11
Matriculants				
Early Assurance Program	0	0	0	0
Early Decision Program	0	0	0	0
Baccalaureate/MD	n/a	n/a	n/a	n/a
MD/PhD	8	0	22	30
Matriculated	181	30	8	**219**

Applications accepted from International Applicants: Yes

Matriculant Demographics: 2007–2008 First Year Class

Men: 115   **Women:** 104

Matriculants' Self-Reported Race/Ethnicity

Mexican American	26	**Korean**	3
Cuban	2	**Vietnamese**	7
Puerto Rican	4	**Other Asian**	20
Other Hispanic	8	**Total Asian**	76
Total Hispanic	40	**Native American**	1
Chinese	20	**Black**	18
Asian Indian	22	**Native Hawaiian**	0
Pakistani	6	**White**	105
Filipino	0	**Unduplicated Number**	
Japanese	1	**of Matriculants**	219

Science and Math Majors: 65%
Matriculants with:
    Baccalaureate degree: 84%
    Graduate degree(s): 5%

Specialty Choice

2003, 2004, 2005 Graduates, Specialty Choice (As reported by program directors to GME Track™)	
Anesthesiology	5%
Emergency Medicine	5%
Family Practice	8%
Internal Medicine	22%
Obstetrics/Gynecology	6%
Orthopaedic Surgery	3%
Pediatrics	12%
Psychiatry	3%
Radiology	8%
Surgery	8%

Financial Information

Source: 2006–2007 LCME I-B survey and 2007–2008 AAMC TSF questionnaire

	Residents	Non-Residents
Total Cost of Attendance	$33,981	$47,081
Tuition and Fees	$12,594	$25,694
Other (includes living expenses)	$20,268	$20,268
Health Insurance (can be waived)	$1,119	$1,119

Average 2007 Graduate Indebtedness: $86,056
% of Enrolled Students Receiving Aid: 85%

Criminal Background Check

This medical school requires a criminal background check prior to matriculation.

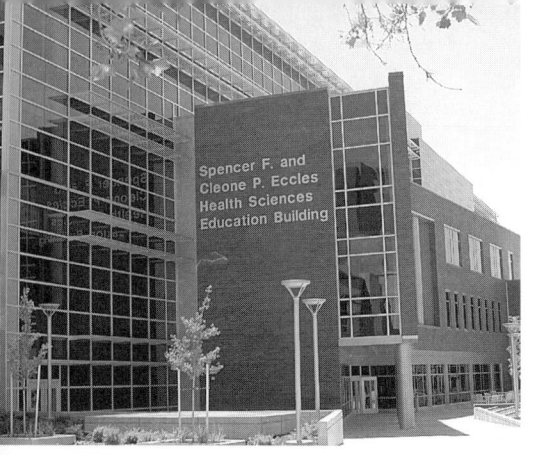

University of Utah
School of Medicine
Salt Lake City, Utah

Office of Admissions
University of Utah School of Medicine
30 North 1900 East Room 1C029
Salt Lake City, Utah 84132-2101
T 801 581 7498   F 801 581 2931

Admissions http://medicine.utah.edu/admissions/
Main http://medicine.utah.edu/
Financial http://medicine.utah.edu/financialaid/
Email deans.admissions@hsc.utah.edu

Public Institution

Dr. David J. Bjorkman, Dean

Dr. Wayne M. Samuelson, Associate Dean for Admissions

Dr. Edward Junkins, Assistant Dean for Diversity & Community Outreach

Dr. A. Lorris Betz, Senior Vice President for Health Sciences, Executive Dean

General Information

A minimum of 75 positions are offered to Utah residents. The school contracts with the State of Idaho to accept eight Idaho residents each year. Approximately 19 positions are offered to nonresidents. Applicants must have ties to Utah or be specifically recognized as a member of a population group underrepresented in the physician workforce. (Africans and African Americans, American Indians, Alaska Natives, Chamorros, Polynesians including Native Hawaiians, Tongans, Samoans, Filipinos, Tahitians, Maoris, Fijians, Niueans, Palauans; Chicanos/as and Latinos/as including Puerto Ricans, Mexican Americans, Central Americans and South Americans), or apply to the M.D./Ph.D. program. M.D./Ph.D. applicants must be U.S. citizens or U.S. permanent residents. Application may be made for three consecutive years. Applicants who have been dismissed from, or on probation or under suspension at, another medical school will not be considered. Transfers are not available unless the transferring student meets all of the following criteria: must be the spouse of a medical school faculty member or of a person accepted into one of the School of Medicine's postgraduate training programs; must be enrolled and in good standing in the third year at a fully LCME-accredited U.S. or Canadian medical school; must have taken Step 1 of the USMLE. The school does not discriminate with respect to applicants' age, color, gender, sexual orientation, race, national origin, religion, status as a person with a disability, or status as a veteran or a disabled veteran. The University of Utah provides reasonable accommodation to known disabilities of applicants.

Mission Statement

The School of Medicine has three major missions: education, research, and clinical service. The three missions are closely interrelated. Each supports and, in turn, benefits from the others. All are considered to be of equal importance.

Curricular Highlights

Community Service Requirement: Optional.
Research/Thesis Requirement: Optional.

The four years of formal medical education constitute but a brief introduction to a broad, deep, and rapidly changing discipline. The mastery of medical knowledge and technical skills requires lifelong self-education. The curriculum is designed to provide students with the knowledge, skills and attitudes necessary to practice medicine.

USMLE

Step 1: Required. Students must record a passing score for promotion.
Step 2: Clinical Skills (CS): Required. Students must record a passing total score to graduate.
Step 2: Clinical Knowledge (CK): Required. Students must record a passing total score to graduate.

Selection Factors

The school's goal is to select the most capable students who will excel in the art and science of medicine. A diverse student body promotes an atmosphere of creativity, experimentation, and discussion that is conducive to learning. Exposure to a variety of perspectives and experiences prepares students to care for patients in every segment of society. The Admissions Committee considers how the applicant balances outside activities and responsibilities with schoolwork to be an indicator of ability to deal with the rigors of life as a physician. The committee is interested in applicants' motivation for attending medical school and their understanding of the medical profession. Commitment to service, ethics, compassion, leadership ability, and communication skills are important characteristics of physicians. Applicants with a science, nonscience, or overall GPA below 3.0 will not

be considered. The minimum score for each section of the MCAT® is 7. If the test is taken more than once within three years of application, the best score for each section will be considered.

Financial Aid

In addition to federal loans, a limited number of institutional loans and scholarships are available. All awards are based on need. Financial aid supplements the contribution of the student and/or family, who are expected to provide the maximum assistance possible.

Information about Diversity Programs

The Office of Diversity and Community Outreach assists in recruiting and graduating a diverse student body. The office presents a series of pre-college and premedical educational outreach programs throughout the state.

Campus Information

Setting

The medical school is situated on the east bench of the Salt Lake Valley with the Wasatch Mountains as a backdrop. Public transportation connects the school with downtown Salt Lake City and surrounding areas.

Enrollment

For 2007, total enrollment was: 414

Special Features

University Hospital is home to many centers and clinics that provide research and specialized care to patients from all over the world.

Housing

Housing is available on and off campus.

Satellite Campuses/Facilities

Rotations are performed at University, VA, and Intermountain Healthcare hospitals including Children's Medical Center. Primary care rotations may be in community settings.

Application Process and Requirements 2009–2010

Primary Application Service: AMCAS
Earliest filing date: June 1, 2008
Latest filing date: November 1, 2008

Secondary Application Required?: Yes
Sent to: Screened applicants
Email: deans.admissions@hsc.utah.edu
Fee: Yes, $100
Fee waiver available: Yes
Earliest filing date: August 2008
Latest filing date: January 2009

Latest MCAT® considered: 2008
Oldest MCAT® considered: 2006

Early Decision Program
School does not have EDP
Applicants notified: n/a
EDP available for: n/a

Regular Acceptance Notice
Earliest date: October 15, 2008
Latest date: Until class is full

Applicant's Response to Acceptance
Offer – Maximum Time: Two weeks

Requests for Deferred
Entrance Considered: Yes

Deposit to Hold Place in Class: Yes
Deposit (Resident): $100
Deposit (Non-Resident): $100
Deposit due: With response to acceptance offer
Applied to tuition: Yes
Deposit refundable: Yes
Refundable by: May 15, 2009

Estimated number of new entrants: 102
EDP: 0, special program: n/a

Start Month/Year: August 2009

Interview Format: Each applicant will have two interviews. Regional interviews available for Idaho applicants.

Other Programs

PREPARATORY PROGRAMS
Postbaccalaureate Program: No
Summer Program: No

COMBINED DEGREE PROGRAMS
Baccalaureate/MD: No
MD/MPH: Yes
http://uuhsc.utah.edu/dfpm/phgroups
MD/MBA: No
MD/JD: No
MD/PhD: Yes
http://uuhsc.med.utah.edu/som/education/mdphd

Premedical Coursework

Course	Req.	Rec.	Lab.	Sems.	Course	Req.	Rec.	Lab.	Sems.
Inorganic Chemistry	•		•	2	Genetics		•		1
Behavioral Sciences		•		1	Humanities	•			1
Biochemistry		•		1	Organic Chemistry	•		•	2
Biology	•			2	Physics	•		•	2
Biology/Zoology		•		1	Psychology		•		1
Calculus		•		1	Social Sciences	•			1
College English	•			2	Diversity	•			1
College Mathematics		•		1	Anatomy		•		1
Computer Science					Cellular Biology		•		1

Selection Factors: 2007 Accepted Applicants

Proportion of Accepted Applicants with Relevant Experience (Data Self-Reported to AMCAS®)		
Community Service/Volunteer		87%
Medically-Related Work		90%
Research		97%

Shaded bar represents accepted scores ranging from the 10th percentile to the 90th percentile. School Median ● National Median ●

Overall GPA	2.0	2.1	2.2	2.3	2.4	2.5	2.6	2.7	2.8	2.9	3.0	3.1	3.2	3.3	3.4	3.5	3.6	(3.7)	3.8	3.9	4.0
Science GPA	2.0	2.1	2.2	2.3	2.4	2.5	2.6	2.7	2.8	2.9	3.0	3.1	3.2	3.3	3.4	3.5	(3.6)	3.7	3.8	3.9	4.0

MCAT® required: Yes, 100% of 2007 accepted applicants took MCAT®

Verbal Reasoning	3	4	5	6	7	8	9	(10)	11	12	13	14	15
Physical Sciences	3	4	5	6	7	8	(9)	10	(11)	12	13	14	15
Biological Sciences	3	4	5	6	7	8	9	(10)	(11)	12	13	14	15
Writing Sample				J	K	L	M	N	O	(P)	(Q)	R	S	T

Acceptance & Matriculation Data for 2007–2008 First Year Class

	Resident	Non-Resident	International	Total
Applied	414	823	33	1270
Interviewed	284	190	0	474
Deferred	1	1	0	2
Matriculants				
Early Assurance Program	0	0	0	0
Early Decision Program	0	0	0	0
Baccalaureate/MD	n/a	n/a	n/a	n/a
MD/PhD	0	2	0	2
Matriculated	75	25	2	**102**

Applications accepted from International Applicants: Yes

Matriculant Demographics: 2007–2008 First Year Class

Men: 70 **Women:** 32

Matriculants' Self-Reported Race/Ethnicity

Mexican American	0	Korean	4
Cuban	0	Vietnamese	1
Puerto Rican	1	Other Asian	2
Other Hispanic	2	Total Asian	19
Total Hispanic	3	Native American	0
Chinese	5	Black	0
Asian Indian	3	Native Hawaiian	0
Pakistani	1	White	82
Filipino	1	Unduplicated Number	
Japanese	3	of Matriculants	102

Science and Math Majors: 68%
Matriculants with:
Baccalaureate degree: 100%
Graduate degree(s): 13%

Specialty Choice

2003, 2004, 2005 Graduates, Specialty Choice (As reported by program directors to GME Track™)	
Anesthesiology	11%
Emergency Medicine	11%
Family Practice	11%
Internal Medicine	10%
Obstetrics/Gynecology	3%
Orthopaedic Surgery	3%
Pediatrics	14%
Psychiatry	2%
Radiology	3%
Surgery	6%

Financial Information

Source: 2006–2007 LCME I-B survey and 2007–2008 AAMC TSF questionnaire

	Residents	Non-Residents
Total Cost of Attendance	$37,480	$55,316
Tuition and Fees	$20,692	$38,528
Other (includes living expenses)	$16,788	$16,788
Health Insurance (can be waived)	$0	$0

Average 2007 Graduate Indebtedness: $123,335
% of Enrolled Students Receiving Aid: 96%

Criminal Background Check

This medical school requires a criminal background check prior to matriculation.

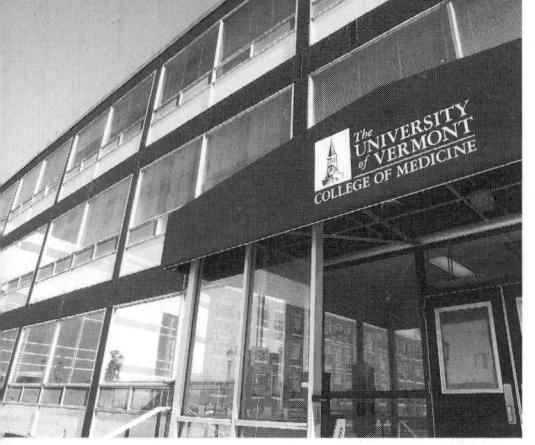

University of Vermont College of Medicine

Burlington, Vermont

The University of Vermont College of Medicine
Office of Admissions, E215 Given Building
89 Beaumont Avenue
Burlington, Vermont 05405
T 802 656 2154   **F** 802 656 9663

Admissions www.med.uvm.edu/Admissions
Main www.med.uvm.edu
Financial www.uvm.edu/financialaid
Email medadmissions@uvm.edu

Public Institution

Dr. Frederick C. Morin, III Dean

Dr. Janice M. Gallant, Associate Dean for Admissions

Dr. Karen Richardson-Nassif, Associate Dean for Faculty and Staff Development and Diversity

Dr. G. Scott Waterman, Associate Dean for Student Affairs

Tiffany Delaney, Director of Admissions

Jeffrey Wallin, Financial Aid Officer

General Information

The University of Vermont College of Medicine is located in Burlington, Vermont, (pop. 40,000). Established in 1822, it is the seventh oldest medical school in the U.S. The education of students remains the principal mission of the College, with teaching hospital partner Fletcher Allen Health Care, adjacent to the College in Burlington. A 100,000 square foot Medical Education Center and Ambulatory Care Center opened in Fall 2005 to serve the College's 400 medical students, 275 residents, and support care for a population base of over 1 million people.

Mission Statement

The overarching goal of our educational program is to provide our students with a knowledge base that will allow them to practice the science and art of medicine in a framework that offers a foundation for lifelong learning.

Curricular Highlights

Community Service Requirement: Optional.
Research/Thesis Requirement: Optional.

The Vermont Integrated Curriculum (VIC) progresses from the study of Foundations of Medicine, both clinical and basic science, to applications in Clinical Clerkship, to senior scholarship and supervised patient management in Advanced Integration. Areas of focus include progressive skill development, health care systems, preventive care, and a greater understanding of applied sciences, particularly genetics, ethics and epidemiology. VIC also places emphasis on professionalism, cultural

competency, scholarly research, teaching skills, and community service.

USMLE

Step 1: Required. Students must record a passing score for graduation, but not promotion.
Step 2: Clinical Skills (CS): Required. Students must record a passing total score to graduate.
Step 2: Clinical Knowledge (CK): Required. Students must record a passing total score to graduate.

Selection Factors

The Committee on Admissions seeks a diverse student body. We look for evidence of excellence accompanied by genuine concern for the welfare of others. Effective interpersonal skills are important, and successful applicants often have a history of service to the community. Selection is based upon a past pattern of academic performance plus an assessment of the applicant's fitness for the study and practice of medicine in terms of aptitude, interests, experience, motivation, leadership abilities, and maturity. Letters of recommendation and a personal interview are required and form an important part of the application process. Students from groups underrepresented in medicine are encouraged to apply. The University of Vermont does not discriminate on the basis of race, color, sex, sexual orientation, religion, age, handicap, national origin, or Vietnam veteran status.

Financial Aid

Financial aid funds are distributed according to relative need for both in and out-of-state students. Entering students are considered for awards on the same basis as those already enrolled. An applicant's financial status has no bearing on the admission determination. All in-state students with financial need are eligible to apply for a $10,000 per year Freeman Scholarship designed to encourage UVM medical graduates to practice in Vermont.

Information about Diversity Programs

The College of Medicine strongly encourages applications from those who have the potential to increase the overall diversity of the class

based on a variety of factors such as economic hardship, first generation college graduates, race, and cultural background.

Campus Information

Setting

Located in Burlington, the University of Vermont College of Medicine, in partnership with Fletcher Allen Health Care, comprises the only academic medical center in the state. Burlington is a vibrant community located on the shores of Lake Champlain, between the Adirondack and Green Mountains. With year-round recreational opportunities, this progressive community has been frequently cited as one of the most livable cities in the U.S. Boston and New York are both within a half-day's drive, and Montreal is just 100 miles north of campus.

Enrollment

For 2007, total enrollment was: 404

Special Features

The University of Vermont College of Medicine is one of only 14 academic medical centers with both a Comprehensive Cancer Center and a General Clinical Research Center.

Housing

While the college does offer limited campus housing options, the majority of medical students find rooms, apartments or houses in the surrounding area via a housing list maintained by the college. Many housing opportunities are within easy walking or bicycling distance from campus.

Satellite Campuses/Facilities

Students have the opportunity to serve clinical rotations in Maine (at the Maine Medical Center in Portland) as well as practice sites in Vermont.

Application Process and Requirements 2009–2010

Primary Application Service: AMCAS
Earliest filing date: June 1, 2008
Latest filing date: November 1, 2008

Secondary Application Required?: Yes
Sent to: All Applicants
Contact: Admissions Office
(802) 656-2154, medadmissions@uvm.edu
Fee: Yes, $85
Fee waiver available: Yes
Earliest filing date: June 15, 2008
Latest filing date: December 30, 2008

Latest MCAT® considered: September 2008
Oldest MCAT® considered: 2005

Early Decision Program
School does have EDP
Applicants notified: October 1, 2008
EDP available for: Both Residents
and Non-Residents

Regular Acceptance Notice
Earliest date: October 16, 2008
Latest date: Until class is full

Applicant's Response to Acceptance
Offer – Maximum Time: Two weeks

Requests for Deferred
Entrance Considered: Yes

Deposit to Hold Place in Class: Yes
Deposit (Resident): $100
Deposit (Non-Resident): $100
Deposit due: With response to acceptance offer
Applied to tuition: Yes
Deposit refundable: Yes
Refundable by: May 15, 2009

Estimated number of new entrants: 110
EDP: 4, special program: 4

Start Month/Year: August 2009

Interview Format: Campus interview with
admissions committee member. Regional
interviews are not available.

Other Programs

PREPARATORY PROGRAMS
Postbaccalaureate Program: Yes
http://learn.uvm.edu/?Page=postbac.html

COMBINED DEGREE PROGRAMS
Baccalaureate/MD: No
MD/MPH: No
MD/MBA: No
MD/JD: No
MD/PhD: Yes, www.med.uvm.edu/mdphd

Premedical Coursework

Course	Req.	Rec.	Lab.	Hrs.
Inorganic Chemistry	•		•	8
Behavioral Sciences		•		
Biochemistry		•		4
Biology	•		•	8
Biology/Zoology				
Calculus				
College English		•		
College Mathematics		•		

Course	Req.	Rec.	Lab.	Hrs.
Computer Science				
Genetics		•		4
Humanities		•		
Organic Chemistry	•		•	8
Physics	•		•	8
Psychology				
Social Sciences		•		
Other				

Selection Factors: 2007 Accepted Applicants

Proportion of Accepted Applicants with Relevant Experience (Data Self-Reported to AMCAS®)		
Community Service/Volunteer		70%
Medically-Related Work		89%
Research		79%

Shaded bar represents accepted scores ranging from the 10th percentile to the 90th percentile. School Median ● National Median ●

Overall GPA	2.0	2.1	2.2	2.3	2.4	2.5	2.6	2.7	2.8	2.9	3.0	3.1	3.2	3.3	3.4	3.5	3.6	(3.7)	3.8	3.9	4.0
Science GPA	2.0	2.1	2.2	2.3	2.4	2.5	2.6	2.7	2.8	2.9	3.0	3.1	3.2	3.3	3.4	3.5	3.6	(3.7)	3.8	3.9	4.0

MCAT® required: Yes, 100% of 2007 accepted applicants took MCAT®

Verbal Reasoning	3	4	5	6	7	8	9	(10)	11	12	13	14	15
Physical Sciences	3	4	5	6	7	8	9	(10)	(11)	12	13	14	15
Biological Sciences	3	4	5	6	7	8	9	(10)	(11)	12	13	14	15
Writing Sample			J	K	L	M	N	O	P	(Q)	R	S	T

Acceptance & Matriculation Data for 2007–2008 First Year Class

	Resident	Non-Resident	International	Total
Applied	102	5626	373	6101
Interviewed	74	478	20	572
Deferred	3	2	0	5
Matriculants				
Early Assurance Program	n/a	n/a	n/a	n/a
Early Decision Program	3	0	0	3
Baccalaureate/MD	n/a	n/a	n/a	n/a
MD/PhD	2	12	1	15
Matriculated	34	72	6	**112**

Applications accepted from International Applicants: Yes

Specialty Choice

2003, 2004, 2005 Graduates, Specialty Choice (As reported by program directors to GME Track™)	
Anesthesiology	7%
Emergency Medicine	11%
Family Practice	7%
Internal Medicine	17%
Obstetrics/Gynecology	6%
Orthopaedic Surgery	2%
Pediatrics	15%
Psychiatry	3%
Radiology	6%
Surgery	7%

Matriculant Demographics: 2007–2008 First Year Class

Men: 54 **Women:** 58

Matriculants' Self-Reported Race/Ethnicity

Mexican American	1	Korean	3
Cuban	1	Vietnamese	4
Puerto Rican	2	Other Asian	0
Other Hispanic	2	Total Asian	16
Total Hispanic	6	Native American	0
Chinese	6	Black	3
Asian Indian	0	Native Hawaiian	0
Pakistani	0	White	85
Filipino	0	Unduplicated Number	
Japanese	4	of Matriculants	112

Science and Math Majors: 58%
Matriculants with:
   Baccalaureate degree: 100%
   Graduate degree(s): 14%

Financial Information

Source: 2006–2007 LCME I-B survey
and 2007–2008 AAMC TSF questionnaire

	Residents	Non-Residents
Total Cost of Attendance	$45,420	$64,960
Tuition and Fees	$27,143	$46,243
Other (includes living expenses)	$18,277	$18,717
Health Insurance (can be waived)	$0	$0

Average 2007 Graduate Indebtedness: $145,409
% of Enrolled Students Receiving Aid: 96%

Criminal Background Check

This medical school requires a criminal background check
prior to matriculation.

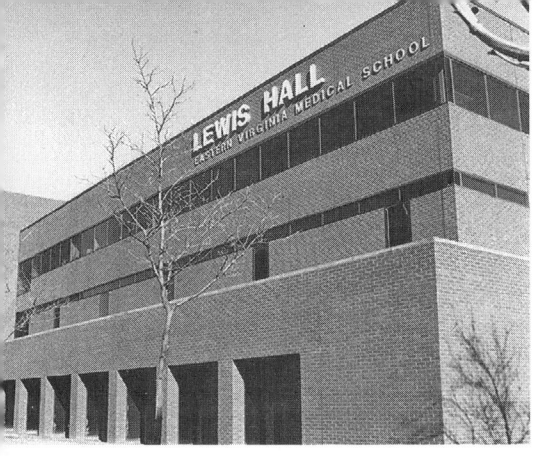

Eastern Virginia Medical School
Norfolk, Virginia

Office of Admissions
Eastern Virginia Medical School
700 W. Olney Road
Norfolk, Virginia 23507-1607
T 757 446 5812   F 757 446 5896

Admissions www.evms.edu/admissions
Main www.evms.edu
Financial www.evms.edu/students/
fin-aid/budgets/md.html
Email nanezkf@evms.edu

Private Institution

Dr. Gerald J. Pepe, Dean and Provost

*Dr. Michael J. Solhaug,
Associate Dean for Admissions*

Susan L. Castora, Director of Admissions

*Gail C. Williams, Assistant Dean for Student
Affairs and Director of Minority Affairs*

Michelle D. Byers, Director of Financial Aid

General Information
Established in 1973 to enhance the quality and diversity of health care throughout the Hampton Roads region, the mission of EVMS is deeply rooted in the education and training of primary care physicians, arming them with the requisite scientific, academic, and humanistic skills most relevant to today's practice of medicine. EVMS provides health care for more than one quarter of Virginia's population as well as neighboring regions of North Carolina.

Mission Statement
EVMS is a private community-based academic institution dedicated to medical and health education, biomedical research, and the enhancement of health care in the Commonwealth of Virginia.

Curricular Highlights
Community Service Requirement: Optional.
Research/Thesis Requirement: Optional.

The first two years focus on clinical medicine through two vehicles: the Theresa A. Thomas Professional Skills Teaching and Assessment Center and a Longitudinal Mentorship with a generalist physician in community practice. Careful coordination between basic sciences and generalist disciplines permits an integrated curriculum. Weekly small-group sessions introduce students to clinical problem-solving. This early introduction to clinical medicine teaches medical history-taking and physical examination along with the application of basic science knowledge to patient care. Third-year clinical clerkships focus on ambulatory care in community-based sites in balance with inpatient care experiences.

In addition to the required clerkships are rotations in substance abuse, geriatrics, and surgical subspecialties. For those interested in generalist medicine, electives are offered in special populations and rural health care, and an elective honors track in generalist medicine. Elective opportunities are available for those interested in research or subspecialty care. Students are graded as Honors, High Pass, Pass, or Fail.

USMLE
Step 1: Required. Students must record a passing score for graduation, but not promotion.
Step 2: Clinical Skills (CS): Required. Students must record a passing total score to graduate.
Step 2: Clinical Knowledge (CK): Required. Students must record a passing total score to graduate.

Selection Factors
EVMS does not discriminate on the basis of sex, race, creed, age, national origin, marital status, or handicap. A supplementary application packet is sent to those applicants receiving a favorable initial screening of their completed AMCAS application. The Admissions Committee considers the entire academic record, including science and overall GPA, MCAT® scores, exposure to the medical field, maturity, character, and motivation. The application fee will be waived if a fee waiver is granted by AMCAS. Preference is given to legal residents of Virginia. EVMS seeks persons with personal and background traits that indicate a high potential for becoming a primary care physician. Applicants who have completed one or more years in a medical school accredited by the LCME can be considered for transfer into the second or third year only to fill vacancies that may arise with the withdrawal of previously enrolled students. All transfers must meet the requirements stated for general admission.

Financial Aid
Scholarships are limited. Loans constitute the majority of aid received. Students may fully meet the costs of medical school at EVMS, providing they meet all federal criteria, meet citizenship requirements, are creditworthy, and maintain satisfactory academic progress. Federal scholarships are available for those interested in primary

care. The Tuition Assistance Grant Program provides annual grants for state residents. Applicants for financial assistance must file the FAFSA and other additional required forms.

Information about Diversity Programs
EVMS is committed to producing a diverse physician workforce to meet the health care needs of the region. Applicants from rural or other underserved regions and those who have been disadvantaged or underrepresented for economic, racial, or social reasons, and who possess the motivation and aptitude required for the study of medicine, are strongly encouraged to apply.

Campus Information
Setting
The EVMS complex includes the Children's Hospital of the King's Daughters and Sentara Norfolk General Hospital. The campus is minutes from downtown shopping areas and cultural attractions.

Enrollment
For 2007, total enrollment was: 448

Special Features
EVMS has numerous Centers of Excellence including the world-renowned Jones Institute for Reproductive Medicine, the Strelitz Diabetes Institute, and the Glennan Center for Geriatric Medicine. The Theresa A. Thomas Professional Skills Teaching and Assessment Center is a leader in the use and training of standardized patients for assessing medical competencies of our students and residents, as well as those from institutes around the world.

Housing
EVMS's Hague Club Apartments offers one-and two-bedroom apartments. Additional housing is located in nearby neighborhoods.

Satellite Campuses/Facilities
EVMS partners with 33 local area hospitals, including Sentara Norfolk General Hospital, the Children's Hospital of the King's Daughters, the U.S. Naval Medical Center in Portsmouth, and the Veterans Affairs Hospital in Hampton.

Application Process and Requirements 2009–2010

Primary Application Service: AMCAS
Earliest filing date: June 1, 2008
Latest filing date: November 15, 2008

Secondary Application Required?: Yes
Sent to: Screened applicants
URL: www.evms.edu/admissions
Fee: Yes, $100
Fee waiver available: Yes
Earliest filing date: July 2008
Latest filing date: January 2009

Latest MCAT® considered: September 2008
Oldest MCAT® considered: 2006

Early Decision Program
School does have EDP
Applicants notified: October 1, 2008
EDP available for: Both Residents and Non-Residents

Regular Acceptance Notice
Earliest date: October 15, 2008
Latest date: Until class is full

Applicant's Response to Acceptance Offer – Maximum Time: Two weeks

Requests for Deferred Entrance Considered: Yes

Deposit to Hold Place in Class: Yes
Deposit (Resident): $100
Deposit (Non-Resident): $100
Deposit due: With response to acceptance offer
Applied to tuition: Yes
Deposit refundable: Yes
Refundable by: May 15, 2009

Estimated number of new entrants: 115
EDP: 2, special program: n/a

Start Month/Year: August 2009

Interview Format: Panel interviews. Regional interviews are not available.

Other Programs

PREPARATORY PROGRAMS
Postbaccalaureate Program: Yes, www.evms.edu/hlthprof/ms-bio-medical/index.html
Summer Program: No

COMBINED DEGREE PROGRAMS
Baccalaureate/MD: Yes
MD/MPH: Yes, www.evms.edu/education/joint-md-mph.htm
MD/MBA: No
MD/JD: No
MD/PhD: No

Premedical Coursework

Course	Req.	Rec.	Lab.	Sems.	Course	Req.	Rec.	Lab.	Sems.
Inorganic Chemistry	•		•	2	Computer Science				
Behavioral Sciences					Genetics				
Biochemistry					Humanities				
Biology	•		•	2	Organic Chemistry	•		•	2
Biology/Zoology					Physics	•		•	2
Calculus					Psychology				
College English					Social Sciences				
College Mathematics					Other				

Selection Factors: 2007 Accepted Applicants

Proportion of Accepted Applicants with Relevant Experience (Data Self-Reported to AMCAS)		
Community Service/Volunteer		70%
Medically-Related Work		89%
Research		78%

Shaded bar represents accepted scores ranging from the 10th percentile to the 90th percentile. School Median ● National Median ●

Overall GPA	2.0	2.1	2.2	2.3	2.4	2.5	2.6	2.7	2.8	2.9	3.0	3.1	3.2	3.3	3.4	3.5	(3.6)	3.7	3.8	3.9	4.0
Science GPA	2.0	2.1	2.2	2.3	2.4	2.5	2.6	2.7	2.8	2.9	3.0	3.1	3.2	3.3	3.4	(3.5)	3.6	3.7	3.8	3.9	4.0

MCAT® required: Yes, 99% of 2007 accepted applicants took MCAT®

Verbal Reasoning	3	4	5	6	7	8	9	(10)	11	12	13	14	15
Physical Sciences	3	4	5	6	7	8	9	(10)	(11)	12	13	14	15
Biological Sciences	3	4	5	6	7	8	9	10	(11)	12	13	14	15
Writing Sample			J	K	L	M	N	O	(P)	(Q)	R	S	T

Acceptance & Matriculation Data for 2007–2008 First Year Class

	Resident	Non-Resident	International	Total
Applied	741	3903	251	4895
Interviewed	336	274	14	624
Deferred	5	0	0	5
Matriculants				
Early Assurance Program	n/a	n/a	n/a	n/a
Early Decision Program	1	0	0	1
Baccalaureate/MD	8	4	0	12
MD/PhD	n/a	n/a	n/a	n/a
Matriculated	72	38	5	**115**

Applications accepted from International Applicants: Yes

Matriculant Demographics: 2007–2008 First Year Class

Men: 53   **Women:** 62

Matriculants' Self-Reported Race/Ethnicity

Mexican American	1	Korean	3
Cuban	0	Vietnamese	2
Puerto Rican	0	Other Asian	3
Other Hispanic	0	Total Asian	24
Total Hispanic	1	Native American	1
Chinese	5	Black	6
Asian Indian	7	Native Hawaiian	0
Pakistani	2	White	81
Filipino	1	Unduplicated Number	
Japanese	2	of Matriculants	115

Science and Math Majors: 68%
Matriculants with:
Baccalaureate degree: 99%
Graduate degree(s): 31%

Specialty Choice

2003, 2004, 2005 Graduates, Specialty Choice
(As reported by program directors to GME Track™)

Anesthesiology	5%
Emergency Medicine	9%
Family Practice	9%
Internal Medicine	18%
Obstetrics/Gynecology	5%
Orthopaedic Surgery	2%
Pediatrics	15%
Psychiatry	3%
Radiology	5%
Surgery	6%

Financial Information

Source: 2006–2007 LCME I-B survey and 2007–2008 AAMC TSF questionnaire

	Residents	Non-Residents
Total Cost of Attendance	$42,345	$61,541
Tuition and Fees	$24,204	$43,400
Other (includes living expenses)	$15,764	$15,764
Health Insurance (can be waived)	$2,377	$2,377

Average 2007 Graduate Indebtedness: $162,255
% of Enrolled Students Receiving Aid: 92%

Criminal Background Check

This medical school requires a criminal background check prior to matriculation.

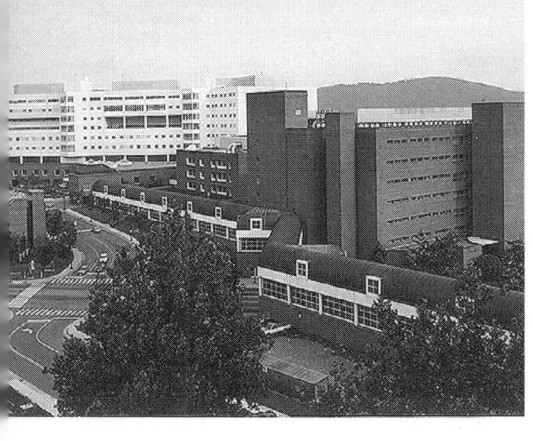

University of Virginia School of Medicine

Charlottesville, Virginia

Medical School Admissions Office
PO Box 800725
University of Virginia School of Medicine
Charlottesville, Virginia 22908
T 434 924 5571   F 434 982 2586

Admissions www.healthsystem.virginia.edu/
internet/admissions
Main www.healthsystem.virginia.edu/internet/som
Financial www.healthsystem.virginia.edu/internet/financial-aid
Email medsch-adm@virginia.edu

Public Institution

Dr. Sharon L. Hostler, Interim Vice President and Dean, School of Medicine

Dr. R.J. Canterbury, Associate Dean for Admissions

Dr. Norm Oliver, Associate Dean for Diversity

Nancy Zimmer, Director of Financial Aid

Lesley L. Thomas, Director of Admissions

General Information

The University of Virginia School of Medicine was opened for instruction in 1825, making it one of the oldest medical schools in the South. Both the School of Medicine and the University of Virginia Hospital are located on the grounds of the University of Virginia in Charlottesville.

Mission Statement

The mission of the University of Virginia School of Medicine is: to educate students to fulfill the need for practitioners and scientists; to provide cost-effective, high-quality patient care at primary, secondary, and tertiary levels; to produce new knowledge required to advance health by conducting research; and, to provide public service as needed by citizens or by public jurisdictions.

Curricular Highlights

Community Service Requirement: Required. Community service learning activities in Year 1.
Research/Thesis Requirement: Optional. A thesis is required for Generalist Scholars only.

The University of Virginia curriculum integrates scientific knowledge, clinical care, and research throughout the entire four years of medical school. The cornerstone of the curriculum is clinical problem solving with the focus on the patient and the physician-patient relationship. Lectures (never more than half a day), self-study from course syllabi and computer-aided instruction provide the factual content necessary for problem solving. Students have three or four afternoons free each week in years 1 and 2 for productive self-study or elective activities. Small-group activities maximize interactions between students and faculty. Basic science concepts are presented in the

context of clinical cases. The Practice of Medicine course in years 1 and 2 teaches professionalism, interviewing skills, physical diagnosis, and ethics in small groups. The elective program of the fourth year offers students the opportunity to pursue their own interests. An innovative clerkship model allows students to tailor their clinical experience to meet their particular interests and needs. Students may choose from a wide variety of electives, including clinical experience, graduate courses, and research activities.

USMLE

Step 1: Required. Students must record a passing score for promotion.
Step 2: Clinical Skills (CS): Required. Students must record a passing total score to graduate.
Step 2: Clinical Knowledge (CK): Required. Students must record a passing total score to graduate.

Selection Factors

All applicants must have completed at least 90 semester hours of course work in a U.S. or Canadian college or university. The Committee on Admissions does not discriminate on the basis of race, gender, sexual preference, creed, national origin, age, or disability. Grades, MCAT® scores, work and volunteer experience, letters of recommendation, and the interview influence committee decisions. The Admissions Committee does not grant regional interviews or interviews by applicant request.

Financial Aid

In addition to Federal Stafford Loans, the University of Virginia School of Medicine provides robust school-funded scholarships and loans to students who demonstrate need via the Free Application for Federal Student Aid (FAFSA). Parental financial information is required for all applicants who wish to receive aid from school funds. Student employment is not encouraged. Financial aid applications are available online at *www.healthsystem.virginia.edu/financialaid* on January 1 or immediately after acceptance. For more information, contact Ms. Nancy Zimmer, financial aid director, at (434) 924-0033.

Information about Diversity Programs

The University of Virginia encourages applications from qualified applicants from groups that are under represented in medicine. Systems in place to facilitate preparation and success of students include: (1) a six-week summer enrichment program; (2) extensive tutorial and other academic support programs upon admission; and (3) need-based and merit-based financial assistance. For more information, please contact Dr. Norm Oliver, Associate Dean for Diversity, at mno3p@virginia.edu.

Campus Information

Setting

The University of Virginia Health System is one of the nation's 100 Top Hospitals with state-of-the-art emergency, operating, and labor and delivery rooms. The medical center is located in the heart of Charlottesville, with significant historical sites located nearby, including Thomas Jefferson's Monticello.

Enrollment

For 2007, total enrollment was: 551

Special Features

The University of Virginia Health System includes the School of Medicine, the University Hospital, and other special centers of excellence, including the Heart Center, Kidney Center, Cancer Center, Transplant Center, and Primary Care Center.

Housing

While there is some limited graduate student housing available, most medical students choose to live in the community close by the medical school and hospital. There are ample housing opportunities in the area, with rents ranging from $300 to $800 per month.

Satellite Campuses/Facilities

During the third-year clinical clerkships, students will spend approximately half their time at the University Health System. They also spend an average of 20 weeks at the Roanoke Memorial Hospital in Roanoke, VA, the Salem Veterans Affairs Hospital, and the Fairfax INOVA Hospital in Fairfax, VA. Housing and meals are provided at offsite clinical locations.

Application Process and Requirements 2009–2010

Primary Application Service: AMCAS
Earliest filing date: June 1, 2008
Latest filing date: November 1, 2008

Secondary Application Required?: Yes
Sent to: All applicants
Contact: Lesley L. Thomas, J.D., (434) 924-5571
llt6p@virginia.edu
Fee: Yes, $80
Fee waiver available: Yes
Earliest filing date: June 1, 2008
Latest filing date: January 5, 2009

Latest MCAT® considered: September 2008
Oldest MCAT® considered: April 2006

Early Decision Program
School does not have EDP
Applicants notified: n/a
EDP available for: n/a

Regular Acceptance Notice
Earliest date: October 15, 2008
Latest date: Until class is full

Applicant's Response to Acceptance
Offer – Maximum Time: Three weeks

Requests for Deferred
Entrance Considered: Yes

Deposit to Hold Place in Class: No
Deposit (Resident): n/a
Deposit (Non-Resident): n/a
Deposit due: n/a
Applied to tuition: n/a
Deposit refundable: n/a
Refundable by: n/a

Estimated number of new entrants: 142
EDP: n/a, special program: n/a

Start Month/Year: August 2009

Interview Format: Two one-on-one, half-hour interviews. Regional interviews are not available.

Other Programs

PREPARATORY PROGRAMS
Postbaccalaureate Program: Yes, www.uvapostbacpremed.info
postbacpremed@virginia.edu
Summer Program: Yes, www.healthsystem. virginia.edu/internet/academic-support/maap1-A.cfm

COMBINED DEGREE PROGRAMS
Baccalaureate/MD: No
MD/MPH: Yes, www.healthsystem.virginia.edu/ internet/hes/mph/mph_home.cfm
MD/MBA: No
MD/JD: No
MD/PhD: Yes, www.healthsystem.virginia.edu/internet/mstp/
Additional Program: Yes, www.healthsystem.virginia.edu/internet/ bio-ethics/MABioethics.cfm

Premedical Coursework

Course	Req.	Rec.	Lab.	Sems.
Inorganic Chemistry	•		•	2
Behavioral Sciences				
Biochemistry				
Biology	•		•	2
Biology/Zoology				
Calculus				
College English				
College Mathematics				

Course	Req.	Rec.	Lab.	Sems.
Computer Science				
Genetics				
Humanities				
Organic Chemistry	•		•	2
Physics	•		•	2
Psychology				
Social Sciences				
Other				

Selection Factors: 2007 Accepted Applicants

Proportion of Accepted Applicants with Relevant Experience (Data Self-Reported to AMCAS®)		
Community Service/Volunteer		71%
Medically-Related Work		91%
Research		85%

Shaded bar represents accepted scores ranging from the 10th percentile to the 90th percentile. School Median ● National Median ●

Overall GPA	2.0	2.1	2.2	2.3	2.4	2.5	2.6	2.7	2.8	2.9	3.0	3.1	3.2	3.3	3.4	3.5	3.6	3.7	(3.8)	3.9	4.0
Science GPA	2.0	2.1	2.2	2.3	2.4	2.5	2.6	2.7	2.8	2.9	3.0	3.1	3.2	3.3	3.4	3.5	3.6	3.7	(3.8)	3.9	4.0

MCAT® required: Yes, 100% of 2007 accepted applicants took MCAT®

Verbal Reasoning	3	4	5	6	7	8	9	(10)	(11)	12	13	14	15
Physical Sciences	3	4	5	6	7	8	9	10	(11)	12	13	14	15
Biological Sciences	3	4	5	6	7	8	9	10	(11)	(12)	13	14	15
Writing Sample			J	K	L	M	N	O	P	(Q)	R	S	T

Acceptance & Matriculation Data for 2007–2008 First Year Class

	Resident	Non-Resident	International	Total
Applied	723	3245	139	4107
Interviewed	186	323	25	534
Deferred	2	2	0	4
Matriculants				
Early Assurance Program	0	0	0	0
Early Decision Program	0	0	0	0
Baccalaureate/MD	n/a	n/a	n/a	n/a
MD/PhD	1	8	0	9
Matriculated	82	59	2	**143**

Applications accepted from International Applicants: Yes

Specialty Choice

2003, 2004, 2005 Graduates, Specialty Choice (As reported by program directors to GME Track™)

Anesthesiology	6%
Emergency Medicine	9%
Family Practice	9%
Internal Medicine	18%
Obstetrics/Gynecology	4%
Orthopaedic Surgery	5%
Pediatrics	11%
Psychiatry	4%
Radiology	6%
Surgery	7%

Matriculant Demographics: 2007–2008 First Year Class

Men: 74   **Women:** 69

Matriculants' Self-Reported Race/Ethnicity

Mexican American	2	Korean	6
Cuban	3	Vietnamese	2
Puerto Rican	2	Other Asian	1
Other Hispanic	5	Total Asian	28
Total Hispanic	12	Native American	0
Chinese	9	Black	8
Asian Indian	8	Native Hawaiian	1
Pakistani	2	White	105
Filipino	0	**Unduplicated Number**	
Japanese	0	**of Matriculants**	143

Science and Math Majors: 71%
Matriculants with:
Baccalaureate degree: 99%
Graduate degree(s): 6%

Financial Information

Source: 2006–2007 LCME I-B survey and 2007–2008 AAMC TSF questionnaire

	Residents	Non-Residents
Total Cost of Attendance	$50,035	$60,035
Tuition and Fees	$31,305	$41,305
Other (includes living expenses)	$16,605	$16,605
Health Insurance (not applicable)	$2,125	$2,125

Average 2007 Graduate Indebtedness: $112,634
% of Enrolled Students Receiving Aid: 90%

Criminal Background Check

This medical school requires a criminal background check prior to matriculation.

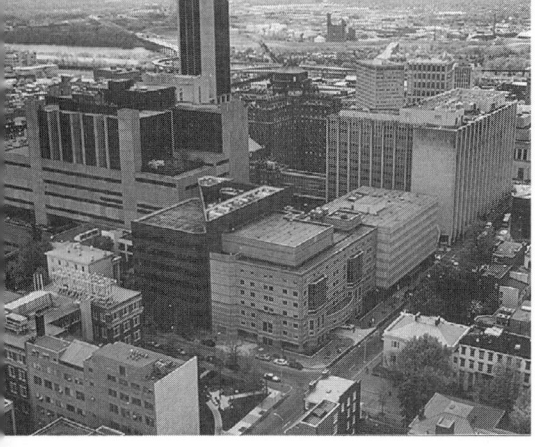

Virginia Commonwealth University
School of Medicine
Richmond, Virginia

Virginia Commonwealth University
School of Medicine
P.O. Box 980565
Richmond, Virginia 23298-0565
T 804-828-9629   **F** 804 828 1246

Admissions www.medschool.vcu.edu/prospective.html
Main www.medschool.vcu.edu
Financial www.medschool.vcu.edu/finaid/
financial.html
Email somume@vcu.edu

Public Institution

Dr. Jerome F. Strauss, III Dean

*Dr. Michelle Whitehurst-Cook,
Associate Dean for Admissions*

*Donna Jackson, Director of Student
Outreach Programs*

*Dr. Glenda Palmer, Asst. Dean of Student
Affairs/Dir. of Financial Aid*

Agnes L. Mack, Director of Admissions

General Information

The School of Medicine, which has been in continuous operation since 1838, is the founding institution of Virginia Commonwealth University. The vitality of VCU's clinical, educational, and research programs is reflected in the caliber of its faculty, the success of its patient care programs, and the level of research funding.

Mission Statement

The mission of the School of Medicine is constant improvement of the quality of health care for citizens of Virginia, using innovative, scholarly activity to create new knowledge, to provide better systems of medical education, and to develop more effective health care methods. The primary aim of the School of Medicine is to provide a diverse academic environment appropriate for the education of its students and continuing education directed toward the needs of practicing physicians.

Curricular Highlights

Community Service Requirement: Optional.
Research/Thesis Requirement: Optional.

The first year is spent studying normal structure and function in a traditional discipline format. The second year emphasizes the pathogenesis of disease and its manifestations and is taught in an organ system manner. Pathogenesis, pathology, pharmacology, and the major manifestations and principles of management are discussed in each of the major body systems. In the longitudinal clinical experience for first and second-year students, students spend two afternoons per month in a small group learning the fundamentals of clinical

medicine. This is supplemented by a clinical experience in the office of a primary care physician two afternoons per month. The clinical experience is integrated with the basic sciences in a way that enhances and enriches students' learning. There is a computer lab with over 40 workstations and a full array of commercial and in-house, faculty-developed educational software. Third-year rotations are at the University and Veterans Affairs Hospitals, with ambulatory care rotations at non-university primary care sites. A select number of students will complete the third and fourth years at the INOVA campus in Northern Virginia. The fourth year is primarily elective time.

USMLE

Step 1: Required. Students must record a passing score for graduation, but not promotion.
Step 2: Clinical Skills (CS): Required. Students must record a passing score in each section to graduate.
Step 2: Clinical Knowledge (CK): Required. Students must record a passing score in each section to graduate.

Selection Factors

Applicants are selected on the basis of their potential as prospective physicians as well as students of medicine. Attributes of character, personality factors, academic skills, and exposure to medicine are considered along with academic performance, GPA, MCAT® scores, letters of recommendation, and personal interviews at the School of Medicine.

Financial Aid

Assistance to students in meeting the cost of their medical education is available in the form of loans and scholarship. Financial counseling is done through the School of Medicine Financial Aid Office. The FAFSA (Free Application for Federal Student Aid) is required of all students who want aid. For need-based scholarship and grant aid the NeedAccess online form should be completed. This information is used to award grants from the Department of Health and Human Services and institutional need-based aid. Completion of these forms will allow the Financial Aid Office to give students an accurate

picture of what their eligibility for aid will be within 48 hours.

Information about Diversity Programs

The office of Student Outreach Programs endeavors to provide support for the school's diverse population. Student Outreach's objectives are to recruit and retain students from disadvantaged or non-traditional backgrounds to an environment conducive for exchange of ideas where students learn from faculty and peers. The main goal of the program is to provide medical school graduates that will best meet the healthcare needs of the state and nation.

Campus Information

Setting

The school is located in downtown Richmond near cultural, historical, and government centers. The medical education buildings are directly across the street from the main hospital.

Enrollment

For 2007, total enrollment was: 734

Special Features

The 750-bed MCV Hospital has both the largest ER and neonatal intensive care units in the state and is one of the largest university-owned medical centers in the U.S. This facility and the full service Veterans and Inova Fairfax Hospitals afford students an unparalleled clinical experience.

Housing

Single student housing is available on campus. Off-campus housing is plentiful, varied in style, and reasonable in cost.

Satellite Campuses/Facilities

There is a regional campus at Inova Hospital, Fairfax, VA, which is used for third and fourth-year training.

Application Process and Requirements 2009–2010

Primary Application Service: AMCAS
Earliest filing date: June 1, 2008
Latest filing date: October 15, 2008

Secondary Application Required?: Yes
Sent to: Screened applicants
Contact: Shenia Tyler
(804) 828-9629
shenia.tyler@vcu.edu
Fee: Yes, $80
Fee waiver available: Yes
Earliest filing date: June 1, 2008
Latest filing date: January 26, 2009

Latest MCAT® considered: August 2008
Oldest MCAT® considered: August 2005

Early Decision Program
School does have EDP
Applicants notified: October 1, 2008
EDP available for: Both Residents
and Non-Residents

Regular Acceptance Notice
Earliest date: October 15, 2008
Latest date: Until class is full

**Applicant's Response to Acceptance
Offer – Maximum Time:** Two weeks

**Requests for Deferred
Entrance Considered:** Yes

Deposit to Hold Place in Class: Yes
Deposit (Resident): $100
Deposit (Non-Resident): $100
Deposit due: With response to acceptance offer
Applied to tuition: Yes
Deposit refundable: Yes
Refundable by: May 15, 2009

Estimated number of new entrants: 192
EDP: 5, special program: n/a

Start Month/Year: August 2009

Interview Format: Single, one-on-one interview
Regional interviews are not available.

Other Programs

PREPARATORY PROGRAMS
Postbaccalaureate Program: Yes,
www.vcu.edu/gradweb
Summer Program: No
Prematriculation workshop: Yes,
Donna Jackson, (804) 828-9629, djackson@vcu.edu

COMBINED DEGREE PROGRAMS
Baccalaureate/MD: Yes,
www.honors.vcu.edu/
MD/MPH: Yes, http://medschool.vcu.edu/
admissions/mdmph.html
MD/MBA: No
MD/JD: No
MD/PhD: Yes, www.vcu.edu/mdphd/
Additional Program: Yes, www.had.vcu.edu

Premedical Coursework

Course	Req.	Rec.	Lab.	Sems.
Inorganic Chemistry	•		•	2
Behavioral Sciences				
Biochemistry				
Biology	•		•	2
Biology/Zoology				
Calculus				
College English	•			2
College Mathematics	•			2

Course	Req.	Rec.	Lab.	Sems.
Computer Science				
Genetics				
Humanities				
Organic Chemistry	•		•	2
Physics	•		•	2
Psychology				
Social Sciences				
Other				

Selection Factors: 2007 Accepted Applicants

Proportion of Accepted Applicants with Relevant Experience (Data Self-Reported to AMCAS)		
Community Service/Volunteer		66%
Medically-Related Work		92%
Research		78%

Shaded bar represents accepted scores ranging from the 10th percentile to the 90th percentile. School Median ● National Median ●

	2.0	2.1	2.2	2.3	2.4	2.5	2.6	2.7	2.8	2.9	3.0	3.1	3.2	3.3	3.4	3.5	3.6	3.7	3.8	3.9	4.0
Overall GPA	2.0	2.1	2.2	2.3	2.4	2.5	2.6	2.7	2.8	2.9	3.0	3.1	3.2	3.3	3.4	3.5	3.6	(3.7)	3.8	3.9	4.0
Science GPA	2.0	2.1	2.2	2.3	2.4	2.5	2.6	2.7	2.8	2.9	3.0	3.1	3.2	3.3	3.4	3.5	(3.6)	3.7	3.8	3.9	4.0

MCAT® required: Yes, 100% of 2007 accepted applicants took MCAT®

Verbal Reasoning	3	4	5	6	7	8	9	(10)	11	12	13	14	15
Physical Sciences	3	4	5	6	7	8	9	(10)	(11)	12	13	14	15
Biological Sciences	3	4	5	6	7	8	9	10	(11)	12	13	14	15
Writing Sample					J	K	L	M	N	O	(P)	(Q)	R	S	T

Acceptance & Matriculation Data for 2007–2008 First Year Class

	Resident	Non-Resident	International	Total
Applied	778	4810	75	5663
Interviewed	351	383	0	734
Deferred	4	2	0	6
Matriculants				
Early Assurance Program	0	0	0	0
Early Decision Program	2	0	0	2
Baccalaureate/MD	12	2	0	14
MD/PhD	2	5	0	7
Matriculated	104	80	0	**184**

Applications accepted from International Applicants: No

Matriculant Demographics: 2007–2008 First Year Class

Men: 96   **Women:** 88

Matriculants' Self-Reported Race/Ethnicity

Mexican American	0	Korean	4
Cuban	0	Vietnamese	4
Puerto Rican	0	Other Asian	7
Other Hispanic	3	Total Asian	50
Total Hispanic	3	Native American	1
Chinese	6	Black	9
Asian Indian	22	Native Hawaiian	1
Pakistani	4	White	123
Filipino	3	Unduplicated Number	
Japanese	1	of Matriculants	184

Science and Math Majors: 69%
Matriculants with:
    Baccalaureate degree: 100%
    Graduate degree(s): 13%

Specialty Choice

2003, 2004, 2005 Graduates, Specialty Choice (As reported by program directors to GME Track™)	
Anesthesiology	4%
Emergency Medicine	5%
Family Practice	7%
Internal Medicine	19%
Obstetrics/Gynecology	6%
Orthopaedic Surgery	2%
Pediatrics	12%
Psychiatry	3%
Radiology	7%
Surgery	7%

Financial Information

Source: 2006–2007 LCME I-B survey
and 2007–2008 AAMC TSF questionnaire

	Residents	Non-Residents
Total Cost of Attendance	$53,563	$67,233
Tuition and Fees	$27,188	$40,858
Other (includes living expenses)	$26,375	$26,375
Health Insurance (can be waived)	$0	$0

Average 2007 Graduate Indebtedness: $136,233
% of Enrolled Students Receiving Aid: 90%

Criminal Background Check

This medical school requires a criminal background check prior to matriculation.

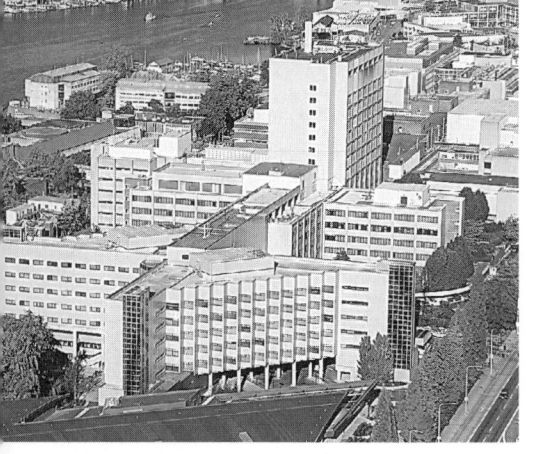

University of Washington School of Medicine

Seattle, Washington

Office of Admissions
Health Sciences Center A-300
Box 356340, University of Washington
Seattle, Washington 98195-6340
T 206 543 7212   F 206 616 3341

Admissions www.uwmedicine.org/Education/
MDProgram/Admissions
Main www.uwmedicine.org
Financial www.uwmedicine.org/Education/
MDProgram/StudentAffairsAndServices/FinancialAid
Email askuwsom@u.washington.edu

Public Institution

Dr. Paul G. Ramsey, Dean

*Dr. Carol C. Teitz, Associate Dean
for Admissions*

*Dr. David Acosta, Associate Dean
for Multicultural Affairs*

Diane Noecker, Financial Aid Officer

Patricia T. Fero, Director of Admissions

General Information

Ranked as the top medical school in training primary care physicians for 14 consecutive years, and first among public medical schools in federal research funding, the UWSOM is dedicated to improving the health of the public by advancing medical knowledge, providing outstanding primary and specialty care to people of the region, and preparing tomorrow's physicians and scientists. Among faculty are 5 Nobel Prize winners, 33 Institute of Medicine members, 30 National Academy of Science members, and 18 Howard Hughes Medicine Institute Investigators. The top-ranked programs in family medicine and rural health are enhanced by 5000 volunteer clinical faculty throughout the WWAMI region. The WWAMI program is a model of community-based training and collaboration in medical education among the states of Washington, Wyoming, Alaska, Montana, and Idaho. The UWSOM is committed to building and sustaining a diverse academic community and to assuring that access to education and training is open to all segments of society.

Mission Statement

The UWSOM has a dual mission 1) meeting the health-care needs of our region, especially by recognizing the importance of primary care and providing service to underserved populations, and 2) advancing knowledge and assuming leadership in the biomedical sciences and academic medicine.

Curricular Highlights

Community Service Requirement: Optional.
Research/Thesis Requirement: Required.

The curriculum in the first two years integrates basic sciences and clinical medicine in both discipline-based and organ-systems courses. Patient contact begins in the first year via community preceptorships and the Introduction to Clinical Medicine course, administered in a college system. The college groups consist of a faculty mentor who guides 24 students for 4 years in acquiring fundamental clinical skills including physical exam and diagnosis, case presentation and write-up, clinical reasoning, communication with patients and colleagues, and professionalism and ethics. Opportunities range from rural or underserved experiences to bench research. Problem based learning, observed standardized clinical examinations (OSCE), and special capstone courses provide transitions from 2nd to 3rd year and from 4th year to residency. Required clerkships leave ample time for electives allowing students to identify and develop diverse career interests. Opportunities are provided for a longitudinal interdisciplinary clerkship and for clerkships in communities across the WWAMI region, as well as international electives. Certificate programs include the Indian Health, Global Health, Hispanic Health and Underserved Pathways.

USMLE

Step 1: Required. Students must record a passing score for promotion.
Step 2: Clinical Skills (CS): Required. Students must record a passing total score to graduate.
Step 2: Clinical Knowledge (CK): Required. Students must record a passing total score to graduate.

Selection Factors

Candidates are considered on the basis of motivation, maturity, integrity, and academic performance. Demonstrated humanitarian qualities, community service, ability to communicate with and relate to a diverse group of individuals, as well as knowledge of issues in health care, ability to think analytically, and intellectual curiosity are important considerations. Strong preference is given to residents of the WWAMI states; less than 5% of the class is from outside the WWAMI region. Applicants with a demonstrated interest in research may apply for the M.D./Ph.D. program (MSTP) regardless of residency. Only U.S.

citizens or permanent residents are considered for either program. Competitive candidates are asked to send additional materials. Matriculation is contingent on the outcome of a criminal background check initiated upon acceptance. Candidates may apply no more than 3 times. Prerequisites are changing for the entering class of 2010.

Financial Aid

Financial status has no bearing on admissions. All applicants for aid must submit data for an analysis of need through FAFSA. Applications are available in January. The application deadline of February 28 must be met, regardless of admission status, in order to receive highest priority for aid; applicants should apply on line (*www.fafsa.ed.gov*) or mail the FAFSA form by mid-February. Most aid is in the form of loans.

Information about Diversity Programs

UWSOM is committed to recruiting, educating, and graduating students from diverse backgrounds. An applicant's background is considered diverse if his/her experience would not ordinarily be well represented in the student body.

Campus Information

Setting

Classrooms and hospitals of the UWSOM are located across five states and run the gamut from primary to tertiary care settings including a level I trauma hospital, and renowned research facilities. Cultural and recreational opportunities abound.

Enrollment

For 2007, total enrollment was: 826

Special Features

A unique aspect of the UWSOM is the WWAMI program of decentralized medical education. Students take a portion of their clinical training at sites away from the UW-Seattle campus. Offers of admission are contingent upon agreement to participate in the WWAMI program.

Housing

On-campus housing is available, but the majority of students live off-campus. Average rent $500-$800/month.

Application Process and Requirements 2009–2010

Primary Application Service: AMCAS
Earliest filing date: June 1, 2008
Latest filing date: November 3, 2008

Secondary Application Required?: Yes
Sent to: Screened applicants
URL: http://depts.washington.edu/mdadmit/secondary/
Contact: Patricia Fero
(206) 543-7212
patf@u.washington.edu
Fee: Yes, $35
Fee waiver available: Yes
Earliest filing date: July 15, 2008
Latest filing date: January 15, 2009

Latest MCAT® considered: September 2008
Oldest MCAT® considered: 2006

Early Decision Program
School does not have EDP
Applicants notified: n/a
EDP available for: n/a

Regular Acceptance Notice
Earliest date: November 1, 2008
Latest date: Until Class is Full

Applicant's Response to Acceptance Offer – Maximum Time: Two weeks before May 15, one week thereafter

Requests for Deferred Entrance Considered: Yes, under special circumstances.

Deposit to Hold Place in Class: No
Deposit (Resident): n/a
Deposit (Non-Resident): n/a
Deposit due: n/a
Applied to tuition: n/a
Deposit refundable: n/a
Refundable by: n/a

Estimated number of new entrants: 216
EDP: n/a, special program: n/a

Start Month/Year: August 2009

Interview Format: A three-member panel interviews each applicant. Only Alaska regional interviews are available.

Other Programs

PREPARATORY PROGRAMS
Postbaccalaureate Program: No
Summer Program: Yes, (206) 685-2489
http://depts.washington.edu/omca/SMDEP/
Prematriculation Program: Yes,
http://depts.washington.edu/omca/PREMAT/

COMBINED DEGREE PROGRAMS
Baccalaureate/MD: No
MD/MPH: Yes, http://depts.washington.edu/
MD/MBA: No
MD/JD: No
MD/PhD: Yes, www.mstp.washington.edu/admissions
(206) 685-0762

Premedical Coursework

Course	Req.	Rec.	Lab.	Sems.
Inorganic Chemistry				
Behavioral Sciences				
Biochemistry		•		1-2
Biology	•			2-4
Biology/Zoology				
Calculus				
College English				
College Mathematics		•		1
Computer Science				

Course	Req.	Rec.	Lab.	Sems.
Genetics		•		
Humanities		•		4
Organic Chemistry				
Physics		•		2
Psychology				
Social Sciences		•		4
Inorganic/Organic Chemistry	•			2-4
'Other' Biology/ Chemistry/Physics	•			2

Selection Factors: 2007 Accepted Applicants

Proportion of Accepted Applicants with Relevant Experience (Data Self-Reported to AMCAS®)		
Community Service/Volunteer		73%
Medically-Related Work		88%
Research		82%

Shaded bar represents accepted scores ranging from the 10th percentile to the 90th percentile. **School Median** ● **National Median** ●

Overall GPA	2.0	2.1	2.2	2.3	2.4	2.5	2.6	2.7	2.8	2.9	3.0	3.1	3.2	3.3	3.4	3.5	3.6	(3.7)	3.8	3.9	4.0
Science GPA	2.0	2.1	2.2	2.3	2.4	2.5	2.6	2.7	2.8	2.9	3.0	3.1	3.2	3.3	3.4	3.5	3.6	(3.7)	3.8	3.9	4.0

MCAT® required: Yes, 100% of 2007 accepted applicants took MCAT®

Verbal Reasoning	3	4	5	6	7	8	9	(10)	11	12	13	14	15
Physical Sciences	3	4	5	6	7	8	9	10	(11)	12	13	14	15
Biological Sciences	3	4	5	6	7	8	9	10	(11)	12	13	14	15
Writing Sample			J	K	L	M	N	O	P	(Q)	R	S	T

Acceptance & Matriculation Data for 2007-2008 First Year Class

	Resident*	Non-Resident	International	Total
Applied	1097	3422	79	4598
Interviewed	732	106	0	838
Deferred	2	0	0	2
Matriculants				
Early Assurance Program	n/a	n/a	n/a	n/a
Early Decision Program	0	0	0	0
Baccalaureate/MD	n/a	n/a	n/a	n/a
MD/PhD	3	9	0	12
Matriculated	176	15	0	**191**

Applications accepted from International Applicants: No
*Resident includes: WA, WY, AK, MT, ID

Matriculant Demographics: 2007–2008 First Year Class

Men: 89 **Women:** 102

Matriculants' Self-Reported Race/Ethnicity

Mexican American	3	Korean	3
Cuban	0	Vietnamese	2
Puerto Rican	3	Other Asian	2
Other Hispanic	5	Total Asian	24
Total Hispanic	9	Native American	2
Chinese	2	Black	2
Asian Indian	6	Native Hawaiian	0
Pakistani	1	White	168
Filipino	3	Unduplicated Number	
Japanese	6	of Matriculants	191

Science and Math Majors: 64%
Matriculants with:
Baccalaureate degree: 99%
Graduate degree(s): 7%

Specialty Choice

2003, 2004, 2005 Graduates, Specialty Choice (As reported by program directors to GME Track™)	
Anesthesiology	10%
Emergency Medicine	8%
Family Practice	15%
Internal Medicine	19%
Obstetrics/Gynecology	7%
Orthopaedic Surgery	3%
Pediatrics	10%
Psychiatry	3%
Radiology	3%
Surgery	7%

Financial Information

Source: 2006–2007 LCME I-B survey and 2007–2008 AAMC TSF questionnaire

	Residents	Non-Residents
Total Cost of Attendance	$35,648	$59,652
Tuition and Fees	$17,425	$41,429
Other (includes living expenses)	$18,223	$18,223
Health Insurance	$0	$0

Average 2007 Graduate Indebtedness: $98,283
% of Enrolled Students Receiving Aid: 90%

Criminal Background Check

This medical school requires a criminal background check prior to matriculation.

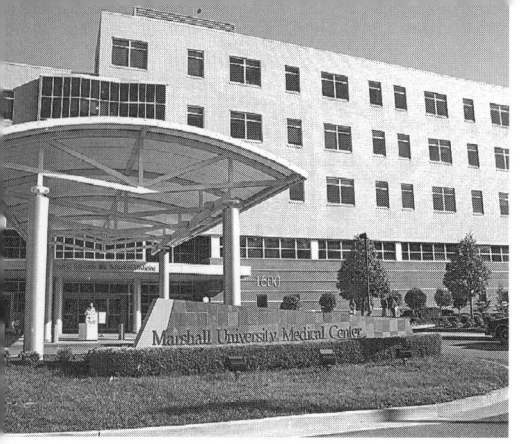

Marshall University
Joan C. Edwards School of Medicine
Huntington, West Virginia

Admissions Office, Marshall University
Joan C. Edwards School of Medicine
1600 Medical Center Drive
Huntington, West Virginia 25701-3655
T 800 544 8514   F 304 691 1744

Admissions http://musom.marshall.edu/admissions
Main http://musom.marshall.edu
Financial www.marshall.edu/sfa
Email warren@marshall.edu

Public Institution

Dr. Charles H. McKown Jr.,
Vice President and Dean

Cynthia A. Warren, Assistant Dean for
Admissions and Student Affairs

Nadine Hamrick, Associate Director of
Student Financial Aid

Dr. Aaron M. McGuffin, Senior Associate Dean
for Medical Education

Dr. Marie C. Veitia, Associate
Associate Dean for Student Affairs

General Information

The Marshall University School of Medicine was developed under the Veterans Administration Medical Assistance and Health Training Act passed by Congress in 1972. The School of Medicine was granted full accreditation and graduated its first class in 1981. The School of Medicine is a community-based program. The school's many affiliations provide the opportunity to experience medical practice in varied settings: a $32 million ambulatory care center, the Veterans Affairs Medical Center, successful rural clinics, highly specialized tertiary-care services in community hospitals, offices of private physicians, and others. Students' educational opportunities are further enhanced by three recently opened facilities: the Edwards Comprehensive Cancer Center, the Robert C. Byrd Biotechnology Science Center and the Byrd Clinical Center, which contains a Clinical Skills Lab.

Mission Statement

The Marshall University School of Medicine has a special mission to respond to the health care needs of West Virginians. We emphasize training in the primary care specialties and encourage graduates to practice in the state's underserved rural areas. Marshall is now tied for first place in the nation in the percentage of graduates who choose to enter family medicine.

Curricular Highlights

Community Service Requirement: Optional.
Research/Thesis Requirement: Optional.

In the first year, the basic science courses of anatomy, physiology, neurosciences, and molecular basis of medicine are supplemented by medical ethics and a clinical interdepartmental course, Introduction to Patient Care, which features students' supervised exposure to direct patient care and covers physical diagnosis and behavioral medicine. Ample unscheduled time during the first year allows students opportunities for independent problem-based, and small-group learning. Beginning in the Fall of 2008, the second year curriculum will become systems based, with emphasis on integration of topics throughout the year using patients as the focal point. All traditional second year disciplines will collaborate to produce integrated teaching and testing to enhance students' understanding of the entirety of a patient's illness. During the third and fourth years, students rotate through clerkships at participating community hospitals and other locations in the clinical fields of medicine, surgery, pediatrics, psychiatry, family practice, obstetrics-gynecology, and emergency medicine. Two months of rural health care at approved sites are required of all students. Twenty-three weeks are devoted to electives in the senior year. A standard letter grading system (A, B, C, D, F) is utilized.

USMLE

Step 1: Required. Students must record a passing score for promotion.
Step 2: Clinical Skills (CS): Required. Students must record a passing total score to graduate.
Step 2: Clinical Knowledge (CK): Required. Students must record a passing total score to graduate.

Selection Factors

There is no discrimination because of race, gender, religion, age, handicap, sexual orientation, or national origin. Qualified members of groups who are underrepresented in medicine are encouraged to apply. Applicants are evaluated on the basis of their academic records, MCAT® scores, recommendations from instructors, and personal qualifications as judged through interviews. Interviews are arranged only by invitation of the Admissions Committee. As a state-assisted institution, the School of Medicine gives preference in selection of students to West Virginia residents. A limited number of positions will be available to well-qualified non-residents from states contiguous to West Virginia or to non-residents who have strong ties to West Virginia. Other non-residents are not considered. Only applicants who are U.S. citizens or who have permanent resident visas are eligible for admission. The School of Medicine considers for transfer admission those applicants who are currently in good standing at an allopathic medical school. Positions are limited by attrition and are rarely available. The residency policy for regular admissions also applies to transfer admissions with the exception that only U.S. citizens are considered.

Financial Aid

The financial needs of the applicant are not a consideration in the admission process. There are a variety of resources for financial assistance available to medical students. The supplemental application fee will be waived for individuals who have been granted an AMCAS fee waiver.

Campus Information

Enrollment
For 2007, total enrollment was: 248

Special Features
Distinguishing features for students at Marshall include options and flexibility and an emphasis on compassion, integrity, leadership, and professionalism. Students determine their own career goals after exploring primary care and specialty rotations at Marshall and other sites, as well as electives, which can include wilderness medicine and international health experiences. Over the past four years, Marshall has become a leader in promoting childhood obesity awareness and intervention through their "Let's Get Moving" program.

Housing
The medical school maintains a list of apartments.

Application Process and Requirements 2009–2010

Primary Application Service: AMCAS
Earliest filing date: June 1, 2008
Latest filing date: November 15, 2008

Secondary Application Required?: Yes
Sent to: State residents
(and those from states bordering WV after review for competitiveness) [NR fee: $100]
Contact: Cynthia A. Warren, (800) 544-8514
warren@marshall.edu
Fee: Yes, $50
Fee waiver available: Yes
Earliest filing date: July 15, 2008
Latest filing date: December 31, 2008

Latest MCAT® considered: September 2008
Oldest MCAT® considered: 2006

Early Decision Program
School does not have EDP
Applicants notified: n/a
EDP available for: n/a

Regular Acceptance Notice
Earliest date: October 15, 2008
Latest date: Until class is full

Applicant's Response to Acceptance Offer – Maximum Time: Two weeks

Requests for Deferred Entrance Considered: Yes

Deposit to Hold Place in Class: No
Deposit (Resident): n/a
Deposit (Non-Resident): n/a
Deposit due: n/a
Applied to tuition: n/a
Deposit refundable: n/a
Refundable by: n/a

Estimated number of new entrants: 75
EDP: n/a, special program: n/a

Start Month/Year: August 2009

Interview Format: Two one-on-one interviews. Regional interviews are not available.

Other Programs

PREPARATORY PROGRAMS
Postbaccalaureate Program: No
Summer Program: No

COMBINED DEGREE PROGRAMS
Baccalaureate/MD: No
MD/MPH: No
MD/MBA: No
MD/JD: No
MD/PhD: Yes,
Richard Niles, Ph.D., (304) 696-7323
niles@marshall.edu

Premedical Coursework

Course	Req.	Rec.	Lab.	Hrs.	Course	Req.	Rec.	Lab.	Hrs.
Inorganic Chemistry	•		•	8	Computer Science				
Behavioral Sciences	•			6	Genetics				
Biochemistry		•			Humanities				
Biology					Organic Chemistry	•		•	8
Biology/Zoology	•		•	8	Physics	•		•	8
Calculus					Psychology				
College English	•			6	Social Sciences	•			6
College Mathematics					Other				

Selection Factors: 2007 Accepted Applicants

Proportion of Accepted Applicants with Relevant Experience (Data Self-Reported to AMCAS®)		
Community Service/Volunteer		58%
Medically-Related Work		67%
Research		61%

Shaded bar represents accepted scores ranging from the 10th percentile to the 90th percentile   School Median ● National Median ●

Overall GPA	2.0	2.1	2.2	2.3	2.4	2.5	2.6	2.7	2.8	2.9	3.0	3.1	3.2	3.3	3.4	3.5	(3.6)	3.7	3.8	3.9	4.0
Science GPA	2.0	2.1	2.2	2.3	2.4	2.5	2.6	2.7	2.8	2.9	3.0	3.1	3.2	3.3	3.4	(3.5)	3.6	3.7	3.8	3.9	4.0

MCAT® required: Yes, 100% of 2007 accepted applicants took MCAT®

Verbal Reasoning	3	4	5	6	7	8	(9)	(10)	11	12	13	14	15
Physical Sciences	3	4	5	6	7	8	(9)	10	(11)	12	13	14	15
Biological Sciences	3	4	5	6	7	8	(9)	10	(11)	12	13	14	15
Writing Sample			J	K	L	M	N	(O)	P	(Q)	R	S	T

Acceptance & Matriculation Data for 2007–2008 First Year Class

	Resident	Non-Resident	International	Total
Applied	189	1733	23	1945
Interviewed	153	79	0	232
Deferred	3	3	0	6
Matriculants				
Early Assurance Program	0	0	0	0
Early Decision Program	0	0	0	0
Baccalaureate/MD	n/a	n/a	n/a	n/a
MD/PhD	0	0	0	0
Matriculated	51	21	0	**72**

Applications accepted from International Applicants: No

Matriculant Demographics: 2007–2008 First Year Class

Men: 33   **Women:** 39

Matriculants' Self-Reported Race/Ethnicity

Mexican American	0	Korean	1
Cuban	0	Vietnamese	1
Puerto Rican	0	Other Asian	0
Other Hispanic	1	Total Asian	9
Total Hispanic	1	Native American	0
Chinese	1	Black	0
Asian Indian	3	Native Hawaiian	0
Pakistani	1	White	63
Filipino	2	Unduplicated Number	
Japanese	0	of Matriculants	72

Science and Math Majors: 75%
Matriculants with:
    Baccalaureate degree: 97%
    Graduate degree(s): 11%

Specialty Choice

2003, 2004, 2005 Graduates, Specialty Choice (As reported by program directors to GME Track™)	
Anesthesiology	5%
Emergency Medicine	4%
Family Practice	17%
Internal Medicine	12%
Obstetrics/Gynecology	6%
Orthopaedic Surgery	2%
Pediatrics	23%
Psychiatry	2%
Radiology	3%
Surgery	6%

Financial Information

Source: 2006–2007 LCME I-B survey and 2007–2008 AAMC TSF questionnaire

	Residents	Non-Residents
Total Cost of Attendance	$35,670	$60,490
Tuition and Fees	$16,110	$40,930
Other (includes living expenses)	$17,556	$17,556
Health Insurance (can be waived)	$2,004	$2,004

Average 2007 Graduate Indebtedness: $128,023
% of Enrolled Students Receiving Aid: 87%

Criminal Background Check

This medical school requires a criminal background check prior to matriculation.

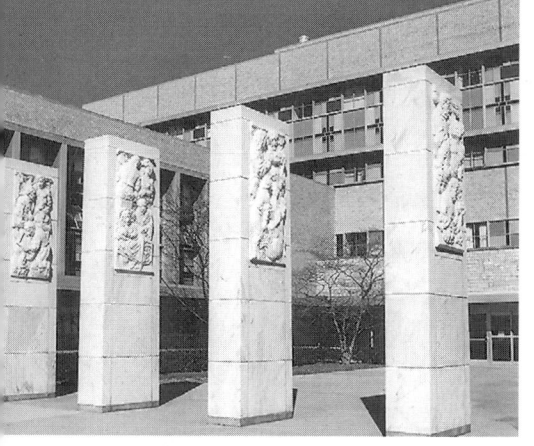

West Virginia University School of Medicine

Morgantown, West Virginia

Office of Student Services
West Virginia University School of Medicine
Health Sciences Center, P.O. Box 9111
Morgantown, West Virginia 26506
T 304 293 2408   **F** 304 293 7814

Admissions www.hsc.wvu.edu/som/students/
aboutSoM/admissionProcess/index.asp
Main www.hsc.wvu.edu/som/
Financial www.hsc.wvu.edu/fin/medbud.htm
Email medadmissions@hsc.wvu.edu

Public Institution

Dr. John E. Prescott, Dean

*Dr. James Helsley, Chair,
Admissions Committee*

*Dr. G. Anne Cather, Associate Dean
for Student Services*

Candace Frazier, Financial Aid Officer

Beth Ann McCormick, Admissions Associate

General Information

WVU has served for more than 100 years as a public institution of health professions education. The Health Sciences Center has more than 1,900 students. The Morgantown campus includes: the Physician Office Center, Ruby Memorial Hospital, Chestnut Ridge Psychiatric Hospital, HealthSouth Regional Rehabilitation Hospital, Mary Babb Randolph Cancer Center, and the WVU Eye Institute. New construction includes the Blanchette Rockefeller Neurosciences Institute, research labs and additions to the Cancer Center. There are three campuses: Morgantown, Charleston, and Eastern Division. Morgantown serves north and central WV with primary and tertiary care. Charleston is the oldest regional medical education campus in the U.S. and serves as a regional referral center for southern WV. Eastern provides a broad, community-based education emphasizing family medicine, primary care, and rural health.

Mission Statement

The mission of the West Virginia University School of Medicine is to improve the health of West Virginians through the education of health professionals, through basic/clinical scientific research and research in rural health care delivery, through the provision of continuing professional education, and through participation in the provision of direct and supportive health care.

Curricular Highlights

Community Service Requirement: Required. 100 hours of service required.
Research/Thesis Requirement: Optional.

The educational program of the School of Medicine provides a strong foundation for any branch of medicine. In the first and second years, study is directed toward the basic medical sciences. The first-year basic science courses are mostly lecture and problem-based learning with computer-based testing. Clinical experiences are introduced in the first year. Summer externships are available. Continued early exposure to patient-oriented instruction occurs throughout the second year. A traditional third-year curriculum gives the student a foundation in general medicine in the major clinical disciplines. The fourth year is composed of requirements (65%) and electives (35%). Many subspeciality requirements are included. Three months of rural rotations are required. International travel scholarships are available.

USMLE

Step 1: Required. Students must record a passing score for promotion.
Step 2: Clinical Skills (CS): Required. Students must record a passing total score to graduate.
Step 2: Clinical Knowledge (CK): Required. Students must record a passing total score to graduate.

Selection Factors

WV residents are given preference for admission. There are available spaces for well-qualified non-residents, especially for those with strong state ties. Admission is based upon scholarship, MCAT® scores, personal qualifications noted on interview, recommendations, community service, leadership, and medical experiences. The school does not discriminate on the basis of race, sex, creed, national origin, age, or handicap. Approximately one third of the students are assigned to clinical years at the Charleston Division and a small number of students are assigned to the Eastern Division.

Financial Aid

A number of scholarship awards are available based on financial need and merit. Multiple loan funds are also available. Students' spouses with reasonable training and experience often find work near the medical school, at WVU, or in Morgantown. Medical students are discouraged from seeking outside employment while enrolled. There is no provision for financial assistance to foreign students.

Information about Diversity Programs

The Health Careers Opportunity Program is available for disadvantaged students or those from groups underrepresented in medicine.

Campus Information

Setting

There are three clinical campuses. The Morgantown campus (*www.morgantown.com*) is a vibrant, active community and the medical, cultural, and commercial hub of the region. It has been named "#1 Dreamtown in America," and "Best Small City In The East." Clinical campuses are also located in the Charleston and Eastern Divisions. Charleston is the state capitol and serves as a hub for business and industry. The Charleston Area Medical Center is the largest in the state and serves as the regional referral center. The Eastern Division is located in the eastern panhandle of the state and serves a large nine-county area. It is associated with two hospitals, the VA system and several health centers.

Enrollment

For 2007, total enrollment was: 428

Special Features

WVU School of Medicine is highly respected for its clinical and rural education. It was a recent recipient of the AAMC Community Service Award. Our computer laptop program provides electronic testing and prepares students well for the USMLE exams. Primary and tertiary care facilities are state-of-the-art, and new construction is currently underway. MPH and International Medicine tracks are available. Community service is required.

Housing

On-campus housing is not available. Affordable housing is available nearby, with average rents of $600-$800/month.

Satellite Campuses/Facilities

Two regional campuses are located at the Charleston (*www.hsc.wvu.edu/charleston*) and Eastern Divisions (*www.hsc.wvu.edu/eastern*) for third and fourth-year clinical rotations.

Application Process and Requirements 2009–2010

Primary Application Service: AMCAS
Earliest filing date: June 1, 2008
Latest filing date: November 1, 2008

Secondary Application Required?: Yes
Sent to: Select applicants by secure email
Contact: Beth Ann McCormick
1-800-543-5650, medadmissions@hsc.wvu.edu
Fee: Yes, $100
Fee waiver available: Yes
Earliest filing date: July 15, 2008
Latest filing date: January 1, 2009

Latest MCAT® considered: September 2008
Oldest MCAT® considered: April 2007

Early Decision Program
School does have EDP
Applicants notified: October 1, 2008
EDP available for: Both Residents
and Non-Residents

Regular Acceptance Notice
Earliest date: October 15, 2008
Latest date: Until class is full

Applicant's Response to Acceptance
Offer – Maximum Time: Two weeks

Requests for Deferred
Entrance Considered: Yes

Deposit to Hold Place in Class: Yes
Deposit (Resident): $100
Deposit (Non-Resident): $100
Deposit due: With response to acceptance offer
Applied to tuition: Yes
Deposit refundable: Yes
Refundable by: May 15, 2009

Estimated number of new entrants: 100
EDP: 10, special program: n/a

Start Month/Year: August 2009

Interview Format: Interview and tour, Morgantown campus. Regional tours can be arranged.

Other Programs

PREPARATORY PROGRAMS
Postbaccalaureate Program: No
Summer Program: No

COMBINED DEGREE PROGRAMS
Baccalaureate/MD: No
MD/MPH: Yes, www.hsc.wvu.edu/som/cmed/degree_programs/md_mph.asp
MD/MBA: No
MD/JD: No
MD/PhD: Yes, www.hsc.wvu.edu/som/resoff/gradprograms/mdphd_main.asp

Premedical Coursework

Course	Req.	Rec.	Lab.	Hrs.
Inorganic Chemistry	•		•	8
Behavioral Sciences				6
Biochemistry		•		4-8
Biology				
Biology/Zoology	•		•	8
Calculus				
College English	•			6
College Mathematics				

Course	Req.	Rec.	Lab.	Hrs.
Computer Science				
Genetics				
Humanities				
Organic Chemistry	•		•	8
Physics	•		•	8
Psychology				
Social Sciences	•			6
Adv and Cell & Molecular Biology		•		4-8

Selection Factors: 2007 Accepted Applicants

Proportion of Accepted Applicants with Relevant Experience (Data Self-Reported to AMCAS®)		
Community Service/Volunteer		64%
Medically-Related Work		84%
Research		66%

Shaded bar represents accepted scores ranging from the 10th percentile to the 90th percentile. **School Median** ● **National Median** ●

Overall GPA	2.0	2.1	2.2	2.3	2.4	2.5	2.6	2.7	2.8	2.9	3.0	3.1	3.2	3.3	3.4	3.5	3.6	3.7	(3.8)	3.9	4.0
Science GPA	2.0	2.1	2.2	2.3	2.4	2.5	2.6	2.7	2.8	2.9	3.0	3.1	3.2	3.3	3.4	3.5	3.6	(3.7)	3.8	3.9	4.0

MCAT® required: Yes, 100% of 2007 accepted applicants took MCAT®

Verbal Reasoning	3	4	5	6	7	8	9	(10)	11	12	13	14	15
Physical Sciences	3	4	5	6	7	8	9	(10)	(11)	12	13	14	15
Biological Sciences	3	4	5	6	7	8	9	(10)	(11)	12	13	14	15
Writing Sample			J	K	L	M	N	(O)	P	(Q)	R	S	T

Acceptance & Matriculation Data for 2007–2008 First Year Class

	Resident	Non-Resident	International	Total
Applied	214	2571	96	2881
Interviewed	138	218	0	356
Deferred	0	0	0	0
Matriculants				
Early Assurance Program	0	0	0	0
Early Decision Program	12	0	0	12
Baccalaureate/MD	n/a	n/a	n/a	n/a
MD/PhD	1	2	0	3
Matriculated	82	26	0	**108**

Applications accepted from International Applicants: Canadian Only

Matriculant Demographics: 2007–2008 First Year Class

Men: 55 **Women:** 53

Matriculants' Self-Reported Race/Ethnicity

Mexican American	0	Korean	2
Cuban	1	Vietnamese	1
Puerto Rican	0	Other Asian	2
Other Hispanic	2	Total Asian	15
Total Hispanic	3	Native American	1
Chinese	1	Black	3
Asian Indian	6	Native Hawaiian	1
Pakistani	2	White	90
Filipino	2	**Unduplicated Number**	
Japanese	0	**of Matriculants**	108

Science and Math Majors: 88%
Matriculants with:
Baccalaureate degree: 95%
Graduate degree(s): 6%

Specialty Choice

2003, 2004, 2005 Graduates, Specialty Choice (As reported by program directors to GME Track™)	
Anesthesiology	6%
Emergency Medicine	4%
Family Practice	10%
Internal Medicine	17%
Obstetrics/Gynecology	7%
Orthopaedic Surgery	3%
Pediatrics	9%
Psychiatry	5%
Radiology	3%
Surgery	9%

Financial Information

Source: 2006–2007 LCME I-B survey and 2007–2008 AAMC TSF questionnaire

	Residents	Non-Residents
Total Cost of Attendance	$35,169	$57,831
Tuition and Fees	$19,204	$41,866
Other (includes living expenses)	$15,965	$15,965
Health Insurance (not applicable)	$0	$0

Average 2007 Graduate Indebtedness: $126,739
% of Enrolled Students Receiving Aid: 93%

Criminal Background Check

This medical school requires a criminal background check prior to matriculation.

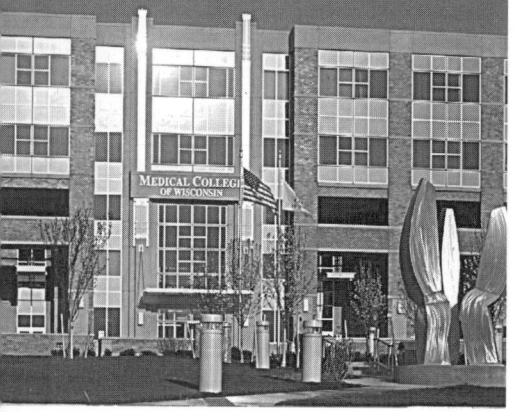

Medical College of Wisconsin
Milwaukee, Wisconsin

Office of Admissions
Medical College of Wisconsin
8701 Watertown Plank Road
Milwaukee, Wisconsin 53226
T 414 456 8246   **F** 414 955 0121

Admissions www.mcw.edu/medicalschool
Main www.mcw.edu
Financial www.mcw.edu/acad/finaid
Email medschool@mcw.edu

Private Institution

Dr. Johnathan Ravdin, Dean and Executive Vice President

Michael T. Istwan, Director of Admissions

Dr. Dawn Bragg, Assistant Dean for Student Affairs – Diversity

Linda L. Paschal, Director of Student Financial Services

General Information

The Medical College of Wisconsin became a private, free-standing school of medicine in 1967. Located on the Milwaukee Regional Medical Campus, it maintains strong relationships and educational programs with institutions statewide. Major affiliated teaching hospitals include Froedtert Hospital, the VA Medical Center, and Children's Hospital of Wisconsin. Area affiliations also include 10 hospitals and a number of health-care facilities.

Mission Statement

The Medical College of Wisconsin is a private, academic institution dedicated to leadership and excellence in advancing the prevention, diagnosis and treatment of disease and injury through: Education: Preparing the physicians and scientists of tomorrow while enhancing the skills of today's health professionals. Discovery: Creating new knowledge in basic, translational and patient based research to improve human health. Patient Care: Providing effective, compassionate, expert care for patients. Community Engagement: Partnering with public and private organizations to enhance learning, research, patient care and the health of the community.

Curricular Highlights

Community Service Requirement: Optional.
Research/Thesis Requirement: Optional. The curriculum provides a foundation for a career in any discipline of medicine. In the first two years, students learn the basic sciences and experience the clinical environment through a mentor course and clinically-related course work in the Clinical Continuum. Clinical topics covered include medical interviewing,

human behavior, information management, ethics, palliative care, physical exam, and health policy. In the third year, students rotate through required clinical clerkships and an optional elective experience to gain exposure to major clinical disciplines. In the fourth year, four one-month rotations are required including two subinternships, one each in a medically- and surgically-oriented specialty, a Medicine rotation, and an Integrated Selective. Five one-month electives are available to senior students. Joint degree programs or an Honors in Research program are available to students with specific research interests. A five-year extended curriculum is available to students who wish to extend their studies over a longer period.

USMLE

Step 1: Required. Students must record a passing score for promotion.
Step 2: Clinical Skills (CS): Required. Students must only record a score.
Step 2: Clinical Knowledge (CK): Required. Students must record a passing total score to graduate.

Selection Factors

Student selection is based on a careful analysis of the suitability for the medical profession. Academic achievement and MCAT® scores are carefully evaluated. Subjective factors include the personal statement, experiences, recommendations and interviews. Interviews are integral, done only at the college and required before acceptance. Applications are reviewed on a rolling basis by date of completion. Interviews are conducted and offers are also made on a rolling basis until the class is filled. Candidates are encouraged to complete the application in a timely fashion. The Medical College of Wisconsin does not discriminate on the basis of race, gender, creed, disability, age, national origin or sexual orientation.

Financial Aid

Most financial assistance, including federal and institutional scholarships and loans, is awarded on basis of need. Financial aid award letters are developed using the Federal Methodology formula. Applicants are encouraged to begin the application process as soon as they are interviewed. To matriculate, a student must provide

a current clean credit report as defined in the College's credit report policy. A student must be a U.S. citizen or eligible non-citizen to receive aid from federal administered programs. International applicants must file proof of financial support before acceptance.

Information about Diversity Programs

The college encourages applications from students of diverse backgrounds. In addition to academic credentials, letters of recommendation, and personal interviews, a student's motivation and educational background are carefully considered. The Office of Academic Affairs/Diversity offers various programs to assist students, demonstrating the college's commitment to their recruitment, retention and graduation.

Campus Information

Setting

Located on the Milwaukee Regional Medical Center Campus, in a suburb seven miles west of downtown Milwaukee, the College offers a safe comfortable environment to live and study, with easy access to the city and its advantages.

Enrollment

For 2007, total enrollment was: 805

Special Features

Froedtert Hospital and Children's Hospital of Wisconsin are nationally ranked, Level One trauma centers. Children's has been selected as one of the ten best Children's Hospital in the country. With over $125 million in grant funds, the College conducted 3000 studies and had 1500 clinical trials in progress during the past year.

Housing

Student housing is not provided. A list of available housing is maintained and students live within easy driving or walking distance of campus.

Satellite Campuses/Facilities

The Milwaukee Regional Medical Campus provides students with the opportunity to complete their clinical requirements at this location.

Application Process and Requirements 2009–2010

Primary Application Service: AMCAS
Earliest filing date: June 1, 2008
Latest filing date: November 1, 2008

Secondary Application Required?: Yes
Sent to: All applicants
Contact: Michael Istwan, (414) 456-8246
mistwan@mcw.edu
Fee: Yes, $70
Fee waiver available: Yes
Earliest filing date: July 1, 2008
Latest filing date: January 31, 2009

Latest MCAT® considered: September 2008
Oldest MCAT® considered: 2006

Early Decision Program
School does have EDP
Applicants notified: October 2008
EDP available for: Both Residents
and Non-Residents

Regular Acceptance Notice
Earliest date: October 15, 2008
Latest date: Until class is full

**Applicant's Response to Acceptance
Offer – Maximum Time:** One Month

**Requests for Deferred
Entrance Considered:** Yes

Deposit to Hold Place in Class: Yes
Deposit (Resident): $100
Deposit (Non-Resident): $100
Deposit due: With acceptance of offer
Applied to tuition: Yes
Deposit refundable: Yes
Refundable by: May 15, 2009

Estimated number of new entrants: 204
EDP: 10, special program: n/a

Start Month/Year: August 2009

Interview Format: Two, thirty-minute
interviews. Regional interviews are not available.

Other Programs

PREPARATORY PROGRAMS
Postbaccalaureate Program: No
Summer Program: No

COMBINED DEGREE PROGRAMS
Baccalaureate/MD: No
MD/MPH: No
MD/MBA: No
MD/JD: No
MD/PhD: Yes, www.mcw.edu/mstp

Premedical Coursework

Course	Req.	Rec.	Lab.	Hrs.
Inorganic Chemistry	•		•	8
Behavioral Sciences				
Biochemistry		•		
Biology	•		•	8
Biology/Zoology				
Calculus		•		
College English	•			6
College Mathematics	•			4

Course	Req.	Rec.	Lab.	Hrs.
Computer Science				
Genetics				
Humanities				
Organic Chemistry	•		•	8
Physics	•			8
Psychology				
Social Sciences				
Other				

Selection Factors: 2007 Accepted Applicants

Proportion of Accepted Applicants with Relevant Experience (Data Self-Reported to AMCAS®)	
Community Service/Volunteer	72%
Medically-Related Work	91%
Research	79%

Shaded bar represents accepted scores ranging from the 10th percentile to the 90th percentile. School Median ● National Median ●

Overall GPA	2.0	2.1	2.2	2.3	2.4	2.5	2.6	2.7	2.8	2.9	3.0	3.1	3.2	3.3	3.4	3.5	3.6	3.7	(3.8)	3.9	4.0
Science GPA	2.0	2.1	2.2	2.3	2.4	2.5	2.6	2.7	2.8	2.9	3.0	3.1	3.2	3.3	3.4	3.5	3.6	(3.7)	3.8	3.9	4.0

MCAT® required: Yes, 100% of 2007 accepted applicants took MCAT®

Verbal Reasoning	3	4	5	6	7	8	9	(10)	11	12	13	14	15
Physical Sciences	3	4	5	6	7	8	9	(10)	(11)	12	13	14	15
Biological Sciences	3	4	5	6	7	8	9	(10)	(11)	12	13	14	15
Writing Sample				J	K	L	M	N	O	(P)	(Q)	R	S	T

Acceptance & Matriculation Data for 2007–2008 First Year Class

	Resident	Non-Resident	International	Total
Applied	600	5770	277	6647
Interviewed	210	531	5	746
Deferred	14	14	0	28
Matriculants				
Early Assurance Program	n/a	n/a	n/a	n/a
Early Decision Program	5	0	0	5
Baccalaureate/MD	n/a	n/a	n/a	n/a
MD/PhD	2	3	0	5
Matriculated	84	119	1	**204**

Applications accepted from International Applicants: Yes

Matriculant Demographics: 2007–2008 First Year Class

Men: 96   **Women:** 108

Matriculants' Self-Reported Race/Ethnicity

Mexican American	5	Korean	4
Cuban	1	Vietnamese	3
Puerto Rican	4	Other Asian	2
Other Hispanic	2	Total Asian	39
Total Hispanic	10	Native American	1
Chinese	7	Black	7
Asian Indian	21	Native Hawaiian	0
Pakistani	2	White	157
Filipino	1	Unduplicated Number	
Japanese	2	of Matriculants	204

Science and Math Majors: 74%
Matriculants with:
Baccalaureate degree: 100%
Graduate degree(s): 5%

Specialty Choice

2003, 2004, 2005 Graduates, Specialty Choice (As reported by program directors to GME Track™)	
Anesthesiology	8%
Emergency Medicine	8%
Family Practice	15%
Internal Medicine	14%
Obstetrics/Gynecology	4%
Orthopaedic Surgery	4%
Pediatrics	10%
Psychiatry	3%
Radiology	5%
Surgery	8%

Financial Information

Source: 2006–2007 LCME I-B survey
and 2007–2008 AAMC TSF questionnaire

	Residents	Non-Residents
Total Cost of Attendance	$46,870	$52,410
Tuition and Fees	$32,515	$38,055
Other (includes living expenses)	$12,051	$12,051
Health Insurance (cannot be waived)	$2,304	$2,304

Average 2007 Graduate Indebtedness: $142,311
% of Enrolled Students Receiving Aid: 95%

Criminal Background Check

This medical school requires a criminal background check prior to matriculation.

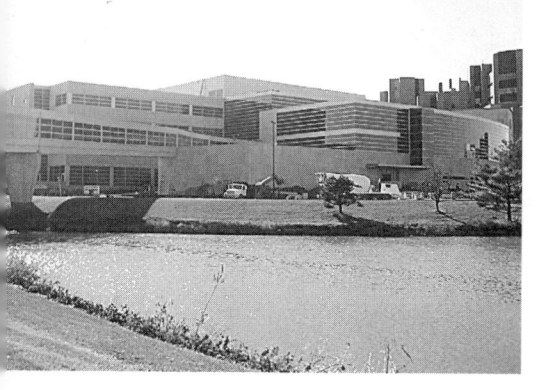

University of Wisconsin School of Medicine and Public Health

Madison, Wisconsin

Admissions Committee
2130 Health Sciences Learning Center
University of Wisconsin School of Medicine
and Public Health
750 Highland Avenue
Madison, Wisconsin 53705-2221
T 608 263 4925 **F** 608 262 4226

Admissions www.med.wisc.edu/education/
admissions
Main www.med.wisc.edu
Financial www.finaid.wisc.edu/
Email medadmissions@mailplus.wisc.edu

Public Institution

Dr. Robert N. Golden, Dean

Lucy J. Wall, Assistant Dean for Admissions

*Dr. Gloria V. Hawkins, Assistant Dean
for Multicultural Affairs*

*Amy J. Schrader, Senior Advisor Student
Financial Services*

General Information

The University of Wisconsin School of Medicine and Public Health has had a four-year program in medicine since 1924 and has the largest research commitment of any school or college on campus, receiving more than $215 million in extramural research support in fiscal 2006. National surveys consistently rank UW Hospital and Clinics among the finest academic medical centers in the United States.

Mission Statement

The University of Wisconsin School of Medicine and Public Health is committed to meeting the health needs of Wisconsin and beyond through excellence in education, research, patient care, and service. The UW School of Medicine and Public Health seeks to be one of the preeminent medical schools by excelling in the creation, integration, and transfer of knowledge through a combination of basic, translational, and clinical research, a greater emphasis on active learning, and consistently outstanding patient care.

Curricular Highlights

Community Service Requirement: Optional.
Research/Thesis Requirement: Optional.

The curriculum introduces students to the generalist practice of medicine by exposing them to community-based settings in the first and second years. There is a focus on active learning; case-based problem-solving; interdisciplinary teaching by basic science and clinical faculty throughout the first and second years; a four-year curriculum that prepares students for either a primary care or specialty career; diverse clinical clerkship experiences around the state, including

inner-city and rural sites; and an eight-week one-on-one preceptorship with an experienced clinician in Year 4. The senior year provides elective opportunities for study at other institutions and abroad. Opportunities for research are available to medical students in individually arranged programs.

USMLE

Step 1: Required. Students must record a passing score for promotion.
Step 2: Clinical Skills (CS): Required. Students must only record a score.
Step 2: Clinical Knowledge (CK): Required. Students must only record a score.

Selection Factors

The Admissions Committee seeks students with diverse backgrounds and interests. Breadth of academic and nonacademic interests and experiences, ability to communicate with others, motivation for medicine, personal characteristics, and intellectual ability are some of the factors considered. Preference is given to residents of Wisconsin. Non-resident applicants compete for relatively few places. Secondary applications and interview invitations are sent to selected applicants.

Financial Aid

All financial aid allocated by the University of Wisconsin School of Medicine and Public Health is awarded on the basis of proven need. Need is calculated as the necessary expenses incurred while attending medical school minus the resources provided to the student by outside agencies, personal resources, and available parental resources. Priority for financial aid, especially grant awards, will be given to students with the greatest need. The major proportion of total financial aid is available in the form of loans.

Information about Diversity Programs

The University of Wisconsin School of Medicine and Public Health is committed to increasing the number of physicians from groups underrepresented in medicine and those showing evidence of socioeconomically and educationally-disadvantaged backgrounds. Applications are encouraged from persons with

socioeconomic disadvantages and from members of groups underrepresented in medicine.

Campus Information

Setting

The University of Wisconsin School of Medicine and Public Health and the Ebling Health Sciences Library are located in the new Health Sciences Learning Center. It is connected to the University of Wisconsin Hospital and Clinics and the School of Pharmacy on the west side of campus. The Learning Center features sophisticated instructional technologies, including advanced digital capabilities throughout its lecture halls, classrooms, clinical training and assessment areas, computing laboratories, and distance education centers. The building was designed to enhance individual and small-group learning.

Enrollment

For 2007, total enrollment was: 647

Special Features

Although students are trained to work in every area of patient care and research, the UW medical degree program has chosen seven areas of medicine on which to focus its resources. These include Aging, Cancer, Cardiovascular and Respiratory Sciences, Neuroscience, Population and Community Health Sciences, Rural Health, and Women's Health. Through programs that are interdisciplinary and translational, the University of Wisconsin School of Medicine and Public Health is at the vanguard of today's medicine and tomorrow's cures.

Housing

Housing information is available at *www.housing.wisc.edu*. Additional private housing is widely available within the city of Madison.

Satellite Campuses/Facilities

The typical UW medical student spends 16 weeks at clinical sites outside Madison and throughout the state of Wisconsin. Other locations are LaCrosse, Marshfield, Green Bay, and Milwaukee teaching hospitals, and community clinics in other cities.

Application Process and Requirements 2009–2010

Primary Application Service: AMCAS
Earliest filing date: June 1, 2008
Latest filing date: November 1, 2008

Secondary Application Required?: Yes
Sent to: Selected applicants
URL: Invitation only
Fee: Yes, $54
Fee waiver available: Yes
Earliest filing date: July 1, 2008
Latest filing date: December 1, 2008

Latest MCAT® considered: September 2008
Oldest MCAT® considered: 2005

Early Decision Program
School does have EDP
Applicants notified: October 1, 2008
EDP available for: Residents only

Regular Acceptance Notice
Earliest date: October 16, 2008
Latest date: Until class is full

Applicant's Response to Acceptance
Offer – Maximum Time: Two weeks

Requests for Deferred
Entrance Considered: Yes

Deposit to Hold Place in Class: No
Deposit (Resident): n/a
Deposit (Non-Resident): n/a
Deposit due: n/a
Applied to tuition: n/a
Deposit refundable: n/a
Refundable by: n/a

Estimated number of new entrants: 160
EDP: 5, special program: 20

Start Month/Year: Mid-August 2009

Interview Format: Selected applicants are invited to interview. Regional interviews are not available.

Other Programs

PREPARATORY PROGRAMS
Postbaccalaureate Program: No
Summer Program: No

COMBINED DEGREE PROGRAMS
Baccalaureate/MD: No
MD/MPH: No
MD/MBA: No
MD/JD: No
MD/PhD: Yes, http://mstp.med.wisc.edu/

Premedical Coursework

Course	Req.	Rec.	Lab.	Sems.
Inorganic Chemistry	•		•	2
Behavioral Sciences		•		
Biochemistry	•			1
Biology				
Biology/Zoology	•		•	1
Calculus		•		
College English				
College Mathematics	•			1
Computer Science				

Course	Req.	Rec.	Lab.	Sems.
Genetics				
Humanities		•		
Organic Chemistry	•			1
Physics	•		•	2
Psychology				
Social Sciences		•		
Statistics	•			1
Advanced level biology	•		•	1

Selection Factors: 2007 Accepted Applicants

Proportion of Accepted Applicants with Relevant Experience (Data Self-Reported to AMCAS®)		
Community Service/Volunteer		67%
Medically-Related Work		85%
Research		81%

Shaded bar represents accepted scores ranging from the 10th percentile to the 90th percentile. **School Median** ● **National Median** ●

Overall GPA 2.0 2.1 2.2 2.3 2.4 2.5 2.6 2.7 2.8 2.9 3.0 3.1 3.2 3.3 3.4 **3.5 3.6 3.7** (3.8) 3.9 4.0
Science GPA 2.0 2.1 2.2 2.3 2.4 2.5 2.6 2.7 2.8 2.9 3.0 3.1 3.2 3.3 **3.4 3.5 3.6 3.7** (3.8) 3.9 4.0

MCAT® required: Yes, 94% of 2007 accepted applicants took MCAT®

Verbal Reasoning 3 4 5 6 7 8 9 (10) 11 12 13 14 15
Physical Sciences 3 4 5 6 7 8 9 10 (11) 12 13 14 15
Biological Sciences 3 4 5 6 7 8 9 10 (11) 12 13 14 15
Writing Sample J K L M N O P (Q) R S T

Acceptance & Matriculation Data for 2007–2008 First Year Class

	Resident	Non-Resident	International	Total
Applied	631	2657	12	3300
Interviewed	459	167	0	626
Deferred	6	2	0	8
Matriculants				
Early Assurance Program	n/a	n/a	n/a	n/a
Early Decision Program	4	0	0	4
Baccalaureate/MD	26	0	0	26
MD/PhD	1	9	0	10
Matriculated	123	32	0	**155**

Applications accepted from International Applicants: No

Matriculant Demographics: 2007–2008 First Year Class

Men: 68   **Women:** 87

Matriculants' Self-Reported Race/Ethnicity

Mexican American	2	Korean	6
Cuban	0	Vietnamese	5
Puerto Rican	0	Other Asian	4
Other Hispanic	3	Total Asian	37
Total Hispanic	5	Native American	0
Chinese	9	Black	6
Asian Indian	14	Native Hawaiian	0
Pakistani	0	White	112
Filipino	2	Unduplicated Number	
Japanese	0	of Matriculants	155

Science and Math Majors: 66%
Matriculants with:
    Baccalaureate degree: 99%
    Graduate degree(s): 10%

Specialty Choice

2003, 2004, 2005 Graduates, Specialty Choice (As reported by program directors to GME Track™)	
Anesthesiology	9%
Emergency Medicine	7%
Family Practice	14%
Internal Medicine	16%
Obstetrics/Gynecology	3%
Orthopaedic Surgery	2%
Pediatrics	16%
Psychiatry	4%
Radiology	5%
Surgery	6%

Financial Information

Source: 2006–2007 LCME I-B survey and 2007–2008 AAMC TSF questionnaire

	Residents	Non-Residents
Total Cost of Attendance	$40,062	$51,186
Tuition and Fees	$22,722	$33,846
Other (includes living expenses)	$15,450	$15,450
Health Insurance (can be waived)	$1,890	$1,890

Average 2007 Graduate Indebtedness: $120,065
% of Enrolled Students Receiving Aid: 96%

Criminal Background Check

This medical school requires a criminal background check prior to matriculation.

Chapter 13

Information About Canadian Medical Schools
Accredited by the LCME and by the CACMS

The 17 medical schools in Canada are members of the Association of Faculties of Medicine of Canada (*www.afmc.ca*) and affiliate members of the AAMC. They participate in the activities of both associations. Canadian medical schools are accredited jointly by the Liaison Committee on Medical Education (*www.lcme.org, LCME*) and the Committee on Accreditation of Canadian Medical Schools (*www.afmc.ca/education-accreditation-e.php*, CACMS). All are M.D. degree-granting schools with high-quality educational programs.

Admission policies and procedures of Canadian schools are similar in many respects to those followed in U.S. schools; thus, many of the suggestions for applicants in chapters 1 through 9 will also apply. Schools vary with respect to the emphasis placed on selection factors, and applicants are encouraged to refer to the individual school entries for additional details.

Fifteen Canadian medical schools offer four-year educational programs; two, McMaster and Calgary, are three-year programs. Some students at the Université de Montréal are admitted into a one-year preparatory program prior to beginning the M.D. curriculum. McGill University's five-year M.D. program includes an initial year that must be completed by graduates of the province of Quebec's Collège d'enseignement général et professionnel (CÉGEP).

Selection Criteria

As reflected in the individual school entries in this chapter, Canadian medical schools vary with respect to the number of years of undergraduate instruction required of applicants. Medical schools also vary with respect to recommended content during pre-medical undergraduate education. Table 13-A shows that physics, inorganic and organic chemistry, biology, biochemistry, humanities, and English are the most common subjects required in undergraduate education by the Canadian medical schools.

Language of Instruction

Three Canadian medical schools — Laval, Montréal and Sherbrooke, all located in the province of Quebec — require students to be fluent in French as all instruction is in that language. Instruction in the other 14 schools is in English, and the University of Ottawa offers the M.D. curriculum in both French and English.

Residency Requirements

In Canada, universities fall under provincial jurisdiction and the majority of places in each faculty of medicine are allocated to permanent residents of the province in which the university is located.

Not all faculties of medicine accept applications from international students. Conversely, some faculties of medicine may reserve positions for international students, possibly as part of agreements with foreign governments and institutions. Statistics compiled by the Association of Faculties of Medicine of Canada (*www.afmc.ca*) show that most medical schools admit international students. In 2006–07, 233 U.S. students applied to Canadian medical schools and recorded a 9.9% success rate. In the same year, 426 non-U.S. international students applied to Canadian medical schools and recorded a 5.6% success rate. The success rate for Canadian applicants was 26.2%. Additional information about Canadian medical schools can be found in the Association of Faculties of Medicine of Canada publication, Admission Requirements of Canadian Faculties of Medicine (2008) (*www.afmc.ca/ publications-admission-2008-e.php*).

Positions filled by international students in Canadian medical schools are not necessarily subsidized by provincial/territorial governments. As such, international students, including U.S. students, may pay higher tuition and fees compared to those of Canadian residents.

TABLE 13-A

Subjects Required by Three or More Canadian Medical Schools, 2009–2010 Entering Class

Required Subject	No. of Schools (n=14)
Physics	6
Inorganic Chemistry	8
Organic Chemistry	8
Biology	7
College English	4
Biochemistry	6
Humanities	3
College Mathematics	3
Calculus	2
Social Sciences	2

NOTE: Figures based on data provided fall 2007. Two of the 17 medical schools (Dalhousie, and McMaster and Western Ontario) did not indicate specific course requirements and are not included in the tabulations.

Academic Record/Suitability

Although an excellent academic record is a very important factor in gaining admission to a Canadian medical school, great deal of effort is expended in assessing applicants' suitability for a medical career based on other factors. Personal suitability is assessed in a variety of ways by the schools; applicants who can demonstrate that they possess the qualities considered important in the practice of medicine may sometimes be admitted even if their academic record is not outstanding. Alternately, applicants with outstanding records who do not possess these qualities may not gain a place in medical school.

Most applicants to Canadian medical schools are interviewed prior to acceptance, so the interview information in Chapter 7 will be useful.

Medical College Admission Test (MCAT®)

Eleven Canadian medical schools require applicants to take the MCAT: Alberta, British Columbia, Calgary, Dalhousie, Manitoba, McGill, Memorial, Queen's, Saskatchewan, Toronto, and Western Ontario.

Other Considerations

Canadian faculties of medicine do not discriminate on the basis of race, religion, or gender in admitting new students. The admission of Aboriginal students (First Nations, Inuit, Métis) is encouraged at several Canadian medical schools, including McGill, Ottawa, Queen's, Western Ontario, Northern Ontario School of Medicine, Saskatchewan, Alberta and British Columbia.

The number of female applicants has risen dramatically in recent years, with correspondingly larger proportions of women in schools' entering classes. Women comprised 57 percent of the 2006–2007 applicant pool, and the success rate for women was slightly higher than that for men. The 2006 entering classes at the 17 Canadian medical schools reporting data about male and female matriculants included 58 percent women and 42 percent men. Overall, 25 percent of applicants received at least one offer of admission.

Expenses/Financial Aid

Tuition and student fees for Canadian and non-Canadian students in the 2007 entering class are provided in Table 13-B and in individual school entries. Expenses vary from school to school and from student to student. Tuition at several Canadian schools is slightly higher for the first year than for successive years. Tuition and fees at all Canadian universities are expected to increase substantially in the next several years.

Some financial aid information is provided in the individual school entries. Eligible Canadian students may apply for a Canadian Student Loan, or they may apply to the Department of Education in their province for a provincial student loan.

Ontario Medical School Application Service (OMSAS)

The Ontario Medical School Application Service (OMSAS) is a non-profit, centralized application service for applicants to the six medical schools in Ontario. OMSAS provides only the application processing service; each medical school is autonomous in reaching its admission decisions. All applications to the Ontario medical schools must be made through OMSAS.

The on-line application, COMPASS. OMSAS, is available in early July. Completed applications must be received at OMSAS by October 1. Official transcripts and references must be received at OMSAS by October 1. Applicants are advised to submit their application and supporting documents prior to the deadline. For the instruction booklet containing information about application procedures and admission requirements, visit *www.ouac.on.ca/omsas/*.

Information Sources

Additional information about admission requirements, the curricula of Canadian medical schools, and medical education in Canada is provided in catalogs available from each school, and can be downloaded free of charge from the AFMC Web site (*www.afmc.ca*). A printed version of Admission Requirements of Canadian Faculties of Medicine can also be ordered from:

TABLE 13-B

Tuition and Student Fees for 2007 – 2008 First-Year Students at Canadian Medical Schools (In Canadian Dollars)

Categories of Students	Range	Average
In-Province	$3,360-$18,146	$11,697*
Canada, Out-of-Province	$7,282-$18,146	$12,979*
Visa	$18,408-$91,686	$34,937*

NOTE: Figures based on data provided fall 2007

* Average In-Province data were derived from all 17 Canadian schools. Average Out-of-Province data were derived from all 17 Canadian schools reporting. Average visa data were derived from eight schools which accept foreign students.

Source: Association of Faculties of Medicine of Canada

The Association of Faculties of Medicine of Canada
265 Carling Avenue, Suite 800
Ottawa, ON K1S 2E1
Canada
(613) 730-0687
Information is also available at
www.afmc.ca.

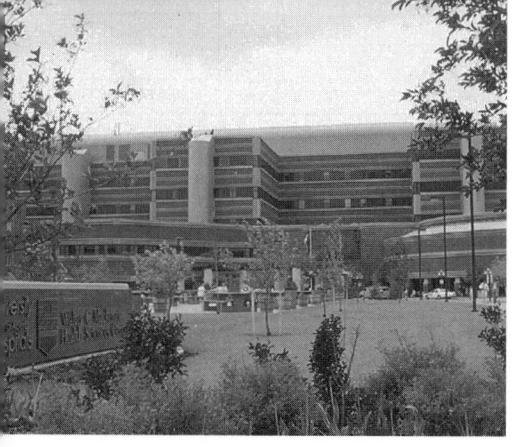

University of Alberta
Faculty of Medicine and Dentistry
Edmonton, Alberta

2-45 Medical Sciences Building
University of Alberta
Faculty of Medicine and Dentistry
Edmonton, Alberta
Canada, T6G 2H7
T 780 492 9524   **F** 780 492 9531

Admissions www.med.ualberta.ca/education/ugme/
Main www.med.ualberta.ca
Financial www.registrar.ualberta.ca/ro.cfm?id=287
Email admission@med.ualberta.ca

Public Institution

Dr. Thomas Marrie, Dean

M. Healey, Admissions Officer

Dr. Marc Moreau, Assistant Dean

General Information

The Faculty of Medicine at the University of Alberta was founded in 1913. The Medical Sciences Building, the Clinical Sciences Building, the Walter C. Mackenzie Health Sciences Centre, and the University of Alberta Hospitals are located on the university campus. Clinical instruction is also given at the Royal Alexandra Hospital, Edmonton General Hospital, Misericordia Hospital, Alberta Hospital, Glenrose Hospital, Cross Cancer Institute, and Grey Nuns Hospital. Counseling services and student health services are available to all University of Alberta students.

Mission Statement

Dedicated to the optimizations of health through scholarship and leadership in our education programs, in fundamental and applied research, and in the prevention and treatment of illness in conjunction with the Capital Health Authority and other partners. Vision: To be nationally and internationally recognized leaders investing in education, research and service, making important contributions to health.

Curricular Highlights

Community Service Requirement: Required.
Rural Family Medicine training.
Research/Thesis Requirement: Optional.

The Faculty of Medicine conducts a fully accredited, four-year program leading to the degree of doctor of medicine. Each of the first two years consists of 33 weeks of instruction, from early September until mid-May. The final two years are conducted as a continuum, during which each student has a four-week holiday period. The first two years of the curriculum are an integrated systems-based program covering the basic and clinical sciences. It is primarily case-based and uses a mixture of lectures and small-group sessions with some problem-based learning. The

last two years are composed of a student internship of at least 56 weeks, during which the student is assigned to hospitals affiliated with the faculty for clinical study and experience, a selective program in medicine and surgery, and an elective program that allows students to develop their own curriculum and spend a minimum of 12 weeks in one or more subject areas of their choice. Throughout the program, emphasis is on self-education; much instruction is on a small-group basis. A graduate training program leading to eligibility for specialist qualifications by the Royal College of Physicians and Surgeons of Canada is offered in most clinical specialties.

USMLE
Step 1: Optional.
Step 2: Clinical Skills (CS): Optional.
Step 2: Clinical Knowledge (CK): Optional.

Selection Factors

The Admissions Committee selects applicants without discrimination to gender, race, religion, or age, and attempts to apply five criteria: undergraduate academic achievement, employment history, extracurricular activities, letters of recommendation, and the MCAT. Final applicants will be required to attend an interview at the University of Alberta at their own expense. Preference is given to Alberta residents. The University of Alberta does not accept applications from international students. Rejected applicants are given the opportunity to reapply for admission. Applicants who have been asked to withdraw or who have been suspended or expelled from any medical school will not usually be considered. There are five positions over the regular quota of 133 for the M.D. program to Aboriginal applicants.

Financial Aid

Loans are available under the Canada Student Loan Plan or the Province of Alberta Loan Plan to Canadian citizens or permanent residents who have been in Canada and in Alberta for 12 months prior to the beginning of the academic term.

Information about Diversity Programs

Five positions each for aboriginal and rural applicants.

Campus Information

Setting

The University of Alberta is in a dynamic city with all amenities of big city living. Edmonton is home to the most expansive urban park in North America. Providing the city with 22 parks, the river valley boasts 1,500 km of trails used for walking, biking, and cross-country skiing. The city boasts sports franchises, one of North America's finest concert halls (the Winspear Centre), a symphony orchestra, a vibrant theatre scene, and a summer packed with major arts and cultural events.

Enrollment

For 2007, total enrollment was: 536

Special Features

Students train in one of Canada's leading clinical, research, and teaching hospitals. The UAH treats more than 700,000 patients annually and is recognized as a national leader in organ and tissue transplant, both in success rates and in transplant volumes. Other major facilities are the Stollery Children's Hospital, Alberta Diabetes Institute and the future Mazankowski Alberta Heart Institute and Lois Hole Women's Pavilion.

Housing

The University of Alberta offers residence service. The two main facilities on campus, the Lister Cenre and HUB Centre, have been updated and have new additions. Information on housing can be found on the University of Alberta, Office of the Registrar and Student Awards, Web site at *www.registrar.ualberta.ca.*

Application Process and Requirements 2009–2010

Primary Application Service: School-specific
Earliest filing date: July 2, 2008
Latest filing date: November 1, 2008

Secondary Application Required?: Yes
Sent to: All applicants
URL: n/a
Fee: Yes, $100
Fee waiver available: No
Earliest filing date: July 2, 2008
Latest filing date: November 15, 2008

Latest MCAT® considered: September 2008
Oldest MCAT® considered: 1991

Early Decision Program
School does have EDP
Applicants notified: May 15, 2009
EDP available for: n/a

Regular Acceptance Notice
Earliest date: May 15, 2009
Latest date: Until class is full

Applicant's Response to Acceptance
Offer – Maximum Time: 10 business days

Requests for Deferred
Entrance Considered: Yes

Deposit to Hold Place in Class: Yes
Deposit (Resident): $1,000
Deposit (Non-Resident): $1,000
Deposit due: With response to acceptance offer
Applied to tuition: Yes
Deposit refundable: No
Refundable by: n/a

Estimated number of new entrant: 144
EDP: 0, special program: n/a

Start Month/Year: August 2009

Interview Format: Multiple Mini Interview (MMI).

Other Programs

PREPARATORY PROGRAMS
Postbaccalaureate Program: No
Summer Program: No

COMBINED DEGREE PROGRAMS
Baccalaureate/MD: No
MD/MPH: No
MD/MBA: No
MD/JD: No
MD/PhD: Yes
www.med.ualberta.ca/research/mdphd.cfm

Premedical Coursework

Course	Req.	Rec.	Lab.	Sems.	Course	Req.	Rec.	Lab.	Sems.
Inorganic Chemistry	•			6	Computer Science				
Behavioral Sciences					Genetics				
Biochemistry	•			3	Humanities				
Biology	•			6	Organic Chemistry	•			6
Biology/Zoology					Physics	•			6
Calculus					Psychology				
College English	•			6	Social Sciences				
College Mathematics					Statistics	•			3

Selection Factors: 2007 Accepted Applicants

Proportion of Accepted Applicants with Relevant Experience (Data Self-Reported to AMCAS®)																					Community Service/Volunteer	100%
																					Medically-Related Work	30%
																					Research	25%

Shaded bar represents accepted scores ranging from the 10th percentile to the 90th percentile   **School Median** ●   **National Median** ●

Overall GPA	2.0	2.1	2.2	2.3	2.4	2.5	2.6	2.7	2.8	2.9	3.0	3.1	3.2	3.3	3.4	3.5	3.6	3.7	(3.8)	3.9	4.0
Science GPA	2.0	2.1	2.2	2.3	2.4	2.5	2.6	2.7	2.8	2.9	3.0	3.1	3.2	3.3	3.4	3.5	3.6	3.7	(3.8)	3.9	4.0

MCAT® required: Yes, 100% of 2007 accepted applicants took MCAT®

Verbal Reasoning	3	4	5	6	7	8	9	(10)	11	12	13	14	15
Physical Sciences	3	4	5	6	7	8	9	10	(11)	12	13	14	15
Biological Sciences	3	4	5	6	7	8	9	10	11	(12)	13	14	15
Writing Sample			J	K	L	M	N	O	P	(Q)	R	S	T

Acceptance & Matriculation Data for 2007–2008 First Year Class

	Resident	Non-Resident	International	Total
Applied	640	634	n/a	1274
Interviewed	308	74	n/a	382
Deferred	0	0	0	0
Matriculants	0	0	0	0
Early Assurance Program	0	0	0	0
Early Decision Program	n/a	n/a	n/a	n/a
Baccalaureate/MD	n/a	n/a	n/a	n/a
MD/PhD	0	0	0	0
Matriculated	133	11	n/a	**144**

Applications accepted from International Applicants: No

Matriculant Demographics: 2007–2008 First Year Class

Men: 69   **Women:** 75

Matriculants' Self-Reported Race/Ethnicity

Mexican American
Cuban
Puerto Rican
Other Hispani
Total Hispanic
Chinese   **DATA NOT COLLECTED**
Asian Indian
Pakistani   Total Asian
Filipino   **Unduplicated Number**
Japanese   **of Matriculants**

Korean
Vietnamese
Other Asian

Science and Math Majors: 85%
Matriculants with:
    Baccalaureate degree: 105
    Graduate degree(s): 6

Specialty Choice

2003, 2004, 2005 Graduates, Specialty Choice

Anesthesiology
Emergency Medicine
Family Practice
Internal Medicine
Obs
Orth   **DATA NOT COLLECTED**
Pedi
Psyc
Radiology
Surgery

Financial Information

	Residents	Non-Residents
Total Cost of Attendance	$7600	n/r
Tuition and Fees	$13,425	n/r
Other (includes living expenses)	n/r	n/r
Health Insurance (can be waived)	n/r	n/r

Average 2007 Graduate Indebtedness: $100,000
% of Enrolled Students Receiving Aid: n/r

Criminal Background Check

This medical school requires a criminal background check prior to matriculation.

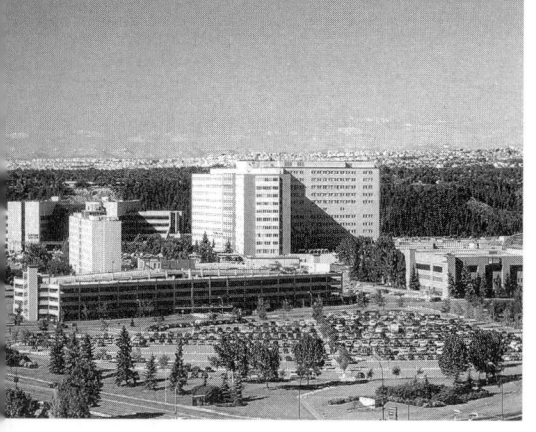

University of Calgary Faculty of Medicine
Calgary, Alberta

Office of Admissions
University of Calgary, Faculty of Medicine
3330 Hospital Drive, N.W.
Calgary, Alberta
Canada, T2N 4N1
T 403 220 4262   **F** 403 210 8148

Admissions www.medicine.ucalgary.ca
Main www.medicine.ucalgary.ca
Financial www.ucalgary.ca/UofC/students/awards
Email ucmedapp@ucalgary.ca

Public Institution

Dr. Thomas Feasby, Dean of Medicine

Adele Meyers, Admissions Officer

Claudia Barrett, Interim Director, Awards and Financial Aid

General Information
The Faculty of Medicine at the University of Calgary accepted its first students in September 1970. In 1972, the Faculty of Medicine moved into its permanent facilities in the Calgary Health Sciences Centre. The centre has been designed to complement the objectives of the faculty's integrated teaching program.

Mission Statement
We wish to be a medical school which is: responsive to community and societal needs; determined to shape the future of society; rooted in basic research and discovery; committed to excellence and pursuit of excellence and to continuous improvement in all endeavours; and committed to innovation and creativity.

Curricular Highlights
Community Service Requirement: Optional. Strongly recommended.
Research/Thesis Requirement: Optional.

The curriculum is based on clinical presentations of the way patients present to physicians. One hundred twenty clinical presentations have been defined, ranging from simple to complex, and they are grouped by body system and human development. The clinical presentation curriculum teaches the basic science and clinical knowledge pertinent to each clinical presentation and provides an approach to the solution of the clinical problems. The Introductory Clinical Skills of Communication and Physical Examination commence in the first weeks of the curriculum. The curriculum maintains an active learning environment with more than 25 percent of scheduled instructional activities spent in small-group, case-based learning sessions.

Students have the opportunity to reinforce in a clinical setting what they have learned in the body systems as they progress through each of the systems. The curriculum also focuses on the relevance of the family and the community in health and disease. The school employs a pass/fail grading system. Each academic year lasts about 11 months. At the end of the three years, students will be granted the M.D. degree. The school's philosophy is to produce generalist physicians who can proceed to further training in specialty, family medicine, or research.

USMLE
Step 1: Optional.
Step 2: Clinical Skills (CS): Optional.
Step 2: Clinical Knowledge (CK): Optional.

Selection Factors
The Admissions Committee selects applicants without discrimination to gender, race, religion, or age, and attempts to apply six criteria: undergraduate academic achievement, employment history, extracurricular activities, an essay, letters of recommendation, and the MCAT®. Final applicants will be required to attend an interview at the University of Calgary at their own expense. Final applicants will also be required to write an on-site essay on a topic assigned by the Admissions Committee. Preference is given to Alberta residents. The University of Calgary does not accept applications from individual international students. Presently, seats for international students are limited to those students who come from institutions/countries with whom the Faculty of Medicine has a formal, contractual agreement. Rejected applicants are given the opportunity to reapply for admission. Applicants who have been asked to withdraw or who have been suspended or expelled from any medical school will not usually be considered.

Financial Aid
The majority of students obtain financial aid through student loans and lines of credit. Because students attend school 11 months each year, summer employment is unlikely, and, therefore, financial support must be sufficient to meet their requirements over the subsequent three years. The student awards officer will provide information about student loans, bursaries, and awards. The financial status of the applicant does not affect acceptance into the program. Students receive a total stipend of $3,420 for the third (final) year.

Campus Information

Setting
The school is located on a hospital site one kilometer from the main university campus.

Enrollment
For 2007, total enrollment was: 400

Special Features
The Heath Sciences Centre offers students state-of-the-art facilities. Students are encouraged to pursue electives in developing countries.

Housing
There are residences on the main campus, as well as apartment buildings and condominiums within walking distance. The average cost per month of a one-bedroom apartment near the hospital is $850.

Satellite Campuses/Facilities
Students have clinical experiences on-site at the Foothills Medical Centre, as well as at two other general hospitals and the children's hospital in Calgary. During the final year, they may rotate through hospitals in smaller centers in the province, in addition to doing electives outside of Alberta.

Application Process and Requirements 2009–2010

Primary Application Service: School-specific
Earliest filing date: July 1, 2008
Latest filing date: October 15, 2008

Secondary Application Required?: No
Sent to: n/a
URL: n/a
Fee: n/a
Fee waiver available: n/a
Earliest filing date: n/a
Latest filing date: n/a

Latest MCAT® considered: September 2008
Oldest MCAT® considered: April 1991

Early Decision Program
School does not have EDP
Applicants notified: n/a
EDP available for: n/a

Regular Acceptance Notice
Earliest date: May 15, 2009
Latest date: Varies

Applicant's Response to Acceptance
Offer – Maximum Time: Fifteen business days

Requests for Deferred
Entrance Considered: Yes

Deposit to Hold Place in Class: Yes
Deposit (Resident): $500
Deposit (Non-Resident): $500
Deposit due: With response to acceptance offer
Applied to tuition: Yes
Deposit refundable: No
Refundable by: n/a

Estimated number of new entrants: 135
EDP: 0, special program: n/a

Start Month/Year: August 2009

Interview Format: A series of short standardized interviews.

Other Programs

PREPARATORY PROGRAMS
Postbaccalaureate Program: No
Summer Program: No

COMBINED DEGREE PROGRAMS
Baccalaureate/MD: No
MD/MPH: Yes
MD/MBA: Yes
MD/JD: No
MD/PhD: Yes, http://gse.myweb.med.ucalgary.ca/x.pro/ModShow/ShowPage/1022
Additional Program: Yes, MD/MSc

Premedical Coursework

Course	Req.	Rec.	Lab.	Sems.
Inorganic Chemistry		•		2
Behavioral Sciences				
Biochemistry		•		2
Biology		•		2
Biology/Zoology				
Calculus		•		1
College English		•		2
College Mathematics				

Course	Req.	Rec.	Lab.	Sems.
Computer Science				
Genetics				
Humanities				
Organic Chemistry		•		2
Physics		•		2
Psychology		•		1
Social Sciences		•		1
Statistics		•		1

Selection Factors: 2007 Accepted Applicants

Proportion of Accepted Applicants with Relevant Experience (Data Self-Reported to AMCAS®)		
Community Service/Volunteer		99%
Medically-Related Work		95%
Research		35%

Shaded bar represents accepted scores ranging from the 10th percentile to the 90th percentile — School Median ● National Median ●

Overall GPA	2.0 2.1 2.2 2.3 2.4 2.5 2.6 2.7 2.8 2.9 3.0 3.1 3.2 3.3 3.4 3.5 (3.6) 3.7 3.8 3.9 4.0
Science GPA	DATA NOT COLLECTED

MCAT® required: Yes, 100% of 2007 accepted applicants took MCAT®

	3	4	5	6	7	8	9	10	11	12	13	14	15
Verbal Reasoning	3	4	5	6	7	8	9	(10)	11	12	13	14	15
Physical Sciences	3	4	5	6	7	8	9	10	(11)	12	13	14	15
Biological Sciences	3	4	5	6	7	8	9	10	(11)	12	13	14	15
Writing Sample			J	K	L	M	N	O	P	(Q)	R	S	T

Acceptance & Matriculation Data for 2007–2008 First Year Class

	Resident	Non-Resident	International	Total
Applied	750	721	0	1471
Interviewed	317	99	0	416
Deferred	3	3	0	6
Matriculants				
Early Assurance Program	0	0	0	0
Early Decision Program	n/a	n/a	n/a	n/a
Baccalaureate/MD	n/a	n/a	n/a	n/a
MD/PhD	9	0	0	9
Matriculated	115	20	0	**135**

Applications accepted from International Applicants: No

Specialty Choice

2003, 2004, 2005 Graduates, Specialty Choice	
Anesthesiology	4
Emergency Medicine	2
Family Practice	37
Internal Medicine	18
Obstetrics/Gynecology	5
Orthopaedic Surgery	5
Pediatrics	4
Psychiatry	11
Radiology	3
Surgery	11

Matriculant Demographics: 2007–2008 First Year Class

Men: 59   **Women:** 76

Matriculants' Self-Reported Race/Ethnicity

Mexican American   Korean
Cuban   Vietnamese
Puerto Rican   Other Asian
Other H
Total Hi   **DATA NOT COLLECTED**
Chinese
Asian In
Pakistani   Total Asian
Filipino   **Unduplicated Number**
Japanese   **of Matriculants**

Science and Math Majors: 80%
Matriculants with:
      Baccalaureate degree: 87%
      Graduate degree(s): 30%

Financial Information

	Residents	Non-Residents
Total Cost of Attendance	$35,000	$66,000
Tuition and Fees	$14,000	$45,000
Other (includes living expenses)	$21,000	$21,000
Health Insurance (can be waived)	$193	$193

Average 2007 Graduate Indebtedness: $100,000
% of Enrolled Students Receiving Aid: 90%

Criminal Background Check

This medical school does not require a criminal background check prior to matriculation.

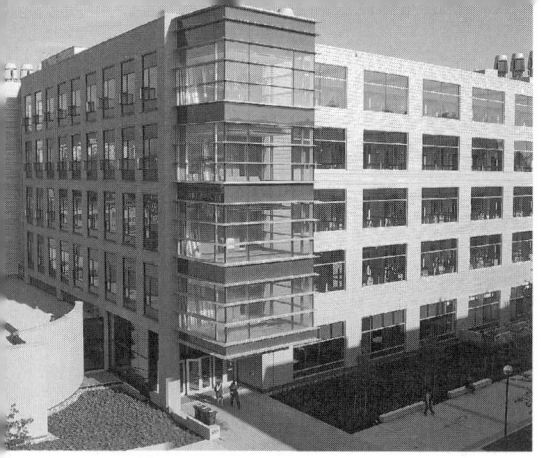

University of British Columbia
Faculty of Medicine
Vancouver, British Columbia

MD Undergraduate Program
Faculty of Medicine, Dean's Office
University of British Columbia
317-2194 Health Sciences Mall
Vancouver, British Columbia
Canada, V6T 1Z3
T 604 822 4482   **F** 604 822 6061

Admissions www.med.ubc.ca/education/md_ugrad/
MD_Undergraduate_Admissions.htm
Main www.med.ubc.ca/home.htm
Financial www.med.ubc.ca/education/md_ugrad/
financial_assistance.htm
Email admissions.md@ubc.ca

Public Institution

Dr. Gavin C.E. Stuart, Dean

Dr. Michael Clifford Fabian, Associate Dean, Admissions

Lori Charvat, Associate Dean, Equity

Bryan Hicks, Student Financial Assistant Officer

Denis Hughes, Director, Admissions

Shelley Small and Joan Munro, Admissions Advisors

General Information
The expansion and distribution of the UBC Faculty of Medicine undergraduate program began in March 15, 2002, creating a partnership in medical education with the University of Northern British Columbia, the University of Victoria, and the regional Health Authorities. The expansion will provide an education model for other Canadian jurisdictions, contribute to meeting federal health care recommendations, and advance BC's economic and educational capacity. The photograph above was provided by Bunting Coady Architects.

Mission Statement
Together, we create knowledge and advance learning that makes a vital contribution to the health of individuals and communities locally, nationally, and internationally.

Curricular Highlights
Community Service Requirement: Required.
Research/Thesis Requirement: Optional.

The program is built on principles of student self-directed learning, integration of biomedical and social sciences, early clinical contact, information management, professional development, and social responsibility. See the UBC Web site for information at *www.med.ubc.ca/education/md_ugrad/Schedule___Courses.htm*.

USMLE
Step 1: Optional.
Step 2: Clinical Skills (CS): Optional.
Step 2: Clinical Knowledge (CK): Optional.

Selection Factors
The selection of candidates for admission to UBC's medical school is governed by guidelines established by the Senate of UBC, and is the responsibility of the Faculty of Medicine Admissions Selection Committee. See the Web site for selection criteria at *www.med.ubc.ca/ education/ md_ugrad/MD_Undergraduate_Admissions/Selection.htm*. The UBC Faculty of Medicine's Associate Dean of Admissions oversees the selection process to ensure that all applicants are given careful consideration without regard to age, gender, sexual orientation, race, ancestry, color, place of origin, family status, physical or mental disability, political belief, religion, or marital or economic status.

Financial Aid
UBC and the Faculty of Medicine are committed to ensuring that financial circumstances are not a barrier to qualified domestic students. Graduates who practice in rural areas are eligible for a number of financial incentives. For information regarding financial aid and awards, please contact the Student Financial Assistance Officer Faculty of Medicine, MD Undergraduate Program by telephone at (604) 875-5834, or toll free at (1-877) 875-7800. Email may be sent to student-finances@medd.med.ubc.ca. Additional information is available at *www.med.ubc.ca/education/md_ugrad/financial_assistance.htm*.

Information about Diversity Programs
The UBC Faculty of Medicine is committed to increasing opportunities for Aboriginal (Status or Non-Status Indians, Treaty, First Nations, Metis, or Inuit) applicants through the Aboriginal Admissions Subcommittee. Contact James Andrew, Aboriginal Programs Coordinator, for more information: at james.andrew@ubc.ca or 604-822-3236. Applicants with disabilities are considered in accordance with UBC's policy on Academic Accommodation for Students with Disabilities. The Northern Medical Program provides an opportunity to complete undergraduate training in a northern regional centre and may be of particular interest to those applicants who come from, or are interested in, rural, remote, or northern communities.

Campus Information

Setting
The University of British Columbia Faculty of Medicine has launched an innovative, distributed medical education program in collaboration with the Government of British Columbia, the University of Northern British Columbia, the University of Victoria, and provincial regional Health Authorities. The first of its kind in Canada, the program creates new opportunities for medical education across BC, almost doubling undergraduate class sizes at sites in the North, on Vancouver Island, in the Fraser Valley, in the BC interior, and in Vancouver.

Enrollment
For 2007, total enrollment was: 256

Special Features
The newly-constructed 40,000 square meter UBC Life Sciences Centre is located on the University of British Columbia campus. It houses basic science departments and teaching and research laboratories, while providing cost-effective sharing of equipment and other resources. The Northern Health Sciences Centre (University of Northern British Columbia campus) and the Medical Sciences Building (University of Victoria campus) use state-of-the-art technology in the delivery of medical education. The buildings contain labs, lecture halls, classrooms, small seminar rooms, and student common areas.

Housing
For detailed information regarding housing, please contact the appropriate program site. For the Island Medical Program, go to *http://imp. uvic.ca/current/affairs/impoffice.php*. For the Northern Medical Program, go to *www.unbc. ca/nmp/nmp.html*. For the Vancouver Fraser Medical Program, go to *www.med.ubc.ca/ education/md_ugrad/student_affairs.htm*.

Satellite Campuses/Facilities
The Island Medical Program (IMP) at the University of Victoria, the Northern Medical Program (NMP) at the University of Northern British Columbia, and the UBC-based Vancouver Fraser Medical Program (VFMP).

Application Process and Requirements 2009–2010

Primary Application Service: School-specific
Earliest filing date: Early June 2008
Latest filing date: Early September 2008

Secondary Application Required?: Yes
Sent to: Applicable applicants
Contact: Admissions Officer, (604) 822-4482, admissions.md@ubc.ca
Fee: No
Fee waiver available: n/a
Earliest filing date: Mid-January 2009
Latest filing date: Early March 2009

Latest MCAT® considered: August 2008
Oldest MCAT® considered: July 2003

Early Decision Program
School does not have EDP
Applicants notified: n/a
EDP available for: n/a

Regular Acceptance Notice
Earliest date: Mid-May 2009
Latest date: Until Class is Full

Applicant's Response to Acceptance Offer – Maximum Time: Varies

Requests for Deferred Entrance Considered: Yes

Deposit to Hold Place in Class: Yes
Deposit (Resident): $300
Deposit (Non-Resident): $300
Deposit due: With response to acceptance offer
Applied to tuition: Yes
Deposit refundable: No
Refundable by: n/a

Estimated number of new entrants: 256
EDP: n/a, special program: n/a

Start Month/Year: August 2009

Interview Format: Multiple Mini-Interview. Regional interviews are not available.

Other Programs

PREPARATORY PROGRAMS
Postbaccalaureate Program: Yes, www.med.ubc.ca/education/md_postgrad.htm
Summer Program: No

COMBINED DEGREE PROGRAMS
Baccalaureate/MD: No
MD/MPH: No
MD/MBA: No
MD/JD: No
MD/PhD: Yes, www.med.ubc.ca/education/md_ugrad/mdphd.htm

Premedical Coursework

Course	Req.	Rec.	Lab.	Hrs.	Course	Req.	Rec.	Lab.	Hrs.
Inorganic Chemistry	•			2	Computer Science				
Behavioral Sciences		•			Genetics				
Biochemistry	•			2	Humanities				
Biology	•			2	Organic Chemistry	•			2
Biology/Zoology					Physics		•		
Calculus					Psychology				
College English	•			2	Social Sciences				
College Mathematics					Other		•		

Selection Factors: 2007 Accepted Applicants

Proportion of Accepted Applicants with Relevant Experience (Data Self-Reported to AMCAS®)		
Community Service/Volunteer		100
Medically-Related Work		50
Research		50

Shaded bar represents accepted scores ranging from the 10th percentile to the 90th percentile. School Median ● National Median ●

Overall GPA	2.0	2.1	2.2	2.3	2.4	2.5	2.6	2.7	2.8	2.9	3.0	3.1	3.2	3.3	3.4	3.5	3.6	(3.7)	3.8	3.9	4.0
Science GPA	2.0	2.1	2.2	2.3	2.4	2.5	2.6	2.7	2.8	2.9	3.0	3.1	3.2	3.3	3.4	3.5	(3.6)	3.7	3.8	3.9	4.0

MCAT® required: Yes, 100% of 2007 accepted applicants took MCAT®

Verbal Reasoning	3	4	5	6	7	8	(9)	10	11	12	13	14	15
Physical Sciences	3	4	5	6	7	8	9	(10)	11	12	13	14	15
Biological Sciences	3	4	5	6	7	8	9	10	(11)	12	13	14	15
Writing Sample			J	K	L	M	N	O	(P)	Q	R	S	T

Acceptance & Matriculation Data for 2007–2008 First Year Class

	Resident	Non-Resident	International	Total
Applied	1081	499	0	1580
Interviewed	603	37	0	640
Deferred	5	0	0	5
Matriculants				
Early Assurance Program	n/a	n/a	n/a	n/a
Early Decision Program	n/a	n/a	n/a	n/a
Baccalaureate/MD	n/a	n/a	n/a	n/a
MD/PhD	4	0	0	4
Matriculated	246	10	0	**256**
Applications accepted from International Applicants: No				

Specialty Choice

2003, 2004, 2005 Graduates, Specialty Choice

Anesthesiology
Emergency Medicine
Family Practice
Internal Medicine
Obst
Orth   **DATA NOT COLLECTED**
Pedia
Psyc
Radiology
Surgery

Matriculant Demographics: 2007–2008 First Year Class

Men: 119   **Women:** 137

Matriculants' Self-Reported Race/Ethnicity

Mexican American   Korean
Cuban   Vietnamese
Puerto Rican   Other Asian
Other H
Total Hi   **DATA NOT COLLECTED**
Chinese
Asian Ir
Pakistan   n/a   Total Asian
Filipino   Unduplicated Number
Japanese   of Matriculants

Science and Math Majors: 84%
Matriculants with:
        Baccalaureate degree: 203
        Graduate degree(s): 39

Financial Information

	Residents	Non-Residents
Total Cost of Attendance	n/c	n/c
Tuition and Fees	$14,566	$14,566
Other (includes living expenses)	n/c	n/c
Health Insurance	n/c	n/c

Average 2007 Graduate Indebtedness: n/c
% of Enrolled Students Receiving Aid: n/c

Criminal Background Check

This medical school requires a criminal background check prior to matriculation.

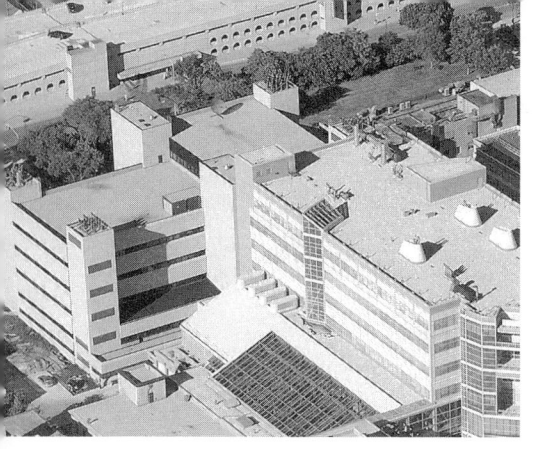

University of Manitoba
Faculty of Medicine
Winnipeg, Manitoba

Chair, Admissions Committee
Faculty of Medicine
University of Manitoba 260-727 McDermot Avenue
Winnipeg, Manitoba
Canada, R3E 3P5
T 204 789 3499   **F** 204 789 3929

Admissions www.umanitoba.ca/medicine/admissions
Main www.umanitoba.ca/medicine
Financial http://umanitoba.ca/admin/financial_services
Email registrar_med@umanitoba.ca

Public Institution

Dr. D. Sandham, Dean

Dr. Fred Aoki, Assistant Dean, Admissions

Ms. Beth Jennings, Student Services Administrator

Sheila Smith, Student Advisor

General Information

Medical education in Manitoba is designed to provide students with the knowledge and experience they need to practice medicine in a profession where new developments in science and public health policy create an ever-changing environment. In the first two years of the program, the subject matter is divided into blocks which cover core concepts in health and medicine, human development, and body systems. Clinical Skills, Problem-Solving, Medical Humanities, Law, Laboratory and Investigative Medicine, Health Equity and Survival Tactics are integrated into the six blocks. The final two years, called the "clerkship," are spent in direct contact with patients and doctors in a clinical setting in which students gain experience with increasing responsibility for patient care and management. General teaching facilities are located in the medical buildings, and facilities for clinical instruction are provided in the teaching hospitals affiliated with the University of Manitoba and in related institutions. The varied settings in which medicine is practiced in Winnipeg and in rural and northern Manitoba also provide students with the opportunity to study community medicine outside the major teaching institutions. For more information on the institution, please visit the Web site.

Mission Statement

The mission of the Faculty of Medicine is to: develop, deliver and evaluate high quality educational programs for undergraduate and postgraduate students of medicine and medical rehabilitation, for graduate students and postdoctoral fellows in basic medical sciences and for physicians to practice; to conduct research and other scholarly enquiry into the basic and applied medical sciences; and to provide advice, disseminate information to health professions and plan for the development and delivery of health care services and to help improve health status and service delivery to the Province of Manitoba and the wider community.

Curricular Highlights
Community Service Requirement: Optional.
Research/Thesis Requirement: Optional.

For information regarding curriculum, scheduling, and enrichment programs, please refer to the links posted at: *www.umanitoba.ca/faculties/medicine/education/undergraduate.html.*

USMLE
Step 1: Optional.
Step 2: Clinical Skills (CS): Optional.
Step 2: Clinical Knowledge (CK): Optional.

Selection Factors
Selection by the Admissions Committee is made on the basis of (1) adjusted grade-point (GPA is calculated on a 4.5 scale); (2) MCAT®; and (3) personal assessment score (PAS). All students must be Canadian citizens or permanent residents of Canada. Preference is given to residents of Manitoba, although a limited number of Out of Province applicants are accepted. Special consideration is given to the Native populations of Manitoba, consistent with efforts made to recruit and retain applicants from the Aboriginal populations, and rural and inner-city areas. For more information, see the Applicant Information Bulletin: *www.umanitoba.ca/faculties/medicine/admissions.*

Financial Aid
Under the Canadian Students Loan Act, Canadians can obtain interest-free loans during their undergraduate course in medicine. Bursaries from the University, the Manitoba Medical College Foundation, and the provincial government are available to deserving students. Applications for these bursaries are available when classes commence. Students may also obtain assistance from the W. K. Kellogg Student Loan Program. Several entrance scholarships are also offered annually.

Information about Diversity Programs
The Health Careers Access Program: University of Manitoba's Access program provides support to persons who have traditionally not had the opportunity for advanced education because of social, economic, or cultural reasons or lack of formal education. This program is exclusive to Aboriginal (Metis, Status, Non-Status, Inuit) residents of Manitoba with a strong interest in becoming a health professional. Sponsorship includes academic and personal support and may include some financial assistance. These programs are funded by Manitoba Education and Training, Advanced Education and Skills Training Division.

Campus Information

Setting
The Faculty of Medicine is located at the Bannatyne Campus. Facilites for instruction are provided there, as well as in the affiliated teaching hospitals; the Institutes and Centres of Cell Biology, Health Policy, Child Health, Cancer Care Manitoba, Cardiovascular Sciences, Spinal Cord Research; St. Boniface General Hospital Research Centre; the National Microbiology Laboratory; and the Institute for Biodiagnostics (NRC).

Enrollment
For 2007, total enrollment was: 372

Housing
On-campus housing is not available at the Bannatyne Campus. However affordable apartments are available nearby. See: *http://umanitoba.ca/student/housing.*

Application Process and Requirements 2009–2010

Primary Application Service: School-specific
Earliest filing date: August 15, 2008
Latest filing date: October 10, 2008

Secondary Application Required?: Yes
Sent to: All applicants
URL: www.umanitoba.ca/medicine/admissions
Fee: Yes, $90
Fee waiver available: No
Earliest filing date: Same as primary application.
Latest filing date: October 10, 2008

Latest MCAT® considered: September 2008
Oldest MCAT® considered: April 2005

Early Decision Program
School does not have EDP
Applicants notified: n/a
EDP available for: n/a

Regular Acceptance Notice
Earliest date: May 15, 2009
Latest date: Until class is full

Applicant's Response to Acceptance
Offer – Maximum Time: Two weeks or as specified in the offer.

Requests for Deferred
Entrance Considered: Yes

Deposit to Hold Place in Class: Yes
Deposit (Resident): $500
Deposit (Non-Resident): $500
Deposit due: With response to acceptance offer
Applied to tuition: Yes
Deposit refundable: No
Refundable by: n/a

Estimated number of new entrants: 100
EDP: n/a, special program: n/a

Start Month/Year: August 25, 2009

Interview Format: Multi-Mini Interview (MMI).

Other Programs
PREPARATORY PROGRAMS
Postbaccalaureate Program: No
Summer Program: Yes, www.umanitoba.ca/medicine/media/EarlyExposureExperienceInfoSheet.pdf

COMBINED DEGREE PROGRAMS
Baccalaureate/MD: Yes, http://umanitoba.ca/medicine/education/undergraduate/preclerkship/bsc_med.html
MD/MPH: No
MD/MBA: No
MD/JD: No
MD/PhD: Yes, Dr. D. Eisenstat, eisensta@cc.umanitoba.ca

Premedical Coursework

Course	Req.	Rec.	Lab.	Hrs.
Inorganic Chemistry				
Behavioral Sciences				
Biochemistry	•			6
Biology		•		
Biology/Zoology		•		
Calculus				
College English				
College Mathematics				

Course	Req.	Rec.	Lab.	Hrs.
Computer Science				
Genetics		•		
Humanities		•		
Organic Chemistry		•		
Physics		•		
Psychology				
Social Sciences		•		
Other				

Selection Factors: 2007 Accepted Applicants

Proportion of Accepted Applicants with Relevant Experience (Data Self-Reported to AMCAS)	DATA NOT COLLECTED

Shaded bar represents accepted scores ranging from the 10th percentile to the 90th percentile — School Median ● National Median ●

Overall GPA	2.0 2.1 2.2 2.3 2.4 2.5 2.6 2.7 2.8 2.9 3.0 3.1 3.2 3.3 3.4 3.5 3.6 3.7 3.8 3.9 (4.0)
Science GPA	DATA NOT COLLECTED

MCAT® required: Yes, 100% of 2007 accepted applicants took MCAT®

Verbal Reasoning	3	4	5	6	7	8	9	(10)	11	12	13	14	15
Physical Sciences	3	4	5	6	7	8	9	10	(11)	12	13	14	15
Biological Sciences	3	4	5	6	7	8	9	10	11	(12)	13	14	15
Writing Sample			J	K	L	M	N	O	P	(Q)	R	S	T

Acceptance & Matriculation Data for 2007–2008 First Year Class

	Resident	Non-Resident	International	Total
Applied	338	619	0	957
Interviewed	248	59	0	307
Deferred	5	0	0	5
Matriculants				
Early Assurance Program	0	0	0	0
Early Decision Program	n/a	n/a	n/a	n/a
Baccalaureate/MD	n/a	n/a	n/a	n/a
MD/PhD	0	0	0	0
Matriculated	90	10	0	**100**

Applications accepted from International Applicants: No

Specialty Choice

2003, 2004, 2005 Graduates, Specialty Choice

Anesthesiology
Emergency Medicine
Family Practice
Internal Medicine
Obste
Ortho   DATA NOT COLLECTED
Pediat
Psychiatry
Radiology
Surgery

Matriculant Demographics: 2007–2008 First Year Class

Men: 50   **Women:** 50

Matriculants' Self-Reported Race/Ethnicity

Mexican American	Korean
Cuban	Vietnamese
Puerto Rican	Other Asian
Other	
Total	DATA NOT COLLECTED
Chine	
Asian Indian	White
Pakistani	Total Asian
Filipino	Unduplicated Number
Japanese	of Matriculants

Science and Math Majors: Data not collected
Matriculants with:
    Baccalaureate degree: 100
    Graduate degree(s): 8

Financial Information

	Residents	Non-Residents
Total Cost of Attendance	n/r	n/r
Tuition and Fees	$7,595	$7,595
Other (includes living expenses)	n/r	n/r
Health Insurance (can be waived)	n/r	n/r

Average 2007 Graduate Indebtedness: $51,900
% of Enrolled Students Receiving Aid: n/r

Criminal Background Check

This medical school requires a criminal background check prior to matriculation.

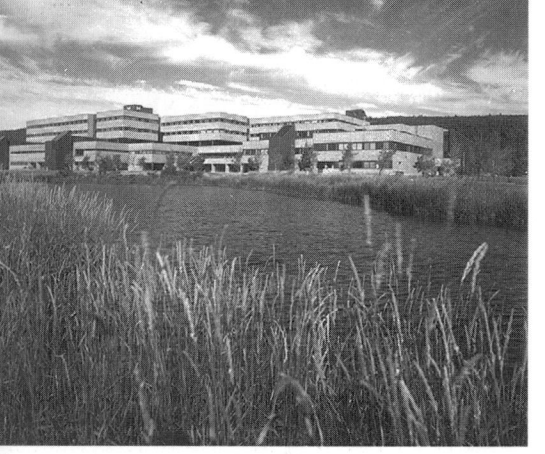

Memorial University of Newfoundland
Faculty of Medicine
St. John's, Newfoundland

Memorial University of Newfoundland
Faculty of Medicine
St. John's, Newfoundland/Labrador
Canada, A1B 3V6
T 709 777 6615   **F** 709 777 8422

Admissions www.med.mun.ca/admissions
Main www.med.mun.ca/med
Financial www.edu.gov.nf.ca/studentaid
Email munmed@mun.ca

Public Institution

Dr. J. Rourke, Dean of Medicine

Janet McHugh, Admissions Officer

Dr. W. Parsons, Assistant Dean for Admissions

General Information

Memorial is the only university in the province of Newfoundland. The university was established as Memorial College in 1925 and incorporated as a university in 1949. In 1959, campus buildings were erected on a 1,000-acre site. There are some 12,000 undergraduates and a faculty of about 1,000 (including visiting professors) working on the campus, which is situated on the periphery of St. John's. The medical school is fully accredited by the Committee on Accreditation of Canadian Medical Schools (CACMS) of the Association of Canadian Medical Colleges and the Canadian Medical Association and the Liaison Committee on Medical Education (LCME) of the Association of American Medical Colleges and the American Medical Association. Thus, the medical school is equivalent in every respect to other medical schools in Canada and the United States. Approved teaching programs for interns and residents are under the direction of the medical school. Research work is being conducted both in the hospitals and in the Health Sciences Centre.

Mission Statement

Our purpose is to enhance the health of people by educating physicians and health scientists, by conducting research in clinical and basic medical sciences and applied health sciences, and by promoting the skills and attitudes of lifelong learning.

Curricular Highlights

Community Service Requirement: Optional.
Research/Thesis Requirement: Optional.

The curriculum, the physical structure, and the administrative organization of the school were planned to allow for maximum cooperation among the various basic science and clinical

disciplines. The M.D. degree is granted upon completion of the fourth year. Canadian students take the LMCC (Medical Council of Canada) Examinations and U.S. students take the USMLE (United States Medical Licensing Examination) Step 1 and Step 2. During the first year of the medical program, students take introductory courses in cell structure and functions, biochemistry, physiology, molecular genetics, pharmacology, microbiology, anatomy, behavioral science, ethics, interviewing skills, and community medicine. In the second half of the first year and the second year, teaching has a systems approach; material from anatomy, physiology, pathology, and clinical medicine is presented in an integrated manner. The third year is a structured clinical clerkship that includes eight weeks of electives, and the fourth year is made up of electives and selectives. Rotations for Rural Medicine take place in the first, third, and fourth years. A pass/fail system is used for grading. Medical students may apply through the Offices of Undergraduate Medical Education and Research/Graduate Studies for the M.D./Ph.D. program.

USMLE
Step 1: Must only record a score.
Step 2: Clinical Skills (CS): Must only record a score.
Step 2: Clinical Knowledge (CK): Optional.

Selection Factors

The school admits students on the basis of residency priority as follows: bona fide residents of Newfoundland and Labrador, of New Brunswick, of Prince Edward Island, of other Canadian provinces, and non-Canadians. In every case, a high academic standard is required. Age by itself is not used as a basis for selection or rejection. However, both age and length of time away from full-time academic studies may be taken into consideration. Normally, the medical school does not accept transfer students from other medical schools. In rare circumstances, a transfer applicant may be considered if there is space available.

Financial Aid

Financial assistance is available to medical students through government student loan programs. Information can be obtained by contacting the Student Affairs Office at: Student Affairs Office, Faculty of Medicine, Memorial University of Newfoundland, St. John's, NL, A1B 3VC; by telephone: (709) 777-6690; or by e-mail: mdray@mun.ca.

Information about Diversity Programs

Although there is no formal affirmative action process at this medical school, the Admissions Committee does take into consideration the background of applicants in making its decisions.

Campus Information

Setting

The Faculty of Medicine is housed with the Health Sciences Centre, Janeway Children's Hospital, H.Bliss Murphy Cancer Centre, Telemedicine Centre, Centre for Offshore and Remote Medicine, and Nursing and Pharmacy Schools.

Enrollment

For 2007, total enrollment was: 240

Special Features

Health services are open to all students on campus.

Housing

On-campus housing for single and married students is provided. In addition, the university maintains a list of approved off-campus accommodations.

Application Process and Requirements 2009–2010

Primary Application Service: School-specific
Earliest filing date: July 2, 2008
Latest filing date: October 15, 2008

Secondary Application Required?: No
Sent to: n/a
URL: n/a
Fee: n/a
Fee waiver available: n/a
Earliest filing date: n/a
Latest filing date: n/a

Latest MCAT® considered: September 2008
Oldest MCAT® considered: 2003

Early Decision Program
School does not have EDP
Applicants notified: n/a
EDP available for: n/a

Regular Acceptance Notice
Earliest date: March 2, 2009
Latest date: Until class is full

Applicant's Response to Acceptance
Offer – Maximum Time: Two weeks

Requests for Deferred
Entrance Considered: Yes

Deposit to Hold Place in Class: Yes
Deposit (Resident): $200
Deposit (Non-Resident): $200
Deposit due: With response to acceptance offer
Applied to tuition: Yes
Deposit refundable: No
Refundable by: n/a

Estimated number of new entrants: 60
EDP: n/a, special program: n/a

Start Month/Year: September 2009

Interview Format: One hour interview with two interviewers. Regional interviews are not available.

Other Programs

PREPARATORY PROGRAMS
Postbaccalaureate Program: No
Summer Program: Yes,
MedQuest, 709-777-6029, mdray@mun.ca

COMBINED DEGREE PROGRAMS
Baccalaureate/MD: No
MD/MPH: No
MD/MBA: No
MD/JD: No
MD/PhD: Yes,
www.med.mun.ca/admissions

Premedical Coursework

Course	Req.	Rec.	Lab.	Sems.	Course	Req.	Rec.	Lab.	Sems.
Inorganic Chemistry		•			Computer Science				
Behavioral Sciences		•			Genetics				
Biochemistry		•			Humanities				
Biology		•			Organic Chemistry		•		
Biology/Zoology					Physics		•		
Calculus		•			Psychology				
College English	•			2	Social Sciences				
College Mathematics		•			Other				

Selection Factors: 2007 Accepted Applicants

Proportion of Accepted Applicants with Relevant Experience (Data Self-Reported to AMCAS®)				Community Service/Volunteer	100%
				Medically-Related Work	75%
				Research	50%

Shaded bar represents accepted scores ranging from the 10th percentile to the 90th percentile ▬ School Median ○ National Median ○

Overall GPA	2.0	2.1	2.2	2.3	2.4	2.5	2.6	2.7	2.8	2.9	3.0	3.1	3.2	3.3	3.4	3.5	3.6	3.7	(3.8)	3.9	4.0
Science GPA									**DATA NOT COLLECTED**												

MCAT® required: Yes, 100% of 2007 accepted applicants took MCAT®

Verbal Reasoning	3	4	5	6	7	8	9	(10)	11	12	13	14	15
Physical Sciences	3	4	5	6	7	8	9	(10)	11	12	13	14	15
Biological Sciences	3	4	5	6	7	8	9	(10)	11	12	13	14	15
Writing Sample			J	K	L	M	N	O	P	(Q)	R	S	T

Acceptance & Matriculation Data for 2008-2009 First Year Class

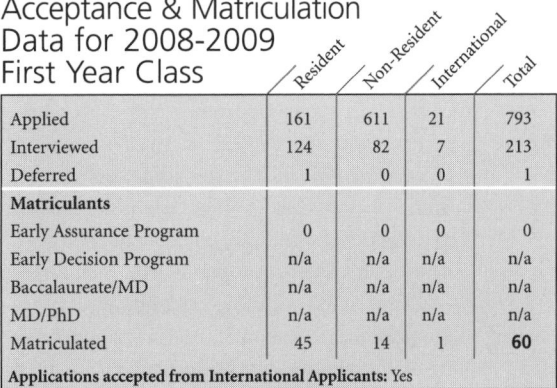

	Resident	Non-Resident	International	Total
Applied	161	611	21	793
Interviewed	124	82	7	213
Deferred	1	0	0	1
Matriculants				
Early Assurance Program	0	0	0	0
Early Decision Program	n/a	n/a	n/a	n/a
Baccalaureate/MD	n/a	n/a	n/a	n/a
MD/PhD	n/a	n/a	n/a	n/a
Matriculated	45	14	1	**60**
Applications accepted from International Applicants: Yes				

Specialty Choice

2003, 2004, 2005 Graduates, Specialty Choice	
Anesthesiology	4%
Emergency Medicine	3%
Family Practice	36%
Internal Medicine	9%
Obstetrics/Gynecology	5%
Orthopedic Surgery	3%
Pediatrics	11%
Psychiatry	10%
Radiology	10%
Surgery	8%

Matriculant Demographics: 2007–2008 First Year Class

Men: 26   **Women:** 34

Matriculants' Self-Reported Race/Ethnicity

Mexican American   Korean
Cuban   Vietnamese
Puerto Rican   Other Asian
Other Hispa...   ...
Total Hispan...
Chinese   **DATA NOT COLLECTED**   ...
Asian Indian
Pakistani
Filipino   **Unduplicated Number**
Japanese   **of Matriculants**

Science and Math Majors: 95%
Matriculants with:
     Baccalaureate degree: 100%
     Graduate degree(s): 4%

Financial Information

	Residents	Non-Residents
Total Cost of Attendance	$27,400	$51,400
Tuition and Fees	$6,250	$30,000
Other (includes living expenses)	$20,988	$20,790
Health Insurance (can be waived)	$162	$610

Average 2007 Graduate Indebtedness: $100,000
% of Enrolled Students Receiving Aid: 80%

Criminal Background Check

This medical school requires a criminal background check prior to matriculation.

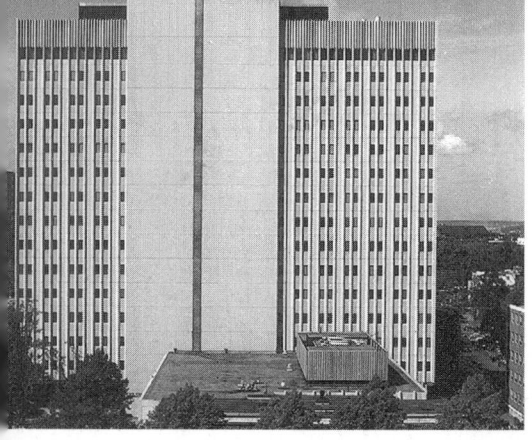

Dalhousie University Faculty of Medicine

Halifax, Nova Scotia

Admissions and Student Affairs
Room C-132, Lower Level
Clinical Research Centre, Dalhousie University
Halifax, Nova Scotia
Canada, B3H 4H7
T 902 494 1874   F 902 494 6369

Admissions http://admissions.medicine.dal.ca
Main www.medicine.dal.ca
Financial http://as01.ucis.dal.ca/staccts/
2006-2007/MD.pdf
Email medicine.admissions@dal.ca

Public Institution

Dr. Harold Cook, Dean

*Dr. Evelyn Sutton, Assistant Dean,
Admissions and Student Affairs*

General Information

Dalhousie University, a privately endowed institution founded in 1838, established the Faculty of Medicine in 1868. The main responsibility of the Faculty of Medicine is to the three Maritime Provinces of Canada (Nova Scotia, New Brunswick, and Prince Edward Island), which have a population of 1.7 million. The teaching hospitals located in the immediate vicinity of the medical school have a total of 2,300 beds covering inpatient and outpatient services in all branches of medicine.

Mission Statement

The Faculty of Medicine, Dalhousie University, strives to benefit society through equal commitment to exemplary patient care, education and the discovery and advancement of knowledge. We aim to create and maintain a learning and research environment of national and international stature, enabling our graduates and us to serve the health needs of the Maritime Provinces and Canada.

Curricular Highlights

Community Service Requirement: Optional.
Research/Thesis Requirement: Optional.

Dalhousie aims to provide a basic education that would permit a graduate to enter any branch of postgraduate training. Medicine One and Two begin in early September and extend through May. Medicine Three begins in late August/early September and ends the following September. Medicine Four begins in late September and extends until the following May. In the first year, students have extensive patient contact hours, with great emphasis on the development of clinical skills. During the first two years, students work in small groups with a tutor. The curriculum is organized around clinical problems to provide an integrated context for students to learn both basic and clinical science, and to

begin the development of clinical reasoning skills. The third and fourth years are predominantly clinical, with third year comprised of 12-week units in the major disciplines. The fourth year is arranged with initial blocks of elective time. Students finish with a unit in Continuing and Preventive Care. Dalhousie offers post-graduate medical trainees university-arranged and university-supervised clinical training which meets national accreditation standards. In all provinces with the exception of Quebec, the basis for licensure for the majority of trainees in a postgraduate training program affiliated with a CACMS/LCME medical school is successful completion of the two-part Medical Council of Canada Qualifying Examination (MCCQE), plus certification by either the College of Family Physicians of Canada or the Royal College of Physicians and Surgeons of Canada. The family medicine program at Dalhousie is a two-year integrated training experience following the M.D., leading to certification by the College of Family Physicians of Canada. Specialty training is conducted in affiliated teaching hospitals in both Halifax and Saint John. Dalhousie University currently holds Royal College approval for 41 specialty training programs. The Faculty of Medicine maintains an active program of continuing medical education for practicing physicians in the Maritime Provinces. Research and graduate education take place in all the basic science departments and in most of the clinical departments.

USMLE

Step 1: Optional.
Step 2: Clinical Skills (CS): Optional.
Step 2: Clinical Knowledge (CK): Optional.

Selection Factors

Sources of information and factors considered by the Admissions Committee include academic requirements, ability as judged on university records and on the MCAT, confidential assessments received from referees of the applicant's choice and from any others the committee may wish to consult, interviews (selected applicants only), and place of residence. Detailed comments and explanations on these selection factors may

be obtained in the Faculty of Medicine Calendar. Dalhousie does not discriminate on the basis of race, sex, creed, national origin, age, or handicap.

Financial Aid

A few entrance scholarships and entrance bursaries are awarded to students in the first year who are residents of the Maritime Provinces. The Dalhousie Medical Alumni Association Entrance Scholarship, the Dr. E. James Gordon Scholarship, and the Halifax Medical Society Entrance Scholarship are available to anyone regardless of residency. A number of bursaries and prizes are available in each year. The university maintains a loan fund, which is interest-free until graduation.

Information about Diversity Programs

Students from groups underrepresented in medicine will be considered on their individual merits. Dalhousie University is an affirmative action and equal opportunity educational institution.

Campus Information

Setting

Dalhousie Medical School plays a direct and vital role in patient care in the Maritimes. Our students and residents experience "distributed learning" in over 100 teaching sites, including tertiary and community hospitals, continuing care facilities and rural physician offices throughout the Maritimes.

Enrollment

For 2007, total enrollment was: Not reported

Housing

University housing and a comprehensive Student Health Service are available.

Application Process and Requirements 2009–2010

Primary Application Service: School-specific
Earliest filing date: September 1, 2008
Latest filing date: October 31, 2008

Secondary Application Required?: No
Sent to: n/a
URL: http://admissions.medicine.dal.ca/application.htm
Fee: n/a
Fee waiver available: n/a
Earliest filing date: n/a
Latest filing date: n/a

Latest MCAT® considered: Not reported
Oldest MCAT® considered: Not reported

Early Decision Program
School does not have EDP
Applicants notified: n/a
EDP available for: n/a

Regular Acceptance Notice
Earliest date: February 27, 2009
Latest date: Varies

Applicant's Response to Acceptance
Offer – Maximum Time: Three weeks

Requests for Deferred
Entrance Considered: No

Deposit to Hold Place in Class: Yes
Deposit (Resident): $200
Deposit (Non-Resident): $200
Deposit due: With response to acceptance offer
Applied to tuition: Yes
Deposit refundable: No
Refundable by: n/a

Estimated number of new entrants: 90
EDP: n/a, special program: n/a

Start Month/Year: August 2009

Interview Format: Interview is a 30 minute interview with a faculty and one student interviewer. Regional interviews are not available.

Other Programs

PREPARATORY PROGRAMS
Postbaccalaureate Program: No
Summer Program: No

COMBINED DEGREE PROGRAMS
Baccalaureate/MD: No
MD/MPH: No
MD/MBA: No
MD/JD: No
MD/PhD: No

Premedical Coursework

Course	Req.	Rec.	Lab.	Hrs.	Course	Req.	Rec.	Lab.	Hrs.
Inorganic Chemistry		•			Computer Science				
Behavioral Sciences					Genetics				
Biochemistry					Humanities		•		
Biology		•			Organic Chemistry		•		
Biology/Zoology					Physics		•		
Calculus					Psychology				
College English					Social Sciences		•		
College Mathematics					Other				

Selection Factors: 2007 Accepted Applicants

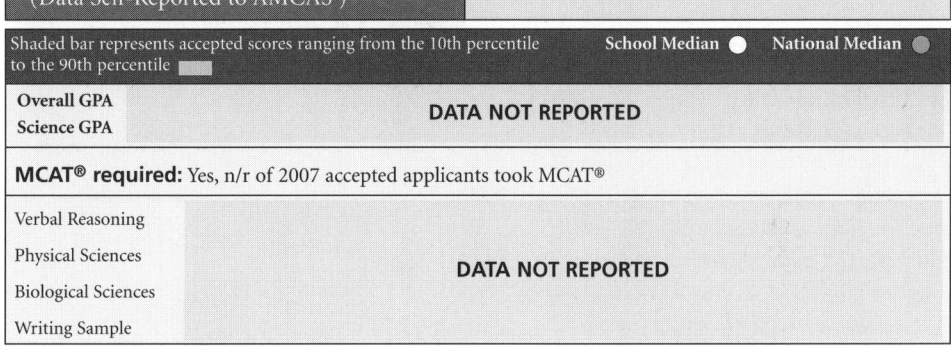

Proportion of Accepted Applicants with Relevant Experience (Data Self-Reported to AMCAS®)	**DATA NOT COLLECTED**

Shaded bar represents accepted scores ranging from the 10th percentile to the 90th percentile. **School Median** ● **National Median** ●

Overall GPA	DATA NOT REPORTED
Science GPA	

MCAT® required: Yes, n/r of 2007 accepted applicants took MCAT®

Verbal Reasoning	DATA NOT REPORTED
Physical Sciences	
Biological Sciences	
Writing Sample	

Acceptance & Matriculation Data for 2007–2008 First Year Class

	Resident	Non-Resident	International	Total
Applied				
Interviewed				
Deferred				
Matriculants				
Early Assurance Program				
Early Decision Program				
Baccalaureate/MD				
MD/PhD				
Matriculated				

DATA NOT REPORTED

Applications accepted from International Applicants: Yes

Specialty Choice

2003, 2004, 2005 Graduates, Specialty Choice
Anesthesiology
Emergency Medicine
Family Practice
Internal Medicine
Obst
Orth
Pedi
Psyc
Radiology
Surgery

DATA NOT COLLECTED

Matriculant Demographics: 2007–2008 First Year Class

Men: 0   **Women:** 0

Matriculants' Self-Reported Race/Ethnicity

Mexican American   Korean
Cuban   Vietnamese
Puerto Rican   Other Asian
Other
Total
Chine   **DATA NOT COLLECTED**
Asian
Pakistan   Total Asian
Filipino   **Unduplicated Number**
Japanese   **of Matriculants**

Science and Math Majors: n/r
Matriculants with:
    Baccalaureate degree: n/r
    Graduate degree(s): n/r

Financial Information

	Residents	Non-Residents
Total Cost of Attendance	n/r	n/r
Tuition and Fees	n/r	n/r
Other (includes living expenses)	n/r	n/r
Health Insurance (not applicable)	n/r	n/r

Average 2007 Graduate Indebtedness: n/r
% of Enrolled Students Receiving Aid: n/r

Criminal Background Check

Criminal background check policy was not reported.

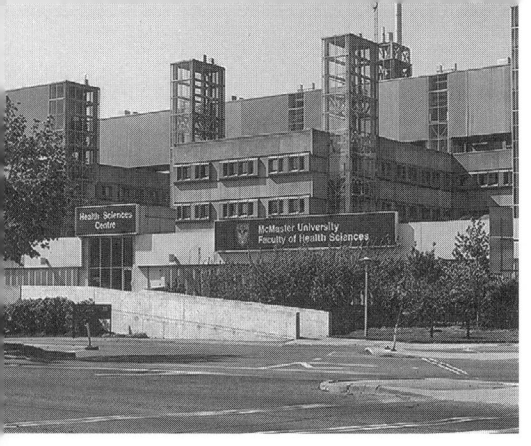

McMaster University, Michael G. DeGroote School of Medicine

Hamilton, Ontario

Michael G. DeGroote School of Medicine
McMaster University
MD Admissions, MDCL 3115
1200 Main Street West
Hamilton, Ontario
Canada, L8N 3Z5
T 905 525 9140 x22235   **F** 905 546 0349

Admissions www.fhs.mcmaster.ca/mdprog/
admissions/admissions.htm
Main www.fhs.mcmaster.ca/mdprog
Financial www.sfas.mcmaster.ca
Email mdadmit@mcmaster.ca

Public Institution

Dr. John Kelton, Dean, and Vice President Health Sciences

Dr. Harold Reiter, Chair, M.D. Admissions

Dr. Alan Neville, Assistant Dean, M.D. Program

Cathy Oudshoorn, M.D. Program Administrator

General Information

The Faculty of Health Sciences at McMaster University offers programs in health sciences education, including undergraduate and post-graduate medical education. The clinical programs use the teaching hospital and extensive ambulatory facilities of the McMaster Division of the Hamilton Health Sciences Corporation, but they also involve clinical teaching units at the major Hamilton hospitals and surrounding community health care centers.

Mission Statement

"Together, Advancing Health Through Learning and Discovery."

Curricular Highlights

Community Service Requirement: Optional.
Research/Thesis Requirement: Optional.

The three-year MD program at McMaster uses an approach to learning that will apply throughout a physician's career. The components have been organized in a logical manner, with early exposure to patients. Flexibility is ensured to allow for the variety of backgrounds and career goals. Graduates of McMaster's Medical Program will have developed the knowledge, ability, and attitudes necessary to qualify for further education in any medical career. The goals for students include the following: the development of competency in problem-based learning and problem-solving, the development of personal characteristics and attitudes compatible with effective health care, the development of clinical and communication skills, and the development of the skills to be a lifelong, self-directed learner and self-reflective practitioner. To achieve these objectives, students are introduced to patients within the first Medical Foundation block of the

curriculum. They are presented with a series of tutorial cases and questions requiring the understanding of principles and data collection. Much of the students' learning occurs within the small-group tutorial. Faculty members serve as tutors or sources of expert knowledge. The medical program is arranged as a pre-clerkship sequence of five Medical Foundations followed by clerkship. A Professional Competencies curriculum runs horizontally across the Foundations and into the clerkship. There are elective opportunities, both in block periods and horizontal electives taken concurrently. The clerkship emphasizes the clinical application of concepts learned in the earlier Foundations and consists of experience in inpatient and ambulatory settings. These include internal medicine, family medicine, emergency medicine, surgery, psychiatry, obstetrics-gynecology, anesthesia, and pediatrics. Students will have the opportunity to work in both teaching hospital and community hospital environments.

USMLE

Step 1: Optional.
Step 2: Clinical Skills (CS): Optional.
Step 2: Clinical Knowledge (CK): Optional.

Selection Factors

Students and members of the community and faculty are involved in the assessment of applicants. The aim is to select students who not only have the necessary academic standards, but who also display characteristics that are deemed to be important for the study and practice of medicine. These include characteristics that suggest sensitivity to the needs of the community; sensitivity to the emotional, psychological, and physical aspects of patients; the ability to detect and solve problems; the ability to learn independently; the ability to function as a member of a small group; and the ability to plan one's career in a way that reflects the needs of the community. Applicants rating highest in academic achievement and in non-cognitive qualities will be invited to the interview. From these applicants, 176 students will be selected for three campuses.

Financial Aid

The M.D. Program and the University Financial Aid Program offer a large bursary program to assist students in financial need. The M.D. Program administers a small loans program for students in further need.

Campus Information

Setting

In 2008, McMaster will have three campuses – the Hamilton campus sits on the main McMaster University campus in Hamilton Ontario; the Waterloo Regional campus, which opened in 2007, is situated in Kitchener, Ontario and the Niagara Regional Campus, located in St. Catharines Ontario.

Enrollment

For 2007, total enrollment was: 458

Special Features

McMaster's undergraduate medical program has become internationally known for its small-group, problem-based learning approach to medical education. Most recently, the school has been renamed in honor of the landmark and generous donation from philanthropist Michael G. DeGroote.

Housing

The McMaster Housing Office maintains a list of affordable housing in the area for students.

Satellite Campuses/Facilities

Tutorial and clinical training opportunities exist at McMaster University and in community hospitals through Central West Ontario. A new satellite campus in Kitchener-Waterloo admitted 15 students in Fall 2007. A second satellite campus opening in 2008 in the Niagara Region will admit 15 students.

Application Process and Requirements 2009–2010

Primary Application Service: OMSAS
Earliest filing date: July 1, 2008
Latest filing date: September 15, 2008

Secondary Application Required?: Yes
Sent to: OMSAS
URL: www.ouac.on.ca/omsas
Fee: Yes, $175
Fee waiver available: No
Earliest filing date: July 1, 2008
Latest filing date: September 15, 2008

Latest MCAT® considered: n/a
Oldest MCAT® considered: n/a

Early Decision Program
School does not have EDP
Applicants notified: n/a
EDP available for: n/a

Regular Acceptance Notice
Earliest date: May 15, 2009
Latest date: Until class is full

Applicant's Response to Acceptance
Offer – Maximum Time: Two weeks

Requests for Deferred
Entrance Considered: Yes

Deposit to Hold Place in Class: Yes
Deposit (Resident): $1,000
Deposit (Non-Resident): $1,000
Deposit due: With acceptance of offer
Applied to tuition: Yes
Deposit refundable: No
Refundable by: n/a

Estimated number of new entrants: 176
EDP: 0, special program: n/a

Start Month/Year: Late August 2009

Interview Format: Multiple mini-interviews. Regional interviews are not available.

Other Programs

PREPARATORY PROGRAMS
Postbaccalaureate Program: No
Summer Program: No

COMBINED DEGREE PROGRAMS
Baccalaureate/MD: No
MD/MPH: No
MD/MBA: No
MD/JD: No
MD/PhD: Yes, https://gradapplication. mcmaster.ca/account/instructions.asp

Premedical Coursework

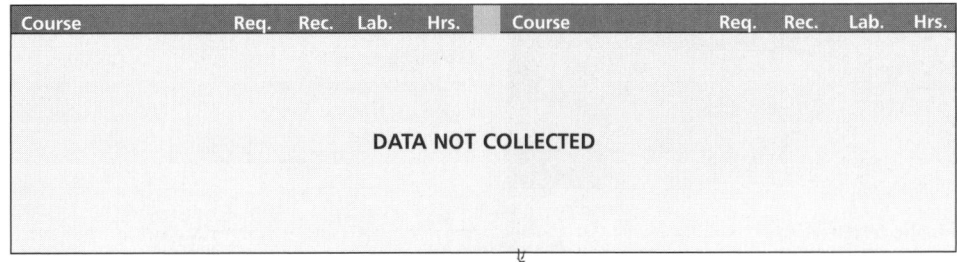

Course	Req.	Rec.	Lab.	Hrs.	Course	Req.	Rec.	Lab.	Hrs.
					DATA NOT COLLECTED				

Selection Factors: 2007 Accepted Applicants

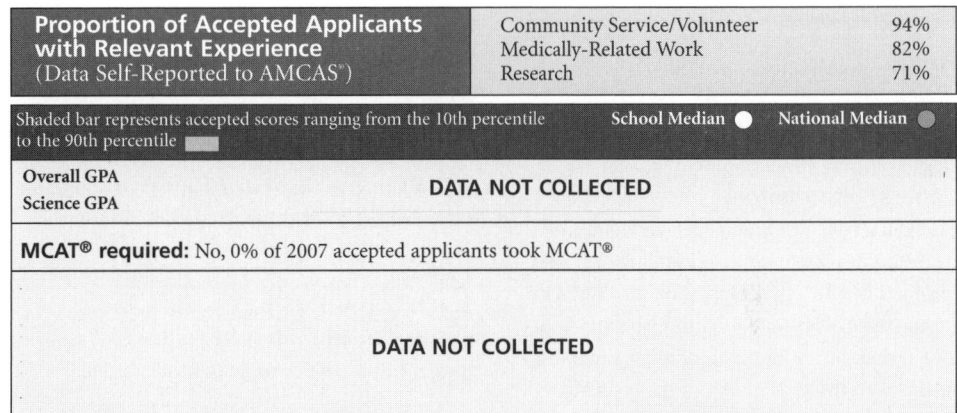

Proportion of Accepted Applicants with Relevant Experience (Data Self-Reported to AMCAS®)		
Community Service/Volunteer		94%
Medically-Related Work		82%
Research		71%

Shaded bar represents accepted scores ranging from the 10th percentile to the 90th percentile. **School Median** ● **National Median** ●

Overall GPA	DATA NOT COLLECTED
Science GPA	

MCAT® required: No, 0% of 2007 accepted applicants took MCAT®

DATA NOT COLLECTED

Acceptance & Matriculation Data for 2007–2008 First Year Class

	Resident	Non-Resident	International	Total
Applied	3814	942	92	4848
Interviewed	492	50	4	546
Deferred	2	0	0	2
Matriculants				
Early Assurance Program	0	0	0	0
Early Decision Program	n/a	n/a	n/a	n/a
Baccalaureate/MD	n/a	n/a	n/a	n/a
MD/PhD	n/a	n/a	n/a	n/a
Matriculated	147	15	2	**164**

Applications accepted from International Applicants: Yes

Specialty Choice

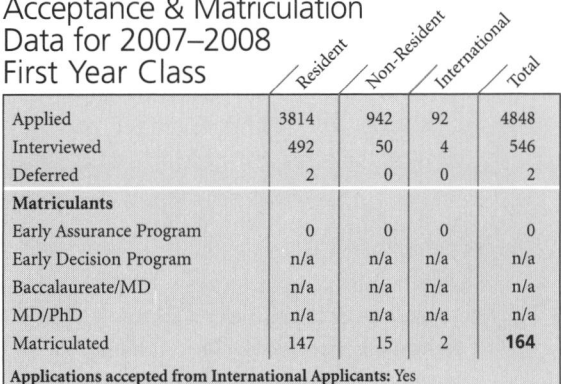

2003, 2004, 2005 Graduates, Specialty Choice

Anesthesiology
Emergency Medicine
Family Practice
Internal Medicine
Obst
Orth
Pedi
Psyc
Radiology
Surgery

DATA NOT COLLECTED

Matriculant Demographics: 2007–2008 First Year Class

Men: 68   **Women:** 96

Matriculants' Self-Reported Race/Ethnicity

Mexican American	Korean
Cuban	Vietnamese
Puerto Rican	Other Asian
Other H...	...rican
Total His...	
Chinese	...aiian
Asian In...	
Pakistan...	...tal Asian
Filipino	Unduplicated Number
Japanese	of Matriculants

DATA NOT COLLECTED

Science and Math Majors: 71%
Matriculants with:
    Baccalaureate degree: 90%
    Graduate degree(s): 10%

Financial Information

	Residents	Non-Residents
Total Cost of Attendance	$20,396	$ 94,137
Tuition and Fees	$17,396	$91,137
Other (includes living expenses)		
Health Insurance (can be waived)		

Average 2007 Graduate Indebtedness: $120,000
% of Enrolled Students Receiving Aid: 90%

Criminal Background Check

This medical school requires a criminal background check prior to matriculation.

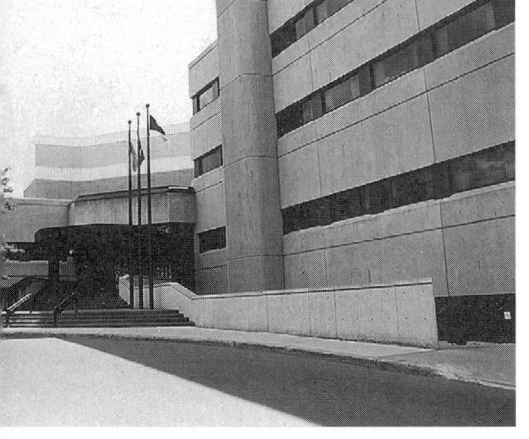

University of Ottawa
Faculty of Medicine
Ottawa, Ontario

Admissions, University of Ottawa
Faculty of Medicine
451 Smyth Road
Ottawa, Ontario
Canada, K1H 8M5
T 613 562 5409   F 613 562 5651

Admissions www.uottawa.ca/whychoose
Main www.medicine.uottawa.ca/eng
Financial www.uottawa.ca/student/englishguide/
1section/finance
Email admissmd@uottawa.ca

Public Institution

Dr. Jacques Bradwejn, Dean

Dr. Richard L. Hebert,
Assistant Dean, Admissions

Dr. Arlington Dungy, Associate Dean,
Alumni and Student Affairs

Nicole Racine, Admissions Officer

General Information

The University of Ottawa received its charter from the province of Ontario in 1866. It was founded by the Missionary Oblates of Mary Immaculate, who were its administrators until 1965, when important structural reforms were introduced through an act of the legislative assembly of the province of Ontario. The management, discipline, and control of the university are free from the restrictions and control of any outside body, whether lay or religious. The Faculty of Medicine was established in 1945.

Mission Statement

We explore, we learn, we care. We develop society's leaders who improve the health of Canadians and communities worldwide. We do this through the integration of education, research, patient care, and technology in an inclusive environment, in both official languages.

Curricular Highlights

Community Service Requirement: Optional.
Research/Thesis Requirement: Optional.

Students acquire the knowledge, skills, and attitudes necessary to recognize, understand, and apply effective, efficient strategies for the prevention and treatment of common and important health problems. Emphasis is placed on self-learning principles, and facts are assimilated in a multidisciplinary fashion, within the context of clinical problems. Lectures and seminars are used to discuss basic concepts. Training occurs in ambulatory, primary, secondary, distributed and tertiary settings. The program emphasizes health promotion and disease prevention and is responsive to individual needs and the health care system. The program fosters the qualities of trust and compassion, communication skills, ethical professional conduct, and patient advocacy. The program is scheduled over four calendar years and is divided into two stages. The preclerkship includes 70 weeks of study of essential bio-medical principles and consists of multi-disciplinary units. Students learn communication and clinical skills in an integrated fashion with the study of body systems. The clerkship, of two years duration, is devoted to clinical rotations; an extended period is available for elective study.

USMLE
Step 1: Optional.
Step 2: Clinical Skills (CS): Optional.
Step 2: Clinical Knowledge (CK): Optional.

Selection Factors

Academic excellence, the detailed autobiographical sketch, and interview rating are the main selection factors used. Academics are measured by an assessment of marks and by a comparison of the applicant's academic record with those of the other applicants. No preference is given to one academic program over another. In selecting its students, the University of Ottawa reserves the right to assess, in the applicant's program, the level of difficulty of the courses and/or their pertinence for future medical studies and the performance achieved by the candidate. The selection is not made by quota. No candidate will be admitted without an interview. It is highly desirable that the candidate who has a broad exposure to biology and physical sciences also have a broad exposure to the arts, humanities, and social sciences. In view of the limited number of places available, a candidate whose GPA is below 3.45 has considerably less chance of being admitted. Sex, race, age, religion, and socioeconomic status play no part in the selection process.

Financial Aid

Students may apply to the Student Financial Aid Office of the university and to their respective provincial governments for loan assistance. The Ontario Medical Association Bursaries and Loan Fund, the Kellogg Foundation Loan Fund, and a special bursaries fund are administered by the Awards Committee of the Faculty. The Association of Professors of the University also provides bursaries. Most of these awards are made on the basis of demonstrable financial need and good academic standing.

Information about Diversity Programs

In 2005, the Faculty established a dedicated admissions program for candidates of Aboriginal ancestry as part of its mission to improve access to better health care for Aboriginal peoples and to better serve society's needs.

Campus Information

Setting

The Faculty of Medicine is located in a building which also houses the Faculty of Health Sciences. The building is located off the main campus within a health sciences complex where a few of the affiliated teaching hospitals are also located. Medical students have access to the many student services on main campus (downtown) through the services of a shuttle.

Enrollment

For 2007, total enrollment was: 591

Special Features

Medical students benefit from a diverse learning environment with a laptop-supported Web-based curriculum and case-based learning (CBL) approach combined with traditional learning methods.

Housing

A good number of medical students live in groups of 2 or 3 and share costs in affordable townhouses in a residential area within close proximity (5 to 10 minutes walking distance) of the campus. The Admissions Office also puts together a housing file of availabilities for newly admitted students' perusal. Housing information (off-campus and residencies) is available at: *www.uottawa.ca/students/housing/*.

Application Process and Requirements 2009–2010

Primary Application Service: OMSAS
Earliest filing date: July 2008
Latest filing date: September 15, 2008

Secondary Application Required?: No
Sent to: n/a
URL: n/a
Fee: n/a
Fee waiver available: No
Earliest filing date: n/a
Latest filing date: n/a

Latest MCAT® considered: Not required
Oldest MCAT® considered: Not required

Early Decision Program
School does not have EDP
Applicants notified: n/a
EDP available for: n/a

Regular Acceptance Notice
Earliest date: May 15, 2009
Latest date: Until class is full

Applicant's Response to Acceptance Offer – Maximum Time: Two weeks

Requests for Deferred Entrance Considered: Yes

Deposit to Hold Place in Class: Yes
Deposit (Resident): $1,000
Deposit (Non-Resident): n/a
Deposit due: with acceptance
Applied to tuition: Yes
Deposit refundable: No
Refundable by: n/a

Estimated number of new entrants: 139
EDP: n/a, special program: n/a

Start Month/Year: September 2009

Interview Format: Semi-structured, 45 minute interviews. Regional interviews are not available.

Other Programs

PREPARATORY PROGRAMS
Postbaccalaureate Program: No
Summer Program: No

COMBINED DEGREE PROGRAMS
Baccalaureate/MD: No
MD/MPH: No
MD/MBA: No
MD/JD: No
MD/PhD: No

Premedical Coursework

Course	Req.	Rec.	Lab.	Sems.
Inorganic Chemistry	•		•	2
Behavioral Sciences				
Biochemistry	•			2
Biology				
Biology/Zoology	•		•	2
Calculus				
College English				
College Mathematics				

Course	Req.	Rec.	Lab.	Sems.
Computer Science				
Genetics				
Humanities	•			2
Organic Chemistry	•		•	2
Physics				
Psychology				
Social Sciences				
Other				

Selection Factors: 2007 Accepted Applicants

Proportion of Accepted Applicants with Relevant Experience (Data Self-Reported to AMCAS®)	**DATA NOT COLLECTED**

Shaded bar represents accepted scores ranging from the 10th percentile to the 90th percentile   School Median ●   National Median ●

	2.0	2.1	2.2	2.3	2.4	2.5	2.6	2.7	2.8	2.9	3.0	3.1	3.2	3.3	3.4	3.5	3.6	3.7	3.8	3.9	4.0
Overall GPA	2.0	2.1	2.2	2.3	2.4	2.5	2.6	2.7	2.8	2.9	3.0	3.1	3.2	3.3	3.4	3.5	3.6	3.7	3.8	(3.9)	4.0
Science GPA	2.0	2.1	2.2	2.3	2.4	2.5	2.6	2.7	2.8	2.9	3.0	3.1	3.2	3.3	3.4	3.5	3.6	3.7	3.8	3.9	4.0

MCAT® required: No

Verbal Reasoning	
Physical Sciences	**DATA NOT COLLECTED**
Biological Sciences	
Writing Sample	

Acceptance & Matriculation Data for 2007–2008 First Year Class

	In Province	Out of Province	International	Total
Applied	2540	816	n/a	3356
Interviewed	n/r	n/r	n/r	516
Deferred	n/r	n/r	n/r	2
Matriculants				
Early Assurance Program	n/a	n/a	n/a	n/a
Early Decision Program	n/a	n/a	n/a	n/a
Baccalaureate/MD	n/a	n/a	n/a	n/a
MD/PhD	n/a	n/a	n/a	n/a
Matriculated	123	16	0	**139**

Applications accepted from International Applicants: No

Specialty Choice

2003, 2004, 2005 Graduates, Specialty Choice

Anesthesiology	
Emergency Medicine	
Family Practice	
Internal Medicine	
Obs	
Orth	**DATA NOT COLLECTED**
Ped	
Psyc	
Radiology	
Surgery	

Matriculant Demographics: 2007–2008 First Year Class

Men: 53   **Women:** 86

Matriculants' Self-Reported Race/Ethnicity

Mexican American	Korean
Cuban	Vietnamese
Puerto Rican	Other Asian
Other	
Total H	
Chines	**DATA NOT COLLECTED**
Asian	
Pakista...	
Filipino	**Unduplicated Number**
Japanese	**of Matriculants**

Science and Math Majors: 60%
Matriculants with:
    Baccalaureate degree: 69%
    Graduate degree(s): 27%

Financial Information

	Residents	Non-Residents
Total Cost of Attendance	n/a	n/a
Tuition and Fees	$15,288	n/a
Incidental fees	$571	n/a
Health Insurance (Voluntary)	$180	n/a

Average 2007 Graduate Indebtedness: n/a
% of Enrolled Students Receiving Aid: n/a

Criminal Background Check

This medical school requires a criminal background check prior to matriculation.

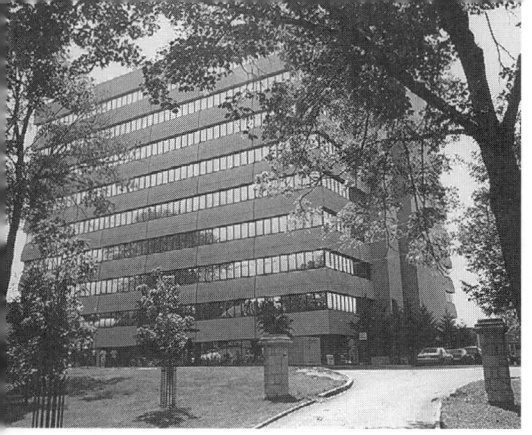

Queen's University Faculty of Health Sciences
School of Medicine
Kingston, Ontario

Admissions Office, Queen's University
School of Medicine
68 Barrie Street
Kingston, Ontario
Canada, K7L 3N6
T 613 533 3307   F 613 533 3190

Admissions http://meds.queensu.ca/undergrad/admissions
Main http://meds.queensu.ca/undergrad/
Financial http://meds.queensu.ca/undergrad/
student_information/financial_awards_or_loans
Email queensmd@queensu.ca

Public Institution

Dr. David Walker, Dean, Faculty of Health Science

Jennifer Saunders, Admissions Officer

Dawna Roney, Manager, Undergraduate Medical Education

Dr. Anthony J. Sanfilippo, Assistant Dean

General Information
The School of Medicine is an integral part of Queen's University. With a legacy of over 150 years of quality teaching and research, the environment and the flexibility of the curriculum complement innovative programs that provide the breadth of training required for practice throughout Canada.

Mission Statement
The mission of Queen's Medicine is to advance our tradition of preparing excellent physicians and leaders in health care. We embrace a spirit of inquiry and innovation in education and research.

Curricular Highlights
Community Service Requirement: Optional.
Research/Thesis Requirement: Optional.

In the four-year curriculum, students are introduced in their first year to communication and physical examination. Clinical Skills runs throughout the curriculum. An eight-week Critical Enquiry elective at the end of the second year provides an opportunity for students to investigate a medical question in depth. Learning formats include lectures, tutorials, seminars, symposia, and problem-based learning.

USMLE
Step 1: Optional.
Step 2: Clinical Skills (CS): Optional.
Step 2: Clinical Knowledge (CK): Optional.

Selection Factors
One hundred students are admitted annually into the first year. Students are selected on the basis of a strong academic record and assessment of personal characteristics considered to be most appropriate for the study of medicine at Queen's University and for the subsequent practice of medicine. Candidates to be invited for an interview are determined based on converted GPA and MCAT results. Members of the Admissions Committee, who will utilize specific guidelines to identify any unusual circumstances, will review applications of those below the cutoff. Candidates who do not make the academic cut based on their undergraduate grade point average, but who have completed graduate work are considered in this group. Candidates meeting the academic requirements are then assessed based on confidential letters of reference, the personal information form, the autobiographic sketch, and the personal interview. These candidates will be ranked for offers and placement on the waiting list. The Admissions Committee does not give preference to applicants who have studied in any particular university program. No preference is shown to applicants at any particular level of training. Place of residence and location of the university where studies have been undertaken are not criteria in selection. Age, gender, race, and religion are not factors considered in the selection process.

Financial Aid
Student financial assistance at Queen's University is offered through merit-based (scholarships) and need-based (bursaries, awards, and work-study) funding. The Student Awards Web site is located at: *www.queensu.ca/registrar/awards*.

Information about Diversity Programs
The Admissions Committee recognizes the critical shortage of aboriginal physicians in Canada and the need to educate more aboriginal physicians to serve as role models and to address the health care needs of Canada's aboriginal people. The committee has developed an alternate process for assessment of aboriginal candidates. Up to a maximum of four qualified aboriginal students per year may be admitted to the M.D. program by the alternate process. Aboriginal candidates may also choose to apply through the regular admission process.

Campus Information

Setting
The campus is located in Kingston, Ontario, a true university town with the benefits of a small community such as affordable cost-of-living, a peaceful waterfront, and minimal traffic and the cultural richness of an urban centre, including acclaimed restaurants, pubs, theatre and music. Kingston is ideally situated between Toronto, Montreal, and Ottawa.

Enrollment
For 2007, total enrollment was: 400

Special Features
Queen's University School of Medicine produces physicians equipped to handle the complex, ever-changing world of 21st-century health care. The curriculum is forward-looking and enhanced by the latest technology, always keeping pace with the newest developments in modern medicine. Small class sizes, frequent interaction with professors, and a strong mentorship program make for a close-knit community at the school. A regional education model allows students to experience a broad range of health-care settings, while exposure to advanced health sciences research nurtures innovation and critical thinking. Early and extensive hands-on clinical experience is another distinctive feature of the program. Queen's offers all the advantages of one of Canada's leading medical schools – including an international reputation for exceptional graduates – in an intimate, supportive learning environment.

Housing
Information on Queen's housing and residence is available at *www.queensu.ca/dsao/housing/ah1.htm* and *https://housing.queensu.ca/residence*. Most medical students prefer to find their own accommodations, generally living within a 15-minute walk from campus.

Satellite Campuses/Facilities
Clinical rotations occur in Kingston teaching hospitals and in affiliated regional sites in Southeastern Ontario.

Application Process and Requirements 2009–2010

Primary Application Service: OMSAS
Earliest filing date: July 2008
Latest filing date: September 15, 2008

Secondary Application Required?: No
Sent to: n/a
URL: n/a
Fee: n/a
Fee waiver available: n/a
Earliest filing date: n/a
Latest filing date: n/a

Latest MCAT® considered: n/r
Oldest MCAT® considered: 1991

**Early Decision Program
School does not have EDP
Applicants notified:** n/a
EDP available for: n/a

**Regular Acceptance Notice
Earliest date:** May 15, 2009
Latest date: Until class is full

**Applicant's Response to Acceptance
Offer – Maximum Time:** Two weeks

**Requests for Deferred
Entrance Considered:** Yes

Deposit to Hold Place in Class: Yes
Deposit (Resident): $1,000
Deposit (Non-Resident): $1,000
Deposit due: With response to firm acceptance
Applied to tuition: Yes
Deposit refundable: No
Refundable by: n/a

Estimated number of new entrants: 100
EDP: n/a, special program: n/a

Start Month/Year: September 2009

Interview Format: Interviews by a team of three interviewers. Regional interviews are not available.

Other Programs

**PREPARATORY PROGRAMS
Postbaccalaureate Program:** No
Summer Program: No

**COMBINED DEGREE PROGRAMS
Baccalaureate/MD:** No
MD/MPH: No
MD/MBA: No
MD/JD: No
MD/PhD: No

Premedical Coursework

Course	Req.	Rec.	Lab.	Sems.
Inorganic Chemistry				
Behavioral Sciences				
Biochemistry				
Biology				
Biology/Zoology				
Calculus				
College English				
College Mathematics				
Computer Science				

Course	Req.	Rec.	Lab.	Sems.
Humanities				
Organic Chemistry				
Physics				
Psychology				
Social Sciences				
Physical Science	•			2
Biological Science	•			2
Social Sciences or Humanities	•			2

Selection Factors: 2007 Accepted Applicants

Proportion of Accepted Applicants with Relevant Experience ✓ (Data Self-Reported to AMCAS®)	
Community Service/Volunteer	50
Medically-Related Work	50
Research	50

Shaded bar represents accepted scores ranging from the 10th percentile to the 90th percentile ▬	School Median ●	National Median ●
Overall GPA Science GPA	DATA NOT COLLECTED	

MCAT® required: Yes, 100% of 2007 accepted applicants took MCAT®

Verbal Reasoning Physical Sciences Biological Sciences Writing Sample	DATA NOT COLLECTED

Acceptance & Matriculation Data for 2007–2008 First Year Class

	Resident	Non-Resident	International	Total
Applied	2305	n/a	n/a	2305
Interviewed	489	n/a	n/a	489
Deferred	1	n/a	n/a	1
Matriculants				
Early Assurance Program	0	0	0	0
Early Decision Program	n/a	n/a	n/a	n/a
Baccalaureate/MD	n/a	n/a	n/a	n/a
MD/PhD	n/a	n/a	n/a	n/a
Matriculated	100	n/a	n/a	**100**

Applications accepted from International Applicants: No

Matriculant Demographics: 2007–2008 First Year Class

Men: 54 **Women:** 46

Matriculants' Self-Reported Race/Ethnicity

Mexican American	**Korean**
Cuban	**Vietnamese**
Puerto Rican	**Other Asian**
Other	
Total H	**DATA NOT COLLECTED**
Chines	
Asian I	
Pakistan	**Total Asian**
Filipino	**Unduplicated Number**
Japanese	**of Matriculants**

Science and Math Majors: 0%
Matriculants with:
 Baccalaureate degree: 0%
 Graduate degree(s): 0%

Specialty Choice

2003, 2004, 2005 Graduates, Specialty Choice	
Anesthesiology	6
Emergency Medicine	5
Family Practice	33
Internal Medicine	12
Obstetrics/Gynecology	4
Orthopaedic Surgery	3
Pediatrics	8
Psychiatry	5
Radiology	3
Surgery	6

Financial Information

	Residents	Non-Residents
Total Cost of Attendance	$14,175	n/r
Tuition and Fees	$14,175	$14,175
Other (includes living expenses)	$810	$810
Health Insurance (not applicable)	n/a	n/a

Average 2007 Graduate Indebtedness: n/r
% of Enrolled Students Receiving Aid: n/r

Criminal Background Check

This medical school requires a criminal background check prior to matriculation.

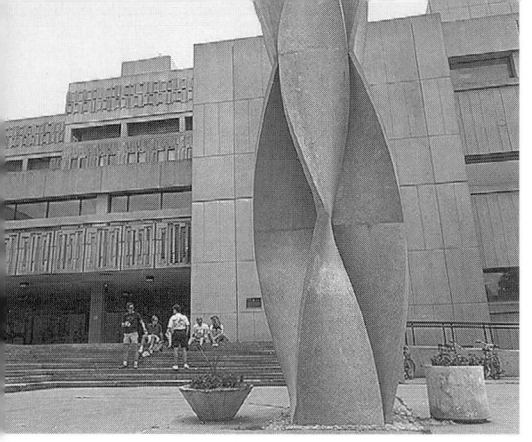

University of Toronto
Faculty of Medicine
Toronto, Ontario

University of Toronto, Faculty of Medicine
Medical Sciences Building, Room 2135
1 King's College Circle
Toronto, Ontario
Canada, M5S 1A8
T 416 978 7928 **F** 416 971 2163

Admissions www.facmed.utoronto.ca/programs/md/
admissions/0809.htm
Main www.facmed.utoronto.ca
Financial www.facmed.utoronto.ca/programs/md/
admissions/finance.htm
Email medicine.admiss@utoronto.ca

Public Institution

Catharine Whiteside, Dean

Dr. M. Shandling, Associate Dean, Admissions and Student Financial Services

David McKnight, Vice Dean, Equity and Professionalism

Bill Gregg, Associate Registrar, Student Financial Services

Deborah L. Coombs, Coordinator, Admissions and Awards

Leslie Taylor, Admissions Officer

General Information
Founded in 1843 as a school of medicine, the University of Toronto's Faculty of Medicine is an integral component of one of North America's largest health science complexes. Through the University of Toronto, the Faculty is affiliated with a network of teaching hospitals and community-based health units that offer the Faculty's students a broad spectrum of educational experiences.

Mission Statement
The Faculty of Medicine has been educating medical students and conducting internationally recognized research for more than 100 years. The school has grown into one of the largest health sciences complexes in North America, with more than 4,500 students in undergraduate and graduate medical education programs, rehabilitation sciences, and graduate study.

Curricular Highlights
Community Service Requirement:
Required. Community placement during a longitudinal course.
Research/Thesis Requirement: Optional.

The four-year curriculum is focused on student-centered learning. The preclerkship phase (approximately 82 weeks) consists of six multidisciplinary courses, each of which is built upon a series of patient-based cases. Selected lectures, seminars, and laboratory exercises will complement small-group, problem-based learning sessions. Following the preclerkship, students spend approximately 78 weeks as clinical clerks. This phase of medical education enables the student to participate in the study and care of patients as a member of a clinical team working in different hospital services. Each rotation includes community experiences as well as elements of problem-based learning and basic science. As part of the clerkship, students spend a total of 18 weeks in elective rotations to allow them to explore areas of medicine of particular interest. During the clerkship, students apply to the Canadian Resident Matching Service to select the program with which they wish to do their postgraduate training. Applications must be submitted in the fall, and students are notified in March as to the program to which they have been matched.

USMLE
Step 1: Optional.
Step 2: Clinical Skills (CS): Optional.
Step 2: Clinical Knowledge (CK): Optional.

Selection Factors
Applicants are judged initially upon their academic and nonacademic records. All applicants are required to take the MCAT®. Selected applicants are invited to appear for an interview in Toronto. Definite preference is given to Canadian residents. A maximum of seven places will be offered to applicants with student visas. Sex, race, and religion are not considered in determining those applicants to whom places are offered. Successful candidates must be deemed by the Admissions Committee to be acceptable in all aspects of the admissions process. This may include cumulative grade-point average, MCAT® scores, reference letters, nonacademic factors, English proficiency, performance on interview, and any other criteria put forward by the faculty.

Financial Aid
Financial aid is available under the Province of Ontario Student Assistance Program, the Canada Student Loan Program, and University of Toronto Faculty of Medicine Bursary and Loan Programs. Applicants are referred to the publications of the University of Toronto for details of the regulations governing these awards. Applicants are advised not to plan to earn money in time-consuming work that may jeopardize their standing during the academic year.

Information about Diversity Programs
The Faculty of Medicine supports mentorship and role-modeling for students from under-represented groups through a number of programs. These include summer mentorship programs organized by the Faculty in collaboration with the Association for the Advancement of Blacks in Health Sciences. These programs include both black and Aboriginal students.

Campus Information

Setting
The Faculty of Medicine provides the only M.D. training program in the Greater Toronto area, with a catchment population of five million people. The school is accessible by subway, and is located in the center of Toronto, one of the world's most culturally diverse cities. The main campus is accessible by public transportation, but students may require private transportation to attend some clinical placements.

Enrollment
For 2007, total enrollment was: 850

Special Features
The University of Toronto's Faculty of Medicine is an integral component of one of North America's largest health science complexes. The Faculty of Medicine provides the only M.D. training program in the Greater Toronto area, providing an extraordinary environment for clinical care, research, and education.

Housing
Limited on-campus housing is available, and affordable housing is available within a short radius. Rents average $500-$1000 per month.

Satellite Campuses/Facilities
Student rotations are divided among nine fully affiliated and eleven partially affiliated teaching hospitals, as well as a large number of community health practices.

Application Process and Requirements 2009–2010

Primary Application Service: OMSAS
Earliest filing date: July 7, 2008
Latest filing date: September 15, 2008

Secondary Application Required?: No
Sent to: n/a
URL: n/a
Fee: n/a
Fee waiver available: n/a
Earliest filing date: n/a
Latest filing date: n/a

Latest MCAT Considered: September 2008
Oldest MCAT Considered: 2003

Early Decision Program
School does not have EDP
Applicants notified: n/a
EDP available for: n/a

Regular Acceptance Notice
Earliest date: May 15, 2009
Latest date: Until class is full

Applicant's Response to Acceptance
Offer – Maximum Time: Normally two weeks from date of offer.

Requests for Deferred
Entrance Considered: No

Deposit to Hold Place in Class: Yes
Deposit (Resident): $1,000
Deposit (Non-Resident): $1,000
Deposit due: With response to acceptance offer
Applied to tuition: Yes
Deposit refundable: No
Refundable by: n/a

Estimated number of new entrants: 224
EDP: 0, special program: n/a

Start Month/Year: August 24, 2009

Interview Format: Forty-five minute interview with faculty and student. Regional interviews are not available.

Other Programs

PREPARATORY PROGRAMS
Postbaccalaureate Program: No
Summer Program: No

COMBINED DEGREE PROGRAMS
Baccalaureate/MD: No
MD/MPH: No
MD/MBA: No
MD/JD: No
MD/PhD: Yes, www.utoronto.ca/mdphd

Premedical Coursework

Course	Req.	Rec.	Lab.	Sems.
Inorganic Chemistry				
Behavioral Sciences				
Biochemistry				
Biology				
Biology/Zoology				
Calculus				
College English				
College Mathematics				
Computer Science				

Course	Req.	Rec.	Lab.	Sems.
Humanities				
Organic Chemistry				
Physics				
Psychology				
Social Sciences				
Life Science	•			4
Humanities or Social Science or a Language	•			2
Statistics		•		1

Selection Factors: 2007 Accepted Applicants

Proportion of Accepted Applicants with Relevant Experience (Data Self-Reported to AMCAS®)		
Community Service/Volunteer		80%
Medically-Related Work		75%
Research		50%

Shaded bar represents accepted scores ranging from the 10th percentile to the 90th percentile   **School Median** ○   **National Median** ○

Overall GPA	2.0	2.1	2.2	2.3	2.4	2.5	2.6	2.7	2.8	2.9	3.0	3.1	3.2	3.3	3.4	3.5	3.6	3.7	3.8	(3.9)	4.0

Science GPA — DATA NOT COLLECTED

MCAT® required: Yes, 100% of 2007 accepted applicants took MCAT®

Verbal Reasoning	3	4	5	6	7	8	9	(10)	11	12	13	14	15
Physical Sciences	3	4	5	6	7	8	9	10	(11)	12	13	14	15
Biological Sciences	3	4	5	6	7	8	9	10	11	(12)	13	14	15
Writing Sample				J	K	L	M	N	O	P	(Q)	R	S	T

Acceptance & Matriculation Data for 2007–2008 First Year Class

	Resident	Non-Resident	International	Total
Applied	3118	n/a	47	3165
Interviewed	483	n/a	4	487
Deferred	0	n/a	n/a	0
Matriculants				
Early Assurance Program	n/a	n/a	n/a	n/a
Early Decision Program	n/a	n/a	n/a	n/a
Baccalaureate/MD	n/a	n/a	n/a	n/a
MD/PhD	5	n/a	n/a	5
Matriculated	222	n/a	2	**224**

Applications accepted from International Applicants: Yes

Specialty Choice

2003, 2004, 2005 Graduates, Specialty Choice	
Anesthesiology	7%
Emergency Medicine	1%
Family Practice	23%
Internal Medicine	21%
Obstetrics/Gynecology	3%
Orthopedic Surgery	5%
Pediatrics	4%
Psychiatry	6%
Radiology	8%
Surgery	4%

Matriculant Demographics: 2007–2008 First Year Class

Men: 97   **Women:** 127

Matriculants' Self-Reported Race/Ethnicity

Mexican American   Korean
Cuban   Vietnamese
Puerto Rican   Other Asian
Other
Total H   **DATA NOT COLLECTED**
Chines
Asian
Pakistan   Total Asian
Filipino   **Unduplicated Number**
Japanese   **of Matriculants**

Science and Math Majors: 97%
Matriculants with:
  Baccalaureate degree: 81.3
  Graduate degree(s): 15.6

Financial Information

	Residents	Non-Residents
Total Cost of Attendance	$36,995	$64,233
Tuition and Fees	$18,145	$45,383
Other (includes living expenses)	$18,850	$18,850
Health Insurance (not applicable)	n/a	n/a

Average 2007 Graduate Indebtedness: $85,033
% of Enrolled Students Receiving Aid: 81%

Criminal Background Check

This medical school requires a criminal background check prior to matriculation.

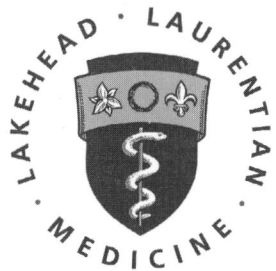

Northern Ontario
School of Medicine

Northern Ontario School of Medicine
Ontario, Canada

West Campus
955 Oliver Rd
Thunder Bay, ON, P7B 5E1
T 807 766 7300
F 807 766 7370

East Campus
935 Ramsey Lake Rd
Sudbury, ON, P3E 2C6
T 705 675 4883
F 705 675 4858

Admissions www.normed.ca/programs/
undergraduate/admissions
Main www.normed.ca
Financial www.normed.ca/programs/undergraduate/
studentaffairs/financialaid
Email nosmadmit@normed.ca

Public Institution

Dr. Roger Strasser, Founding Dean

Julie Pacifico, Admissions Officer

Dr. Joel Lanphear, Associate Dean, Undergraduate Medical Education

Dr. Blair Schoales, Assistant Dean, Admissions

General Information
The Northern Ontario School of Medicine is the first new medical school in Canada in the 21st century. It is the Faculty of Medicine of Laurentian University, Sudbury, and of Lakehead University, Thunder Bay. With main campuses in Thunder Bay and Sudbury, the school has multiple teaching and research sites distributed across Northern Ontario, including large and small communities.

Mission Statement
The Northern Ontario School of Medicine is a pioneering faculty of medicine working to the highest international standards. Its overall mission is to educate skilled physicians and undertake health research suited to community needs. In fulfilling this mission NOSM will become a cornerstone of community health care in Northern Ontario.

Curricular Highlights
Community Service Requirement: Optional.
Research/Thesis Requirement: Optional.

Grounded in Northern Ontario, our four-year M.D. program provides students with a unique mix of learning opportunities in a diverse range of sites, including Aboriginal and Francophone communities. Patient-Centered Medicine (PCM) was chosen as the major underlying concept of health and medicine in the development of the M.D. program. PCM is a comprehensive clinical method with six interactive components supported by substantial and growing research evidence. PCM links well to Learner-Centered Education (LCE), which was chosen as the underlying concept of education for the medical school. Throughout the four-year program, the curriculum is organized around five themes: 1. Northern and Rural Health, 2. Personal and Professional Aspects of Medical Practice, 3. Social and Population Health, 4. The Foundations of Medicine, and 5. Clinical Skills in Healthcare. The focus of the Northern Ontario School of Medicine program is on graduating skilled physicians who are ready and able to pursue further training and clinical practice anywhere, but who will have a special affinity for, and comfort in, Northern Ontario. The curriculum is highly integrated, with students undertaking most learning in small-group, patient-centered Case-Based Learning. The cases present complex real-life scenarios, which present people in their home/family/community context. In addition to small-group learning, students participate in hands-on practical classes, self-directed learning, and clinical education in a range of different health service and community settings. Through the mix of themes and different learning modalities, the program covers core curricula, ensuring that students gain a strong grounding in the basic medical sciences, the humanities, social and behavioral sciences, and clinical medicine. Clinical education starts at the beginning of the program and occurs in a diverse range of settings.

USMLE
Step 1: Optional
Step 2: Clinical Skills (CS): Optional
Step 2: Clinical Knowledge (CK): Optional

Selection Factors
Applications that meet the minimum requirement are assigned a score based on the grade point average, the autobiographic sketch and school submission questions, and context. Context is primarily based on place(s) of residence of one year or more. Advantage is given to those applicants from within Northern Ontario, rural and remote areas in the rest of Canada, and Aboriginal and Francophone applicants. Based on the total application score, the top-ranked candidates are invited to participate in the admission interviews. The final selection for admission is based on a combination of the total application and interview scores. Check our website for current information.

Financial Aid
Financial assistance is available to medical students through provincial and federal student loan programs. The Northern Ontario School of Medicine also has bursaries and other awards available for students enrolled in the medical program.

Information about Diversity Programs
Aboriginal applicants are given modest advantage in the application process. Aboriginal applicants can select either the General or Aboriginal Admission Stream. A minimum of 2 program seats are designated for Aboriginal students.

Campus Information

Setting
The Northern Ontario School of Medicine is the Faculty of Medicine of both Lakehead University in Thunder Bay, Ontario and Laurentian University in Sudbury, Ontario. Two new buildings, one on each campus, house the medical school.

Enrollment
For 2007, total enrollment was: 56

Housing
On campus housing is available through our host universities, Lakehead and Laurentian University.

Satellite Campuses/Facilities
While the majority of the first two years will be spent in either Thunder Bay or Sudbury, students will spend a month at the end of the first year in an Aboriginal community. In the second year, there will be two placements of six weeks in rural and remote communities throughout Northern Ontario. The majority of third year will be spent in the small urban and large rural communities of Northern Ontario. The Clinical Clerkship in the 4th year is primarily in hospitals of Thunder Bay, Sudbury, and other large urban northern center.

Application Process and Requirements 2009–2010

Primary Application Service: OMSAS
Earliest filing date: July 2008
Latest filing date: October 1, 2008

Secondary Application Required?: No
Sent to: n/a
URL: n/a
Fee: No
Fee waiver available: n/a
Earliest filing date: n/a
Latest filing date: n/a

Latest MCAT® considered: not required
Oldest MCAT® considered: not required

Early Decision Program
School does not have EDP
Applicants notified: n/a
EDP available for: n/a

Regular Acceptance Notice
Earliest date: May 2009
Latest date: Until class is full

Applicant's Response to Acceptance Offer – Maximum Time: Two weeks

Requests for Deferred Entrance Considered: Yes

Deposit to Hold Place in Class: Yes
Deposit (Resident): $1,000
Deposit (Non-Resident): $1,000
Deposit due: n/r
Applied to tuition: Yes
Deposit refundable: No
Refundable by: n/a

Estimated number of new entrants: 56
EDP: n/a, special program: n/a

Start Month/Year: August 2009

Interview Format: Multiple mini-interviews. Regional interviews are not available.

Other Programs

PREPARATORY PROGRAMS
Postbaccalaureate Program: No
Summer Program: No

COMBINED DEGREE PROGRAMS
Baccalaureate/MD: No
MD/MPH: No
MD/MBA: No
MD/JD: No
MD/PhD: No

Premedical Coursework

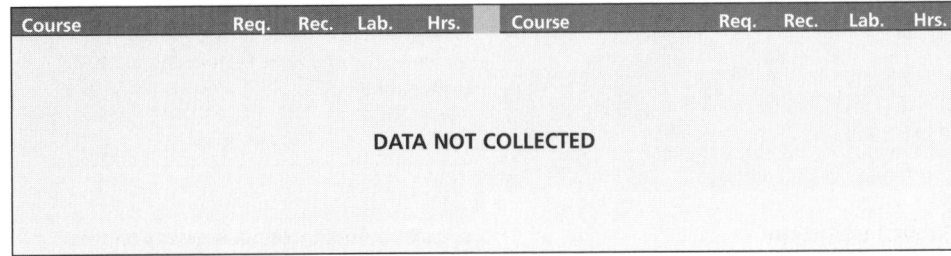

Course	Req.	Rec.	Lab.	Hrs.	Course	Req.	Rec.	Lab.	Hrs.
				DATA NOT COLLECTED					

Selection Factors: 2007 Accepted Applicants

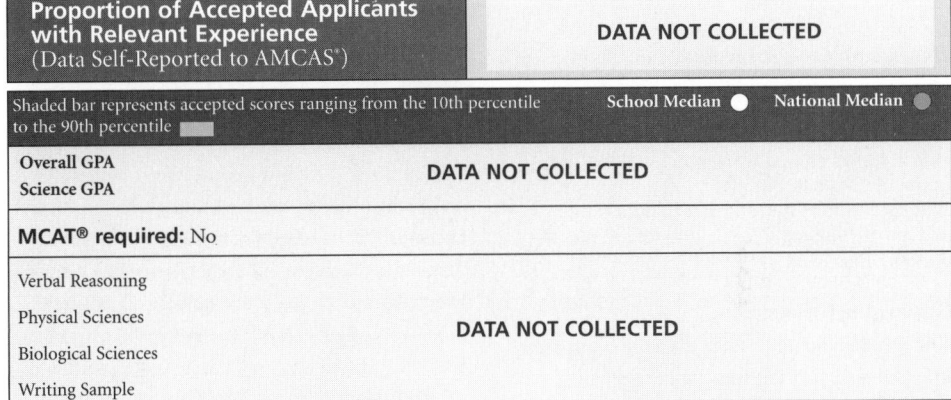

Proportion of Accepted Applicants with Relevant Experience (Data Self-Reported to AMCAS®)	DATA NOT COLLECTED

Shaded bar represents accepted scores ranging from the 10th percentile to the 90th percentile. School Median ● National Median ●

Overall GPA	DATA NOT COLLECTED
Science GPA	

MCAT® required: No

Verbal Reasoning	
Physical Sciences	DATA NOT COLLECTED
Biological Sciences	
Writing Sample	

Acceptance & Matriculation Data for 2007–2008 First Year Class

	Resident	Non-Resident	International	Total
Applied	n/r	n/r	n/r	2274
Interviewed	n/r	n/r	n/r	408
Deferred	0	0	0	0
Matriculants				
Early Assurance Program	0	0	0	0
Early Decision Program	n/a	n/a	n/a	n/a
Baccalaureate/MD	n/a	n/a	n/a	n/a
MD/PhD	n/a	n/a	n/a	n/a
Matriculated	n/r	n/r	n/r	**56**

Applications accepted from International Applicants: No

Matriculant Demographics: 2007–2008 First Year Class

Men: 16   **Women:** 40

Matriculants' Self-Reported Race/Ethnicity

Mexican American	Korean
Cuban	Vietnamese
Puerto Rican	Other Asian
Other	
Total	
Chinese	DATA NOT COLLECTED
Asian	
Pakist	
Filipino	Unduplicated Number
Japanese	of Matriculants

Science and Math Majors: n/a
Matriculants with:
    Baccalaureate degree: 56
    Graduate degree(s): 14

Specialty Choice

2003, 2004, 2005 Graduates, Specialty Choice

Anesthesiology
Emergency Medicine
Family Practice
Internal Medicine
Obst...
Orth...   DATA NOT COLLECTED
Pedi...
Psych...
Radiology
Surgery

Financial Information

	Residents	Non-Residents
Total Cost of Attendance	n/r	n/r
Tuition and Fees	$15,450	$15,450
Other (includes living expenses)	$1,750	n/r
Health Insurance	n/a	n/a

Average 2007 Graduate Indebtedness: n/a
% of Enrolled Students Receiving Aid: n/a

Criminal Background Check

This medical school requires a criminal background check prior to matriculation.

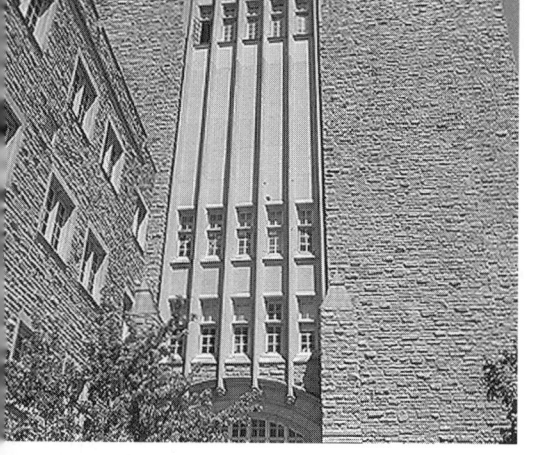

The University of Western Ontario, Schulich School of Medicine & Dentistry

London, Ontario

Admissions & Student Affairs
Schulich School of Medicine & Dentistry
The University of Western Ontario
London, Ontario
Canada, N6A 5C1
T 519 661 3744   F 519 850 2958

Admissions www.schulich.uwo.ca/education/
admissions/medicine
Main www.schulich.uwo.ca
Financial n/a
Email admissions.medicine@schulich.uwo.ca

Public Institution

Dr. Carol P. Herbert, Dean

Dr. Francis Chan, Associate Dean, Admissions & Student Affairs

Dr. Barbara Lent, Associate Dean for Equity/Gender Issues and Faculty Health

Dr. Tom Scott, Associate Dean, Windsor Program

Pamela Bere, Manager, Admissions & Student Affairs and Equity/Gender Issues and Faculty Health

General Information

The Schulich School of Medicine & Dentistry at The University of Western Ontario (Western) has a long tradition of excellence, beginning with the founding of the medical school in 1881. The School is home to more than 1,800 faculty and 2,700 students in medicine, dentistry, medical sciences, graduate and postgraduate training. Western is one of Canada's oldest post-secondary institutions and is committed to providing the best student experience among Canada's leading research-intensive universities.

Mission Statement

The Schulich School of Medicine & Dentistry provides outstanding education within a research-intensive environment where tomorrow's physicians, dentists, and health researchers learn to be socially responsible leaders in the advancement of human health.

Curricular Highlights

Community Service Requirement: Required.
Research/Thesis Requirement: Optional.
Programs of Study: Beginning in Fall, 2008, the Doctor of Medicine program will be offered from two home sites – London, Ontario and Windsor, Ontario. Twenty-four students each year will complete all of their academic studies on the campus of the University of Windsor and graduate from The University of Western Ontario. The new Windsor initiative is a partnership between Western, the University of Windsor and London and Windsor hospitals. Curriculum and clinical training will be equivalent at both sites. The

undergraduate curriculum is patient-centered in content and student-centered in delivery. It is designed to provide students with an opportunity to acquire the knowledge, skills, and attitudes required to advance to postgraduate training leading to clinical practice, research, or other medical careers. The format is a blend of lectures, laboratory experience, small-group problem-based learning sessions, and supervised clinical experiences. The curriculum in first and second year provides students with solid grounding in the basic and clinical sciences. System-based courses include: Introduction to Medicine, Blood & Oncology, Digestive System & Nutrition, Emergency Care, Endocrine & Metabolism, Heart & Circulation, Infection & Immunity, Musculoskeletal System, Respiration & Airways, Neurosciences, Eye, & Ear, Psychiatry & Behavioral Sciences, Reproduction, and Urinary System. Students are also introduced to Community Health and have numerous opportunities for community involvement. The Clinical Methods courses span two years. During the first year, students participate in patient contact emphasizing a patient-centered approach. During third-year Clerkships, students become active members of clinical care teams in family medicine, medicine, obstetrics and gynecology, pediatrics, psychiatry, and surgery. Under faculty and senior resident supervision, clerks are given graded responsibility in the diagnosis, investigation, and management of patients in hospital, clinic, and outpatient settings. All third-year students are required to complete a community Clinical Clerkship in a region outside London or Windsor for a minimum of four weeks through Schulich's Southwestern Ontario Medical Education Network, to ensure students at all levels gain an understanding and experience of the practice of medicine from both a rural/regional and a tertiary care/urban perspective. Fourth-year Clinical Electives are arranged entirely by the student in any area of medicine. After completion of the Clinical Electives, students return in February for the Transition Period, to complete advanced learning opportunities in basic and clinical sciences. This permits students to further integrate the basic and clinical aspects of medicine in light of their clinical experience.

USMLE

Step 1: Optional.
Step 2: Clinical Skills (CS): Optional.
Step 2: Clinical Knowledge (CK): Optional.

Selection Factors

Admission consideration is based on academic achievement, MCAT scores, and a personal interview score. Only those applicants deemed competitive will be selected for an interview.

Financial Aid

The Schulich School of Medicine & Dentistry makes financial assistance for students in need a top priority.

Information about Diversity Programs

Schulich Medicine has designated three seats in each entering class for First Nations, Metis, and Inuit students who provide proof of Indigenous status or ancestral Indigenous origin.

Campus Information

Setting

Western is located in London, Ontario (approximately halfway between Toronto, Ontario and Detroit, Michigan). The Windsor-based portion of the MD program operates from the campus of the University of Windsor, just across the border from Detroit.

Enrollment

For 2007, total enrollment was: 553

Special Features

The Schulich School of Medicine & Dentistry is one of Canada's top centers for medical research and education, with more than $140 million annually in research funding and 49 accredited postgraduate specialty programs.

Housing

For housing information, see:
www.has.uwo.ca/housing/offcampus/index.htm.

Regional/Satellite Campuses/Facilities:

The Windsor-based portion of the MD Program is situated on the campus of the University of Windsor.

Application Process and Requirements 2009–2010

Primary Application Service: OMSAS
Earliest filing date: July 2008
Latest filing date: September 2008

Secondary Application Required?: No
Sent to: n/a
URL: n/a
Fee: No
Fee waiver available: No
Earliest filing date: n/a
Latest filing date: n/a

Latest MCAT® considered: September 2008
Oldest MCAT® considered: 2003
Early Decision Program
School does not have EDP
Applicants notified: n/a
EDP available for: n/a

Regular Acceptance Notice
Earliest date: May 2009
Latest date: Until class is full

Applicant's Response to Acceptance
Offer – Maximum Time: Two weeks

Requests for Deferred
Entrance Considered: No

Deposit to Hold Place in Class: Yes
Deposit (Resident): $1,000
Deposit (Non-Resident): $1,000
Deposit due: With response form
Applied to tuition: Yes
Deposit refundable: No
Refundable by: n/a

Estimated number of new entrants: 147
EDP: 0, special program: n/a

Start Month/Year: September 2009

Interview Format: One physician, one community person, one senior medical student. Regional interviews are not available.

Other Programs

PREPARATORY PROGRAMS
Postbaccalaureate Program: No
Summer Program: No

COMBINED DEGREE PROGRAMS
Baccalaureate/MD: No
MD/MPH: No
MD/MBA: No
MD/JD: No
MD/PhD: Yes,
www.schulich.uwo.ca/medicine/md_phd/index.php
ADDITIONAL PROGRAM
www.eng.uwo.ca/undergraduate/
ProgramInformation/program_information.htm

Premedical Coursework

Course	Req.	Rec.	Lab.	Sems.	Course	Req.	Rec.	Lab.	Sems.
Inorganic Chemistry					Genetics				
Behavioral Sciences					Humanities				
Biochemistry					Organic Chemistry				
Biology					Physics				
Biology/Zoology					Psychology				
Calculus					Social Sciences				
College English					Other 1				
College Mathematics					Other 2				

Selection Factors: 2007 Accepted Applicants

Proportion of Accepted Applicants with Relevant Experience (Data Self-Reported to AMCAS®)		
Community Service/Volunteer	100%	
Medically-Related Work	70%	
Research	25%	

Shaded bar represents accepted scores ranging from the 10th percentile to the 90th percentile ▪ **School Median** ● **National Median** ●

Overall GPA	2.0	2.1	2.2	2.3	2.4	2.5	2.6	2.7	2.8	2.9	3.0	3.1	3.2	3.3	3.4	3.5	3.6	(3.7)	3.8	3.9	4.0
Science GPA	2.0	2.1	2.2	2.3	2.4	2.5	2.6	2.7	2.8	2.9	3.0	3.1	3.2	3.3	3.4	3.5	3.6	(3.7)	3.8	3.9	4.0

MCAT® required: Yes, 100% of 2007 accepted applicants took MCAT®

Verbal Reasoning	3	4	5	6	7	8	9	(10)	11	12	13	14	15
Physical Sciences	3	4	5	6	7	8	9	(10)	11	12	13	14	15
Biological Sciences	3	4	5	6	7	8	9	(10)	11	12	13	14	15
Writing Sample			J	K	L	M	N	O	P	(Q)	R	S	T

Acceptance & Matriculation Data for 2007–2008 First Year Class

	Resident	Non-Resident	International	Total
Applied	2300	n/r	n/a	2300
Interviewed	445	n/r	n/a	445
Deferred	n/r	n/r	0	0
Matriculants				
Early Assurance Program	0	0	0	0
Early Decision Program	n/a	n/a	n/a	n/a
Baccalaureate/MD	n/a	n/a	n/a	n/a
MD/PhD	8	n/r	n/a	8
Matriculated	n/r	n/r	n/r	**147**

Applications accepted from International Applicants: No

Matriculant Demographics: 2007–2008 First Year Class

Men: 75   **Women:** 72

Matriculants' Self-Reported Race/Ethnicity

Mexican American	Korean
Cuban	Vietnamese
Puerto Rican	Other Asian
Other Hispa	
Total Hispar	
Chinese	**DATA NOT COLLECTED**
Asian Indian	
Pakistani	~~Total Asian~~
Filipino	**Unduplicated Number**
Japanese	**of Matriculants**

Science and Math Majors: 86%
Matriculants with:
    Baccalaureate degree: 100%
    Graduate degree(s): 8%

Specialty Choice

2003, 2004, 2005 Graduates, Specialty Choice	
Anesthesiology	8
Emergency Medicine	13
Family Practice	47
Internal Medicine	18
Obstetrics/Gynecology	5
Orthopaedic Surgery	5
Pediatrics	4
Psychiatry	4
Radiology	4
Surgery	7

Financial Information

	Residents	Non-Residents
Total Cost of Attendance	n/r	n/r
Tuition and Fees	$16,527	$16,527
Other (includes living expenses)	$16,050	$16,050
Health Insurance	n/a	n/a

Average 2007 Graduate Indebtedness: $120,000
% of Enrolled Students Receiving Aid: 50%

Criminal Background Check

This medical school requires a criminal background check prior to matriculation.

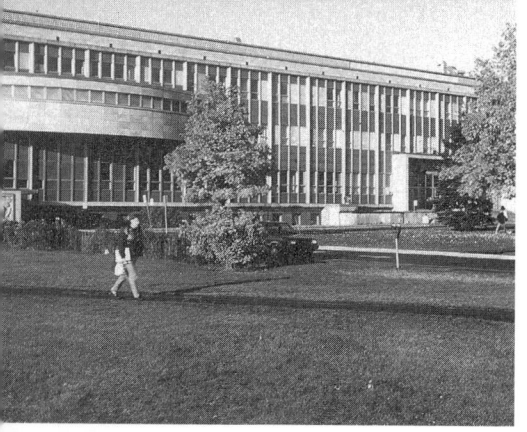

Université Laval
Faculty of Medicine
Quebec, Quebec

Admissions Committee
Universite Laval Faculty of Medicine
Quebec, Quebec
Canada, G1K 7P4
T 418 656 2131 x2492   **F** 418 656 2733

Admissions www.reg.ulaval.ca/p4.html
Main www.fmed.ulaval.ca
Financial www.bbaf.ulaval.ca/bbaf/entree.htm
Email admission@fmed.ulaval.ca

Public Institution

Dr. Pierre J. Durand, Dean

Dr. Evens Villeneuve, Admission Committee Chairman

Guy Labrecque Sr., Admission Committee

General Information

Universite Laval was established by a Royal Charter in 1852 granted by Queen Victoria. It was named after Monseigneur de Laval, first bishop of Quebec. For more than 150 years, the medical school has been dedicated to the formation of health professionals through high standard teaching programs and research activities. Research opportunities are provided in all the basic sciences and in many fields of clinical investigation. The clinical teaching is provided through a network of affiliated health institutions. Residence accommodations are provided for many students. There is a University Health Service for students, as well as vocational guidance, and counseling services.

Mission Statement

The overall goal of the program is to assure a theoretical and clinical formation which prepares students for practicing medicine competently in a contemporary health system, with emphasis on an approach which is scientific, ethical, global, and humanistic. In addition, the program strives to prepare students for a lifetime of continued learning.

Curricular Highlights

Community Service Requirement: Optional.
Research/Thesis Requirement: Optional.

The curriculum aims to prepare students to undertake any career in medicine. During the first two years, the program provides early introduction to clinical problems and interdepartmental teaching by both basic science and clinical faculty. This part of the curriculum is designed to be flexible and can be spread over three calendar years. The basic clinical clerkships are given in the third and fourth years and provide a basic exposure to each major clinical discipline, including family medicine. Both faculty and students monitor the curriculum.

USMLE

Step 1: Optional.
Step 2: Clinical Skills (CS): Optional.
Step 2: Clinical Knowledge (CK): Optional.

Selection Factors

Preference is given to applicants from the province of Quebec. Admission requirements for application from Quebec colleges (CEGEP) and universities include a standardized autobiographical note and a two-hour group session called Assessment by Simulation (APS). This test evaluates different personal characteristics of the candidates. A few outstanding French-speaking candidates are admitted from other Canadian provinces and the United States. These candidates are selected on the basis of different parameters: scholastic achievement, interview, and curriculum vitae. Sex, race, religion, age, and socioeconomic status are not considered in the selection process.

Financial Aid

Financial aid is available to Quebec residents through the Bursaries Division of the Provincial Ministry of Education. Summer scholarships of $4,200 to $5,000 are also available to students who wish to devote their vacation period to research. There is no financial assistance for foreign applicants.

Information about Diversity Programs

Laval University School of Medicine, associated with other Quebec medical schools, is working on a program focused on integrating more aboriginal students.

Campus Information

Setting

The medical school is located in Quebec, a city famous for its walled old city center. Public transportation is widely available and makes travel very easy. Quebec is a lively French city with abundant cultural activities. There are several public parks, cultural institutions, cinemas, shopping areas, and natural areas. The city is surrounded by lakes, rivers, and mountains and enjoys four distinct seasons. Water and snow activities are easily accessible.

Enrollment

For 2007, total enrollment was: 209

Special Features

The medical school has a international exchange program for talented students. Laval has reciprocity agreements with several countries, including Cuba, Peru, Nicaragua, India, Mali, Senegal, and China. The program has two stages: first, five to six weeks of observation and second, three months of medical training.

Housing

Universite Laval boasts four residences with 2,400 Internet-equipped, comfortable rooms. Three of the residences are equipped with modern communal kitchens. For more information, see *www.ulaval.ca/sres* or call the Residence Office at (418) 656-2921 or email sres@sres.ulaval.ca.

Regional/Satellite Campuses/Facilities:

Students rotate among several general and specialized hospitals and affiliated ambulatory care centers. Locations are spread throughout the city and in several towns in the eastern part of the province of Quebec.

Application Process and Requirements 2009–2010

Primary Application Service: School-specific
Earliest filing date: November 15, 2008
Latest filing date: March 1, 2009 (Quebec colleges), February 1, 2009 (all others)

Secondary Application Required?: No
Sent to:
URL: n/a
Fee: n/a
Fee waiver available: No
Earliest filing date: n/a
Latest filing date: Same as primary application

Latest MCAT® considered: n/a
Oldest MCAT® considered: n/a

Early Decision Program
School does not have EDP
Applicants notified: n/a
EDP available for: n/a

Regular Acceptance Notice
Earliest date: May 22, 2009
Latest date: Until class is full

Applicant's Response to Acceptance Offer – Maximum Time: May 21, 2009

Requests for Deferred Entrance Considered: No

Deposit to Hold Place in Class: No
Deposit (Resident): n/a
Deposit (Non-Resident): n/a
Deposit due: n/a
Applied to tuition: n/a
Deposit refundable: n/a
Refundable by: n/a

Estimated number of new entrants: 209
EDP: n/a, special program: n/a

Start Month/Year: September 2009

Interview Format: Six ten-minute role-playing sessions and one 30-minute group session (APS).

Other Programs

PREPARATORY PROGRAMS
Postbaccalaureate Program: Yes
Summer Program: No
Additional: Three Month International Study Abroad
Guy Labrecque, (418) 656-2131 #2492
guy.labrecque@fmed.ulaval.ca

COMBINED DEGREE PROGRAMS
Baccalaureate/MD: Yes, Dr. Joan Glenn
(418) 656-2131 #2492, joan.glenn@fmed.ulaval.ca
MD/MPH: No
MD/MBA: No
MD/JD: No
MD/PhD: Yes, Dr. Lucie Rochefort
(418) 656-2131 #5709
lucie.rochefort@fmed.ulaval.ca

Premedical Coursework

Course	Req.	Rec.	Lab.	Hrs.
Inorganic Chemistry	•		•	1
Behavioral Sciences				
Biochemistry	•			1
Biology	•		•	2
Biology/Zoology			•	
Calculus	•			
College English				
College Mathematics	•			2

Course	Req.	Rec.	Lab.	Hrs.
Computer Science				
Genetics				
Humanities				
Organic Chemistry	•		•	1
Physics	•		•	3
Psychology				
Social Sciences				
Other				

Selection Factors: 2007 Accepted Applicants

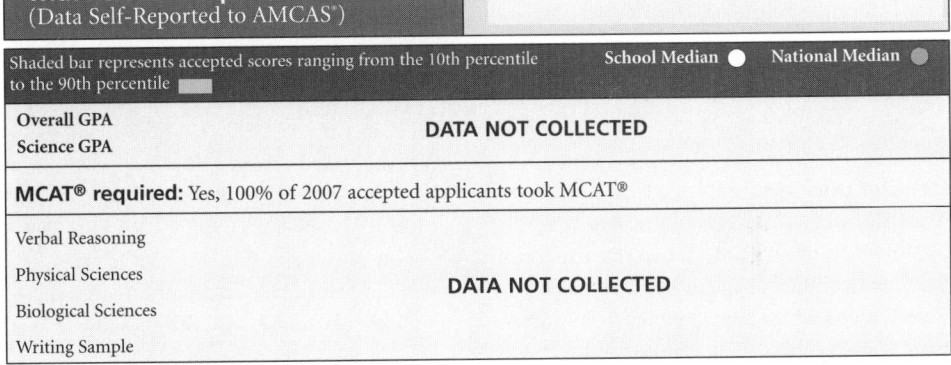

Proportion of Accepted Applicants with Relevant Experience (Data Self-Reported to AMCAS®)	**DATA NOT COLLECTED**

Shaded bar represents accepted scores ranging from the 10th percentile to the 90th percentile   School Median ●   National Median ●

Overall GPA	
Science GPA	**DATA NOT COLLECTED**

MCAT® required: Yes, 100% of 2007 accepted applicants took MCAT®

Verbal Reasoning	
Physical Sciences	
Biological Sciences	**DATA NOT COLLECTED**
Writing Sample	

Acceptance & Matriculation Data for 2007–2008 First Year Class

	Resident	Non-Resident	International	Total
Applied	1584	56	73	1713
Interviewed	n/r	n/r	n/r	n/r
Deferred	n/r	n/r	n/r	n/r
Matriculants				
Early Assurance Program	0	0	0	0
Early Decision Program	n/a	n/a	n/a	n/a
Baccalaureate/MD	n/a	n/a	n/a	n/a
MD/PhD	n/a	n/a	n/a	n/a
Matriculated	204	3	1	**208**

Applications accepted from International Applicants: Yes

Specialty Choice

2003, 2004, 2005 Graduates, Specialty Choice
Anesthesiology
Emergency Medicine
Family Practice
Internal Medicine
Ob:
Ort   **DATA NOT COLLECTED**
Ped
Psy
Radiology
Surgery

Matriculant Demographics: 2007–2008 First Year Class

Men: 59   **Women:** 149

Matriculants' Self-Reported Race/Ethnicity

Mexican American	**Korean**
Cuban	**Vietnamese**
Puerto Rican	**Other Asian**
Other Hispanic	**Native American**
Total Hispanic	**Black**
Chinese	**Native Hawaiian**
Asian Indian	**White**
Pakistani	**Total Asian**
Filipino	**Unduplicated Number**
Japanese	**of Matriculants** 208

Science and Math Majors: 80%
Matriculants with:
Baccalaureate degree: 42%
Graduate degree(s): 3%

Financial Information

	Residents	Non-Residents
Total Cost of Attendance	n/r	n/r
Tuition and Fees	n/r	n/r
Other (includes living expenses)	n/r	n/r
Health Insurance (can be waived)	n/r	n/r

Average 2007 Graduate Indebtedness: n/r
% of Enrolled Students Receiving Aid: n/r

Criminal Background Check

This medical school does not require a criminal background check prior to matriculation.

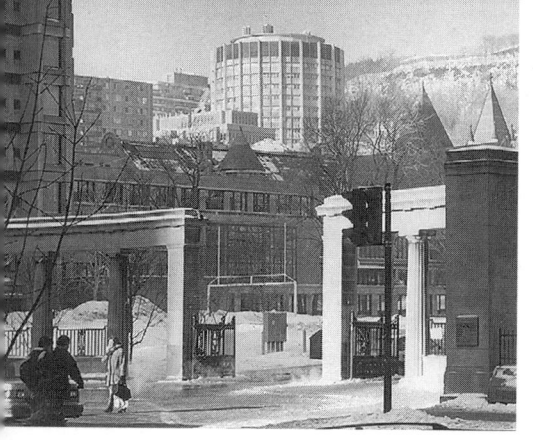

McGill University Faculty of Medicine
Montréal, Quebec

Admissions Office
McGill University Faculty of Medicine
3655 Promenade Sir William Osler
Montréal, Quebec
Canada, H3G 1Y6
T 514 398 3517   **F** 514 398 4631

Admissions www.medicine.mcgill.ca/admissions
Main www.mcgill.ca/medicine/
Financial www.mcgill.ca/student-aid/
Email admissions.med@mcgill.ca

Public Institution

Dr. Richard I. Levin, Dean

Dr. Joyce Pickering, Associate Dean, Medical Education & Student Affairs

France Drolet, Director of Admissions

Judy Stymest, Director of Scholarships and Student Aid

Michel Dansereau, Admissions Officer

General Information
The Faculty of Medicine, established in 1829, is a foundation of medicine in Canada. Clinical facilities include four major teaching hospitals, several affiliated hospitals, specialized centers, and research units. In the Québec health care system, all patients are available for medical student teaching, giving McGill graduates extensive clinical exposure. McGill's Faculty of Medicine is accredited by the LCME, allowing American students to return to the U.S. for residency.

Mission Statement
The advancement of learning through teaching, scholarship, and service to society by offering to outstanding undergraduate and graduate students the best education available; by carrying out scholarly activities judged to be excellent when measured against the highest international standards; and by providing service to society in well-suited ways by virtue of academic strengths. Within this context, the mission of the Faculty of Medicine is to pursue internationally significant scholarship and to provide undergraduate, graduate, and professional programs of the highest academic quality in order to contribute to the well-being of mankind.

Curricular Highlights
Community Service Requirement: Optional.
Research/Thesis Requirement: Optional.

The curriculum has two central themes. The basic sciences and scientific methodology are pillars of medical knowledge and the physician assumes two complementary roles: those of a professional and a healer, referred to as Physicianship. The program utilizes a variety of teaching and evaluation methods, emphasizing small-group teaching. There are four components: The Basis of Medicine covers the basic sciences, with opportunities for hands-on labs, including cadaver dissection. Computer-assisted and on-line instruction is available. Small-group sessions are designed to provide clinical relevance. The Introduction to Clinical Medicine provides a clinical experience in most of the core disciplines. Students are assigned to small groups and provided many opportunities to refine their clinical skills, under supervision, not having responsibility for patient care. The Clerkships start with the Core Clerkship rotations (family medicine rotations are undertaken in both urban and rural sites), followed by Senior Clerkship rotations in Surgical Sub-specialties, Emergency Medicine, and Geriatrics with opportunities for Clinical Electives and/or Research. All clerkships provide extensive clinical contact, under supervision. Optional participation in seminars where the basic sciences are reinforced. The Physicianship program is longitudinal over the four years and focuses on the professional and healer roles. It teaches the main elements of the clinical method, including observation, skillful listening, medical history-taking, physical examination, reasoning, and hypothesis generation. In a longitudinal physician apprenticeship module, all students are assigned, in small groups, to a faculty member. This module provides for mentoring and assists students in their transition from lay-manship to physicianship. All students must successfully complete the Medical Council of Canada exam (MCC-QE-I), USMLE Step 2 CK, or a McGill Exit exam to graduate.

USMLE
Step 1: Optional. Students must only record a score.
Step 2: Clinical Skills (CS): Required. Students must record a passing total score to graduate.
Step 2: Clinical Knowledge (CK): Required. Students must record a passing total score to graduate.

Selection Factors
Student selection is based upon academic achievement, personal characteristics and accomplishments, and MCAT scores. Graduate degrees are taken into account, but the undergraduate degree and GPA hold the most weight. Successful applicants tend to have overall GPAs and Science GPAs of 3.5+ and an MCAT total of 30 or more. Competitive applicants are invited for interviews following which the overall components of the application process are reviewed by committee. Admission decisions are final and are not subject to appeal.

Financial Aid
The McGill Student Aid Office assists students with the financial resources necessary to help cover the cost of school. The website gives information about government aid programs, McGill loans and bursaries, scholarship funding, debt management, individualized budget counseling, and the Work-Study program.

Information about Diversity Programs
All candidates are reviewed without regard to ethnic, religious, linguistic, or socio-cultural background.

Campus Information

Setting
The campus spans 80 acres of downtown Montréal, home to countless cultures and festivities. The campus is within walking distance of major hospitals, advanced teaching facilities, shops, and housing, as well as atop Mount-Royal, the city's central park and natural forest.

Enrollment
For 2007, total enrollment was: 690

Special Features
Major teaching facilities: the Douglas Mental Health University Institute, McGill University Health Centre, Sir Mortimer B. Davis/Jewish General Hospital, St. Mary's Hospital and the McGill Medical Simulation Centre.

Housing
Three styles of housing are available. Wonderful off-campus housing is also available. For more information, see: *www.mcgill.ca/residences/ or /offcampus/.*

Application Process and Requirements 2009–2010

Primary Application Service: School-specific
Earliest filing date: September 1, 2008
Latest filing date: November 15, 2008
non-residents; January 15, 2009: residents

Secondary Application Required?: No
Sent to: n/a
URL: www.medicine.mcgill.ca/admissions/
Fee: No, $80
Fee waiver available: No
Earliest filing date: n/a
Latest filing date: n/a

Latest MCAT® considered: September 2008
Oldest MCAT® considered: January 2006

Early Decision Program
School does have EDP
Applicants notified: Refer to
www.medicine.mcgill.ca/admissions/ for details
EDP available for: Both residents
and non-residents

Regular Acceptance Notice
Earliest date: Mid-February 2009
Latest date: Until Class is Full

Applicant's Response to Acceptance
Offer – Maximum Time: Two weeks

Requests for Deferred
Entrance Considered: Yes

Deposit to Hold Place in Class: Yes
Deposit (Resident): $500
Deposit (Non-Resident): $500
Deposit due: With response to acceptance offer
Applied to tuition: Yes
Deposit refundable: Yes
Refundable by: May 15, 2009: non-residents;
June 15, 2009: residents

Estimated number of new entrants: 172
EDP: n/a, special program: 7

Start Month/Year: Mid-August 2009

Interview Format: Two individual interviews.
Regional interviews are not available.

Other Programs

PREPARATORY PROGRAMS
Postbaccalaureate Program: No
Summer Program: No

COMBINED DEGREE PROGRAMS
Baccalaureate/MD: No
MD/MPH: No
MD/MBA: Yes,
www.medicine.mcgill.ca/admissions
MD/JD: No
MD/PhD: Yes,
www.medicine.mcgill.ca/admissions

Premedical Coursework

Course	Req.	Rec.	Lab.	Hrs.
Inorganic Chemistry	•		•	6
Behavioral Sciences				
Biochemistry		•		
Biology	•		•	6
Biology/Zoology				
Calculus				
College English				
College Mathematics				
Computer Science				

Course	Req.	Rec.	Lab.	Hrs.
Genetics				
Humanities				
Organic Chemistry	•		•	3
Physics	•		•	6
Psychology				
Social Sciences				
Cell/Molecular Biology		•		
Statistics		•		

Selection Factors: 2007 Accepted Applicants

Proportion of Accepted Applicants with Relevant Experience (Data Self-Reported to AMCAS®)	DATA NOT COLLECTED

Shaded bar represents accepted scores ranging from the 10th percentile to the 90th percentile ▪   School Median ● National Median ●

	2.0	2.1	2.2	2.3	2.4	2.5	2.6	2.7	2.8	2.9	3.0	3.1	3.2	3.3	3.4	3.5	3.6	3.7	3.8	3.9	4.0
Overall GPA	2.0	2.1	2.2	2.3	2.4	2.5	2.6	2.7	2.8	2.9	3.0	3.1	3.2	3.3	3.4	3.5	3.6	(3.7)	3.8	3.9	4.0
Science GPA	2.0	2.1	2.2	2.3	2.4	2.5	2.6	2.7	2.8	2.9	3.0	3.1	3.2	3.3	3.4	3.5	3.6	(3.7)	3.8	3.9	4.0

MCAT® required: Yes, 54% of 2007 accepted applicants took MCAT®

	3	4	5	6	7	8	9	10	11	12	13	14	15
Verbal Reasoning	3	4	5	6	7	8	9	(10)	11	12	13	14	15
Physical Sciences	3	4	5	6	7	8	9	10	11	(12)	13	14	15
Biological Sciences	3	4	5	6	7	8	9	10	11	(12)	13	14	15
Writing Sample			J	K	L	M	N	O	P	(Q)	R	S	T

Acceptance & Matriculation Data for 2007–2008 First Year Class

	Resident	Non-Resident	International	Total
Applied	696	530	151	1377
Interviewed	319	49	41	409
Deferred	2	0	0	2
Matriculants				
Early Assurance Program	n/a	n/a	n/a	n/a
Early Decision Program	0	0	0	0
Baccalaureate/MD	n/a	n/a	n/a	n/a
MD/PhD	3	2	0	5
Matriculated	156	9	7	**172**

Applications accepted from International Applicants: Yes

Specialty Choice

2003, 2004, 2005 Graduates, Specialty Choice	
Anesthesiology	3
Emergency Medicine	3
Family Practice	20
Internal Medicine	22
Obstetrics/Gynecology	3
Orthopaedic Surgery	2
Pediatrics	10
Psychiatry	2
Radiology Diagnostic	4
Surgery General	7

Matriculant Demographics: 2007–2008 First Year Class

Men: 83   **Women:** 89

Matriculants' Self-Reported Race/Ethnicity

Mexican American   Korean
Cuban   Vietnamese
Puerto Rican   Other Asian
Other
Total H   DATA NOT COLLECTED
Chines
Asian I
Pakista...
Filipino   **Unduplicated Number**
Japanese   **of Matriculants**

Science and Math Majors: 80%
Matriculants with:
     Baccalaureate degree: 54%
     Graduate degree(s): 8%

Financial Information

	Residents	Non-Residents
Total Cost of Attendance	n/r	$5,1784
Tuition and Fees	$3,565	$10,499 (Canadian)
Other (includes living expenses)	$2,480	$2,519 (Canadian)
Health Insurance (can be waived)	$693	n/a

Average 2007 Graduate Indebtedness: $n/r
% of Enrolled Students Receiving Aid: n/a

Criminal Background Check

This school does not require a criminal background check prior to matriculation.

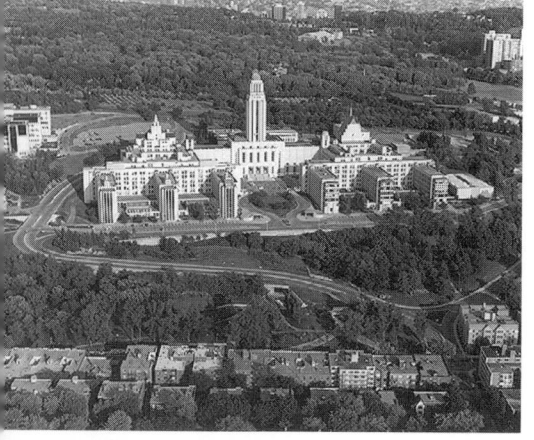

Université de Montréal School of Medicine

Montréal, Quebec

Committee on Admission
Université de Montréal School of Medicine
P.O. Box 6128, Station Centre-Ville
Montréal Quebec H3C 3J7
T 514 343 6265   **F** 514 343 6629

Admissions www.med.umontreal.ca/etudes/admission.htm
Main www.med.umontreal.ca
Financial n/a
Email admmed@ere.umontreal.ca

Public Institution

*Dr. Jean-Lucien Rouleau,
Dean of Faculty of Medicine*

*Dr. Christian Bourdy, President
of Admission Committee*

*Dr. Raymond Lalande, Vice Dean,
Undergraduate Studies*

General Information

The Faculty of Medicine of the Université de Montréal can be traced back to a school first established in Montréal in 1843 and incorporated in 1845 under the name of Ecole de Medecine et de Chirurgie de Montréal. In 1891 the school merged with the Faculty of Medicine of the Montréal Branch of Laval University, which had been founded in 1877. In 1920, by an act of the Quebec legislature, the Montréal branch of Laval University was granted its independence, and the school of medicine became known by its present name. All instruction is in French, and clinical instruction is carried out at 14 affiliated teaching hospitals and research centers.

Mission Statement

The Faculty of Medicine of the Université de Montréal seeks through its undergraduate medical program to provide a general preparation so that students will be able to enter postgraduate training in either family medicine or a medical specialization or fields related to research, teaching, or health care management.

Curricular Highlights

Community Service Requirement: Optional.
Research/Thesis Requirement: Optional.

In September 1993, a new four-year curriculum came into effect. It consists of two years (70 weeks) of problem-based learning during which students are exposed to biomedical and psychosocial sciences basic to medicine. Courses are interdisciplinary and system-based. Introduction to clinical skills takes place in a continuous fashion throughout those two preclinical years. Clinical exposure begins with Year 1. Fourty-five hours of electives are mandatory during the first two years.

The third and fourth years consist of an 80-week clerkship. In the new curriculum, formal lecturing is reduced to a minimum and replaced by active methods, especially problem-based learning and small-group discussion. A premedical year devoted to basic biological and behavioral sciences is restricted to students having just graduated from the provincial colleges of general and professional education (CEGEP). Students who have completed one to three years at the university level in humanities are also eligible for the premedical year. Residency training in the teaching hospitals is under the responsibility of the Faculty of Medicine. Various courses and symposia are organized by the continuing medical education division.

USMLE

Step 1: Optional.
Step 2: Clinical Skills (CS): Optional.
Step 2: Clinical Knowledge (CK): Optional.

Selection Factors

Candidates accepted must be either Canadian citizens or landed immigrants, but due consideration will be given to French-speaking applicants from other provinces of Canada. Selection of candidates is competitive and based on a global score derived from scholastic records and an interview. Interviews, conducted on the site of the medical school, are granted to about one-quarter of the applicants on the basis of their scholastic records. This interview can be eliminatory. For candidates holding a Ph.D. degree, performance in research may constitute an important selection factor. No consideration is given to race, sex, creed, or age.

Financial Aid

Financial aid is available to students through the Bursaries Division of the Department of Education, the Kellogg Foundation Loan Fund, the Scholarships and Loan Committee of the university, and the Jean Frappier Fund. Summer scholarships are also available.

Campus Information

Setting

The medical school is located in the main campus in downtown Montréal, which can be reached by buses and subways. University and community-based hospitals associated with the University are spread in the downtown area and suburbs.

Enrollment

For 2007, total enrollment was: 1217

Housing

On-campus housing is available.

Satellite Campuses/Facilities

Since 2004, there is a regional campus in Trois-Rivières, located 125 kilometers east of Montréal. Each year, thirty-two students start medical school on Trois-Rivières campus most of them at the pre-medical level. The currula at the Montréal campus and Trois-Rivières campus are identical. Clinical training will be done in community hospital in the Mauricie region.

Application Process and Requirements 2009–2010

Primary Application Service: School-specific
Earliest filing date: December 1, 2008
Latest filing date: January 15, 2009

Secondary Application Required?: No
Sent to: n/a
URL: n/a
Fee: No
Fee waiver available: No
Earliest filing date: n/a
Latest filing date: n/a

Latest MCAT® considered: Not required
Oldest MCAT® considered: Not required

Early Decision Program
School does not have EDP
Applicants notified: n/a
EDP available for: n/a

Regular Acceptance Notice
Earliest date: April 11, 2009
Latest date: Until class is full

Applicant's Response to Acceptance
Offer – Maximum Time: Two weeks

Requests for Deferred
Entrance Considered: No

Deposit to Hold Place in Class: Yes
Deposit (Resident): $200
Deposit (Non-Resident): $200
Deposit due: With response to acceptance offer
Applied to tuition: Yes
Deposit refundable: No
Refundable by: n/a

Estimated number of new entrants: 265
EDP: n/a, special program: n/a

Start Month/Year: August 2009

Interview Format: Individual and group interviews conducted. Regional interviews are not available.

Other Programs

PREPARATORY PROGRAMS
Postbaccalaureate Program: No
Summer Program: No

COMBINED DEGREE PROGRAMS
Baccalaureate/MD: No
MD/MPH: No
MD/MBA: No
MD/JD: No
MD/PhD: Yes

Premedical Coursework

Course	Req.	Rec.	Lab.	Hrs.	Course	Req.	Rec.	Lab.	Hrs.
Inorganic Chemistry	•				Computer Science				
Behavioral Sciences					Genetics				
Biochemistry					Humanities				
Biology	•				Organic Chemistry	•			
Biology/Zoology					Physics	•			
Calculus					Psychology				
College English					Social Sciences				
College Mathematics	•								

Selection Factors: 2007 Accepted Applicants

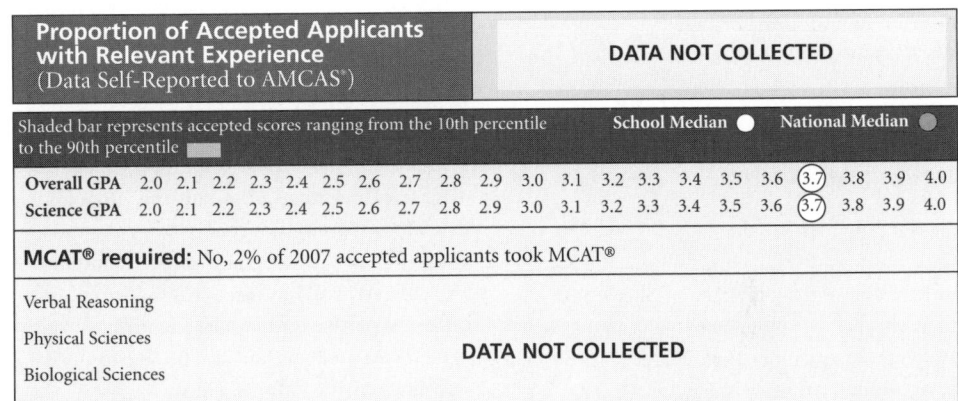

	Proportion of Accepted Applicants with Relevant Experience (Data Self-Reported to AMCAS®)	DATA NOT COLLECTED

Shaded bar represents accepted scores ranging from the 10th percentile to the 90th percentile. School Median ● National Median ●

	2.0	2.1	2.2	2.3	2.4	2.5	2.6	2.7	2.8	2.9	3.0	3.1	3.2	3.3	3.4	3.5	3.6	3.7	3.8	3.9	4.0
Overall GPA																		(3.7)			
Science GPA																		(3.7)			

MCAT® required: No, 2% of 2007 accepted applicants took MCAT®

Verbal Reasoning	
Physical Sciences	DATA NOT COLLECTED
Biological Sciences	
Writing Sample	

Acceptance & Matriculation Data for 2007–2008 First Year Class

	Resident	Non-Resident	International	Total
Applied	1891	37	188	2116
Interviewed	785	7	4	796
Deferred	0	0	0	0
Matriculants				
Early Assurance Program	0	0	0	0
Early Decision Program	n/a	n/a	n/a	n/a
Baccalaureate/MD	n/a	n/a	n/a	n/a
MD/PhD	0	0	0	0
Matriculated	265	4	1	**270**

Applications accepted from International Applicants: Yes

Specialty Choice

2003, 2004, 2005 Graduates, Specialty Choice

Anesthesiology
Emergency Medicine
Family Practice
Internal Medicine
Obst...
Orth... **DATA NOT COLLECTED**
Pedi...
Psyc...
Radiology
Surgery

Matriculant Demographics: 2007–2008 First Year Class

Men: 88 **Women:** 182

Matriculants' Self-Reported Race/Ethnicity

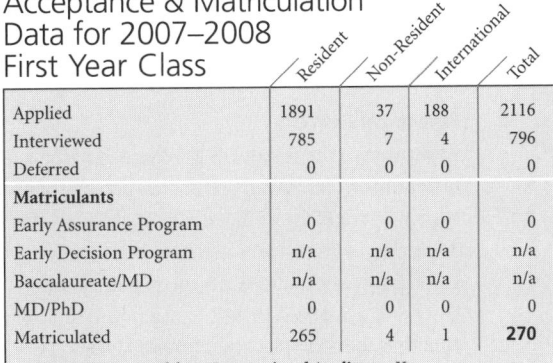

Mexican American	Korean
Cuban	Vietnamese
Puerto Rican	Other Asian
Other	
Total	
Chine	**DATA NOT COLLECTED**
Asian	
Pakist	
Filipino	**Unduplicated Number**
Japanese	**of Matriculants**

Science and Math Majors: 65%
Matriculants with:
 Baccalaureate degree: 35
 Graduate degree(s): 1

Financial Information

	Residents	Non-Residents
Total Cost of Attendance	n/r	n/r
Tuition and Fees	$4,000	$23,000
Other (includes living expenses)	$2,000	$2,000
Health Insurance (can be waived)	n/r	n/r

Average 2007 Graduate Indebtedness: $25,000
% of Enrolled Students Receiving Aid: n/r

Criminal Background Check

This school does not require a criminal background check prior to matriculation.

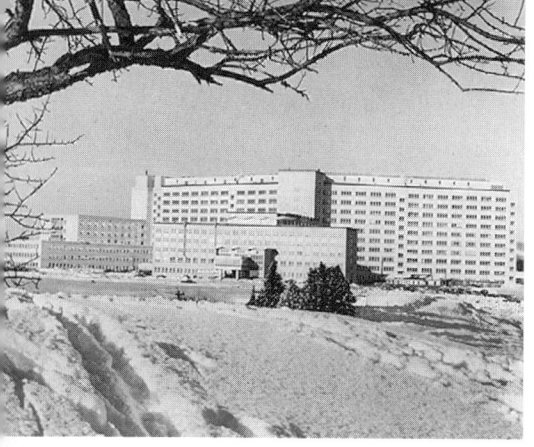

University of Sherbrooke
Faculty of Medicine
Sherbrooke, Quebec

Admission Office, University of Sherbrooke
Faculty of Medicine and Health Sciences
3001, 12e Avenue Nord
Sherbrooke, Quebec
Canada, J1H 5N4
T 819 564 5208   F 819 820 6809

Admissions www.usherbrooke.ca/
doctorat_medecine
Main www.usherbrooke.ca
Financial www.usherbrooke.ca/jetudie/financement
Email Admission-Med@USherbrooke.ca

Public Institution

Dr. Rejean Hebert, Dean

Dr. Daniel J.Cote, Chair, Admissions Committee

Dr. Jocelyne Faucher, Vice Dean, Student Affairs

*Dr. Paul Grand 'Maison, Vice Dean,
Undergraduate Medical Education*

Dr. Guy Waddell, MD Program Director

General Information
Officially founded in February 1961, the Faculty of Medicine at the University of Sherbrooke is a French-speaking institution. It admitted its first students in September 1966. The Faculty opened two outside campuses in September 2006 and offers its whole MD program in a distributed approach. The first is located in Saguenay, the central city of Quebec peripheral region. The second one is located in Moncton, the central French speaking city in the province of New Brunswick. Students complete the program either in the central campus in Sherbrooke (144 -148 admitted students,) or in Moncton (24 students,) or in Saguenay (24 students).

Mission Statement
Improved health and well-being of people and populations through education, research, clinical services, and knowledge transfer.

Curricular Highlights
Community Service Requirement: Optional.
Research/Thesis Requirement: Optional.

The MD degree is granted after successful completion of the four-year course. Teaching is given through small-group problem-based learning in an integrated and system-based curriculum. Audiovisual facilities, seminars, small-group discussions, panels, field work, and case studies are used extensively. Teaching of clinical skills starts during the first month of the program and is offered through a continuous and integrated program throughout the preclinical years. Community-based education is a major characteristic of the clerkship. The clerkship is 18 months long. Clinical training starts with the

winter trimester of the third year. Clerkship rotations are offered in a network of primary to tertiary health care institutions located in urban, suburban, peripheral, rural and remote areas in the Province of Québec and New-Brunswick which offer complementary experience to the students. Each student must spend at least 1/3 of their clerkship in community-based settings. Postgraduate programs are available in most clinical disciplines including community health. A joint MD/MSc program is offered to students who are enrolled in he MD program with outstanding academic records. Its objective is to form physicians who will have achieved a scientific approach of medicine and who will also be able to pursue scientific activities among a team.

USMLE
Step 1: Optional.
Step 2: Clinical Skills (CS): Optional.
Step 2: Clinical Knowledge (CK): Optional.

Selection Factors
Admission to the Faculty of Medicine is based primarily on ability and premedical achievement, as demonstrated by a students' academic records. A learning skills test is included in the selection. University candidates from the province of Quebec are required to participate in the Multiple Mini Interviews (MMI) in addition to the other admission criteria. One hundred and sixty-five places are reserved for applicants from the province of Quebec (3 of these positions may be filled by French speaking students coming from western Canadian provinces and Territories). In addition, 24 places are reserved for applicants from New Brunswick, one place is available for an applicant from Prince Edward Island, and three places are available for applicants from Nova Scotia. One place is available for applicants from Newfoundland. One to six places are available for Canadian Forces candidates. One place is available for a qualified foreign applicant with a student visa. In 2007, 196 students entered into the program. The same number should enter the program for 2008-2009 academic year. Applicants must be fluent in both written and spoken French.

Financial Aid
Financial aid is available to resident students through the Bursaries Division of the Provincial Ministry of Education, the Scholarships and Loans Committee of the university, and a few private foundations.

Campus Information

Setting
The Faculty's main campus is located on the Health Sciences Campus of the University in a joint building with the 425-bed University Hospital and major Research Center.

Enrollment
For 2007, total enrollment was: 696

Satellite Campuses/Facilities
The Saguenay outside site is located at the Universite du Quebec a Chicoutimi and at the Chicoutimi regional Hospital. The Moncton site is located at the Universite de Moncton and partners with Hospital Georges L. Dumont, the French speaking regional hospital in Moncton.

Application Process and Requirements 2009–2010

Primary Application Service: School-specific
Earliest filing date: Applications accepted year round.
Latest filing date: Students from Quebec University, other Canadian provinces and foreign students: January 15, 2009; Quebec College students: March 1, 2009
Secondary Application Required?: No
Sent to: n/a
URL: n/a
Fee: Yes, $70
Fee waiver available: No
Earliest filing date: n/a
Latest filing date: n/a

Latest MCAT® considered: not required
Oldest MCAT® considered: not required

Early Decision Program
School does not have EDP
Applicants notified: n/a
EDP available for: n/a

Regular Acceptance Notice
Earliest date: May 2009
Latest date: Varies

Applicant's Response to Acceptance Offer – Maximum Time: Varies. 1-15 days, depending on when the acceptance notice is sent.

Requests for Deferred Entrance Considered: No

Deposit to Hold Place in Class: Yes
Deposit (Resident): $200
Deposit (Non-Resident): $200
Deposit due: With response to acceptance offer
Applied to tuition: Yes
Deposit refundable: No
Refundable by: n/a

Estimated number of new entrants: 196
EDP: n/a, special program: n/a

Start Month/Year: August 2009

Interview Format: The process includes a learning skills test. Regional interviews are not available.

Other Programs

PREPARATORY PROGRAMS
Postbaccalaureate Program: No
Summer Program: No

COMBINED DEGREE PROGRAMS
Baccalaureate/MD: No
MD/MPH: No
MD/MBA: No
MD/JD: No
MD/PhD: Yes, Dr Claude Asselin, www.usherbrooke.ca/doctorat_medecine (819) 564-5276, Claude.Asselin@USherbrooke.ca
MD-M.Sc master degrees: Yes, www.usherbrooke.ca/doctorat_medecine Dr. Claude Asselin, (819) 564-5276, Claude.Asselin@USherbrooke.ca

Premedical Coursework

Course	Req.	Rec.	Lab.	Sems.
Inorganic Chemistry	•			
Behavioral Sciences		•		
Biochemistry				
Biology	•		•	2
Biology/Zoology				
Calculus	•			
College English				
College Mathematics	•		•	2

Course	Req.	Rec.	Lab.	Sems.
Computer Science				
Genetics				
Humanities		•		
Organic Chemistry	•		•	3
Physics	•		•	3
Psychology		•		
Social Sciences		•		
Other				

Selection Factors: 2007 Accepted Applicants

Proportion of Accepted Applicants with Relevant Experience (Data Self-Reported to AMCAS®)		
Community Service/Volunteer		0
Medically-Related Work		0
Research		0

Shaded bar represents accepted scores ranging from the 10th percentile to the 90th percentile   School Median ●   National Median ●

Overall GPA Science GPA	**DATA NOT COLLECTED**
MCAT® required: No	

Verbal Reasoning	
Physical Sciences	**DATA NOT COLLECTED**
Biological Sciences	
Writing Sample	

Acceptance & Matriculation Data for 2007–2008 First Year Class

	Resident	Non-Resident	International	Total
Applied	1538	109	86	1733
Interviewed	685	79	1	765
Deferred	0	0	0	0
Matriculants				
Early Assurance Program	0	0	0	0
Early Decision Program	n/a	n/a	n/a	n/a
Baccalaureate/MD	n/a	n/a	n/a	n/a
MD/PhD	n/a	n/a	n/a	n/a
Matriculated	163	30	1	**194**

Applications accepted from International Applicants: Yes

Specialty Choice

2003, 2004, 2005 Graduates, Specialty Choice
Anesthesiology
Emergency Medicine
Family Practice
Internal Medicine
Obst...
Orth... **DATA NOT COLLECTED**
Pedia...
Psych...
Radiology
Surgery

Matriculant Demographics: 2007–2008 First Year Class

Men: 75   **Women:** 119

Matriculants' Self-Reported Race/Ethnicity

Mexican American   Korean
Cuban   Vietnamese
Puerto Rican   Other Asian
Other H...
Total Hi...   **DATA NOT COLLECTED**
Chinese...
Asian I...
Pakistan...   Total Asian
Filipino   **Unduplicated Number**
Japanese   **of Matriculants**

Science and Math Majors: n/a
Matriculants with:
       Baccalaureate degree: 14%
       Graduate degree(s): 1%

Financial Information

	Residents	Non-Residents
Total Cost of Attendance	$10495 - 15090	$26910 - 31900
Tuition and Fees	$3330 - 3830	$8500 - 9900
Other (includes living expenses)	$550/month	$550/month
Health Insurance (not applicable)	n/a	n/a

Average 2007 Graduate Indebtedness: $25,000
% of Enrolled Students Receiving Aid: 50%

Criminal Background Check

This medical school does not require a criminal background check prior to matriculation.

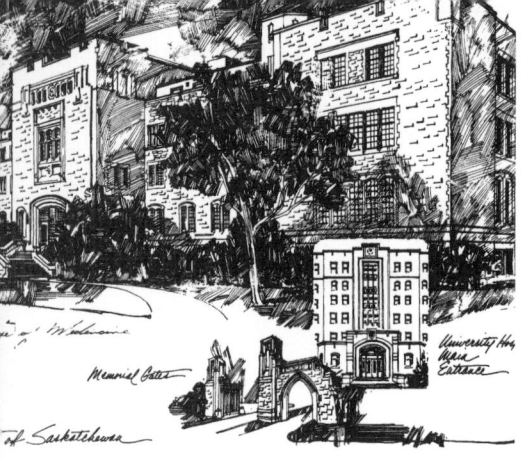

University of Saskatchewan
College of Medicine

Saskatoon, Saskatchewan

Admissions
University of Saskatchewan College of Medicine
A204 Health Sciences Bld, 107 Wiggins Rd
Saskatoon, Saskatchewan
Canada, S7N 5E5
T 306 966 8554   F 306 966 2601

Admissions www.medicine.usask.ca/admissions
Main www.medicine.usask.ca
Financial www.usask.ca/calendar/scholarships
Email med.admissions@usask.ca

Public Institution

Dr. William L. Albritton, Dean

Dr. Barry Ziola, Director, Admissions & Student Affairs

Heather Mandeville, Administrative Coordinator, Admissions & Student Affairs

General Information

The University of Saskatchewan began teaching medical students in a two-year medical sciences program in 1926. The present college was introduced in 1953, with a four-year curriculum leading to the M.D. degree. In 1968, the curriculum changed to five years with a one-year premedical university requirement. The curriculum reverted to a four-year program in 1988 with a minimum two-year premedical requirement. Clinical teaching is based at the Royal University, St. Paul's, and Saskatoon City Hospitals in Saskatoon, and the Plains Health Centre and General Hospital in Regina. Students also complete rotations in Saskatchewan Health Regions. The class size will increase over the next couple years; 80 students will be accepted in 2008, 88 students in 2009, with further possible expansions to 100 students.

Mission Statement

The College of Medicine is a departmentalized collegial unit of the University of Saskatchewan. The mission is to improve health through excellence in education, research, and clinical care.

Curricular Highlights

Community Service Requirement: Optional.
Research/Thesis Requirement: Optional.

The College of Medicine provides a curriculum leading to the general professional education of the physician; graduates may select careers in family medicine, specialty practice, or research. The current curriculum was launched in the fall of 1997. Phase A (31 weeks) provides students with an overview of the basic science disciplines appropriate to the study of medicine, as well as an introduction to professional skills (including primary clinical skills) within the context of developing the patient-doctor relationship. This phase includes a two-week clinical experience done in one of the Saskatchewan Health Districts. Phase B (33 weeks) enables students to acquire specific knowledge in those subjects bridging the basic and clinical sciences and to enhance basic clinical skills. Phase C (15 weeks), enables learning of the principles and methods in core clinical knowledge and linking courses. Phase D (64 weeks) of clinical clerkships provides an opportunity to apply the knowledge, skills, and attitudes students have acquired to the management of patients. Provision is made for clinical electives. Learning in the basic and clinical sciences has been organized by body systems with a problem-solving emphasis.

USMLE

Step 1: n/a
Step 2: Clinical Skills (CS): n/a
Step 2: Clinical Knowledge (CK): n/a

Selection Factors

The Admissions Committee considers academic ability and personal qualities assessed through scholastic records, letters of recommendation, and results of an interview. All eligible candidates are interviewed during a weekend in March.

Financial Aid

Various loan funds and scholarships are available. A limited number of bursaries enable students to engage in research between the end of one academic year and the beginning of another.

Information about Diversity Programs

There is an Aboriginal Access Program for Canadian residents of Aboriginal ancestry. For more information, contact the Admissions office.

Campus Information

Setting

Our medical school is situated on 755 hectares of land, in the heart of the city of Saskatoon on the scenic bank of the South Saskatchewan River. Much of the original architecture remains from the University's opening in 1909, and grey-stone buildings ornamented with garrets and turrets are a monument of fine craftsmanship. The University of Saskatchewan has the largest collection of health sciences in Canada.

Enrollment

For 2007, total enrollment was: 248

Housing

As a student at the U of S, you have several options for finding appropriate, affordable housing. Students may choose from both on- and off-campus accommodations. Living in residence offers the opportunity to meet people from all colleges and cultures and you will become more familiar with the opportunities offered at university, both social and academic. To find out more about housing and residence at the U of S, please visit *http://explore.usask.ca/about/housing/.*

Satellite Campuses/Facilities

The University of Saskatchewan College of Medicine has a distributive learning environment in which a number of clinical educational experiences take place in a number of Saskatchewan Health Regions and teaching hospitals. Students will be assigned to a core set of rotations centered either in the Saskatoon Health Region or in the Regina/Qu'Appelle Health Region.

Application Process and Requirements 2009–2010

Primary Application Service: School-specific
Earliest filing date: July 1, 2008
Latest filing date: November 1, 2008

Secondary Application Required?: No
Sent to: n/a
URL: www.medicine.usask.ca/admissions
Fee: n/a
Fee waiver available: n/a
Earliest filing date: n/a
Latest filing date: n/a

Latest MCAT® considered: September 2008
Oldest MCAT® considered: April 2004

Early Decision Program
School does not have EDP
Applicants notified: May 15, 2009
EDP available for: n/a

Regular Acceptance Notice
Earliest date: May 15, 2009
Latest date: Until Class is Full

**Applicant's Response to Acceptance
Offer – Maximum Time:** Two weeks

**Requests for Deferred
Entrance Considered:** Yes

Deposit to Hold Place in Class: Yes
Deposit (Resident): $500
Deposit (Non-Resident): $500
Deposit due: With response to acceptance offer
Applied to tuition: Yes
Deposit refundable: No
Refundable by: n/a

Estimated number of new entrant: 88
EDP: 0, special program: n/a

Start Month/Year: August 2009

Interview Format: Multiple Mini Interview.
Regional Interviews are not available.

Other Programs

PREPARATORY PROGRAMS
Postbaccalaureate Program: No
Summer Program: No

COMBINED DEGREE PROGRAMS
Baccalaureate/MD: No
MD/MPH: No,
MD/MBA: No
MD/JD: No
MD/PhD: Yes, www.medicine.usask.ca/research/
clinical_programs

Premedical Coursework

Course	Req.	Rec.	Lab.	Hrs.
Inorganic Chemistry	•		•	3
Behavioral Sciences				
Biochemistry	•			6
Biology	•		•	6
Biology/Zoology				
Calculus				
College English	•			6
College Mathematics				

Course	Req.	Rec.	Lab.	Hrs.
Computer Science				
Genetics				
Humanities		•		
Organic Chemistry	•		•	3
Physics	•		•	6
Psychology				
Social Sciences	•			6
Other				

Selection Factors: 2007 Accepted Applicants

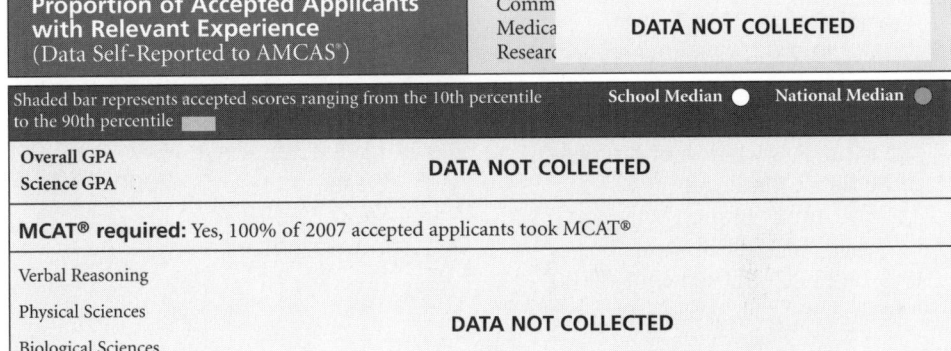

Proportion of Accepted Applicants with Relevant Experience (Data Self-Reported to AMCAS®)

Community, Medical, Research: DATA NOT COLLECTED

Shaded bar represents accepted scores ranging from the 10th percentile to the 90th percentile. School Median / National Median

Overall GPA / Science GPA: DATA NOT COLLECTED

MCAT® required: Yes, 100% of 2007 accepted applicants took MCAT®

Verbal Reasoning / Physical Sciences / Biological Sciences / Writing Sample: DATA NOT COLLECTED

Acceptance & Matriculation Data for 2007–2008 First Year Class

	Resident	Non-Resident	International	Total
Applied	197	371	n/a	568
Interviewed	185	42	n/a	227
Deferred	0	0	n/a	0
Matriculants				
Early Assurance Program	n/a	n/a	n/a	n/a
Early Decision Program	n/a	n/a	n/a	n/a
Baccalaureate/MD	n/a	n/a	n/a	n/a
MD/PhD	n/a	n/a	n/a	n/a
Matriculated	n/a	n/a	n/a	**80**

Applications accepted from International Applicants: No

Specialty Choice

2003, 2004, 2005 Graduates, Specialty Choice

Anesthesiology
Emergency Medicine
Family Practice
Internal Medicine
Obst...
Orth... DATA NOT COLLECTED
Pedi...
Psyc...
Radiology
Surgery

Matriculant Demographics: 2007–2008 First Year Class

Men: 39   **Women:** 29

Matriculants' Self-Reported Race/Ethnicity

Mexican American	n/a	Korean	n/a
Cuban	n/a	Vietnamese	n/a
Puerto Rican	n/a	Other Asian	n/a
Other			/a
Total			/a
Chinese	DATA NOT COLLECTED		/a
Asian			/a
Pakist...			/a
Filipin...			
Japanese	n/a	of Matriculants	60

Science and Math Majors: n/a
Matriculants with:
  Baccalaureate degree: 23%
  Graduate degree(s): 2%

Financial Information

	Residents	Non-Residents
Total Cost of Attendance	n/r	n/r
Tuition and Fees	$11,460	n/r
Other (includes living expenses)	n/r	n/r
Health Insurance (can be waived)	n/a	n/a

Average 2007 Graduate Indebtedness: n/r
% of Enrolled Students Receiving Aid: n/r

Criminal Background Check

This medical school does not require a criminal background check prior to matriculation.

Resources for Other Health Careers

1. **American Association of Colleges of Osteopathic Medicine**
   5550 Friendship Boulevard, Suite 310
   Chevy Chase, MD 20815-7231
   (301) 968-4100; www.aacom.org

2. **American Association of Colleges of Pharmacy**
   1426 Prince Street
   Alexandria, VA 22314-2815
   (703) 739-2330; *www.aacp.org*

3. **American Association of Colleges of Podiatric Medicine**
   15850 Crabbs Branch Way, Suite 320
   Rockville, MD 20855-4307
   (800) 922-9266; (301) 948-9760
   info@aacpm.org; *www.aacpm.org*

4. **American Association of Dental Schools**
   1400 K Street, N.W., Suite 1100
   Washington, D.C. 20005
   (202) 289-7201; *www.adea.org*

5. **Association of American Veterinary Medical Colleges**
   1101 Vermont Avenue, N.W., Suite 301
   Washington, D.C. 20005-3521
   (202) 371-9195
   hbenedict@aavmc.org; *www.aavmc.org*

6. **Association of Schools and Colleges of Optometry**
   6110 Executive Boulevard, Suite 420
   Rockville, MD 20852
   (301) 231-5944
   admini@opted.org; *www.opted.org*

7. **Association of Schools of Public Health**
   1101 15th Street, N.W., Suite 910
   Washington, D.C., 20005
   (202) 296-1099
   info@asph.org; *www.asph.org*

Publications for the Health Professions

1. 300 Ways to Put Your Talent to Work in the Health Field

Single copy, $15 member,
$18.00 non-member
National Health Council
1730 M Street, N.W., Suite 500
Washington, D.C. 20036
(202) 785-3910;
www.nationalhealthcouncil.org/
pubs/pub_list.htm

2. Autsin, L., What's Holding You Back? 8 Critical Choices for Women's Success

$14.00
Basic Books, 2000
www.perseusbooksgroup.com/basic/
home.jsp

3. Bickel, J., Women in Medicine: Getting In, Growing & Advancing

$36.95
Sage, 2000
(805) 499-9774; www.sagepub.com

4. Educational Survival Skills Study Guide

Free
Office of Statewide Health
Planning and Development
Health Professions Career
Opportunity Program
1600 Ninth Street, Room 441
Sacramento, CA 95814
www.oshpd.ca.gov/HWDD/pdfs/
StudySkills.pdf

5. Financial Advice and Health Careers Resources Directory for Students

Free
Office of Statewide Health
Planning and Development
Health Professions Careers
Opportunity Program
1600 Ninth Street, Room 441
Sacramento, CA 95814
www.oshpd.ca.gov/HWDD/pdfs/
FinancialAdvice.pdf

6. The Journal for Minority Medical Students

$20.00, published quarterly
Spectrum Unlimited
630 Goldpoint Trace
Woodstock, GA 30189
(800) 661-3319, (504) 433-5040

7. Kaltreider, Nancy B., Dilemmas of a Double Life, Women Balancing Careers and Relationship

$44.95
Jason Aronson, Inc., 1997
(800) 462-6420;
www.rowmanlittlefield.com/Catalog/

8. Minorities in Medicine: A Guide for Premedical Students

Free
Office of Statewide Health Planning
and Development
Health Professions Career
Opportunity Program
1600 Ninth Street, Room 441
Sacramento, CA 95814
www.oshpd.ca.gov/HWDD/pdfs/
MinoritiesMedicine.pdf

9. Minority Student Opportunities in United States Medical Schools

$15.00, published bi-annually
Association of American
Medical Colleges
2450 N Street, N.W.
Washington, D.C. 20037
(202) 828-0416;
www.aamc.org/publications

10. More, E.S., Restoring the Balance: Women Physicians and the Profession of Medicine, 1850-1995.

$62.00 hardcover, $29.50 paperback
Harvard University Press, 2000
www.hup.harvard.edu

11. Need a Lift? College Financial Aid Handbook

$3.00, plus shipping
The American Legion
P.O. Box 1050
Indianapolis, IN 46206
888-453-4466;
www.emblem.legion.org

12. The Student Guide

U.S. Department of Education Federal
Student Aid Information Center
P.O. Box 84
Washington, D.C. 20044-0084
(800) 4-FED-AID, (800) 433-3243
http://studentaid.ed.gov/students/
attachments/siteresources/Funding
EduBeyondHighSchool_0809.pdf

13. Time Management for Students

Free
Office of Statewide Health
Planning and Development
Health Professions Career
Opportunity Program
1600 Ninth Street, Room 441
Sacramento, CA 95814
www.oshpd.ca.gov/HWDD/pdfs/
TimeManagement.pdf

14. Wear, D. (Ed), Women in Medical Education: An Anthology of Experience

$22.50 hardcover, $21.95 paperback
SUNY Press, 1996
www.sunypress.edu/details.asp?id=53512

15. The Young Scientist: A Career Guide for Underrepresented Science Graduates

$5.00, published annually
Spectrum Unlimited
630 Goldpoint Trace
Woodstock, GA 30189
(800) 661-3319, (504) 433-5040

You can change the face of medicine.

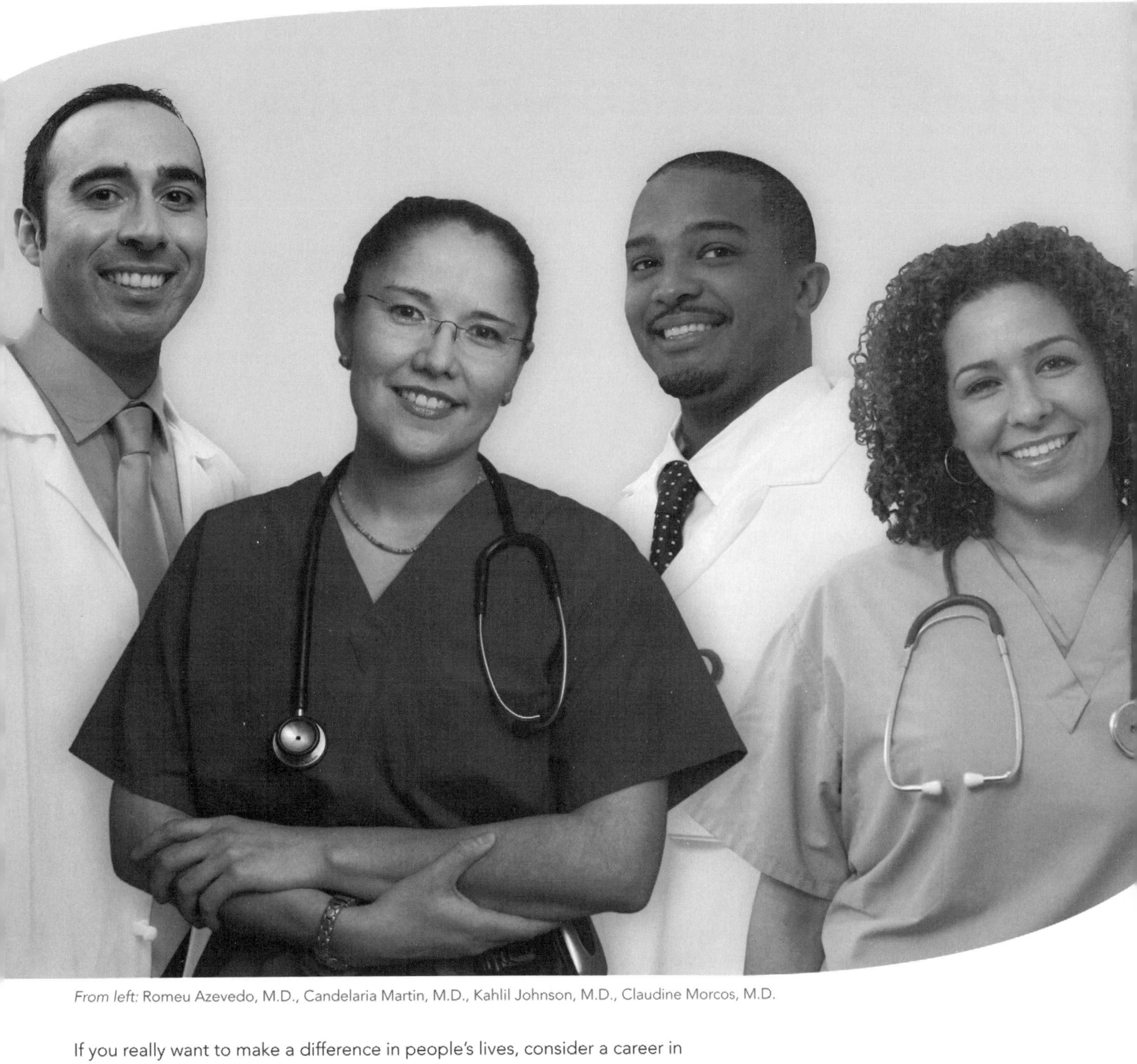

From left: Romeu Azevedo, M.D., Candelaria Martin, M.D., Kahlil Johnson, M.D., Claudine Morcos, M.D.

If you really want to make a difference in people's lives, consider a career in medicine. Too many African Americans, Latinos/as, and Native Americans don't get the care they need. Help us change this reality. Log on to **AspiringDocs.org™**, a new resource from the Association of American Medical Colleges, to learn more.

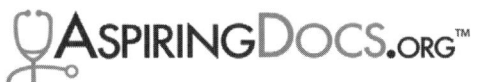

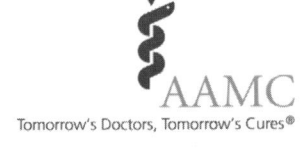

Tomorrow's Doctors, Tomorrow's Cures®

© 2006 AAMC

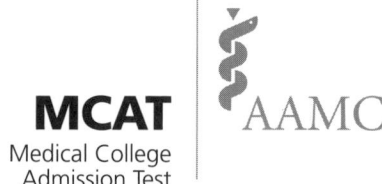
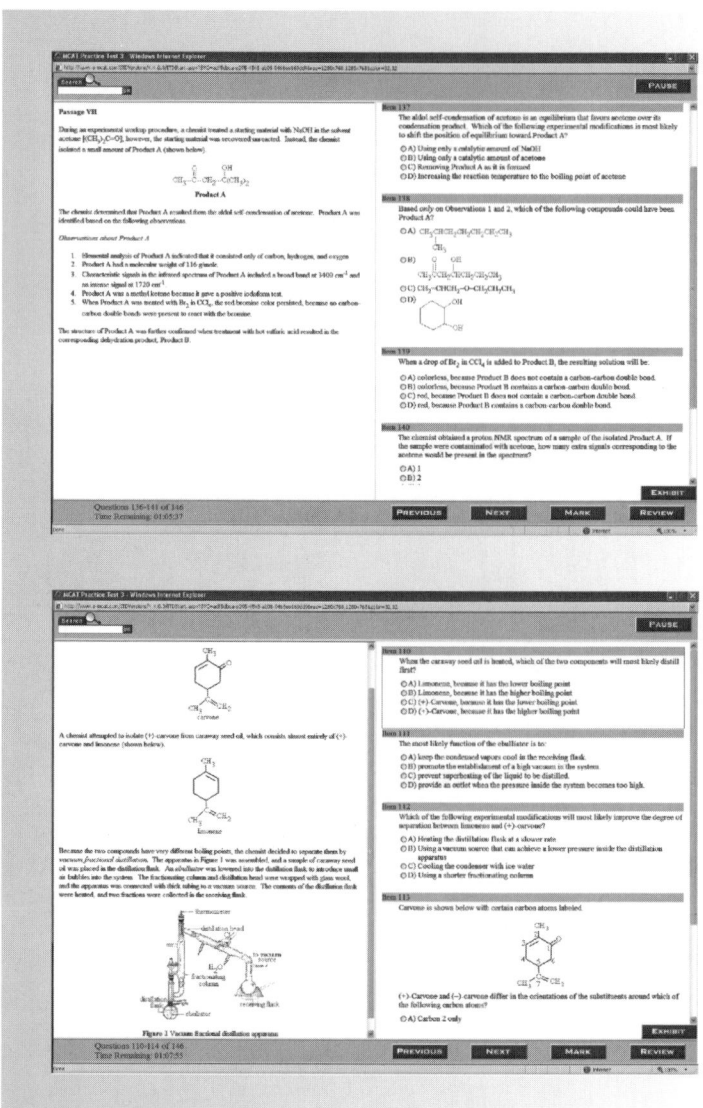

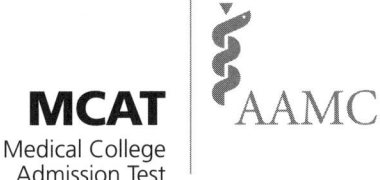

Your ONLY online source for authentic MCAT items

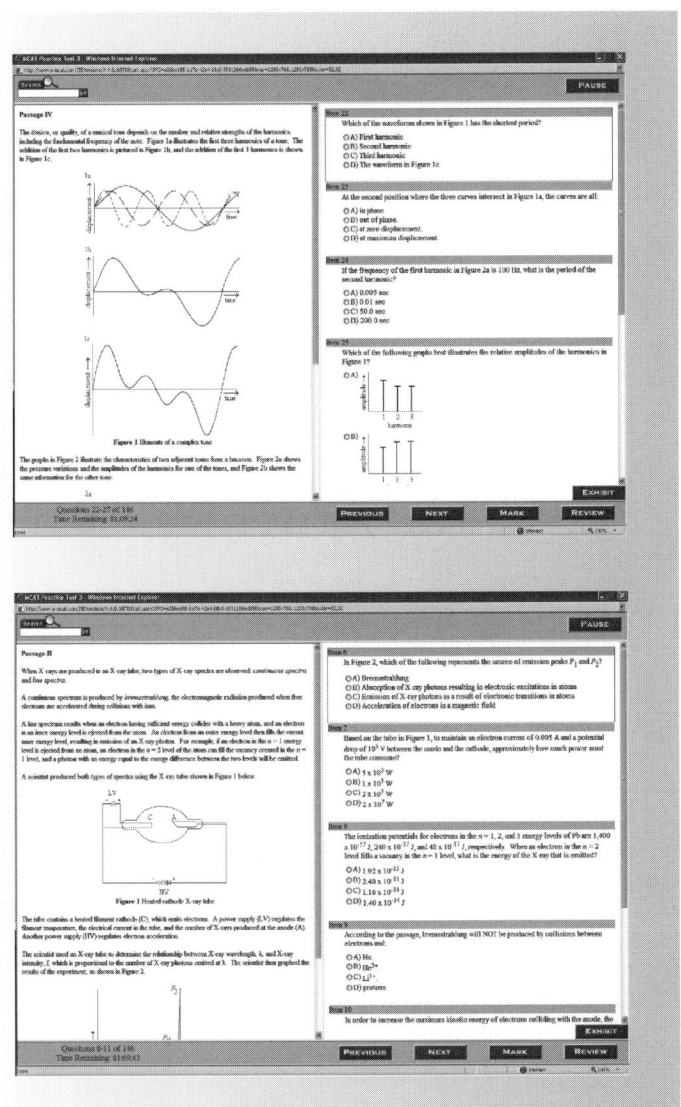

"This was a great tool for me. There is no better way to prepare for the MCAT than by taking actual tests."

An MCAT examinee comments on MCAT Practice Online.

Online practice tests require a valid email account and IE V5.0, AOL V6.0, Netscape 7.1, or Mozilla 1.0.

Please call the Customer Service and Order Fullfillment Department at 202.828.0416 for information on bulk orders and discounts.